Scaphoid Fractures: Evidence-Based Management

Scaphoid Fractures: Evidence-Based Management

GEERT A. BUIJZE, MD PHD
Hand and Upper Extremity Fellow
Department of Orthopaedic Surgery
Academic Medical Center
University of Amsterdam
Amsterdam, The Netherlands

JESSE B. JUPITER, MD
Past President
American Shoulder and Elbow Surgeons
Hansjoerg Wyss/AO Professor
Harvard Medical School
Visiting Orthopedic Surgeon
Massachusetts General Hospital
Yawkey Center
Boston, MA, United States

ELSEVIER

ELSEVIER

3251 Riverport Lane
St. Louis, Missouri 63043

SCAPHOID FRACTURES: EVIDENCE-BASED MANAGEMENT ISBN: 978-0-323-48564-7

Notices

Knowledge and best practice in this field are constantly changing. As new research and experience broaden our understanding, changes in research methods, professional practices, or medical treatment may become necessary.

Practitioners and researchers must always rely on their own experience and knowledge in evaluating and using any information, methods, compounds, or experiments described herein. In using such information or methods they should be mindful of their own safety and the safety of others, including parties for whom they have a professional responsibility.

With respect to any drug or pharmaceutical products identified, readers are advised to check the most current information provided (i) on procedures featured or (ii) by the manufacturer of each product to be administered, to verify the recommended dose or formula, the method and duration of administration, and contraindications. It is the responsibility of practitioners, relying on their own experience and knowledge of their patients, to make diagnoses, to determine dosages and the best treatment for each individual patient, and to take all appropriate safety precautions.

To the fullest extent of the law, neither the Publisher nor the authors, contributors, or editors, assume any liability for any injury and/or damage to persons or property as a matter of products liability, negligence or otherwise, or from any use or operation of any methods, products, instructions, or ideas contained in the material herein.

Content Strategist: Kayla Wolfe
Content Development Specialist: Kristen Helm
Project Manager: Deepthi Unni
Designer: Gopalakrishnan Venkatraman

Last digit is the print number: 9 8 7 6 5 4 3 2 1

This book is dedicated to Sam.

List of Contributors

Editors

Geert A. Buijze, MD, PhD
Hand and Upper Extremity Fellow
Department of Orthopaedic Surgery
Academic Medical Center
University of Amsterdam
Amsterdam, The Netherlands

Jesse B. Jupiter, MD
Past President
American Shoulder and Elbow Surgeons
Hansjoerg Wyss/AO Professor
Harvard Medical School
Visiting Orthopedic Surgeon
Massachusetts General Hospital
Yawkey Center
Boston, MA, United States

Authors

Rohit Arora, MD
Professor of Trauma Surgery
Vice Director
Department of Trauma Surgery
Medical University Innsbruck
Innsbruck, Austria

Gregory I. Bain, MBBS, FRACS, PhD
Professor of Orthopaedic Hand and Upper Extremity Surgery
Flinders University
Adelaide, SA, Australia
Department of Orthopaedic Surgery
Flinders Medical Centre
Department of Orthopaedic Surgery and The Biomechanics & Implants Research Group
Flinders University
Adelaide, SA, Australia

Frank J.P. Beeres, MD, PhD
Luzern Canton Hospital
Luzern, Switzerland

Mohit Bhandari, MD, PhD, FRCSC
Professor
Orthopedic Trauma Surgeon
Division of Orthopaedic Surgery
McMaster University
Center for Evidence Based Orthopaedics
Hamilton, ON, Canada

Anders Björkman, MD, PhD
Department of Hand Surgery
Skane University Hospital
Lund University
Sweden

Bastiaan N.P. de Boer, BSc
Department of Orthopaedic Surgery
Academic Medical Center
University of Amsterdam
Amsterdam, The Netherlands

Michael J. Botte, MD
Co-Director
Hand Rehabilitation Surgery Section
Division of Orthopaedic Surgery
Scripps Clinic;
Chief
Orthopaedic Foot and Ankle Surgery
San Diego VA Healthcare System;
Clinical Professor
Department of Orthopaedic Surgery
University of California, San Diego
School of Medicine;
San Diego, CA, United States

Peter R.G. Brink, MD, PhD
Department of Trauma Surgery
Maastricht University Medical Centre
Maastricht, The Netherlands

Geert A. Buijze, MD, PhD
Hand and Upper Extremity Fellow
Department of Orthopedic Surgery
Academic Medical Center
University of Amsterdam
Amsterdam, The Netherlands

Anne Eva J. Bulstra, MD
PhD Candidate
Department of Orthopaedic Surgery
Academic Medical Center and University of Amsterdam
Amsterdam, The Netherlands
PhD Research Fellow
Department of Orthopaedic Surgery
Flinders Medical Center & Flinders University
Adelaide, SA, Australia

Raúl M. Casas Contreras, MD
Hospital Barros Luco Trudeau
Santiago, Chile

Michel Chammas, MD, PhD
Hand and Upper Extremity Unit
Lapeyronie University Hospital
Montpellier Cedex 5, France

Pierre E. Chammas
Hand and Upper Extremity Unit
Lapeyronie University Hospital
Montpellier Cedex 5, France

Georgios Christopoulos, MD
Klinik für Radiologie
Rhön-Klinikum
Bad Neustadt, Germany

Martin Clementson, MD, PhD
Department of Hand Surgery
Skåne University Hospital
Malmö, Sweden

Joris P. Commandeur, MD
Luzern Canton Hospital
Luzern, Switzerland

Timothy A. Coughlin, BMBS, BMedSci, MRCS
Specialist Registrar
Trauma & Orthopaedics
Queen's Medical Centre
Nottingham, Great Britain

Joseph Dias, MBBS, FRCS (Orth), MD
Academic Team of Musculoskeletal Surgery (AToMS)
Undercroft, Leicester General Hospital
Leicester, United Kingdom

Job N. Doornberg, MD, PhD
Trauma Fellow
Flinders Medical Centre
Adelaide, SA, Australia
Postdoc Research Fellow
Department of Orthopaedic Surgery
Academisch Medisch Centrum
Amsterdam, The Netherlands

Tessa Drijkoningen, MD
Department of Plastic, Reconstructive, and Hand Surgery
Academic Medical Center
University of Amsterdam
Amsterdam-Zuidoost, The Netherlands

Andrew D. Duckworth, BSc (Hons), MBChB, MSc, FRCSEd (Tr&Orth), PhD
Specialty Registrar (StR) and Clinical Research Fellow
Edinburgh Orthopaedic Trauma Unit
Royal Infirmary of Edinburgh
Edinburgh, United Kingdom

Diego L. Fernandez, MD
Professor of Orthopedic Surgery
Department of Orthopedic Surgery Lindenhof Hospital
Bern, Switzerland

Daren P. Forward, MA, FRCS, DM
Consultant Orthopaedic Trauma Surgeon
Queen's Medical Centre
Nottingham University Hospitals NHS Trust
Nottingham, United Kingdom

Markus Gabl, MD
Department of Trauma Surgery
Medical University Innsbruck
Innsbruck, Austria

Michael R. Gale, MA, MBBChir, FRCS (Tr&Orth)
Specialist Registrar
Trauma & Orthopaedics
Queen's Medical Centre
Nottingham, Great Britain

Kanai Garala, BSc (Hons), MBChB (Hons), MRCS, DipMedEd
University Hospitals Coventry and Warwickshire
Coventry, United Kingdom

Marc Garcia-Elias, MD, PhD
Institut Kaplan
Barcelona, Spain

William B. Geissler, MD
Department of Orthopedic Surgery
University Mississippi Medical Center
Jackson, MS, United States

Nicholas Goddard, MB, FRCS
Department of Orthopaedics
Royal Free Hospital
London, United Kingdom

Michael B. Gottschalk, MD
Assistant Professor Hand and Upper Extremity
Director of Clinical Research
Department of Orthopaedic Surgery
Emory University School of Medicine
Dunwoody, GA, United States

Mathilde Gras, MD
Institut de la Main, Clinique BIZET
Paris, France

Ruby Grewal, MD, MSc, FRCSC
Associate Professor
Roth|McFarlane Hand and Upper Limb Clinic
St Joseph's Health Center
Division of Orthopedic Surgery
University of Western Ontario
London, ON, Canada

Pascal F.W. Hannemann, MD, PhD
Department of Trauma Surgery
Maastricht University Medical Centre
Maastricht, The Netherlands

Jan-Ragnar Haugstvedt, MD, PhD
Department of Orthopaedics
Divison of Hand Surgery
Østfold Hospital
Moss, Norway

Steven L. Henry, MD
Department of Surgery and Perioperative Care
Dell Medical School at the University of Texas at Austin
Austin, TX, United States

Pak-Cheong Ho, MBBS, FRCS, FHKAM (Orthopaedic Surgery), FHKCOS
Consultant and Chief
Division of Hand and Microsurgery
Department of Orthopaedics & Traumatology
Prince of Wales Hospital
Sha Tin, Hong Kong
Honorary Clinical Associate Professor
Department of Orthopaedics & Traumatology
The Chinese University of Hong Kong
Sha Tin, Hong Kong

M. Jake Hamer, MD
Co-Director
Hand and Microvascular Surgery Section
Division of Orthopaedic Surgery
Scripps Clinic
San Diego, CA, United States
Scripps Clinic
Division of Orthopaedic Surgery
San Diego, CA, United States

Herman Johal, MD, MPH, PhD(C), FRCSC
Clinical Scholar
Orthopedic Trauma Surgeon
Division of Orthopaedic Surgery
McMaster University
Center for Evidence Based Orthopedics
Hamilton, ON, Canada

Nicholas A. Johnson, MBCHB, FRCS
Specialty Registrar
Academic Team of Musculoskeletal Surgery
University Hospitals of Leicester NHS Trust
Leicester, United Kingdom

Peter Jørgsholm, MD, PhD
Hand Surgery Clinic
Mølholm Private Hospital
Vejle, Kerteminde, Denmark, Department of Hand Surgery
Skåne University Hospital
Malmö, Sweden

Sanjeev Kakar, MD, MRCS
Professor of Orthopaedic Surgery
Mayo Clinic
Rochester, MN, United States

Dr. Karlheinz Kalb, MD
Klinik für Handchirurgie
Rhön-Klinikum
Bad Neustadt, Germany

Tobias Kastenberger, MD
Department of Trauma Surgery
Medical University Innsbruck
Innsbruck, Austria

Joseph S. Khouri, MD
University of Rochester Medical Center
Section of Plastic & Reconstructive Surgery
Rochester, NY, United States

Jong-Pil Kim, MD
Department of Orthopedic Surgery
College of Medicine
Department of Kinesiology and Medical Science
Graduate School
Dankook University
Cheonan, Korea

Hebe D. Kvernmo, MD, PhD, MHA
Senior Consultant/Professor in Hand- and Orthopedic Surgery
Hand Surgery Unit
Orthopedic Department
University Hospital of North-Norway
UiT-Arctic University of Norway
Tromsø, Norway

Steve K. Lee, MD
Hand and Upper Extremity Service
Hospital for Special Surgery
New York, NY, United States
Weill Medical College of Cornell University
New York, NY, United States
New York-Presbyterian Hospital
New York, NY, United States

Shai Luria, MD
Department of Orthopaedic Surgery
Hadassah Medical Organization
Kiryat Hadassah
Jerusalem, Israel

Wouter H. Mallee, MD
Department of Orthopaedic Surgery
Academic Medical Center of Amsterdam
Amsterdam, The Netherlands

Christophe L. Mathoulin, MD
Institut de la Main, Clinique BIZET
Paris, France

Geert Meermans, MD
Bravis Hospital
Bergen op Zoom, The Netherlands

Hisao Moritomo, MD
Department of Physical Therapy
Osaka Yukioka College of Health Science
Ibaraki-Shi, Osaka, Japan

Jaydeep Moro, MD, FRCSC
Clinical Assistant Professor
Upper Extremity Surgeon
Division of Orthopaedic Surgery
McMaster University
St. Joseph's Hospital
Hamilton, ON, Canada

Kunihiro Oka, MD
Health Care Center
Osaka University and Department of Orthopaedic Surgery
Osaka University Graduate School of Medicine
Suita, Osaka, Japan

Diana M. Ortega Hernández, MD
Centro Médico Teknon
Barcelona, Spain

Lorenzo L. Pacelli, MD
Assistant Director
Division of Orthopaedic Surgery
Scripps Clinic
San Diego, CA, United States

Emmanuella Peraut, MD
Hand and Upper Extremity Unit
Lapeyronie University Hospital
Montpellier Cedex 5, France

Martijn Poeze, MD, PhD
Department of Trauma Surgery
Maastricht University Medical Centre
Maastricht, Netherlands

Karl-Josef Prommersberger, MD, PhD
Professor
Klinik für Handchirurgie
Rhön-Klinikum
Bad Neustadt, Germany

Schneider K. Rancy, BA
Hand and Upper Extremity Service
Hospital for Special Surgery
New York, NY, United States

Steven J. Rhemrev, MD, PhD
Medical Center Haaglanden
Den Haag, The Netherlands

David Ring, MD, PhD
Department of Surgery and Perioperative Care
Dell Medical School at the University of Texas at Austin
Austin, TX, United States

Marieke G.A. de Roo, MD
Department of Plastic, Reconstructive and Hand Surgery
Department of Biomedical Engineering and Physics
Academic Medical Center (AMC)
University of Amsterdam
Amsterdam, The Netherlands

Eliana B. Saltzman, BA
Hand and Upper Extremity Service
Hospital for Special Surgery
New York, NY, United States
Department of Education
Icahn School of Medicine at Mount Sinai
New York, NY, United States

Gernot Schmidle, MD
Department of Trauma Surgery
Medical University Innsbruck
Innsbruck, Austria

Rainer Schmitt, MD, PhD
Professor
Klink für Diagnostische und Interventionelle Radiologie
Herz- und Gefäß-Klinik GmbH
Bad Neustadt, Germany
Institut für Diagnostische und Interventionelle Radiologie
Universitätsklinikum Würzburg
Bad Neustadt, Germany

Yonatan Schwarcz, MD
Department of Orthopaedic Surgery
Hadassah Medical Organization
Kiryat Hadassah
Jerusalem, Israel

Alexander Y. Shin, MD
Professor
Orthopedic Surgery and Neurosurgery
Mayo Clinic
Department of Orthopaedic Surgery
Rochester, MN, United States

Faiz S. Shivji, BMBS, BMedSci, MRCS
Specialist Registrar
Trauma & Orthopaedics
Queen's Medical Centre
Nottingham, Great Britain

Harvinder Singh, MBBS, MS (Orth), FRCS (Orth), PhD
Leicester General Hospital
Leicester, United Kingdom

Simon D. Strackee, MD, PhD
Department of Plastic, Reconstructive and Hand Surgery
Academic Medical Center (AMC)
University of Amsterdam
Amsterdam, The Netherlands

Geert J. Streekstra, PhD, Ir.
Department of Biomedical Engineering and Physics
Department of Radiology
Academic Medical Center (AMC)
University of Amsterdam
Amsterdam, The Netherlands

Jason A. Strelzow, MD
Department of Surgery
Roth|McFarlane Hand & Upper Limb Center at The University of Western Ontario
London, ON, Canada

Paul W. ten Berg, MD
Department of Plastic, Reconstructive, and Hand Surgery
Academic Medical Center
University of Amsterdam
Amsterdam-Zuidoost, The Netherlands

Michael A. Thompson, MD
Co-Director
Hand and Microvascular Surgery Section
Division of Orthopaedic Surgery
Scripps Clinic
San Diego, CA, United States

Niels Thomsen, MD, PhD
Department of Hand Surgery
Skåne University Hospital
Malmö, Sweden

Wing-lim Tse, MBChB, MRCS, FRCSEd (Orth), FHKAM (Orthopaedic Surgery), FHKCOS
Department of Orthopaedics & Traumatology
The Chinese University of Hong Kong
Sha Tin, Hong Kong

Arthur Turow, MBBS
Department of Orthopaedic Surgery
Flinders Medical Centre
SA, Adelaide, Australia

Matthias Vanhees, MD, PhD
Department of Orthopaedic Surgery
Monica Hospital
Deurne, Belgium

Frederik Verstreken, MD
Department of Orthopaedic Surgery
Monica Hospital
Deurne, Belgium

Maarten J. de Vos, MD, PhD
Department of Orthopaedic Surgery
Tergooi Hospital
Hilversum, The Netherlands

Scott W. Wolfe, MD
Chief Emeritus
Hand and Upper Extremity Service
Hospital for Special Surgery
Professor of Orthopedic Surgery
Weill Medical College of Cornell University
New York, NY, United States
New York-Presbyterian Hospital
New York, NY, United States

Wing-Yee C. Wong, MBChB, MRCS, FRCSEd (Orth), FHKAM (Orthopaedic Surgery), FHKCOS
Department of Orthopaedics & Traumatology
The Chinese University of Hong Kong
Sha Tin, Hong Kong

Foreword

The scaphoid is a small bone with a bad attitude. From early in our orthopedic/plastic surgical training we are taught to suspect a scaphoid fracture and immobilize the wrist of any patient who presents with a history of trauma and snuffbox tenderness. This is because the consequences of a missed fracture and a subsequent scaphoid nonunion are so dire. Of all the bones in our skeleton, this small bone demands much more attention than one would expect based on its diminutive stature. The scaphoid's contribution to the architecture and function of the wrist, however, cannot be overemphasized. The past practice of experiential learning and expert witness are still integral to our training, but the emergence of evidenced based medicine (EBM) has ushered in a new era in practice management. To this end, this timely book by Geert Buijze, MD, PhD, and Jesse Jupiter, MD, exemplifies the utility and essential nature of EBM when treating scaphoid injuries. Regional and international practice patterns no longer solely dictate our approach to fracture management. Specialized outcome instruments and Level I scientific evidence have taken their proper place in the treatment algorithm to help guide us through the bewildering maze of seeming contradictions in the literature.

Dr. Buijze has assembled an international group of experts to shepherd us through the treatment of scaphoid injuries from acute fractures to nonunions to salvage procedures. Each chapter reflects both the experience of this distinguished group of authors and a literature review section that summarizes the relevant peer reviewed publications that support their conclusions. Dr. Buijze is to be congratulated for assembling and guiding this group of experts to produce a comprehensive and coherent evidence-based guide to the treatment of scaphoid injuries, and he has rightly taken his place among them as a preeminent scholar in this field.

David J. Slutsky, MD
Hand and Wrist Institute
Torrance, CA
Chief of Reconstructive Hand Surgery
Orthopedics
Harbor-UCLA Medical Center
Torrance, CA

Preface

Small Bone—Big Deal: From the "painful snuffbox" of a suspicious scaphoid to the "bloody challenge" of an avascular nonunion, day in day out we deal with scaphoid injuries in clinics around the world. And from the nervous emergency medicine intern overcarefully treating a suspected fracture to the experienced hand surgeon brainstorming on salvage options for a failed humpback repair, everyone has his/her own challenges in managing scaphoid fractures. This book is intended to anyone dealing with scaphoid fractures: all who are eager to keep up-to-date with the newest evidence on both diagnosis and treatment of simple fractures as well as creative state-of-the-art solutions for managing more complex cases—such as inventive open grafting techniques for failed screw fixation and minimal invasive techniques for perilunate injuries—the whole spectrum.

The purpose of this book is to enhance your practice by bringing you the best of both worlds: *Evidence-Based Management* and *Expert-Based Opinion* combined. The innovative resultant format is what we like to label as *Best Practice*. While each chapter's core content is evidence-based management, it is encompassed by panels with practical expert-based content: case scenarios introducing key dilemmas engaging the reader to seek for the best solution and expert-based practice algorithms, step-by-step illustrated techniques, and pearls and pitfalls from pioneers in the field.

We are grateful to all 83 contributing authors from 20 countries around the world for investing their valuable spare time seeking the best available evidence and providing us with their highly valued experience to maximize the book's potential for the clinician. We are also indebted to Dr. David Slutsky for pitching the idea for this sequel of his original chef-d'oeuvre "The Scaphoid." Moreover, this book could not have been realized without the disciplined work and always optimistic support of editorial manager Mrs. Erika Mokarian, developmental editor Mrs. Kristen Helm, and project manager Mrs. Deepthi Unni.

As clinicians, we also face ludic challenges such as explaining our friends and relatives the whole deal about scaphoid fractures as you hear them thinking out loud: "But it's such a small bone, why all the fuss about breaking it or not?" Well, simply because you don't want to miss it—nor maltreat it. Just like a gastrointestinal surgeon wouldn't want to miss an occult appendicitis. In fact, as the scaphoid forms the pivotal link between the proximal and distal rows, disruption of its integrity can lead to severe carpal instability, ultimately leading to the feared advanced collapse wrist. Perhaps it's useful to illustrate and analyze this more from a historical perspective before the era of evidence-based management.

After a classic FOOSH—fall on the outstretched hand—a young adult male sustained an occult scaphoid waist fracture in 1956 (Fig. 1). Lacking adequate

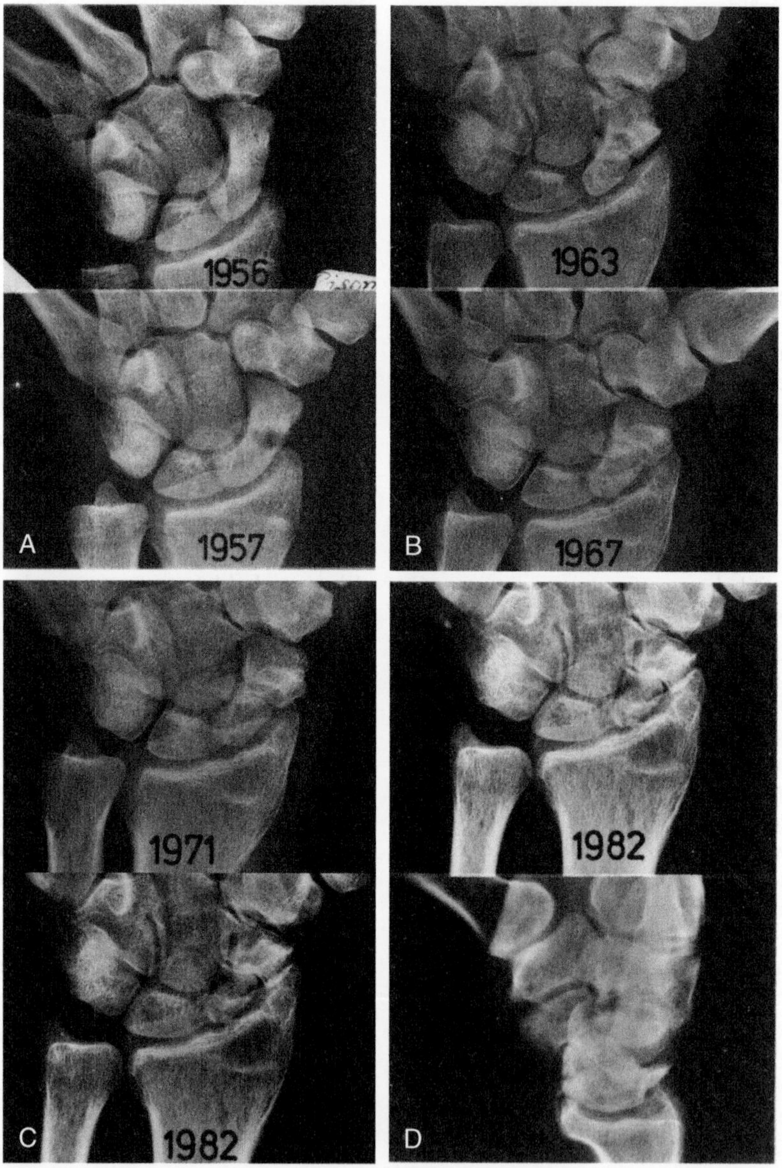

FIG. 1 **(A)** A young adult male sustained an occult scaphoid waist fracture in 1956 after a classic FOOSH—fall on the outstretched hand. The diagnosis of a nonunited fractured at 1-year follow-up (1957). **(B)** The nonunion progressed over the next 10 years (1963–67). **(C)** Over the subsequent 4 years (1971), degeneration progressed toward the proximal scaphocapitate articulation consistent with a stage-2 SNAC wrist. **(D)** The final stage-3 SNAC wrist became apparent during the following 11 years (1982) with progressive pan-scaphoid arthritis and a clear dorsal intercalated segment instability. (From Buijze GA. Scaphoid Fractures : Anatomy, Diagnosis and Treatment. University of Amsterdam, Netherlands 2012, with permission)

treatment, the diagnosis of a nonunited fracture only became apparent at 1-year follow-up (1957). As surgical reconstructive management had just been introduced by McLaughlin in those days and had not yet been established as standard of care around the world, a conservative management was adopted. Nonetheless, the nonunion progressed over the next 10 years (1963–67) to what we now define as a stage-1 scaphoid nonunion advanced collapse (SNAC) wrist. At this stage, osteoarthritis only affected the cartilage of the tip of the radial styloid and distal scaphoid fragment. Over the subsequent 4 years (1971), degeneration progressed toward the proximal scaphocapitate articulation consistent with a stage-2 SNAC wrist. The final stage-3 SNAC wrist became apparent during the following 11 years (1982) with progressive panscaphoid arthritis and a clear dorsal intercalated segment instability.

Now you may question: "Is this scaphoid beyond repair?" Hopefully this book will provide an evidence-based answer to that question but, surely, this case will awake your enthusiasm to keep improving your management of scaphoid fractures—from the early diagnostics of occult fractures to the delayed treatment of recalcitrant nonunions. For each challenge you may face, you can browse this book to help guide you toward *Evidence-Based Management* and enhance your *Best Practice* of the entire spectrum of scaphoid fractures.

Geert A. Buijze, MD, PhD
Department of Orthopaedic Surgery
Academic Medical Center
University of Amsterdam
Amsterdam, The Netherlands

Jesse B. Jupiter, MD
Past President, American Shoulder and Elbow Surgeons
Hansjoerg Wyss/AO Professor
Harvard Medical School
Visiting Orthopedic Surgeon
Massachusetts General Hospital
Yawkey Center Suite 2100
Boston, MA

Contents

CHAPTER 1

Using Evidence to Manage Scaphoid Fractures

STEVEN L. HENRY, MD • DAVID RING, MD, PHD

KEY POINTS

- Habits make us comfortable amidst uncertainty, but evidence helps ensure that our habits provide optimal treatment.
- Medicine has inherent uncertainties and patients and surgeons are nearly always managing probabilities. Scientific techniques such as Bayes-adjusted diagnostic performance characteristics and latent class analysis can be used to describe and quantify these probabilities.
- Given the inherent uncertainties, it's important to account for informed patient preferences based on values such as tolerance of risk, desire to avoid surgery, and urgency of return to activity.

INTRODUCTION

Like most surgeons, we hand surgeons are products of our apprenticeship, doing things the way we were taught or the way that has worked for us over the years. Understandably, after a decade of toiling in medical school, residency, and fellowship, when we are finally ready to do surgery on our own, our desire is to *do*, to hone the technical skills we spent so much of our lives acquiring. For as smart as we are, we are fundamentally doers more than philosophers, and by the time we finish training, it is much easier (and more profitable) to do than to think.

However, as comfortable as habit can be, the one constant in life is change. Now, with the shift toward alternative payment strategies, such as bundled payments, we will be pressured to justify everything we do with scientific evidence. It's hard to wrap one's head around the implications of this shift, but it may be seismic, forcing us to start over in our treatment strategy for many conditions that we can currently treat almost reflexively. (You have tennis elbow—here's a cortisone shot! You have trapeziometacarpal arthritis—you need an LRTI!)

As comfortable as habit can be, the one constant in life is change.

Scaphoid fractures are a great place to start on our quest for evidence-based practice. It's a common yet vexing injury and the subject of a bewildering number of studies. Indeed, with multiple scaphoid studies appearing monthly in our various journals, the idea of an evidence-based textbook may seem almost oxymoronic, as it is possible that the information in this book may be, at least incrementally, out of date by the time you are reading it. However, from a broad perspective, this book will have longstanding value as a roadmap to the pivotal issues in the management of scaphoid fractures and how evidence can inform and improve treatment.

DIAGNOSIS OF TRUE FRACTURES AMONG SUSPECTED FRACTURES

One pivotal issue we can explore is the most basic—what is the most appropriate way to diagnose a scaphoid fracture? An undiagnosed and undertreated scaphoid waist or proximal pole fracture is at risk for nonunion, which leads to wrist arthrosis and exposes doctors to litigation. Consequently, in litigious cultures such as the United States, doctors tend to practice defensively and send patients with wrist tenderness after a fall for sophisticated imaging (CT or MRI) to "rule out" a fracture, although the rate

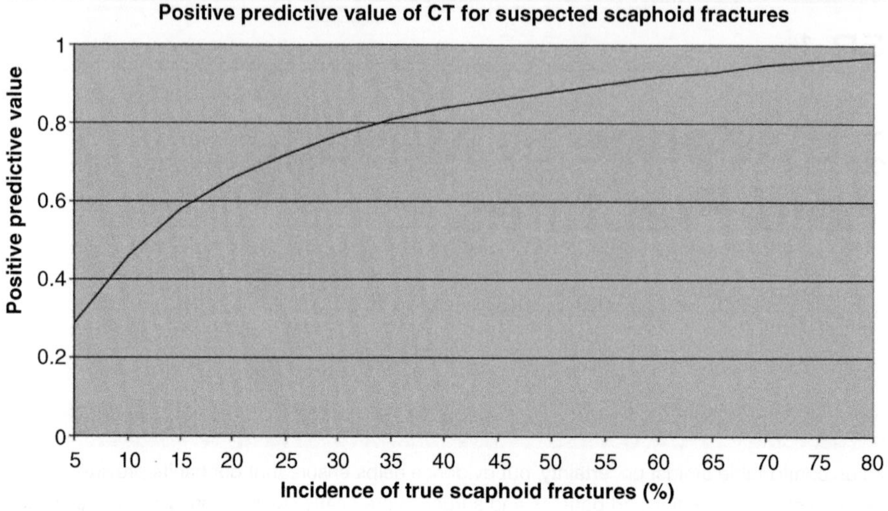

FIG. 1.1 In a low prevalence environment, even an accurate test can have a relatively low positive predictive value. (From Ring D, Lozano-Calderón S. Imaging for suspected scaphoid fracture. *J Hand Surg*. 2008;33(6):956; with permission.)

of true fractures among suspected fractures in this situation may be as low as 1 in 20.[1] The rate of true fractures is higher in less litigious cultures such as the Netherlands. However, although CT or MRI may be quite sensitive in identifying fractures, they may not be very specific because they often identify signal changes that can be misinterpreted as a fracture, even in uninjured people, let alone in patients who have fallen and might have changes in the bone that don't constitute a fracture at risk for nonunion (e.g., a bone bruise). Using Bayes' theorem, if the true incidence of scaphoid fracture in this situation is 5%, and MRI is 99% sensitive and 94% specific for fracture, the probability that a patient with a "positive" MRI has a true fracture is only 46%; in other words, it would be more likely that this patient with a "positive" MRI does *not* have a fracture! Thus, in this low prevalence environment, even a very sensitive and specific test may have a relatively low positive predictive value (Fig. 1.1).[2] In this sense, we can see why relying on sophisticated imaging to make the diagnosis is not always beneficial, as it could easily lead to overtreatment.

Of course, estimating the true sensitivity and specificity of CT and MRI is itself problematic because there is no consensus reference standard for a true scaphoid fracture. Many of us think that because MRI produces such good images, it must be the reference standard. However, MRI has false positives (Fig. 1.2).[3] Most studies trying to establish the value of MRI have used radiographs obtained 6 weeks after injury as the reference standard; because diagnosis of a fracture on radiographs is the problem we are trying to solve, this has obvious drawbacks.

There are other areas of hand surgery where there is no consensus reference standard—carpal tunnel syndrome and compartment syndrome, just to name two. In the absence of a consensus reference standard, we can use latent class analysis to incorporate multiple factors (patient characteristics, injury mechanism, symptoms, signs, and test results) that together define the probability of a specific diagnosis.[4] Thus, the way forward to improve diagnosis of true scaphoid fractures among suspected fractures may be to hold off on sophisticated imaging until there is sufficient probability of a true fracture based on these factors. Groups of such factors can also define probabilities using what is termed a clinical prediction rule.[5] Several clinical prediction rules are proposed for this problem, but none is in wide use, perhaps because each uses tests or interventions that are unfamiliar to many of us (e.g., pain with ulnar deviation of the wrist).

Current evidence suggests that we should cast or splint until physical and radiographic examinations bring the probability of true fracture to the level that is

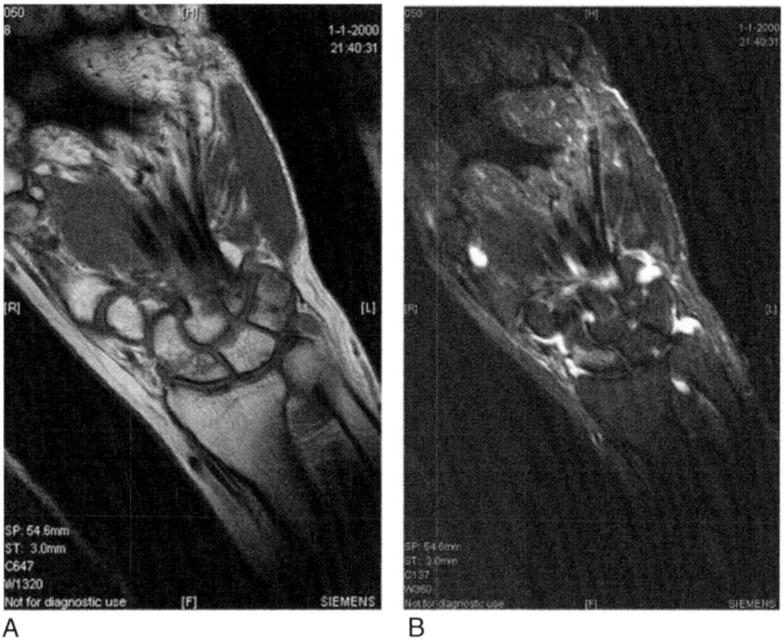

FIG. 1.2 False-positive MRI in healthy volunteer on a **(A)** T1 sequence and **(B)** T2 sequence. (From De Zwart AD, Beeres FJ, Ring D, et al. MRI as a reference standard for suspected scaphoid fractures. *Br J Radiol*. 2012;85(1016):1101; with permission.)

either acceptably low to proceed, as if there is no fracture, or acceptably high that more sophisticated imaging will not be misleading. This applies to a large number of people with disproportionate symptoms and limitations seen in emergency rooms. Time to get settled, experience some improvement, and be evaluated by a specialist will resolve the concern for potential scaphoid fracture in the vast majority of such patients. Individuals that have a strong preference to return to activity as soon as possible can take the risk of overdiagnosis (and overtreatment) that accompanies MRI to benefit from its high negative predictive value, returning to work or play if the scan is normal. At this point, improved assessment of patient factors to generate more accurate probabilities of fracture has greater potential to improve management than more sophisticated imaging, which might simply increase detection of minor abnormalities unrelated to true fracture that distract and mislead us.

DIAGNOSIS OF DISPLACEMENT AND FRACTURE INSTABILITY

The greatest risk factor for nonunion of a scaphoid waist fracture is fracture displacement. Diagnosis of displacement is imperfect on radiographs, but there can also be uncertainty about what constitutes displacement on CT.

Standard axial, sagittal, and coronal cuts are usually oblique to the long axis of the scaphoid and the fracture line, making interpretation difficult. However, obtaining cuts in the proper plane (perpendicular to the fracture line) can also be very difficult. The reference standard for displacement might be operative exposure, including midcarpal arthroscopy. However, there are fractures that are mobile on direct visualization that are nondisplaced on CT, and it's not clear that well-aligned mobile fractures are at greater risk of nonunion.[6]

Again, with current best evidence, we can only approximate diagnosis of displacement and instability. Future investigation can be aimed at improving our ability to generate accurate probabilities of displacement, better understand the prognosis of instability without displacement, and determine the optimal ways to determine patient preferences for treatment based on these factors.

CLASSIFICATION

Some classification systems are detailed, separating the scaphoid into several areas.[7] Careful analysis of imaging techniques suggests that the vast majority of fractures are waist fractures that may look deceivingly distal or proximal based on radiographic technique and wrist positioning. Distal tubercle fractures are usually benign and can be treated symptomatically. Proximal pole fractures are uncommon but can be more troublesome. Investigation should build on these observations, applying the science of reliability and accuracy of diagnosis of distal tubercle, waist, and proximal pole fractures.

TREATMENT

Humans tend to see things in terms of contests. What's better: operative or nonoperative treatment of a scaphoid waist fracture? The evidence will probably never identify a "best" treatment that applies to everyone. Evidence defines probabilities of various outcomes and adjusts treatment options. We can present these to patients in ways they can understand, as well as ways that get them past their first impression that might be based on misconceptions, toward preferences based on their core values. For instance, a person in pain might feel they need to fix the problem for everything to be OK. Once presented with the evidence in a way that is calming and creates an appreciation of all the treatment options, that same person might realize that their preference is to avoid surgery if at all possible.

Another example is, because nondisplaced waist fractures reliably heal with adequate protection, the primary allure of a percutaneous screw is reduced time in a cast. As evidence demonstrates that less cumbersome protection for a shorter duration is adequate,[8] the appeal of surgery may decline.

DIAGNOSIS OF UNION

Evidence regarding the reliability and accuracy of diagnosis of union is also important. Some patients want to return to activity, but the radiographic appearance makes us cautious. Others are sore and protective even when their radiographs suggest healing is advancing.

What is the best approach? Does CT scanning improve the reliability and accuracy of diagnosis of union? It's not clear that it does.[9] Can we safely let people put it to the test (resume normal activity) based on a probability that the fracture should be healed? Given the health benefits of resuming meaningful activity during a painful and draining recovery process (i.e., fostering resiliency), we should err on the side of returning to normality, rather than using small probabilities of adverse outcomes to justify overprotection, prolonged limitations, and unnecessary treatment. Evidence can help determine the advantages and disadvantages of various approaches and how to best present them to patients so that they can make choices consistent with their values and preferences.

DIAGNOSIS OF VASCULARITY AND TREATMENT OF NONUNION

Many of our treatments for scaphoid nonunion address vascularity of the proximal pole of the scaphoid. However, it's not clear that we can reliably and accurately diagnose vascularity on imaging or even on direct inspection in the operating room. Furthermore, it's not clear that avascularity affects outcomes with nonvascularized grafts or that vascularized grafts improve outcomes.

As with so much in modern medicine, there is a gradual tendency to use ever more sophisticated and intricate techniques with little evidence of a meaningful benefit to patients. If we involved patients more dispassionately in these decisions, we suspect we would see diminished appeal of lengthy surgery with increasing donor site morbidity.

NATURAL HISTORY AND SALVAGE PROCEDURES

What's going to happen to someone with a persistent fracture line with or without a loose screw, but reasonable alignment of the scaphoid? Will the screw loosen or move further causing harm? Will the wrist develop arthrosis? We've all seen patients—and Herbert included them in his classification—who appear to have stable, fibrous unions. When deciding on additional treatment, it would be useful to have a measure of the probabilities of various outcomes with or without treatment.

How quickly will a wrist with scaphoid nonunion, humpback deformity, and carpal instability progress to arthrosis? At what point is the arthrosis progression established and unresponsive to realignment and healing of the scaphoid? If there is visible radioscaphoid arthritis on radiographs, does that make attempts at scaphoid union unhelpful? Is there an amount of time, or number of surgeries, beyond which trying to heal the scaphoid is unhelpful?

These questions are important because once the discussion moves from modification of disease (attempt to heal the scaphoid to prevent or slow arthrosis) to palliation and salvage, there is plenty of breathing room. If we do all we can to help patients adapt to the situation, they may be able to put off or avoid salvage procedures. The contention that delay will diminish the result of a salvage procedure seems unlikely and exposes a surgical bias that risks overutilization. Salvage is about being as comfortable and capable as possible, and the evidence is clear that capability, comfort, and calm have less to do with disease than with resiliency.

CONCLUSION

There are so many questions to be answered about the scaphoid; we could almost be paralyzed by the uncertainty. Our habits and principles have served a purpose in providing a recipe for care, but it is crucial that we stay curious and identify evidence to help adjust our habits. The healthiest decisions are informed by evidence rather than misconceptions.

REFERENCES

1. Mallee WH, Wang J, Poolman RW, et al. Computed tomography versus magnetic resonance imaging versus bone scintigraphy for clinically suspected scaphoid fractures in patients with negative plain radiographs. *Cochrane Database Syst Rev*. 2015;(6):CD010023.
2. Ring D, Lozano-Calderon S. Imaging for suspected scaphoid fracture. *J Hand Surg Am*. 2008;33(6):954–957.
3. De Zwart AD, Beeres FJ, Ring D, et al. MRI as a reference standard for suspected scaphoid fractures. *Br J Radiol*. 2012;85(1016):1098–1101.
4. Buijze GA, Mallee WH, Beeres FJ, et al. Diagnostic performance tests for suspected scaphoid fractures differ with conventional and latent class analysis. *Clin Orthop Relat Res*. 2011;469(12):3400–3407.
5. Duckworth AD, Buijze GA, Moran M, et al. Predictors of fracture following suspected injury to the scaphoid. *J Bone Joint Surg Br*. 2012;94(7):961–968.
6. Buijze GA, Jorgsholm P, Thomsen NO, et al. Diagnostic performance of radiographs and computed tomography for displacement and instability of acute scaphoid waist fractures. *J Bone Joint Surg Am*. 2012;94(21):1967–1974.
7. Ten Berg PW, Drijkoningen T, Strackee SD, Buijze GA. Classifications of acute scaphoid fractures: a systematic literature review. *J Wrist Surg*. 2016;5(2):152–159.
8. Geoghegan JM, Woodruff MJ, Bhatia R, et al. Undisplaced scaphoid waist fractures: is 4 weeks' immobilization in a below-elbow cast sufficient if a week 4 CT scan suggests fracture union? *J Hand Surg Eur Vol*. 2009;34(5):631–637.
9. Buijze GA, Wijffels MM, Guitton TG, et al. Interobserver reliability of computed tomography to diagnose scaphoid waist fracture union. *J Hand Surg Am*. 2012;37(2):250–254.

CHAPTER 2

Principles of Evidence-Based Management of Scaphoid Fractures

HERMAN JOHAL, MD, MPH, PHD(C), FRCSC • JAYDEEP MORO, MD, FRCSC • MOHIT BHANDARI, MD, PHD, FRCSC

KEY POINTS

- Evidence-based management requires the combination of the best evidence with patient values and provider preferences to make treatment decisions.
- The practice of evidence-based management involves the formulation of question, acquisition of related literature, appraisal of study quality, and the appropriate application of research findings to individual patients.
- Evidence-based management does not strictly depend on the results of randomized controlled trials, but more accurately involves the informed and effective use of all types of evidence.

THE ERA OF EVIDENCE-BASED MEDICINE

Traditionally, the approach to clinical problem-solving has relied on the practice of "evidence-based medicine," by which decisions were based primarily on professional authority, pathophysiologic rationale, and experience.[1] This approach was heavily influenced by opinion and fraught with bias, leading to an environment of unsystematic assemblage and propagation of literature to support the intuition of prominent authors. In contrast to this paradigm, "evidence-based medicine" shifted the focus to the conscientious and judicious use of the current best available evidence.[2]

> Bias is a systematic tendency to produce an outcome that differs from the underlying truth. There are many sources of bias that clinicians need to identify, and interpretation of the literature with "enlightened skepticism" is fundamental to an evidence-based approach.

A quick search using Google Scholar for the term "evidence-based medicine" reveals approximately 1,060,000 results, over 20,000 of which focus on orthopedics. Considering the relatively recent introduction of these concepts, we are amidst an era of change in the way we approach clinical problems. The term "evidence-based medicine" was first coined in 1991 by Dr. Gordon Guyatt, and it described a set of principles developed by Dr. David Sackett and fellow clinical epidemiologists from McMaster University.[3] Evidence-based medicine begins with the clear delineation of clinically important questions, followed by a thorough, systematic search of the literature for relevant articles, and critical appraisal of the available evidence for both quality and applicability to the question.[4] The approach culminates in the balanced

PANEL 1
Case Scenarios

CASE 1

A 30-year-old male recreational soccer player presented to the fracture clinic with complaints of right wrist pain following a fall on the outstretched hand the day prior. Initial radiographs show an undisplaced midwaist scaphoid fracture (Fig. 2.1A–C).

CASE 2

A 22-year-old male patient presents to the emergency room complaining of wrist pain after falling off a motorcycle. Initial radiographs show an undisplaced proximal pole fracture of the scaphoid (Fig. 2.2A–C).

How can you come to an evidence-based decision in the management of each of these patients' injuries?

What is the role of patients and provider preferences, practice environment, and current literature in the end treatment chosen?

application of the best available evidence as part of clinical decision-making, in concert with clinician expertise and judgment as well as patient preferences and values (Fig. 2.3). Since its introduction, the concepts of evidence-based medicine have permeated all clinical fields, including hand surgery. "Evidence-based orthopedics" has applied these concepts to musculoskeletal conditions and adapted them to the unique challenges associated with the objective assessment of surgical interventions and the nature of the available literature.[1,5,6] An evidence-based approach to surgical management cannot rely solely on the results of the relatively few randomized controlled trials (RCTs) that exist,[7] but instead must incorporate the results from various study designs represented in the hierarchy of evidence (Fig. 2.4).

Hand surgery and, particularly, fractures of the scaphoid have garnered the attention of numerous publications over the years, mostly of retrospective design, the subject of frequent misinterpretation.[8] This raises concerns for the inaccurate propagation of lower quality evidence, which may lead to errors in the management of patients with these complex injuries. An understanding of the principles of

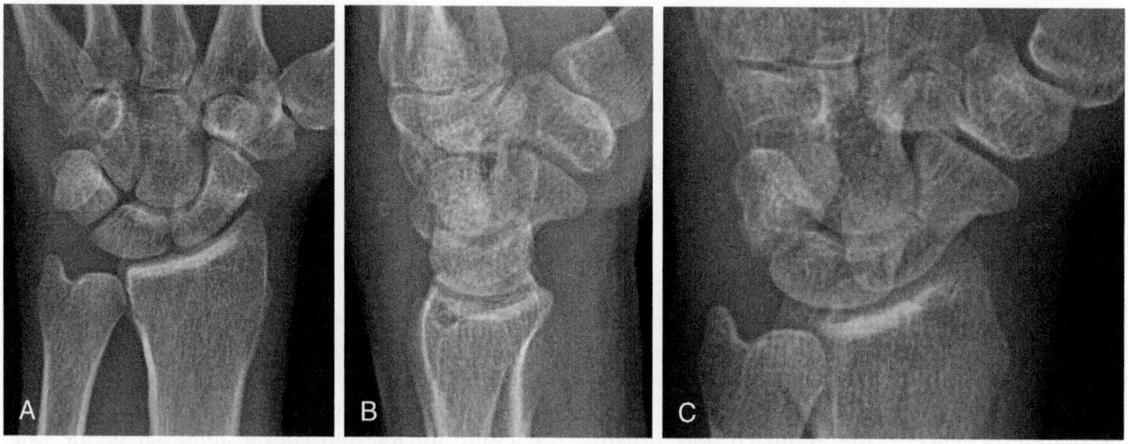

FIG. 2.1 **(A)** anteriorposterior (AP) and **(B)** lateral wrist and **(C)** scaphoid radiographs of Case 1—a 30-year-old male with an undisplaced midwaist scaphoid fracture.

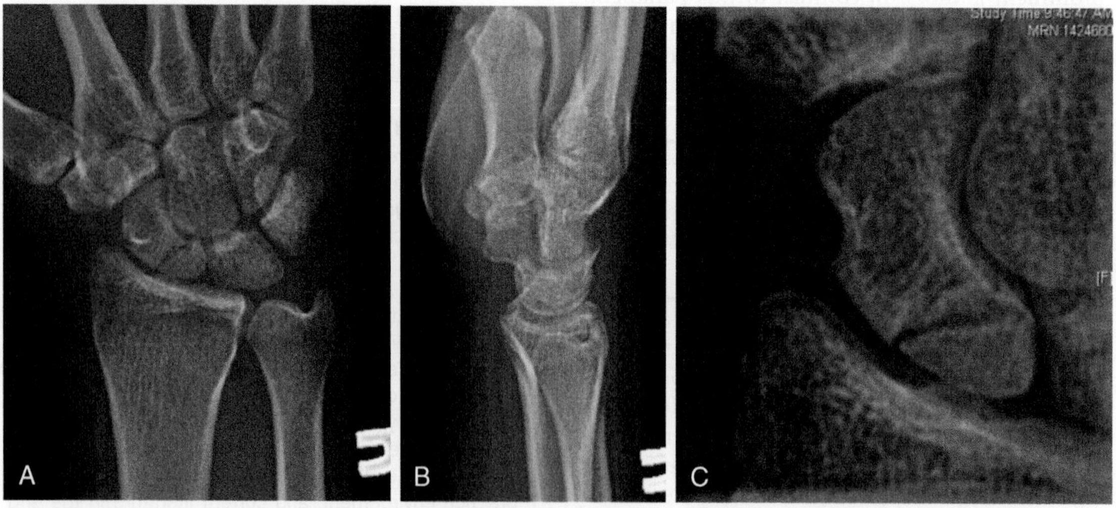

FIG. 2.2 **(A)** AP and **(B)** lateral wrist and **(C)** scaphoid radiographs of Case 2—a 22-year-old male with an undisplaced proximal pole scaphoid fracture.

evidence-based management and hierarchy of evidence, along with knowledge of the study design, quality, and presentation of results, will aid surgeons in interpreting and applying the best available evidence to treatment.

Principles of Evidence-Based Management

The key principles of evidence-based management can best be summarized by the evidence pathway (Fig. 2.5):

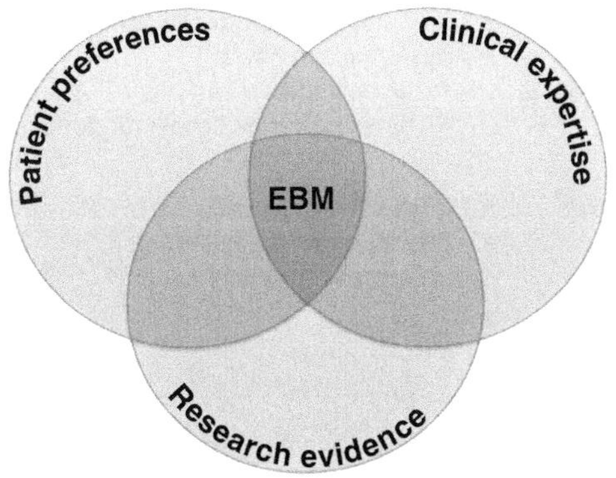

FIG. 2.3 The trillium model of evidence-based medicine (EBM).

1. *Assess:* The pathway begins by clinicians understanding the importance of a clinical issue that is affecting patients and outcomes.
2. *Ask:* With respect to the clinical issue, the provider must formulate a research question that will form the foundation for a structured literature search. This will outline the patient population, intervention, comparator, and outcomes of interest and is known as the PICO framework.
3. *Acquire:* Perform an objective, systematic search to obtain pertinent evidence from databases and other sources (including bibliographies, relative research conference abstracts, and content experts).

> Commonly used databases to perform literature searches include the National Library of Medicine (Medline/Pubmed, https://www.ncbi.nlm.nih.gov/pubmed), EMBASE (www.embase.elsevier.com), and the Cochrane Library (www.cochranelibrary.com).

4. *Appraise:* Critically appraise the evidence to evaluate where the study fits into the hierarchy of evidence, assess if the results are valid with respect to the methodological quality and clinical relevance.

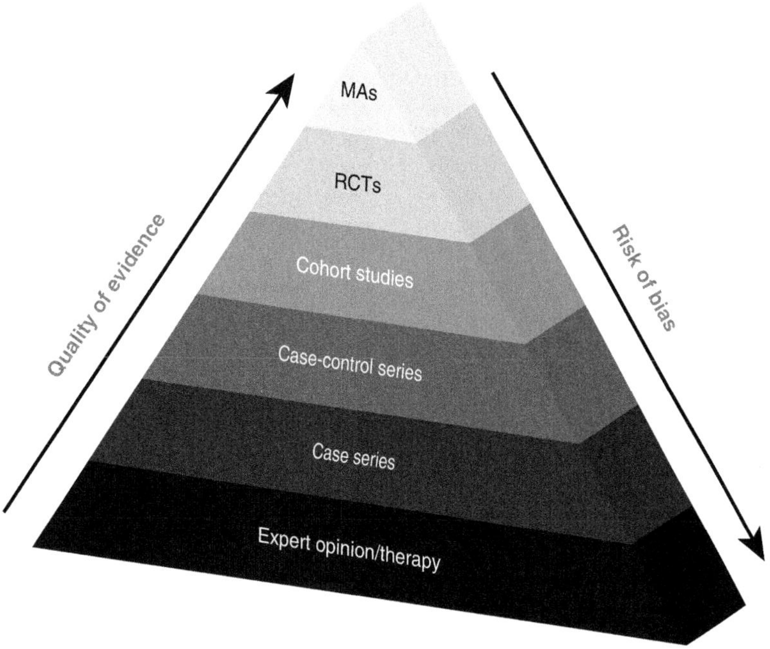

FIG. 2.4 The hierarchy of evidence depicts that, as one moves from the bottom to top, the rigor of the research design improves, which corresponds with an increase in the quality of evidence and a decrease in the influence of bias. *MA*, metaanalysis; *RCT*, randomized controlled trial.

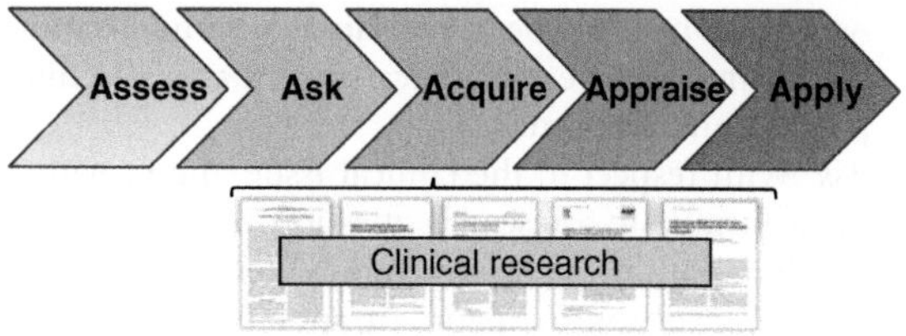

FIG. 2.5 The steps of the evidence pathway.

5. *Apply:* The collected and evaluated evidence is applied in conjunction with patient preferences and provider expertise.

Using this framework when making treatment decisions in the management of scaphoid fractures will allow surgeons to deliver evidence-based solutions in the face of conflicting literature of varying quality, which can then be applied in line with patient values and clinical settings. The tools required to take this approach will be described throughout the remainder of this chapter and will equip the reader to knowledgeably interpret and apply the rest of this text.

HIERARCHY OF EVIDENCE AND QUALITY

For the busy clinician, routinely sifting through the seemingly endless mountain of literature, appraising all of the articles and synthesizing the results to apply the "best available evidence" may be a daunting task.[9] Hierarchies of evidence facilitate an approach to the literature for clinicians by providing a measure of quality.[10] They generally rank research studies in order of methodological rigor and susceptibility to the inclusion of bias; more rigorous, methodologically sound studies are less likely to have bias impact the validity of their findings. This places RCTs at the top of the hierarchy, followed by controlled observational studies in the middle, and uncontrolled case series/expert opinion at the bottom (Fig. 2.4). These rankings can be categorized into levels of evidence, a grading system introduced by Dr. Sackett, that has been widely adopted across specialties and journals.[10,11] Table 2.1 outlines the application of these levels of evidence as they apply to studies of therapeutic interventions, which make up the majority of the evidence in the scaphoid fracture literature.[10] Inherent to an understanding of the hierarchy of evidence is a familiarity with the merits of the various study designs and impact had on overall quality.

RCTs exist at the top of the hierarchy and traditionally represent the standard to which other study types are compared.[12] Although relatively rare across the landscape of surgical literature, their use is growing because of their ability to mitigate the influence of bias in comparison with the other designs. They involve the random allocation of eligible patients to either an intervention (new treatment) or control arm (standard or no treatment). This eliminates the influence of selection bias by balancing the distribution of known and unknown prognostic factors among the treatment arms. However, randomization alone does not protect these studies from other flaws that can compromise study quality and move an RCT from Level I quality of evidence down to Level II. Other key methodological features of RCTs include allocation concealment, blinding, avoidance of expertise bias, minimization of attrition, and analysis of results using the intent-to-treat principle.[13]

TABLE 2.1
Levels of Evidence for Therapeutic Investigations

Level I	• Randomized controlled trial:
	  • showing significant difference
	  • showing no significant difference, but with narrow confidence intervals
	• Systematic review of Level I randomized controlled trials

Level II	• Prospective cohort study
	• Low-quality randomized controlled trial
	• Systematic review of:
	  • Level II trials
	  • heterogeneous Level I randomized controlled trials

Level III	• Case-control study • Retrospective cohort study • Systematic review of Level III studies
Level IV	• Case series • with either no or historical control group
Level V	• Expert opinion

Adapted from Sackett DL. Rules of evidence and clinical recommendations on the use of antithrombotic agents. *Chest*. 1989;95(suppl 2):3S; with permission.

Allocation concealment—The investigators enrolling patients are unable to determine which treatment arm the next patient will be assigned to. Acceptable methods include central (Internet- or telephone-based) allocation or the use of sequentially numbered, sealed, opaque envelopes. Methods susceptible to bias include the use of chart numbers, odd/even dates, or unsealed envelopes.

Blinding—The participants of interest are unaware of which treatment arm the patient has been allocated to. Groups that can be blinded include patients, clinicians, outcome collectors, outcome adjudicators, data analysts, and manuscript writers. The more groups that are blinded, the less likelihood there is of performance or detection bias due to knowledge of treatment allocation.

Expertise bias—The differential ability of a clinician to apply the intervention or procedure due to skill or prior beliefs. This may occur when a surgeon is asked to perform a procedure that they either are not proficiently trained in or think it is not effective compared with the alternative treatment arm.

Attrition—The loss of patients to follow-up to the point where the final cohort may no longer represent the original cohort. Traditional thresholds have required at least 80% of patients to be included at final follow-up. Bias may occur if those who drop out of a trial systematically differ from those who remain.

Intent-to-treat principle—The analysis of patient outcomes by the treatment group to which they were allocated to, regardless of whether this was the treatment which they actually received. This form of analysis preserves the power imparted by randomization to balance the distribution of known and unknown factors among the treatment groups.

Despite RCTs representing the highest level of evidence, they may not be feasible or appropriate for the assessment of particular interventions. Particularly, for the investigation of potentially harmful exposures, rare outcomes, or outcomes that develop over a long period, RCTs may be prohibitive based on ethical grounds or the resources required. Observational study designs allow patient or provider preferences to determine which treatment (or exposure) group the patient is in. Although lower in the hierarchy of evidence because of the impact of selection bias, these study designs serve as a valuable tool in providing answers to questions that RCTs cannot. For instance, in the investigation of the relationship between smoking and nonunion in scaphoid fractures, it is unethical to randomize patients to either smoking or nonsmoking arms, and it would be more appropriate to observe the rates of nonunion among patients who have made the decision to smoke (or not) for themselves.[14]

Within observational trial designs, several study types exist. Cohort studies involve the comparison of patients who are exposed to a risk factor (or treatment) to unexposed patients, who are then followed to determine the rate of occurrence of an outcome of interest.[12] To be considered as higher level evidence, cohort studies can be prospective, which ensures more rigorous data collection and patient follow-up, as well as facilitates the investigation of multiple outcomes over time. However, this design typically requires a large number of patients followed over a prolonged period, which may still pose feasibility challenges.[13] Retrospective cohort studies similarly involve the identification of exposed and unexposed patients; however, it is done by looking at past records and identifying outcomes that have already occurred. Although these are considerably less time and resource intensive compared with prospective designs, they lack control over the measure of outcomes and are prone to additional sources of bias, such as recall bias.[13]

Prospective trial designs begin at a specified point when patients are either exposed or unexposed. These patients are then followed forward in time to evaluate the impact of the exposure(s) on the outcomes of interest. Retrospective trial designs involve looking backward from the present into past records to identify patient outcomes and exposures.

The case-control study is a specific type of retrospective observational design where a group of patients are identified who have already developed an outcome of interest (cases) and are matched to a similar group of patients who did not develop the outcome (controls). These groups are then assessed by looking back in time for differences in previous exposures to risk factors that are possibly associated with the outcome.[12,13] This is a particularly efficient design when assessing multiple risk factors, rare outcomes, or outcomes that develop over a prolonged period, such as degeneration associated with scaphoid nonunion advanced collapse.[15] However, these still suffer from the limitations of retrospective study designs and data collection outlined above.

Recall bias is the differential likelihood of patients or providers to report an exposure in the setting of an adverse event or poor outcome.

Case reports and case series are descriptive study designs that involve detailed profiles of one or several patients. They are near the bottom of the hierarchy of evidence because they do not have an unexposed control group for comparison, and therefore conclusions cannot be made with respect to causal associations between exposures and outcomes, which is the major limitation of their design. Additionally, case series and case reports tend to describe the experience of a single surgeon or center and, therefore, have limited generalizability to other practice settings. However, these studies still play a role in the reporting of rare events, in new techniques, or in the generation of hypothesis that may drive research questions amenable to investigation with more rigorous, higher quality study designs.

Generalizability refers to the ability to apply the findings of a study to a larger group of similar individuals.

Lastly, systematic reviews and metaanalysis represent overviews that employ an organized, reproducible, and objective approach to the collection and synthesis of data from several studies. Metaanalyses have the additional ability to combine the results of the studies identified to increase the sample size and provide a single, pooled estimate of the treatment effect.[12] These features place them high up in the hierarchy of evidence; however, their overall level of evidence is dependent on the quality of studies included for analysis. Therefore, a metaanalysis of Level I RCTs ranks at the very top of the hierarchy, whereas those that include lower quality RCTs or observational studies rank further down in terms of quality and level of evidence. Additionally, confidence in the effect estimate from a metaanalysis is dependent on the limitation of heterogeneity among the included trials. If the study characteristics and results across the included trials are consistent and precise, then the reader can be confident in the overall estimate of effect produced and can use these results to make well-informed, evidence-based management decisions. Although conventional metaanalyses quantify the effectiveness of two interventions based on head-to-head (direct) comparisons, for many conditions, multiple treatment options exist that may not have all been directly compared in the literature. The recent emergence of network metaanalyses deals with this issue, as they allow the use of both direct and indirect comparisons to quantify the relative effectiveness more than two treatment options.[16,17] While these are more complex in their analysis and pooling methodology, similar principles can be applied to their interpretation and application.

Effect estimate (or effect size) is the difference in outcomes between the intervention and control groups.

Heterogeneity refers to differences in patients or differences in the results across multiple studies.

Precision refers to the width of confidence intervals surrounding an estimate of effect. The narrower this interval is, the more precise the estimate.

PRESENTATION OF RESEARCH FINDINGS

Once studies have be identified and assessed with respect to their quality, their results have to be accurately interpreted to form the basis for treatment recommendations. Box 2.1 provides a summary of commonly reported measures of treatment effects, using an example of an RCT that compared open reduction and internal fixation (ORIF) with a Herbert screw to treatment in a below elbow cast for acute, nondisplaced scaphoid fractures.[18]

Absolute risk is, perhaps, the more straightforward measure to understand. In the trial identified, the absolute risk for nonunion in the ORIF group is 3.1% (1 of 32), and the absolute risk of nonunion in the cast-treatment group is 6.7% (2 of 30).[18] Another terminology used to describe the absolute risk in the control group includes baseline risk or control event rate.[1] To describe the actual effect of treatment, the absolute risk reduction (or risk difference) can be used. This expresses the difference in absolute risk between the intervention and control groups and represents the proportion of patients that were able to avoid an unfavorable outcome due to the intervention. In the case of ORIF and the treatment of undisplaced scaphoid fractures, the absolute risk reduction is 3.5%.

The relative risk (risk ratio) represents the proportion of baseline risk that is still present following treatment with the intervention.[1] A relative risk of 1.0 indicates no difference in risk between the intervention and control groups. For the example given, the relative risk of nonunion after being treated with ORIF is 1 of 32 divided by 2 of 30 (risk in the control group), or 0.469. This could be interpreted as, for patients with undisplaced scaphoid fractures, the risk of nonunion in patients treated with ORIF is 0.469 (or 46.9%) of the risk of nonunion in patients treated with a cast. Most commonly, dichotomous results are reported as the relative risk reduction, which is the proportion of baseline risk that is eliminated by the intervention.[1] It can be obtained by either subtracting the relative risk from 1 or dividing the absolute risk reduction by the baseline risk. Again, in the example given, the relative

BOX 2.1
Measures of Treatment Effect

Standard 2 x 2 table

	Outcome Yes (+)	Outcome No (–)
Intervention (Y)	a	b
Control (X)	c	d

Absolute risk *of outcome*
Intervention = a/(a+b) = Y
Control = c/ (c+d) = X

Example 2 x 2 table (data from Saeden, 2001 – for nondisplaced scaphoid fractures)

	Nonunion Yes (+)	Nonunion No (–)
ORIF with Herbert screw	1	31
Below elbow cast	2	28

Absolute risk of nonunion
ORIF = 1/(1+31) = 3.1%
Cast = 2/(2+28) = 6.7%

Absolute risk reduction (ARR)—difference in risk between the control and intervention groups.
$ARR = [c/(c+d)] - [a/(a+b)] = X - Y.$
Example: $ARR = [2/(2+28)] - [1/(1+31)] = 3.5\%$

Relative risk or risk reduction (RR)—ratio in risk in the intervention group (Y) to risk in the control group (X)
$RR = Y/X.$
Example: $RR = [1/(1+31)]/[2/(2+28)] = 0.469.$

Relative risk reduction (RRR)—the percent reduction in risk in the intervention group compared with the control group.
$RRR = 1 - RR = (1 - X/Y) \times 100\%$ or $[(X - Y)/X] \times 100\%$
Example: $RRR = 1 - 0.469 \times 100\% = 53\%$

risk reduction equates to 0.531 (or 53%), which means that treatment of undisplaced scaphoid fractures with ORIF reduced the risk of nonunion by 53% relative to treatment with a below elbow cast.

Dichotomous outcomes describe “yes” or “no” events that either occur or do not (such as infection, nonunion, avascular necrosis, or death). This is in contrast to continuous outcomes that can theoretically take on any value; however, practically, these outcomes take on any value with an upper and lower limit.

Note the difference in interpretation between the relative risk reduction and absolute risk reduction. In the example given, the relative risk reduction of nonunion by 53% with ORIF appears to be quite striking; however, when accounting for the baseline risk, this results in an absolute risk reduction of only 3.5% (from 6.7% in the control group to 3.1% in the intervention group). This raises the question of how much a difference in the effect size would be meaningful in clinical practice. For both dichotomous and continuous outcomes, the most common reference point for the interpretation of patient-reported outcomes, such as pain and physical function, is the minimal clinical important difference, which describes the smallest change in the outcome of interest that informed patients would perceive as important, either beneficial or harmful, and that would lead the patient or clinician to consider a change in management.[19,20] The distinction between absolute and relative effects, as well as interpretation of the effect size in the clinical context, are important to keep in mind when reviewing the results reported in the literature.

All the above outcomes are presented as single-point estimates from the example study, each of which indicates that ORIF may have a beneficial effect in the prevention of nonunion compared with treatment in casts alone. However, these represent only one estimate of the truth. Because of variation among any sample selected (i.e., the 62 patients in the example study) and the overall population of patients with the clinical problem (i.e., all patients with undisplaced scaphoid fractures), the true treatment effect may be either smaller or larger than the one reported in the literature. Confidence intervals (CIs) can reveal a plausible range of values for the entire population of patients from whom the study sample was selected.[1] These are most influenced by the sample size, as well as the number of events in each group for dichotomous outcomes, or standard deviation for continuous ones. Using Saeden's reported data,[18] the treatment effect estimates with 95% CI for nonunion would be an absolute risk reduction of 3.5% (95% CI: 7%–14%) and a relative risk of 0.47 (95% CI: 0.04–4.91). The negative sign preceding the lower bound of the 95% CI for absolute risk reduction indicates a possible 7% increase in the risk of nonunion for the ORIF group compared with the casting group. Similarly, with respect to the relative risk, the upper bound greater than 1.0 indicates that ORIF may result in a risk of nonunion up to 4.91 times that of cast treatment. Together, these wide CIs indicate that we do not have enough evidence to confidently declare that ORIF is truly better than cast treatment in the prevention of nonunion following undisplaced scaphoid fractures.

Presenting results with both point estimates and CIs provides clinicians with a possible treatment effect estimate as well as a range of plausible effect estimates within which the true effect may lie. This concept was demonstrated through an examination of the effect of sample size on the results and interpretation of the Study to Prospectively evaluate Reamed Intramudulary Nails in patients with Tibial fractures (SPRINT).[21] Following completion of the study, the authors went back to evaluate the effect estimate and CIs at incremental enrollment points, until the final sample size of 1226 patients was reached (Fig. 2.6). They show that, as the sample size increased, the CI became more narrow. Although the ultimate effect estimate was within the bounds of the initial CI, the precision of the final estimate allows for meaningful conclusions to be made with respect to the use of reamed nailing for closed fractures.[21] This illustrates that the more patients that are included to inform effect estimates (i.e., the greater the sample size between single and pooled evidence), the more likely these estimates are to represent the truth.

A precise CI that does not overlap the bounds of "no effect" (i.e., relative risk of 1) helps define whether the results can be interpreted as being statistically significant. However, as discussed, these estimates are based on the events from single samples of patients that

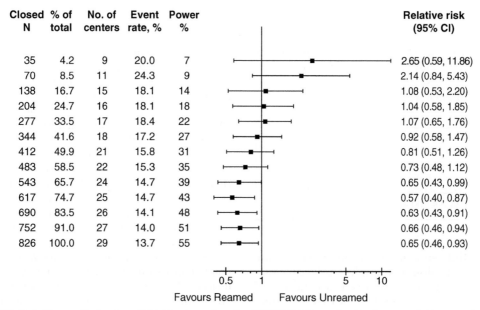

Closed N	% of total	No. of centers	Event rate, %	Power %	Relative risk (95% CI)
35	4.2	9	20.0	7	2.65 (0.59, 11.86)
70	8.5	11	24.3	9	2.14 (0.84, 5.43)
138	16.7	15	18.1	14	1.08 (0.53, 2.20)
204	24.7	16	18.1	18	1.04 (0.58, 1.85)
277	33.5	17	18.4	22	1.07 (0.65, 1.76)
344	41.6	18	17.2	27	0.92 (0.58, 1.47)
412	49.9	21	15.8	31	0.81 (0.51, 1.26)
483	58.5	22	15.3	35	0.73 (0.48, 1.12)
543	65.7	24	14.7	39	0.65 (0.43, 0.99)
617	74.7	25	14.7	43	0.57 (0.40, 0.87)
690	83.5	26	14.1	48	0.63 (0.43, 0.91)
752	91.0	27	14.0	51	0.66 (0.46, 0.94)
826	100.0	29	13.7	55	0.65 (0.46, 0.93)

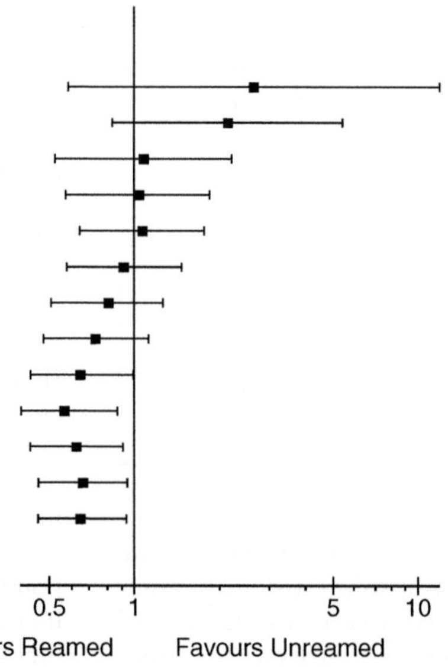

FIG. 2.6 The results for closed tibial fractures from the SPRINT trial examined by incremental increase in the sample size. (From SPRINT Investigators, Bhandari M, Tornetta P, et al. (Sample) size matters! An examination of sample size from the SPRINT trial study to prospectively evaluate reamed intramedullary nails in patients with tibial fractures. *J Orthop Trauma*. 2013;27(4):183–188; with permission.)

are meant to be representative of the entire population. It is important to recognize that spurious events may have occurred among the sample, and (particularly when only relatively few events occur) if these events had not occurred, the overall conclusion of the study would be different. This describes the concept of study "fragility," which can be measured using the "fragility index."[22] The literature from several areas of orthopedic surgery have been examined to assess the impact of fragility on overall results and have shown that the statistical significance of conclusions hinged on the occurrence (or nonoccurrence) of as few as two events.[23,24]

> The fragility index is the minimum number of patients per treatment group that would have to change from having a dichotomous outcome event (i.e., nonunion) to not having the event (or vice versa) for study results to go from statistically significant to nonsignificant.

Lastly, as clinicians scour the literature in an attempt to collect evidence surrounding a particular clinical scenario, often times they will encounter studies that primarily set out to answer a question with a population broader than the one of interest. These studies may go on to provide subgroup analysis to provide information on individual subsets of patients. Although these may seemingly meet the goal of meeting clinicians' needs for data on specific population, caution needs to be taken when interpreting these results.[25] To determine the credibility of subgroup analysis, several questions need to be answered (Table 2.2).[26] These questions pertain to the timing of analysis relative to the hypothesis, number of subgroup hypothesis tested, comparisons within studies (rather than between studies), the magnitude and statistical significant of the subgroup difference, consistency of the subgroup differences across studies, and the support of external evidence.[25,26] Although these analyses can often be hypothesis-generating and prompt further research questions, however, using them to support clinical decision-making should be done carefully. Thinking beyond the simple presentation of point estimates of effect, and incorporating the concepts of CIs, fragility, and subgroup credibility, equips clinicians with an understanding of the accuracy and robustness of results. This informs the certainty to which results can be applied, which, combined with quality assessments, provide the basis to make recommendations for management decisions.

TABLE 2.2
Guidelines to Assess the Credibility of Subgroups

Criteria	Question
Timing	Was the hypothesis made a priori (i.e., did it proceed the analysis)? • Was the subgroup variable a characteristic that was measured at baseline or following randomization?
Hypothesis	Was the hypothesis for subgroup effect one of many or a small number hypothesis tested?
Nature of comparison	Is the effect suggested based on comparisons done within the same study or between different studies?
Effect size	Is the size of the subgroup effect large? Was the direction of the effect hypothesized a priori?
Statistical significance	Was the difference in subgroups statistically significant? • Do tests for interaction suggest a low likelihood that the differences can be explained by chance? • Is the subgroup effect independent?
Consistency	Is the interaction consistent across other studies?
External evidence	Is the hypothesized subgroup difference supported by external evidence?

Data from Sun X, Briel M, Walter SD, et al. Is a subgroup effect believable? Updating criteria to evaluate the credibility of subgroup analyses. *BMJ*. 2010;340:c117.

MAKING RECOMMENDATIONS

When considering whether to proceed with an intervention, accounting for the above factors is vital, along with a balance of the associated benefits and for a given intervention. Often times, this requires a careful systematic search for and appraisal of the best evidence as already outlined in this chapter, combined with the judgment of content experts. To add objectivity to the process of making treatment decisions, the GRADE Working Group at McMaster University has provided a structured approach and grading system that outlines the factors that need to be considered prior to making one of eight possible alphanumeric grades of recommendation, which summarize both the strength and quality of the evidence.[1,27] Fig. 2.7 depicts the process of ranking the quality of the evidence into one of four

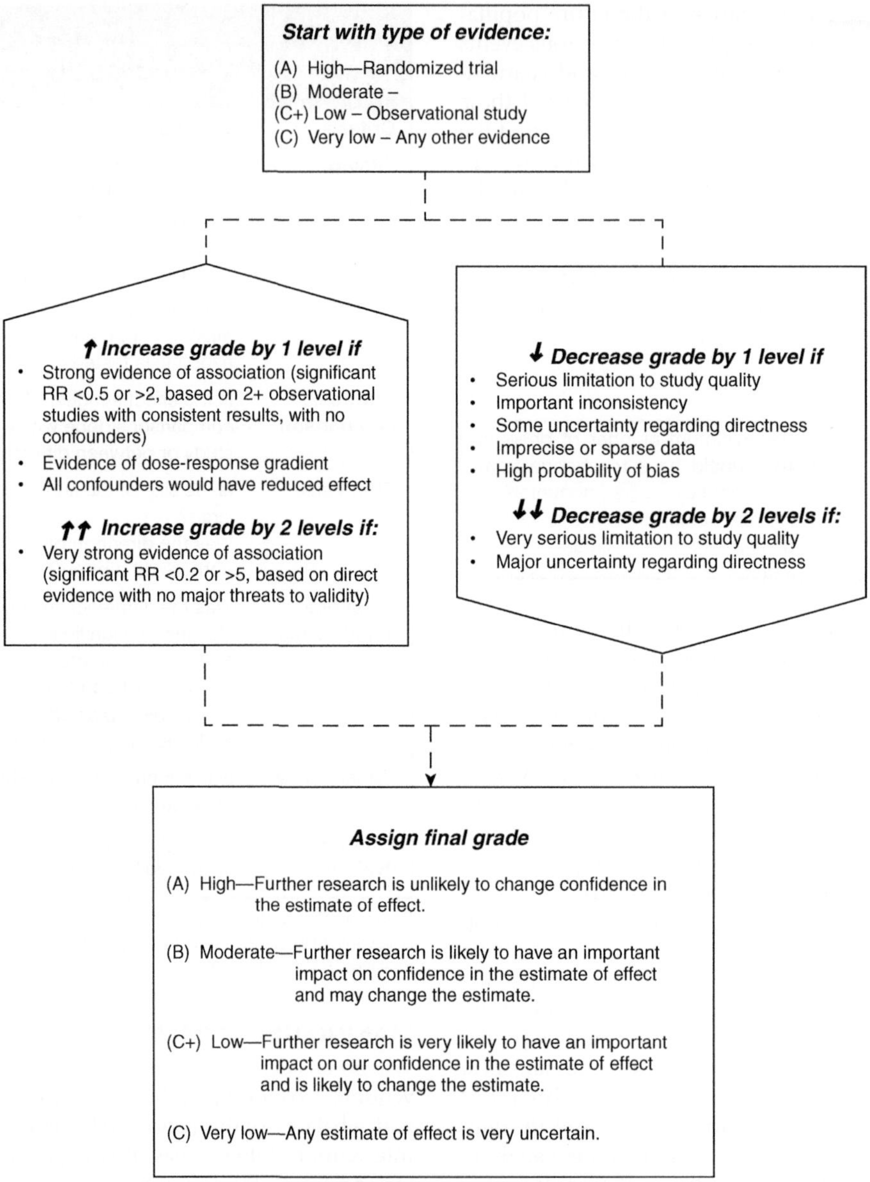

FIG. 2.7 Assigning grades based on the quality of evidence on the GRADE Working Group system. (Data from Guyatt G, Oxman AD, Akl EA, et al. GRADE guidelines: 1. Introduction-GRADE evidence profiles and summary of findings tables. *J Clin Epidemiol*. 2011;64(4):383–394.)

rankings: "high" (A), "moderate" (B), "low" (C+), or "very low" (C). An RCT will start off as "high"-quality evidence, whereas observational studies (cohorts and case controls) will start off as "low"-quality evidence. The quality grade is then either increased or decreased based on the characteristics of the evidence. The strength of the recommendation is based on the overall balance of risks and benefits, as determined by experts, and will determine whether an intervention is given a Grade 1 or Grade 2 rating. If experts are very certain that the benefits do (or do not) outweigh the harms associated with an intervention, they can give a Grade 1 recommendation.[1] If there is uncertainty surrounding the magnitude of benefit and harms, as well as their impact

TABLE 2.3
The GRADE Working Group Categories for Recommendation

Grade	Clarity of Risk/ Benefit	Supporting Evidence Methodology	Strength of Recommendation	Implications
1A	Clear	Randomized controlled trials without important limitations	Strong recommendation	Can apply to most patients in most circumstances without reservation
1B	Clear	Randomized controlled trials with important limitations (inconsistent results and methodological flaws)	Strong recommendation	Likely to apply to most patients
1C+	Clear	Indirect evidence from extrapolated randomized controlled trials or overwhelming evidence from observational evidence	Strong recommendation	Can apply to most patients in most circumstances
1C	Clear	Observational studies	Intermediate strength	May change when stronger evidence is available
2A	Unclear	Randomized controlled trials without important limitations	Intermediate strength	Best treatment choice may differ depending on circumstances and patient/societal values
2B	Unclear	Randomized controlled trials with important limitations (inconsistent results and methodological flaws)	Weak recommendation	Alternative approached likely to be better for some patients under some circumstances
2C+	Unclear	Indirect evidence from extrapolated randomized controlled trials or overwhelming evidence from observational evidence	Weak recommendation	Best treatment choice may differ depending on circumstances and patient/societal values
2C	Unclear	Observational studies	Very weak recommendation	Other alternatives may be equally reasonable

Data from Schünemann HJ, Bone L. Evidence-based orthopaedics: a primer. *Clin Orthop Relat Res*. 2003;413:117–132.

relative to one another, a weaker Grade 2 recommendation is made.[1] Grade 1 recommendations provide strong evidence to inform treatment decisions, whereas Grade 2 recommendations provide an opportunity for the incorporation of patient and provider values to guide management. Together, the strength and quality recommendation categories from GRADE (Table 2.3) facilitate an approach to evidence-based management and will provide guidance for clinicians to the challenging issues surrounding the treatment of scaphoid fractures throughout the following sections. Panel 2 completes the case scenario from the beginning of the chapter and outlines how evidence-based management can be put into action for the management of scaphoid fractures, using the best available evidence.[28-32]

CONCLUSION

Critics of an evidence-based approach tend to misunderstand its purpose and process. Although it places a focus on the use of RCTs to avoid errors associated with bias, it emphasizes the consideration of different types of evidence as appropriate and acknowledges that they offer important information to inform decision-making. Observational studies play a particularly prominent role in evidence-based management when higher level evidence is nonexistent or not feasible to obtain. The overall recommendations are made in light of the evidence that has been included and any limitations it brings. This, in turn, leaves room for the incorporation of patient values and provider experience into the decision-making process.

PANEL 2
The Evidence-Based Medicine Approach Applied

CASES 1 AND 2

Assess: The optimal management for undisplaced scaphoid fractures has been the subject of considerable debate. There have been advocates for internal fixation of these injuries; however, it is unknown whether surgery improves clinically relevant patient outcomes.

Ask: In patients with acute undisplaced scaphoid fractures, what is the effect of internal fixation versus casting on the rates of union, return to activity, grip strength, and range of motion? (PICO format)

Acquire: Several systematic reviews on the topic were identified that were relevant to this clinical question.[28–32] The reviews by Bhandari,[28] Grewal,[29] and Buijze[32] address undisplaced scaphoid fractures as a whole, whereas Ram[30] focuses on fractures of the waist and Eastley[31] on fractures of the proximal pole.

Appraise: The metaanalyses addressing the issue of undisplaced scaphoid waist fractures limited their inclusion to RCTs; however, these trials had some methodological limitations and were, therefore, considered Level II evidence.[28–31] The metaanalysis addressing undisplaced proximal pole fractures included RCTs, as well as cohort studies and case series, and is therefore considered lower down on the hierarchy (Level IV).[32]

Apply: Bhandari, Grewal, Buijze, and Ram all overlapped in the trials they included to assess undisplaced fractures of the scaphoid waist.[28–31] They separately concluded that there were no differences between internal fixation and cast treatment with respect to nonunion rates, grip strength, and range of motion, but there was a significantly earlier return to work in the internal fixation group. Grewal, Buijze, and Ram went on to emphasize that the possible complications and costs of surgery were not to be underestimated and that, with equivocal outcomes in the objective measures, the benefits imparted by subjectively quicker return to activity may only be limited to a few patients.[29,31] Together, all recommended an aggressively conservative approach as a Grade 2B recommendation, with consideration of surgical treatment for improvement in function outcomes and return to work as a 2C recommendation.

With respect to undisplaced proximal pole fractures, Eastley found that there was a 34% baseline risk of nonunion for those treated conservatively, which was 7.5 times that of fractures that were more distal. Based on limited evidence, the authors recommend offering surgical fixation to patients with these injuries but, overall, emphasize a thorough inclusion of patient and provider input into the final treatment decision.[20] Overall, this would constitute a Grade 2C recommendation.

ACT

Case 1

There was a discussion with the patient regarding nonoperative and operative treatment options. This patient did not have a need for early use of his hand and wrist. Thus, nonoperative management was implemented, and this patient's fracture went on to heal uneventfully with nonoperative care (Fig. 2.8A–C)

Case 2

In discussing the treatment options with this patient, it was emphasized that the more proximally the scaphoid is fractured, the higher the nonunion risk. Thus, acute operative management was agreed on. This patient underwent acute ORIF via a dorsal approach (Fig. 2.9A and B) and went onto heal at 3 months postoperatively with radiography and CT follow-up imaging (Fig. 2.10A–D).

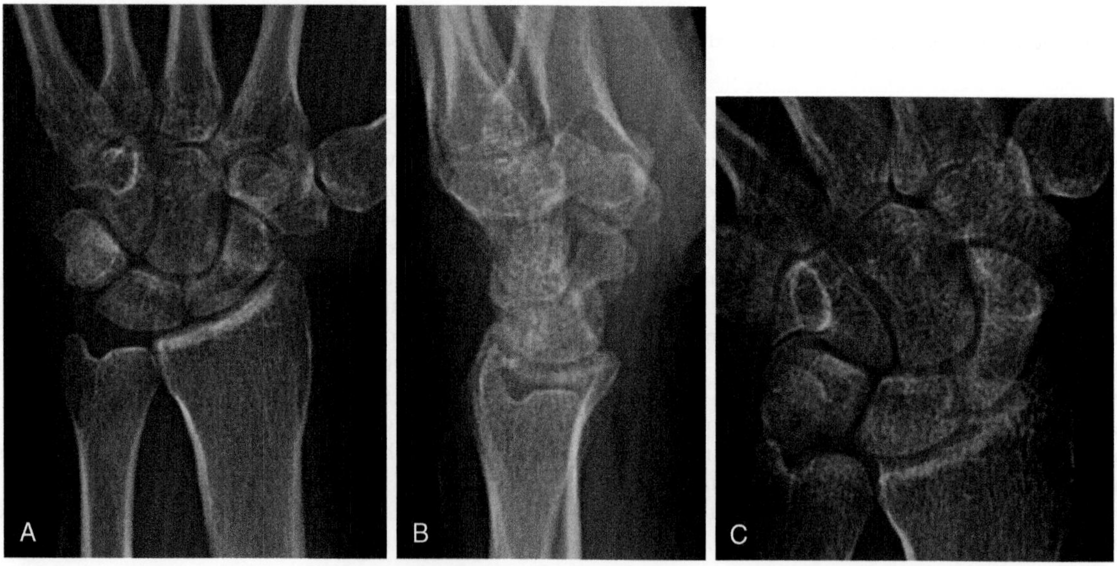

FIG. 2.8 Final follow-up **(A)** AP and **(B)** lateral wrist and **(C)** scaphoid radiographs of Case 1, which went on to uneventful healing with nonoperative management.

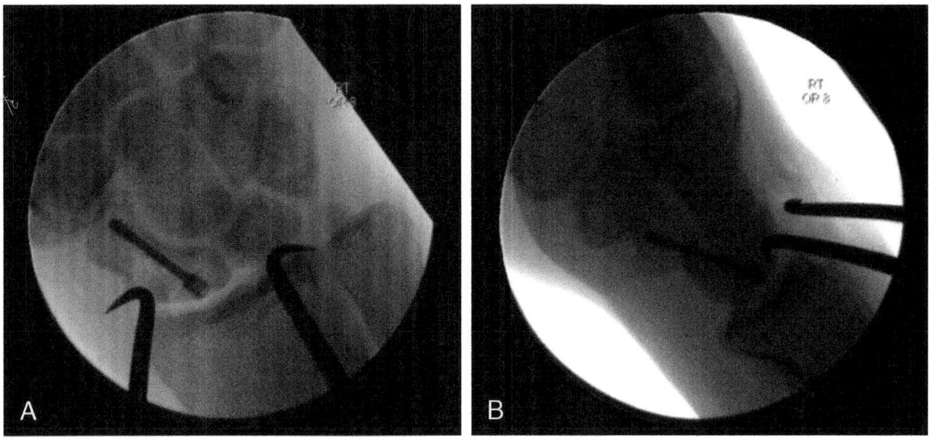

FIG. 2.9 Intraoperative **(A)** AP and **(B)** lateral wrist of Case 2, which received internal fixation with a dorsally placed, anterograde Herbert screw.

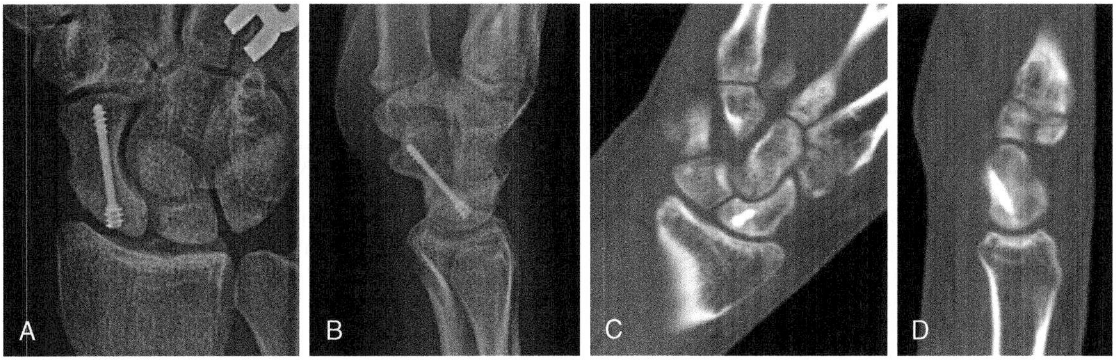

FIG. 2.10 Final follow-up **(A)** AP and **(B)** lateral wrist radiographs as well as select **(C)** coronal and **(D)** sagittal CT cuts of Case 2, which show uneventful healing following internal fixation.

REFERENCES

1. Schünemann HJ, Bone L. Evidence-based orthopaedics: a primer. *Clin Orthop Relat Res*. 2003;413:117–132. http://dx.doi.org/10.1097/01.blo.0000080541.81794.26.
2. Sackett DL, Rosenberg WM, Gray JA, Haynes RB, Richardson WS. Evidence based medicine: what it is and what it isn't. *BMJ*. 1996;312(7023):71–72.
3. Guyatt GH. Evidence-based medicine. *ACP J Club*. 1991. http://dx.doi.org/10.7326/ACPJC-1991-114-2-A16.
4. Bhandari M, Giannoudis PV. Evidence-based medicine: what it is and what it is not. *Injury*. 2006;37:302–306.
5. Devereaux PJ, McKee MD, Yusuf S. Methodologic issues in randomized controlled trials of surgical interventions. *Clin Orthop Relat Res*. 2003;413:25–32. http://dx.doi.org/10.1097/01.blo.0000080539.81794.54.
6. Hartz A, Marsh JL. Methodologic issues in observational studies. *Clin Orthop Relat Res*. 413:33–42. http://dx.doi.org/10.1097/01.blo.0000079325.41006.95.
7. Obremskey WT, Pappas N, Attallah-Wasif E, Tornetta P, Bhandari M. Level of evidence in orthopaedic journals. *J Bone Joint Surgery Am Vol*. 2005;87(12):2632–2638. http://dx.doi.org/10.2106/JBJS.E.00370.
8. Buijze GA, Weening AA, Poolman RW, Bhandari M, Ring D. Predictors of the accuracy of quotation of references in peer-reviewed orthopaedic literature in relation to publications on the scaphoid. *J Bone Joint Surg Br*. 2012;94(2):276–280. http://dx.doi.org/10.1302/0301-620X.94B2.
9. Atkins D, Best D, Briss PA, et al. Grading quality of evidence and strength of recommendations. *BMJ*. 2004;328(7454):1490. http://dx.doi.org/10.1136/bmj.328.7454.1490.
10. Wright JG, Swiontkowski MF, Heckman JD. Introducing levels of evidence to the journal. *J Bone Joint Surgery Am Vol*. 2003;85-A(1):1–3.
11. Sackett DL. Rules of evidence and clinical recommendations on the use of antithrombotic agents. *Chest*. 1989;95(2 suppl):S2–S4.

12. Guyatt G, Rennie D, Meade M, Cook D. Users' guides to the medical literature: a manual for evidence-based clinical practice. *JAMA Arch J.* 2008.
13. Brighton B, Bhandari M, Tornetta III P, Felson DT. Hierarchy of evidence: from case reports to randomized controlled trials. *Clin Orthop Relat Res.* 2003;413:19–24. http://dx.doi.org/10.1097/01.blo.0000079323.41006.12.
14. Little CP, Burston BJ, Hopkinson-Woolley J, BURGE P. Failure of surgery for scaphoid non-union is associated with smoking. *J Hand Surg Br.* 2006;31(3):252–255. http://dx.doi.org/10.1016/j.jhsb.2005.12.010.
15. Mack GR, Bosse MJ, Gelberman RH, Yu E. The natural history of scaphoid non-union. *J Bone Joint Surgery Am Vol.* 1984;66(4):504–509.
16. Foote CJ, Chaudhry H, Bhandari M, et al. Network meta-analysis: users' guide for surgeons: Part I – credibility. *Clin Orthop Relat Res.* 2015:1–6. http://dx.doi.org/10.1007/s11999-015-4286-x.
17. Chaudhry H, Foote CJ, Guyatt G, et al. Network meta-analysis: users' guide for surgeons: Part II – certainty. *Clin Orthop Relat Res.* 2015:1–7. http://dx.doi.org/10.1007/s11999-015-4287-9.
18. Saedén B, Törnkvist H, Ponzer S, Höglund M. Fracture of the carpal scaphoid. A prospective, randomised 12-year follow-up comparing operative and conservative treatment. *J Bone Joint Surg Br.* 2001;83(2):230–234.
19. Jaeschke R, Singer J, Guyatt GH. Measurement of health status: Ascertaining the minimal clinically important difference. *Control Clin Trials.* 1989;10(4):407–415.
20. Johnston BC, Thorlund K, Schünemann HJ, et al. Improving the interpretation of quality of life evidence in meta-analyses: the application of minimal important difference units. *Health Qual Life Outcomes.* 2010;8:116. http://dx.doi.org/10.1186/1477-7525-8-116.
21. SPRINT Investigators, Bhandari M, Tornetta P, et al. (Sample) size matters! an examination of sample size from the SPRINT trial study to prospectively evaluate reamed intramedullary nails in patients with tibial fractures. *J Orthop Trauma.* 2013;27(4):183–188. http://dx.doi.org/10.1097/BOT.0b013e3182647e0e.
22. Walsh M, Srinathan SK, McAuley DF, et al. The statistical significance of randomized controlled trial results is frequently fragile: a case for a Fragility Index. *J Clin Epidemiol.* 2014;67(6):622–628. http://dx.doi.org/10.1016/j.jclinepi.2013.10.019.
23. Evaniew N, Files C, Smith C, et al. The fragility of statistically significant findings from randomized trials in spine surgery: a systematic survey. *The Spine J.* 2015;15(10):2188–2197. http://dx.doi.org/10.1016/j.spinee.2015.06.004.
24. Khan M, Evaniew N, Gichuru M, et al. The fragility of statistically significant findings from randomized trials in sports surgery: a systematic survey. *Am J Sports Med.* 2016. http://dx.doi.org/10.1177/0363546516674469.
25. Ghert M, Petrisor B. Subgroup analyses: when should we believe them? *J Bone Joint Surg Am Vol.* 2012;1(suppl 94):61–64. http://dx.doi.org/10.2106/JBJS.L.00272.
26. Sun X, Briel M, Walter SD, Guyatt GH. Is a subgroup effect believable? Updating criteria to evaluate the credibility of subgroup analyses. *BMJ.* 2010;340(mar30 3):c117. http://dx.doi.org/10.1136/bmj.c117.
27. Guyatt G, Oxman AD, Akl EA, et al. GRADE guidelines: 1. Introduction. *J Clin Epidemiol.* 2011;64(4):383–394. http://dx.doi.org/10.1016/j.jclinepi.2010.04.026.
28. Bhandari M, Hanson BP. Acute nondisplaced fractures of the scaphoid. *J Orthop Trauma.* 2004;18(4):253–255.
29. Grewal R, King GJW. An evidence-based approach to the management of acute scaphoid fractures. *J Hand Surg Am Vol.* 2009;34(4):732–734. http://dx.doi.org/10.1016/j.jhsa.2008.12.027.
30. Ram AN, Chung KC. Evidence-based management of acute nondisplaced scaphoid waist fractures. *J Hand Surg Am Vol.* 2009;34(4):735–738. http://dx.doi.org/10.1016/j.jhsa.2008.12.028.
31. Eastley N, Singh H, Dias JJ, Taub N. Union rates after proximal scaphoid fractures; meta-analyses and review of available evidence. *J Hand Surg Eur Vol.* 2013;38(8):888–897. http://dx.doi.org/10.1177/1753193412451424.
32. Buijze GA, Doornberg JN, Ham JS, Ring D, Bhandari M, Poolman RW. Surgical compared with conservative treatment for acute nondisplaced or minimally displaced scaphoid fractures: a systematic review and meta-analysis of randomized controlled trials. *J Bone Joint Surg Am Vol.* 2010;92(6):1533–1544. http://dx.doi:10.2106/JBJS.I.01214.

CHAPTER 3

Anatomy of the Scaphoid Bone and Ligaments

ANNE EVA J. BULSTRA, MD • JOB N. DOORNBERG, MD, PHD • GEERT A. BUIJZE, MD, PHD • GREGORY I. BAIN, MBBS, FRACS, PHD

KEY POINTS

- The scaphoid articulates with five adjacent bones through a largely cartilaginous surface and features a complex network of ligamentous attachments, making it a unique and key component of the wrist.
- Variations in this anatomy, osseous and more importantly ligamentous, are likely to result in distinct kinematic patterns of the scaphoid, thus playing an important role in carpal (in)stability in both normal and injured wrists.
- In current literature no consensus has been reached on the description and classification of scaphoid anatomy and its variations.
- The inconsistency in ligament classification is due to the complexity of identifying and delineating complex soft tissue structures in cadaver dissections, as well as interindividual variability.

CASE 1
A Patient with Ulnar Carpal Translocation

A 34-year-old man injured his right dominant hand during a bicycle accident, falling onto an outstretched hand. His wrist is painful and swollen. Radiographs show no fracture or dislocation and are interpreted as normal. One month later, the patient complains of persistent wrist pain. Careful reevaluation of the radiographs reveals a subtle ulnar translocation of the radiocarpal joint (Fig. 3.1).

What pathoanatomic characteristic accounts for both the clinical presentation and radiologic findings in this patient?

IMPORTANCE OF THE PROBLEM

The scaphoid has characteristic anatomic features: it has a complex relation to surrounding structures through numerous ligamentous attachments and up to 80% of the scaphoid bony surface is covered with cartilage.[1–3] The interpretation and description of scaphoid anatomy has proven controversial in current literature. Consensus is specifically lacking on the anatomy and classification of the ligaments attaching to the scaphoid.[2] Variations in this anatomy result in distinct kinematic patterns of the scaphoid.[3] Clarification of the ligamentous anatomy will thus enhance our understanding of the role of the scaphoid in carpal stability, for example clarifying the different collapse patterns following scaphoid fractures. Furthermore, it will contribute to our radiographic diagnosis and interpretation of ligamentous injuries.

MAIN QUESTION

What are current concepts on osseous and ligamentous scaphoid anatomy and what (in)consistencies exist in the anatomic description in current literature?

Current Opinion

The scaphoid and its ligamentous attachments play an important role in carpal stability.[1–4] Various classification systems exist to describe the anatomy of the scaphoid and the ligaments attached to it. To date, a universal description and classification system of the ligamentous anatomy has not been accepted.

Finding the Evidence

This chapter is an update of authors' previous systematic literature review on scaphoid osseous and ligamentous anatomy, using similar methodology[2]:

1. Online search
   - Medline: *ligament**[Title] AND (*carp** [Title] OR *scaph** [Title] OR *wrist* [Title]).
   - All original descriptions of the anatomy, morphology of the scaphoid, and/or ligaments available in full-text copy were included.
   - Articles that were not in English, French, Italian, Dutch, German, or Spanish were not included. Personal communications, letters, or meeting proceedings were excluded.
2. Manual search for book chapters
   - Screening of reference lists of all selected articles using the same inclusion and exclusion criteria was performed.

Quality of the Evidence

Current knowledge of scaphoid anatomy is based on both in vitro studies—cadaver dissections—and in vivo studies—imaging techniques. The evidence aggregated in this chapter is predominantly based on macroscopic dissections[1,5-19] combined with few arthroscopic[20] and magnetic resonance imaging studies.[17,21,22] No standardized criteria for evaluating the quality of such studies exist. The most important constraint in identifying ligamentous anatomy is the difficulty of delineating complex soft tissue structures in cadaver dissections, with risk of creating "iatrogenic" anatomy in complex fibrous structures. This may account for the variability in anatomy reported. In addition, interindividual variability in ligament insertion and morphology exists.[2] The variety in individual anatomy can only be explored through larger studies on cadaver specimens.

FINDINGS

Osseous Anatomy

The scaphoid bone has a characteristic and irregular "boat-shaped" form (i.e., Latin *scaphoides* for bowl or boat shaped).[3,4,23] It is the largest bone of the proximal carpal row and is aligned on an oblique axis at 45 degrees to the long axis of the wrist, in both radial and volar directions.[3] Computed tomography (CT) reconstructions along this oblique axis are proven to be more accurate to detect an occult scaphoid fracture than standardized CT reconstructions in frontal,

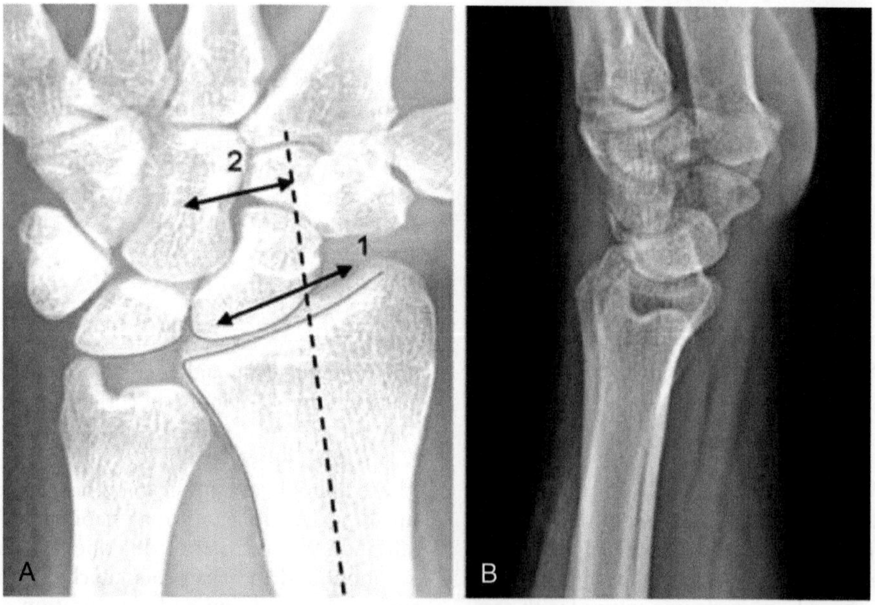

FIG. 3.1 **Posttraumatic Ulnar Translocation of the Radiocarpal Joint. (A)** The interval designated by *line 1* demonstrates an increased distance between the radial styloid and scaphoid. Here, the scaphoid seems positioned in the lunate fossa. The interval designed by *line 2* indicates an increased distance between a line drawn centrally through the radius and through the center of the capitate. The distance is more than the average 5.7 ± 1.4 mm, indicating ulnar translocation of the carpus.[52] (From Rutgers M, Jupiter J, Ring D. Isolated posttraumatic ulnar translocation of the radiocarpal joint. *J Hand Microsurg*. 2009;1(2):108–112; with permission.)

sagittal, and axial planes.[24,25] The scaphoid forms an important link between the proximal and distal carpalia, as it is the only bone to cross both carpal rows.[17,20]

Three-dimensional anatomic imaging of cadavers using CT and cryomicrotome imaging revealed a mean scaphoid surface of 1503 ± 17 mm^2.[1] Approximately 75% of this surface is covered with cartilage, articulating with five adjacent bones.[26] Traditionally four distinct anatomic regions of the scaphoid bone can be differentiated: (1) the proximal pole; (2) the distal pole; (3) the tubercle; and (4) the waist. A substantial variety of shapes has been described and classified[27] (Box 3.1).

BOX 3.1
Morphometric features and a variety in osseous anatomy

Although four distinct anatomic regions (proximal pole, distal pole, tubercle, and waist) can typically be differentiated, a substantial variety in shapes exists. An anatomic study on cadavers by Ceri et al. demonstrated the tubercle and a dorsal sulcus (Fig. 3.4) to be present in all scaphoid specimens, whereas other features were often absent. A great variation in waist circumference, tubercle size, and sulcus width was also reported.[27]

Proximal pole and articulations

Proximally, the biconvex dorsally sloped scaphoid surface articulates with the scaphoid fossa of the distal radius (Fig. 3.2A–D). The orientation of the scaphoid fossa is 11 °volar and 21 ° ulnar to the long axis of the radius, thus preventing dorsal and radial translation of the scaphoid.[28,29] This "dorsal lip" of the distal radius, covering the proximal pole of the scaphoid, makes a dorsal (percutaneous) approach for scaphoid fixation technically challenging.[30] On the proximal ulnar side, a flat and semilunate area of the scaphoid forms an articulation with the lunate bone[28,29] (Fig. 3.2C). The scapholunate articulation plays an important role in wrist kinematics, in which the lunate acts as a proximal anchor to the scaphoid, restrained by the scapholunate interosseous ligament (SLIO).[3]

Distal pole and articulations

Distally, the convex surface forms the scapho-trapezio-trapezoid (STT) joint, articulating with the trapezoid and the trapezium on the ulnodorsal and radiovolar sides, respectively[28,29] (Fig. 3.2A–D). The distal scaphoid surface has a cartilaginous ridge, dividing the articulation into the two facets of the STT joint.[26,28,29] Osteoarthrosis is commonly seen in this articulation, resulting in extension of the joint.[3] Anatomic variations in the shape of the distal articular surface, as described by Moritomo et al., may lead to divergent carpal kinematics contributing to

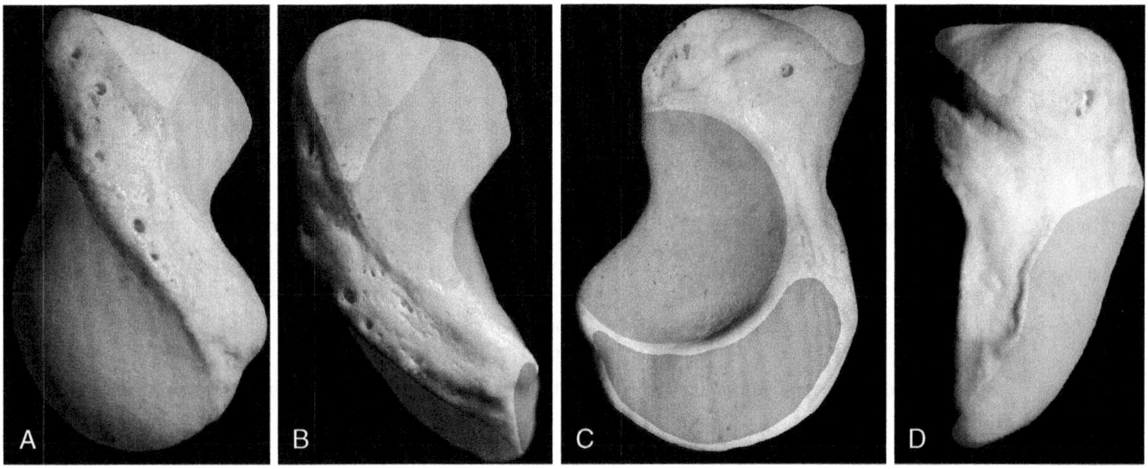

FIG. 3.2 **Osseous Anatomy and Articulations of the Scaphoid.** **(A)** Radial, **(B)** dorsal, **(C)** ulnar, and **(D)** volar views of the scaphoid and its articular surfaces color coded for contact with the distal radius (green), trapezium (yellow), trapezoid (orange), capitate (blue), and lunate (red). The bottom of each image represents the proximal and the top represents the distal end. Note the vascular foramina in the regions of the radiodorsal ridge and the tubercle. (From Buijze GA, Lozano-Calderon SA, Strackee SD, et al. Osseous and ligamentous scaphoid anatomy: Part I. A systematic literature review highlighting controversies. *J Hand Surg*. 2011;36(12):1929; with permission.)

degenerative changes.[14] Studies have suggested a direct association between scaphoid alignment, the extent to which the trapezium and trapezoid cover the scaphoid surface and the development of degenerative changes.[14]

On the ulnar distal side, the concave surface accommodates the proximal radial part of the capitate[28,29] (Fig. 3.2C). This concave facet may be elongated and shallow, when associated with a rotating scaphoid (type 1), or round and deep as seen in a flexing scaphoid (type 2)[31] (Box 3.2, Fig. 3.3). Yazaki et al. described capitate morphology to vary from flat to V-shaped, articulating with type 1 and type 2 scaphoids, correspondingly.[32]

BOX 3.2
Rotating (Type 1) and Flexing (Type 2) Scaphoids

Fogg et al. classified two subtypes of the scaphoid based on different kinematics resulting from alternative ligamentous insertions and articulations: a type 1 rotating scaphoid and a type 2 flexing scaphoid. A type 1 scaphoid has a single dorsal ridge oriented obliquely across the waist. A type 2 scaphoid has three similarly oriented ridges, which are located lower along the scaphoid waist. Each type is associated with specific alternative ligamentous attachments and articulations, resulting in distinct kinematic patterns. Table 3.1 summarizes the differences in ligamentous attachments. The ligament morphology of a type 1 or type 2 scaphoid allows the scaphoid to either rotate or flexion around its axis, respectively[31] (Fig. 3.3).

Scaphoid tubercle

The volar side of the scaphoid is largely nonarticulate. It constitutes a depressed irregular zone on its proximal side and the tubercle, pointing radiovolarly, on its distal side. Various ligamentous attachments, including the flexor retinaculum, the flexor carpi radialis tendon sheath, the STT ligament, and a small portion of the origin of the abductor pollicis brevis attach to the distal tubercle.[12,26,33,34]

Scaphoid waist

The scaphoid waist acts as a point of attachment for the joint capsule and various ligaments.[12,26] Radial artery branches course into the scaphoid through dorsal foramina located on the scaphoid waist.[26,33] The ridges located obliquely across the scaphoid waist function as points of attachment of the dorsal joint capsule, dorsal intercarpal ligaments, and bundles of the radioscaphocapitate ligament (Fig. 3.4).

Vascular Anatomy

Approximately 70%–80% of the intraosseous vascularity and the vascularity of the entire proximal pole is supplied by the radial artery branches entering through the dorsoradial ridge of the scaphoid.[35] There is substantial variation in the anatomy of the arteries

TABLE 3.1
Summary of Osseous and Ligamentous Variations in Wrists With Rotating (Type 1) and Flexing (Type 2) Scaphoids

	Scaphoid Type	Rotating (Type 1)	Flexing (Type 2)
	Scaphotrapezial ligament	Distally based "V" with narrow scaphoid attachment	Proximally based "V" with broad scaphoid attachment
Distal pole	*Scaphocapitate ligament*	Long to allow rotation	Short (axis of flexion)
	Scaphocapitate articulation	Shallow capitate fossa, flat-type capitate	Deep capitate fossa, "V"-shaped capitate
Scaphoid waist	*Dorsal intercarpal ligament*	Attached to trapezium, not scaphoid	Attached to scaphoid
	Radioscaphocapitate ligament	Not attached to scaphoid	Scaphoid attachment
Proximal pole	*Scapholunate articulation*	To lunate with single distal facet	To lunate with distal double facet
Kinematics		Rotation around long axis of scaphoid	Flexion-extension around axis of scaphocapitate ligament
Radiology	*Lunate* *CT distance* *Scaphoid nonunion*	Single distal facet <2 mm DISI deformity	Double distal facet >4 mm No carpal collapse

CT distance, minimum distance between the capitate and triquetrum on an anteroposterior radiograph; *DISI*, dorsal intercalated segment instability.
From Watts AC, McLean JM, Fogg Q, et al. Scaphoid anatomy. In: Slutsky DJ, Slade JF, editors. *The Scaphoid*. New York: Thieme; 2011; with permission.

entering the dorsal scaphoid cortex[27,31] (Fig. 3.4). About 20%–30% of the scaphoid is vascularized by volar branches of the radial artery, entering through the vascular foramina located on the depressed volar side of the scaphoid.[35] Detailed vascular anatomy is described in Chapter 4.

Ligament Anatomy

The ligaments attached to the scaphoid play a critical role in wrist kinematics and carpal stability, as exemplified by type 1 rotating and type 2 flexing scaphoid bones.[31,36] Buijze et al. demonstrated approximately $131 \pm 14\,mm^2$ of the scaphoid surface to be covered by ligamentous attachments, accounting for $9 \pm 0.9\%$ of the total surface.[1] Numerous classification systems for carpal ligaments have been described. To date, the most commonly used classification is the classification by Berger and Landsmeer. This nomenclature will therefore be used as a guideline in this chapter (Box 3.3).[5–7,20,26] Table 3.2 summarizes the variations in ligamentous anatomy described in this chapter.

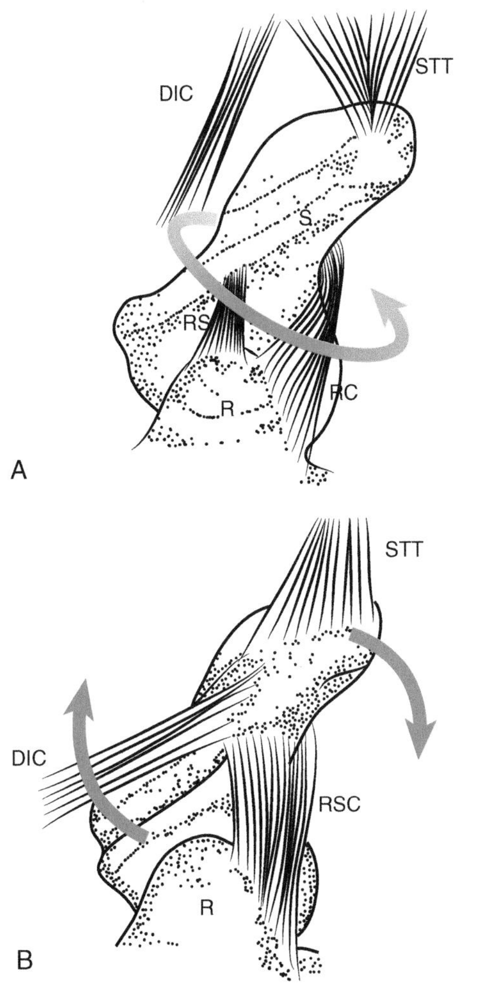

FIG. 3.3 **(A) Type 1 (Rotating) and (B) Type 2 (Flexing) Scaphoids.** *DIC*, dorsal intercarpal; *RC*, radiocapitate; *RS*, radioscaphoid; *RSC*, radioscaphocapitate; *STT*, scapho-trapezio-trapezoid; *R*, radius; *S*, scaphoid. (From Fogg QA. Scaphoid variation and an anatomical basis for variable carpal mechanics. Adelaide: University of Adelaide, Dept. of anatomical sciences; 2004:1:48; with permission.)

Volar ligaments

Radioscaphocapitate ligament. The radioscaphocapitate (RSC) ligament originates from the volar side of the radial styloid and inserts on the volar central part of the capitate head[29,37] (Figs. 3.5,3.7, and 3.8). The RSC acts as a fulcrum around which the scaphoid rotates.[3] The presence of a large number of mechanoreceptors suggests a mechanical and proprioceptive role.[38] Separate bundles of the RSC have been described to insert on multiple locations on the scaphoid, such as the radial side of the scaphoid waist and tubercle. Fogg described the RSC ligament to attach to the waist of type 2 scaphoids only; whereas in type 1 scaphoids the RSC ligament is believed to "bypass" the scaphoid with attachments to the radial styloid and capitate only[31] (Fig. 3.3). A study using cryomicrotome images of eight cadavers by Buijze et al. showed a small bundle of the RSC to attach onto the proximal edge of the scaphoid tubercle[1] (Fig. 3.8). The RSC is commonly reported to form interdigitations with surrounding ligaments, including the ulnocapitate, triquetrocapitate, and volar scaphotriquetral ligament. This interdigitation forms the arcuate ligament, also known as the deltoid, palmar distal V, or Weitbrechts oblique ligament.[39–41] Many variations of this interdigitation have been reported.[17,21]

Long radiolunate ligament. According to general consensus, the long radiolunate (LRL) originates ulnar to the RSC ligament on the volar rim. It then courses over the anterior pole of the scaphoid and inserts on the lunate and triquetrum[15,19,42] (Fig. 3.5). The LRL is sometimes referred to as radiolunotriquetral ligament.[12,39]

Volar scaphotriquetral ligament. The existence of the volar scaphotriquetral ligament (vScTq) remains controversial. Its presence has only been described by two studies.[17,21] Authors have inconsistently described the ligament as both a separate entity[21] and as part of other ligament attachments, such as the arcuate ligament.[17] In cadaver dissections, Buijze et al.

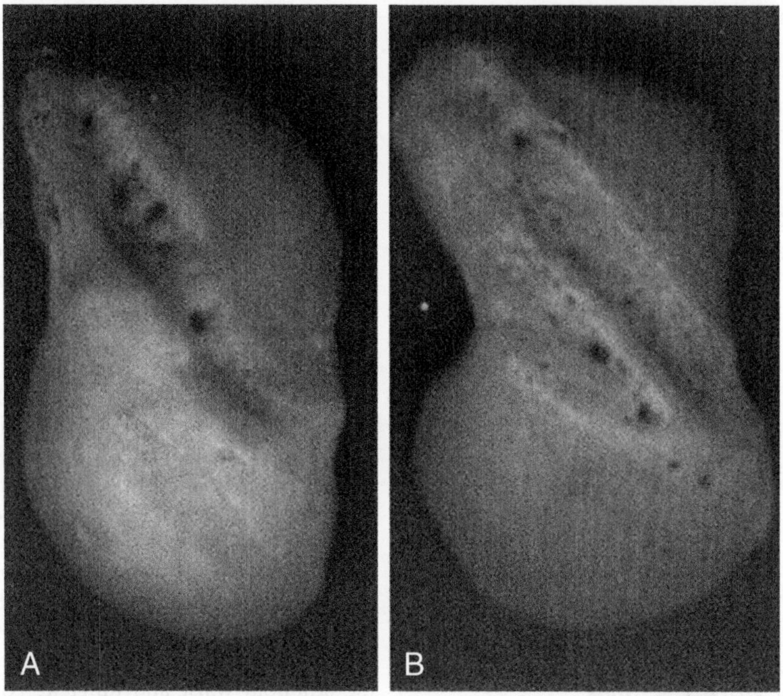

FIG. 3.4 **Variations in the Anatomy of the Dorsal Scaphoid Cortex.** Note the variation in the dorsal sulcus and its vascular foramina. **(A)** Main dorsal sulcus. **(B)** Two separate sulci. (From Ceri N, Korman E, Gunal I, et al. The morphological and morphometric features of the scaphoid. *J Hand Surg (Br.)*. 2004;29(4):396; with permission.)

BOX 3.3
Berger's Ligament Classification and Nomenclature

Berger's classification is based on the localization of the ligaments within the carpus and their organization within the joint capsule. The name of each ligament refers to the proximal (origin) and distal (insertion) attachment (Figs. 3.5A and 3.6A).

recognized the vScTq as part of the arcuate ligament, rather than a separate ligament.[1]

Radioscapholunate ligament. The radioscapholunate (RSL) ligament originates on the volar rim of the distal radius and inserts on the proximal edge of the scaphoid and lunate[1–3] (Fig. 3.5). It is one of the smallest extrinsic ligaments and lacks organized fascicular collagen bundles.[5,6,11] It is therefore considered a relatively weak structure. Some authors consider it a mesocapsular structure rather than a ligament.[6,11] Studies have revealed it to support abundant vascular and neural networks, including arterioles from the radial carpal arch and anterior interosseous nerve endings.[11,37] The RSL ligament courses along the interfossal ridge between the scaphoid and lunate fossa. During arthroscopy it will therefore cover the volar component of the SLIO.[3] Several authors regard the RSL ligament as a reinforcement of this volar component.[6,12,43] RSL ligament rupture is associated with SLIO ligament injury.[44]

Scaphocapitate ligament. The scaphocapitate (ScC) is a large capsular ligament originating from the distal pole of the scaphoid. It transverses obliquely to insert on the radial half of the volar capitate surface (Figs. 3.5A and 3.7A). It is the thickest scaphoid ligament.[14,15] The ScC has the largest attachment surface area to the scaphoid bone—approximately 40% of the total surface area of scaphoid attachments—covering almost the entire ulnar part of the tubercle.[1] The ScC ligament is part of the scaphotrapezial ligament and is considered an important stabilizer of the midcarpal joint, restraining the distal pole of the scaphoid.[3,10] In individuals with a rotating scaphoid, the ScC ligament is typically longer, allowing for rotation of the bone.[3]

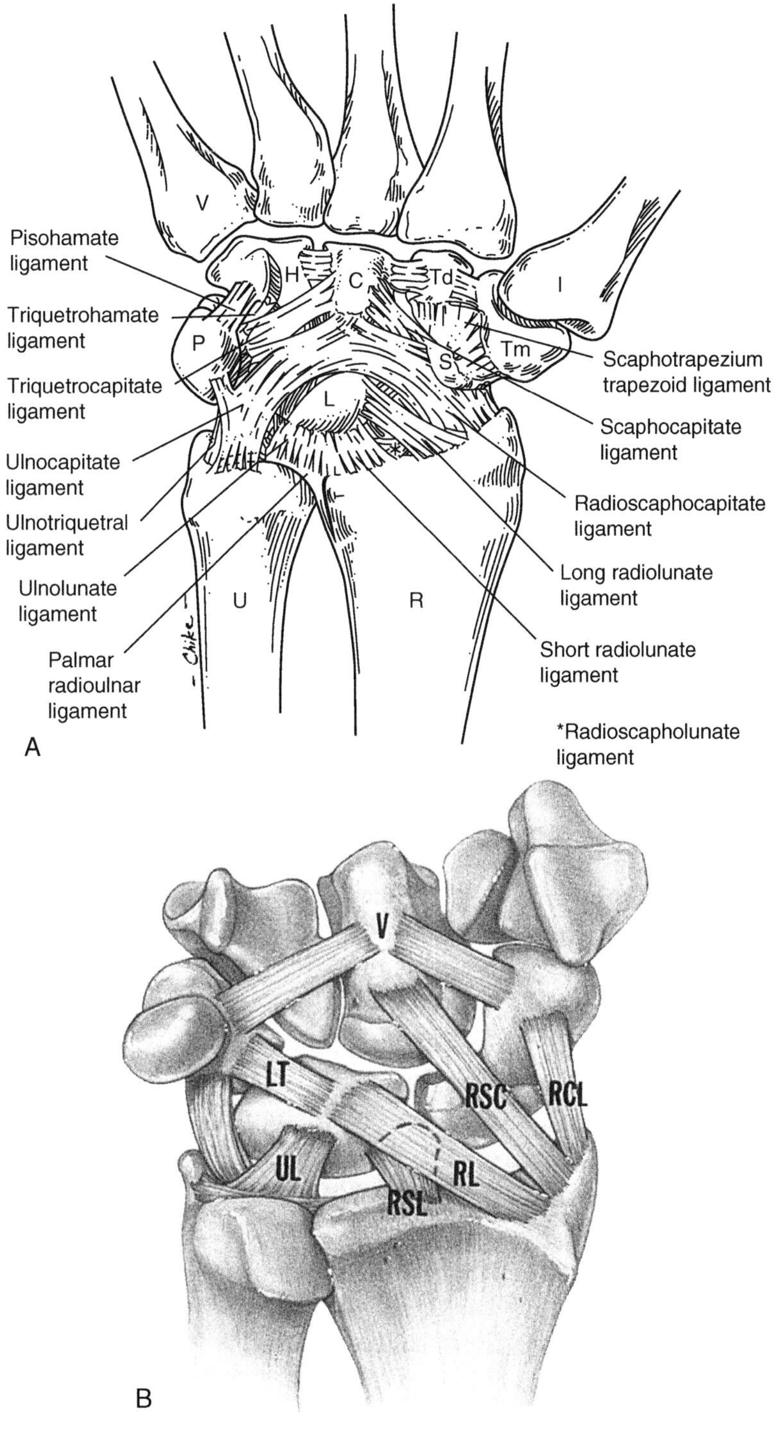

FIG. 3.5 Volar Ligaments of the Scaphoid. **(A)** Volar carpal ligaments according to Berger. *U*, ulna; *R*, radius; *P*, pisiforme; *L*, lunate; *S*, scaphoid; *Tm*, trapezium; *Td*, trapezoid; *C*, capitate; *H*, hamate. **(B)** Volar carpal ligaments according to Taleisnik. Note the presence of radial collateral ligament. *RCL*, radial collateral ligament; *RSC*, radioscaphocapitate; *RSL*, radioscapholunate; *RL*, radiolunate; *UL*, ulnolunate; *LT*, lunotriquetral. ((A) From William P. Coomey, ed. The Wrist. Diagnosis and Operative Treatment. Ligament anatomy. St. Louis, MO: Elsevier Mosby-Year Book, 1998:79; vol. 1; with permission and (B) Courtesy of Elizabeth Martin/Taleisnik J, ed. The Wrist. New York: Churchill Livingstone,1985; with permission.)

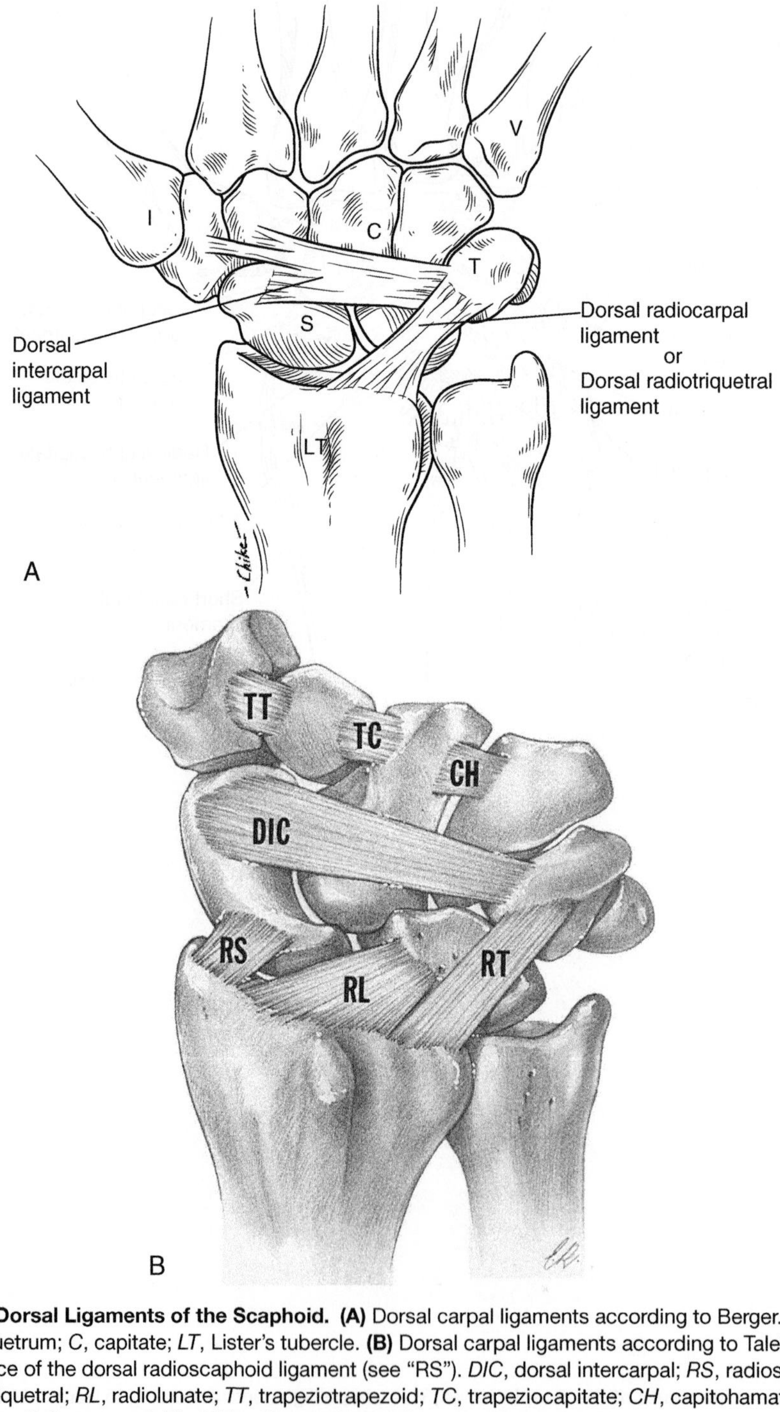

FIG. 3.6 **Dorsal Ligaments of the Scaphoid. (A)** Dorsal carpal ligaments according to Berger. *S*, scaphoid; *T*, triquetrum; *C*, capitate; *LT*, Lister's tubercle. **(B)** Dorsal carpal ligaments according to Taleisnik. Note the presence of the dorsal radioscaphoid ligament (see "RS"). *DIC*, dorsal intercarpal; *RS*, radioscaphoid; *RT*, radiotriquetral; *RL*, radiolunate; *TT*, trapeziotrapezoid; *TC*, trapeziocapitate; *CH*, capitohamate. ((A) From William P. Coomey, ed. The Wrist. Diagnosis and Operative Treatment. Ligament anatomy. St. Louis, MO: Elsevier Mosby-Year Book, 1998:79; vol. 1; with permission and (B) From Taleisnik J, ed. The Wrist. New York: Churchill Livingstone, 1985; with permission.)

TABLE 3.2
Consistency and Controversies in Scaphoid Ligamentous Attachments in Literature

Ligament	Generally Accepted	Controversial
RSC	Origin at the radial styloid Insertion on the volar capitate	Separate vScTq ligament[17,21] Separate vRSc ligament[21] Separate SC portion No insertion on the scaphoid[21]
RCL	Most radial carpal structure	Separate ligament[13,19,44] Part of RSC ligament[39,40] Radiodorsal origin[13] Radiovolar origin[19,44] Insertion(s)[13,19,44] RCL does not exist
LRL	No insertion on the scaphoid	LRL is also called RLTq[12,39,44]
RSL	All attachment areas	Histologically no true ligament[6,7,11,20]
SLIO	Dorsal, proximal, and volar portions	Dimensions of the three portions[5,50]
DRC	Origin at the distal radius Insertions on lunate and triquetrum	Location of the origin on the distal radius[12,13,15,39,40,44,49] Dorsal radioscaphoid ligament[19,28] No insertion on the scaphoid[12,13,15,39,40,44,49]
DIC	Origin at the dorsoradial triquetrum Insertion on the dorsoradial ridge of the scaphoid Varying additional insertion(s) on the lunate, trapezium, trapezoid and/or capitate	Insertion on the volar scaphoid[13] No insertion on the scaphoid[44] No insertion on the trapezium, lunate or capitate[37,39]
STT	Two or more bundles originating at volar distal pole of scaphoid with an insertion on the trapezium	Additional insertion on trapezoid[15,26,39] No insertion on trapezoid[8,10,14,19]
ScC	Origin at the volar distal pole of the scaphoid Insertion on the radiovolar capitate	No controversies
TCL	Extraarticular structure Origin at the hook of hamate and pisiform and insertion on the volar trapezial ridge and scaphoid tubercle	Flexor retinaculum and TCL are different entities[9,16,18] TCL is the midportion of the flexor retinaculum[9,16]

DIC, dorsal intercarpal; *DRC*, dorsal radiocarpal; *LRL*, long radiolunate; *RCL*, radial collateral ligament; *RSC*, radioscaphocapitate; *RSL*, radioscapholunate; *ScC*, scaphocapitate; *vScTq*, volar scaphotriquetral ligament; *SLIO*, scapholunate interosseous ligament; *STT*, scapho-trapezio-trapezoid; *TCL*, transverse carpal ligament; *vRSc*, volar radioscaphoid; *SC*, scaphocapitate; *RLTq*, radiolunotriquetral.
From Buijze GA, Lozano-Calderon SA, Strackee SD, et al. Osseous and ligamentous scaphoid anatomy: Part I. A systematic literature review highlighting controversies. *J Hand Surg*. 2011;36(12):1931; with permission.

The scapho-trapezio-trapezoid ligament. The STT ligament comprises two or more bundles originating on the ulnar, volar, and radial edges of the distal pole of the scaphoid bone (distal to the RSC attachment)[15,26,39]. Some studies describe two distinguishable bundles. Others report two separate ligaments inserting onto the trapezium and trapezoid: the scapotrapezium (ScTm) and scaphotrapezoid (ScTd) ligament, respectively.[15,26,39] (Figs. 3.5A and 3.7A) The STT ligament, particularly the ScTm, functions as a stabilizer of the scaphoid and STT joint, inhibiting excessive flexion of the scaphoid.[45] In type 1 scaphoids, the ScTm attachment on the scaphoid apex is narrower than its insertion on the trapezium, rendering a V-shaped ligament allowing for rotation at the base of the V. In type 2 scaphoids a reversed V-shaped ScTm ligament is found, with a broad-based attachment to the scaphoid[31] (Fig. 3.3).

The presence of the ScTd ligament as a separate entity is controversial and has not been reported by

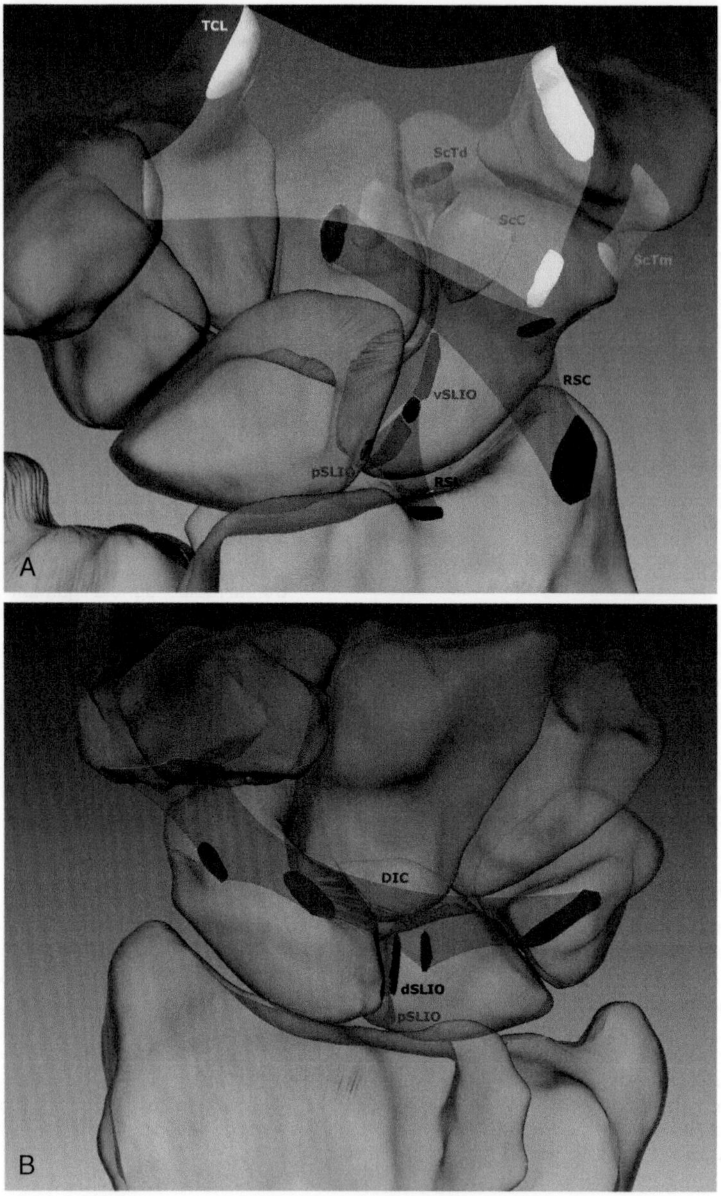

FIG. 3.7 **(A) Volar and (B) Dorsal Views of the Three-Dimensional Representation of the Wrist, Showing the Scaphoid Ligaments and Its Attachments.** *DIC*, dorsal intercarpal; *pSLIO*, proximal portion of the scapholunate interosseous ligament; *dSLIO*, distal portion of the scapholunate interosseous ligament; *RSC*, radioscaphocapitate; *RSL*, radioscapholunate; *ScC*, scaphocapitate; *ScTd*, scaphotrapezoid; *ScTm*, scapotrapezium; *TCL*, transverse carpal ligament; *vSLIO*, volar portion of the scapholunate interosseous ligament. (From Buijze GA, Dvinskikh NA, Strackee SD, et al. Osseous and ligamentous scaphoid anatomy: Part II. Evaluation of ligament morphology using three-dimensional anatomical imaging. *J Hand Surg*. 2011;36(12):1942; with permission.)

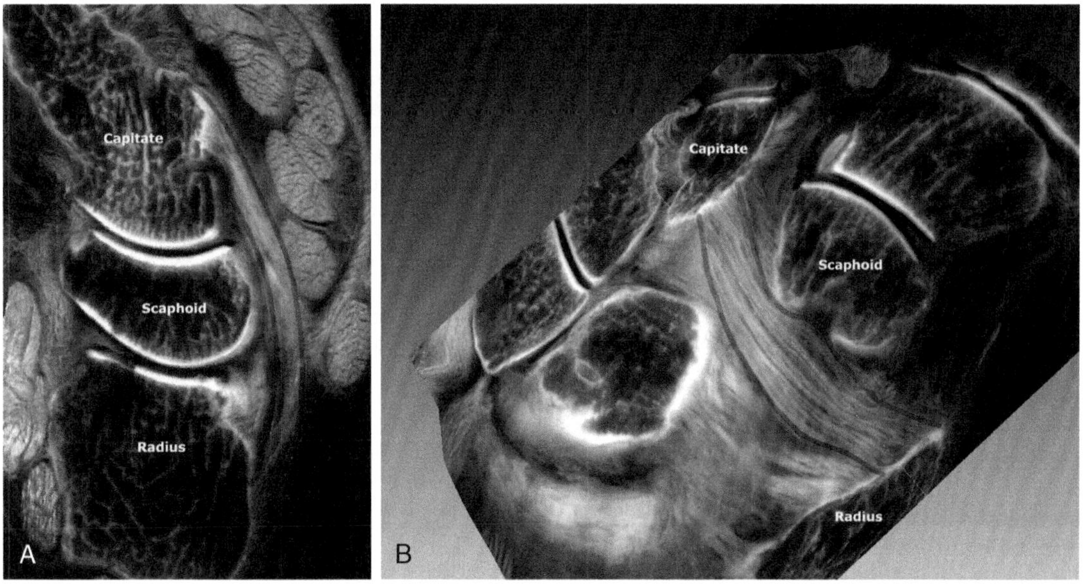

FIG. 3.8 **Cryomicrotome Image of a Right Wrist. (A)** An oblique sagittal plane through the estimated center of the radioscaphocapitate ligament and **(B)** a curved coronal surface fitted through this curved ligament, orthogonal to the oblique sagittal plane, to visualize its entire course from origin to insertion. The *red lines* indicate the margins of the ligament, used to indicate its thickness and width. Several ligament bundles deviate from the main ligament, directing radial to its attachment on the scaphoid. (From Buijze GA, Dvinskikh NA, Strackee SD, et al. Osseous and ligamentous scaphoid anatomy: Part II. Evaluation of ligament morphology using three-dimensional anatomical imaging. *J Hand Surg*. 2011;36(12):1938; with permission.)

all studies. In cadaver studies using three-dimensional imaging, it was identified as the narrowest and thinnest scaphoid ligament.[1]

Transverse carpal ligament. The transverse carpal ligament (TCL) is an extracapsular structure originating ulnarly on the hamate and pisiform. It inserts onto the entire volar trapezoidal ridge and the scaphoid[8,15,16,18] (Fig. 3.7A). The TCL is described as the widest ligament attached to the scaphoid and forms the roof of the flexor carpi radialis tunnel. It is the middle part of the three portions (proximal, mid, and distal) comprising the flexor retinaculum.[9,16] Rupture of the TCL significantly disrupts scaphoid kinematics.[46,47]

Radial collateral ligament. The radial collateral ligament (RCL) is a controversial structure. Some studies report it as a separate ligament,[13,19,33,44] connecting the scaphoid to the distal radius. Others describe it as a bundle of the RSC or even deny its existence.[39,40] Buijze et al. did not identify any volar or dorsal radioscaphoid ligament. Instead, a capsular-like structure bypassing the scaphoid radiodorsally was found.[1]

Dorsal ligaments

Dorsal intercarpal ligament. The dorsal intercarpal (DIC) ligament originates from the dorsoradial part of the triquetrum.[1-3,48] Many variations on the insertion of the ligament have been described (Figs. 3.6 and 3.7B). In type 2 scaphoids the DIC ligament is described to insert onto the proximal crest of the waist.[3,31] Consistently, Buijze et al. reported its insertion on the dorsoradial ridge of the proximal and waist region.[1] In type 1 scaphoids, however, the DIC ligament reaches the margin STT complex, without attaching onto the scaphoid[31] (Fig. 3.3). The DIC ligament forms a lateral configuration with the dorsal radiocarpal (DRC) ligament, formerly described at the dorsal V ligament. Together they restrain ulnar drift of the carpus.[14,33,37] Additional insertions on the lunate, trapezium, trapezoid, and/or capitate vary greatly.[1] Although the DIC ligament is a weak capsular structure, it functions as a stabilizer, restraining the dorsal proximal pole of the capitate. A proprioceptive role is suggested through the presence of numerous posterior interosseous nerve endings.[38] In type 2 scaphoids, the additional insertion of the ligament onto the waist may provide additional stability, possibly reducing the risk of carpal collapse into a dorsal intercalated segment instability deformity.[14]

Dorsal radiocarpal ligament. The DRC ligament is most commonly described to originate from the distal radius and to insert onto the lunate and triquetrum.[2] Controversy exists on its relation with the scaphoid. Some studies describe a thin ligamentous fiber coverage of the proximal scaphoid, providing dorsal stability without insertion.[13,49] Others describe no coverage or insertion of the ligament on the scaphoid bone at all.[12,13,15,21,39,44,49] Three-dimensional imaging of eight cadaver specimens showed no attachment to the scaphoid.[1]

Scapholunate interosseous ligaments

Scapholunate interosseous ligament. The SLIO ligament is a C-shaped ligament spanning the perimeter of the scapholunate joint[1] (Fig. 3.7B). It divides the radiocarpal joint from the lunate facet. Along with the lunotriquetral ligament, it separates the radiocarpal from the midcarpal joints.[3] Tearing of the SLIO ligament will result in leakage of contrast into the midcarpal joint, when injected into the radiocarpal joint. This does not confirm carpal instability, however.[3]

The SLIO ligament is described to consist of three interconnecting bundles: a dorsal, proximal, and volar portion.[5,50] Minor inconsistencies consist regarding the dimensions of these bundles. The dorsal portion is generally considered the thickest and most crucial portion of the SLIO ligament.[51] It courses from the dorsal lunate horn to the ulnar-dorsal region of the proximal edge of the scaphoid. The most proximal portion of the SLIO ligament is considered the widest but weakest portion of the SLIO ligament. The volar portion courses obliquely between the proximal pole of the scaphoid and the lunate. Along with the proximal bundle, it contributes to the rotational stability of the scapholunate joint.[51]

RECOMMENDATIONS

- A consistent description and classification of both osseous and ligamentous scaphoid anatomy is strongly advised to enhance our understanding of scaphoid kinematics.
- Berger's classification of scaphoid ligaments constitutes the most detailed subdivision of ligaments and the most independent ligaments of all classifications.[2,26,37,39]

> **CASE 1**
> **A Patient with Ulnar Carpal Translocation—Continued**
>
> The ulnar translocation seen on the radiographs is the key diagnostic feature. Commonly also referred to as "ulnar drift," it is in this case the result of disruption of the radioscaphocapitate and LRL ligament. The patient is operated and an avulsion of the volar capsule of the distal radius with disruption of the two ligaments is confirmed. The joint is realigned and stabilized using Kirschner wires. The ligament origins are attached onto the volar distal radius using suture anchors.

- Classifying morphologic scaphoid subtypes and their correlated kinematic patterns—for instance, by classifying flexing and rotating scaphoids[3,31]—will allow these variations to be employed as a basis for carpal mechanics.
- Further cadaver studies are required to explore the variations in scaphoid anatomy and its clinical relevance in terms of carpal stability.

CONCLUSION

A substantial variety in both osseous and ligamentous scaphoid anatomy has been described in literature. Consensus is specifically lacking on scaphoid ligamentous attachments. Variations in anatomic features are known to result in distinct kinematic patterns. A thorough knowledge and consistent description of scaphoid anatomy—and more importantly its associated carpal mechanics—are therefore of crucial importance to understanding the role of the scaphoid in carpal stability in both normal and injured wrists.

REFERENCES

1. Buijze GA, Dvinskikh NA, Strackee SD, Streekstra GJ, Blankevoort L. Osseous and ligamentous scaphoid anatomy: Part II. Evaluation of ligament morphology using three-dimensional anatomical imaging. *J Hand Surg Am.* 2011;36(12):1936–1943.
2. Buijze GA, Lozano-Calderon SA, Strackee SD, Blankevoort L, Jupiter JB. Osseous and ligamentous scaphoid anatomy: Part I. A systematic literature review highlighting controversies. *J Hand Surg Am.* 2011;36(12):1926–1935.
3. Watts ACMJM, Fogg Q, Bain GI. Scaphoid anatomy. In: Slutsky DJ, ed. *The Scaphoid.* New York: Thieme; 2011:22–30.
4. Tueting J. Scaphoid anatomy. In: Yao J, ed. *Scaphoid Fractures and Nonunions.* Switzerland: Springer International Publishing; 2015.

5. Berger RA. The gross and histologic anatomy of the scapholunate interosseous ligament. *J Hand Surg Am.* 1996;21(2):170–178.
6. Berger RA, Blair WF. The radioscapholunate ligament: a gross and histologic description. *Anat Rec.* 1984;210(2): 393–405.
7. Berger RA, Kauer JM, Landsmeer JM. Radioscapholunate ligament: a gross anatomic and histologic study of fetal and adult wrists. *J Hand Surg Am.* 1991;16(2):350–355.
8. Bettinger PC, Linscheid RL, Berger RA, Cooney 3rd WP, An KN. An anatomic study of the stabilizing ligaments of the trapezium and trapeziometacarpal joint. *J Hand Surg Am.* 1999;24(4):786–798.
9. Cobb TK, Dalley BK, Posteraro RH, Lewis RC. Anatomy of the flexor retinaculum. *J Hand Surg Am.* 1993;18(1):91–99.
10. Drewniany JJ, Palmer AK, Flatt AE. The scaphotrapezial ligament complex: an anatomic and biomechanical study. *J Hand Surg Am.* 1985;10(4):492–498.
11. Hixson ML, Stewart C. Microvascular anatomy of the radioscapholunate ligament of the wrist. *J Hand Surg Am.* 1990;15(2):279–282.
12. Mayfield JK, Johnson RP, Kilcoyne RF. The ligaments of the human wrist and their functional significance. *Anat Rec.* 1976;186(3):417–428.
13. Mizuseki T, Ikuta Y. The dorsal carpal ligaments: their anatomy and function. *J Hand Surg Br.* 1989;14(1):91–98.
14. Moritomo H, Viegas SF, Nakamura K, Dasilva MF, Patterson RM. The scaphotrapezio-trapezoidal joint. Part 1: An anatomic and radiographic study. *J Hand Surg Am.* 2000;25(5):899–910.
15. Nanno M, Patterson RM, Viegas SF. Three-dimensional imaging of the carpal ligaments. *Hand Clin.* 2006;22(4): 399–412 (abstract v).
16. Pacek CA, Chakan M, Goitz RJ, Kaufmann RA, Li ZM. Morphological analysis of the transverse carpal ligament. *Hand (N Y).* 2010;5(2):135–140.
17. Sennwald GR, Zdravkovic V, Oberlin C. The anatomy of the palmar scaphotriquetral ligament. *J Bone Joint Surg Br.* 1994;76(1):147–149.
18. Stecco C, Macchi V, Lancerotto L, Tiengo C, Porzionato A, De Caro R. Comparison of transverse carpal ligament and flexor retinaculum terminology for the wrist. *J Hand Surg Am.* 2010;35(5):746–753.
19. Taleisnik J. The ligaments of the wrist. *J Hand Surg Am.* 1976;1(2):110–118.
20. Berger RA. Arthroscopic anatomy of the wrist and distal radioulnar joint. *Hand Clin.* 1999;15(3):393–413. vii.
21. Smith DK. Volar carpal ligaments of the wrist: normal appearance on multiplanar reconstructions of three-dimensional Fourier transform MR imaging. *AJR Am J Roentgenol.* 1993; 161(2):353–357.
22. Smith DK. Dorsal carpal ligaments of the wrist: normal appearance on multiplanar reconstructions of three-dimensional Fourier transform MR imaging. *AJR Am J Roentgenol.* 1993;161(1):119–125.
23. Wolfe P, Hotchkiss K. In: 6th ed. *Green's Operative Hand Surgery.* vol. 1. Churchill Livingstone; 2010.
24. Mallee W, Doornberg JN, Ring D, van Dijk CN, Maas M, Goslings JC. Comparison of CT and MRI for diagnosis of suspected scaphoid fractures. *J Bone Joint Surg Am.* 2011;93(1):20–28.
25. Mallee WH, Doornberg JN, Ring D, et al. Computed tomography for suspected scaphoid fractures: comparison of reformations in the plane of the wrist versus the long axis of the scaphoid. *Hand (N Y).* 2014;9(1): 117–121.
26. Berger RA. The anatomy of the scaphoid. *Hand Clin.* 2001; 17(4):525–532.
27. Ceri N, Korman E, Gunal I, Tetik S. The morphological and morphometric features of the scaphoid. *J Hand Surg Br.* 2004;29(4):393–398.
28. Taleisnik J. *The Bones of the Wrist.* New York: Churchill Livingstone; 1985.
29. Williams PLW, Osteology R. *Gray's Anatomy.* 37th ed; 1989:153–201.
30. Adamany DC, Mikola EA, Fraser BJ. Percutaneous fixation of the scaphoid through a dorsal approach: an anatomic study. *J Hand Surg Am.* 2008;33(3):327–331.
31. Fogg Q. *Scaphoid Varation and an Anatomical Basis for Variable Carpal Mechanics.* Adelaide: Department of anatomical sciences, University of Adelaide; 2004.
32. Yazaki N, Burns ST, Morris RP, Andersen CR, Patterson RM, Viegas SF. Variations of capitate morphology in the wrist. *J Hand Surg Am.* 2008;33(5):660–666.
33. Bogumill G. *Anatomy of the Wrist. The Wrist and its Disorders.* Philadelphia: WB Saunders; 1988:14–26.
34. Botte MJ. *Skeletal Anatomy. Surgical Anatomy of the Hand and Upper Extremity.* Philadelphia: Lippincott Williams & Wilkins; 2003:3–91.
35. Gelberman RHM. The vascularity of the scaphoid bone. *J Hand Surg.* 1980:508–513.
36. McLean JM, Turner PC, Bain GI, Rezaian N, Field J, Fogg Q. An association between lunate morphology and scaphoid-trapezium-trapezoid arthritis. *J Hand Surg Eur Vol.* 2009; 34(6):778–782.
37. Berger RA, G-E M. General anatomy of the wrist. In: An KNBRA, Cooney WP, eds. *Biomechanics of the Wrist Joint.* New York: Springer-Verlag; 1991:1–22.
38. Tomita K, Berger EJ, Berger RA, Kraisarin J, An KN. Distribution of nerve endings in the human dorsal radiocarpal ligament. *J Hand Surg Am.* 2007;32(4):466–473.
39. Berger RA. The ligaments of the wrist. A current overview of anatomy with considerations of their potential functions. *Hand Clin.* 1997;13(1):63–82.
40. Sennwald S. *The Wrist.* Berlin: Springer-Verlag; 1987.
41. Weitbrecht J. *Syndesmologia sive historia ligamentorum corporis humani, quam secundum observationes antaomicas concinnavit en figuris et objecta recetnia adumbratis illustravit.* Petropoli, Petersburg: Academy of Sciences; 1742.
42. Berger RA, Landsmeer JM. The palmar radiocarpal ligaments: a study of adult and fetal human wrist joints. *J Hand Surg Am.* 1990;15(6):847–854.
43. D L. *The wrist and its disorders.* Philadelphia: WB Saunders; 1988.

44. Zancolli EEP. *The Carpus. Atlas of Surgical Anatomy of the Hand.* Singapore: Churchill Livingstone; 1992:416–430.
45. Boabighi A, Kuhlmann JN, Kenesi C. The distal ligamentous complex of the scaphoid and the scapho-lunate ligament. An anatomic, histological and biomechanical study. *J Hand Surg Br.* 1993;18(1):65–69.
46. Ishiko T, Puttlitz CM, Lotz JC, Diao E. Scaphoid kinematic behavior after division of the transverse carpal ligament. *J Hand Surg Am.* 2003;28(2):267–271.
47. Tengrootenhuysen M, van Riet R, Pimontel P, Bortier H, Van Glabbeek F. The role of the transverse carpal ligament in carpal stability: an in vitro study. *Acta Orthop Belg.* 2009;75(4):467–471.
48. Compson JP, Waterman JK, Heatley FW. The radiological anatomy of the scaphoid. Part 1: Osteology. *J Hand Surg Br.* 1994;19(2):183–187.
49. Viegas SF, Yamaguchi S, Boyd NL, Patterson RM. The dorsal ligaments of the wrist: anatomy, mechanical properties, and function. *J Hand Surg Am.* 1999;24(3): 456–468.
50. Nagao S, Patterson RM, Buford Jr WL, Andersen CR, Shah MA, Viegas SF. Three-dimensional description of ligamentous attachments around the lunate. *J Hand Surg Am.* 2005;30(4):685–692.
51. Berger RA, Imeada T, Berglund L, An KN. Constraint and material properties of the subregions of the scapholunate interosseous ligament. *J Hand Surg Am.* 1999;24(5): 953–962.
52. DiBenedetto MR, Lubbers LM, Coleman CR. A standardized measurement of ulnar carpal translocation. *Arch Orthop Trauma Surg.* 1990;122(3):179–181.

CHAPTER 4

Vascular Supply to the Scaphoid

MICHAEL J. BOTTE, MD • MICHAEL A. THOMPSON, MD •
LORENZO L. PACELLI, MD • M. JAKE HAMER, MD

KEY POINTS

- The scaphoid has a relatively limited vascular supply because the majority of the surface is covered with articular cartilage, areas void of vascular leases. Vessels enter the scaphoid only through the limited areas of soft tissue attachment, which include (1) a dorsal ridge of vascular attachments in the midportion of the dorsal scaphoid, and (2) attachments on the palmar aspect at the distal scaphoid tubercle.
- The main vascular supply to the scaphoid is through vessels that originate from the radial artery and enter the scaphoid at the midscaphoid dorsal ridge. These dorsal ridge vessels then continue in an intraosseous retrograde direction (distal to proximal and dorsal to palmar), to supply 70%–80% of the proximal scaphoid. Fractures of the waist or proximal scaphoid may disrupt these vessels and render the more proximal portion of the scaphoid avascular.
- The vascular supply to the distal portion of the scaphoid is from branches that originate from the radial artery that enter through the distal palmar tubercle of the scaphoid. These vessels supply the distal 20%–30% of the scaphoid, and because of the more extensive vascular coverage, fractures of the distal scaphoid and tubercle usually heal more rapidly and without sequela.

IMPORTANCE OF THE PROBLEM

The vascular supply to the scaphoid is unique, including the location and limited attachments of the leash of dorsal ridge vessels and the usual retrograde intraosseous course of these vessels. The vascular anatomy helps explain the relatively high occurrence of nonunion and osteonecrosis, as well as the relatively long healing times of proximal fractures. Time required for healing usually increases as the fracture location becomes more proximal because of the more sequentially limited vascularity of the proximal scaphoid.

These vascular anatomical aspects will also help guide a surgeon operatively in protecting the valuable dorsal ridge vessels when a dorsal approach is used or when internal fixation is placed in the vicinity of the vessels.

MAIN QUESTION

Which vascular supply is essential to scaphoid fracture healing?

Current Opinion

Current opinion agrees as to the importance of the dorsal ridge vessels, including the correlation of scaphoid fracture location to fracture healing. The more proximal the fracture, the more limited the vascularity to the proximal pole. Subsequently, the more proximal fractures are associated with longer healing times, higher incidence of delayed or nonunion, and the higher potential for development of osteonecrosis.

Finding the Evidence

- Pubmed: "scaphoid bone" or "scaphoid" AND "vascular*".
- Bibliography of eligible articles.
- Only articles written in English were included.

Quality of the Evidence

The anatomy and cadaver studies are basic science studies, thus do not exactly fit evaluation of quality of evidence used in clinical studies. Many of these anatomic studies used new techniques for their time, and several authors developed or augmented anatomic techniques specifically to answer questions regarding scaphoid vascularity. These techniques included injection studies using India ink or Wards blue latex, used digestion techniques of Spalteholz, and required meticulous cadaver dissection.[13-18] The consistent findings and similar results would indicate a high degree of quality of technique. Of note, the Spalteholz technique is subject to critique because it probably reflects the largest vessels that would fill with the relatively thick dye.

Additionally, the conclusions were based on a relatively limited number of specimens.

FINDINGS

The scaphoid is unique in that a major portion of its external surface area is covered with articular cartilage. This results in limited areas for soft tissue attachments. Because the vascular structures enter only through these soft tissue attachments, the vascularity of the scaphoid is also relatively limited. This limited vascularity has clinical implications in fracture healing, osteonecrosis, and the development of Preiser disease.[1–10] Similar osseous structures that are largely covered with articular cartilage and thus have limited vascularity (and similar clinical problems of nonunion and osteonecrosis) include the lunate, femoral head, talus, and tarsal navicular.[6,7]

Basic science anatomic studies have led to an understanding of the unique vascularity of the scaphoid. These cadaver studies show the importance of the dorsal vascular supply to the scaphoid and the intraosseous retrograde flow of the proximal vessels. These findings correlate well with clinical studies on scaphoid fractures union rates and help explain difference in healing rates with location of the fracture.[1–12]

Vascular studies were performed as early as 1910 with Preiser and Lexer. These early anatomic studies consisted of injection studies in cadavers followed by dissection techniques. Preiser suspected the occurrence of osteonecrosis was due to disruption of the vascular supply to the scaphoid.

In 1938, Obletz and Halbstein studied scaphoid nutrient foramina.[1] In 13% of 297 scaphoids, there were no noted foramina proximal to the waist. In 14%, dorsal foramen were located distal to the waist. In 27%, foramina were located proximal to the waist but within 2–3 mm of the midsection the bone. In the remaining 59%, the vascular foramina were located directly over the dorsal waist.[1]

Early additional authors felt the scapholunate ligament may provide vascularity to the scaphoid. Lutzeler (1932), Travaglini,[13] and Barber[14] noted vessels in the dorsal scapholunate ligament and attributed vascularity of the proximal pole through the scapholunate ligament.[13–14] Barber based his conclusions on eight cadaver specimens injected with barium sulfate and clearing the scaphoids with the Spalteholz technique. He noted three groups of vessels entering at various intervals along the dorsal ridge and branching to supply the tuberosity and proximal pole. He did not find any vessels entering the scaphoid through its palmar surface.[14]

Later studies by Gelberman[15] using injected specimens with Wards blue latex demonstrated vessels in the both the dorsal and palmar scapholunate ligaments, but the vessels consistently did not penetrate the scaphoid or supply any vascularity to the proximal pole. It was concluded that the scapholunate ligaments do not supply vascularity to the scaphoid.

Grettve[16] studied five cadaver specimens, noted small vessels entering the scaphoid through the radial vessels, and suspected the major blood supply to the scaphoid came from the dorsum.

The external vascularity was then described in detail by Gelberman and Mennon and by Teleisnik.[15,17] Fifteen cadaver forearm specimens were studied by Gelberman and Mennon. Vascular injection of the cadaver limbs using Wards blue latex solution was used. The injected specimens were refrigerated to allow consolidation of the latex. The soft tissues were digested to allow visualization and evaluation of the external vascular supply. Taleisnik and Kelly performed similar studies with 11 cadaver studies, using a technique of injection of the radial artery with India ink and barium sulfate followed by dissection of the scaphoid blood vascular structures under magnification. In both studies, the scaphoids were treated and cleared by the Spalteholz method. This rendered the scaphoid translucent and allowed visualization of the internal vascularity.

The scaphoid was found by Gelberman and Menon to receive its vascular supply primarily from the radial artery.[15] The radial artery supplies two major vascular sources, one through the scaphoid dorsal surface and the other through its palmar surface. These vessels enter the scaphoid cortex through ligamentous attachments in the nonarticular surface areas. Taleisnik found similar results, although the terminology and naming of the vessels was slightly different.[17] Taleisnik described three major vessels to the scaphoid: the laterovolar, dorsal, and distal vessels. They concluded that the laterovolar vessels were the largest and provided most of the blood supply to the proximal two-thirds of the bone. The intraosseous vascular patterns in their study were well demonstrated because of the use of freshly amputated limbs. On studying the major vessels of their cleared specimens, it was apparent that their laterovolar vessels were similar to the dorsal ridge vessels described by Gelberman and Mennon. Their distal vessels were similar to Gelberman's tuberosity vessels.

External Vascularity

Based on anatomic studies as noted earlier, the vascularity of the scaphoid can be described and summarized[13–19] (Figs. 4.1–4.4) (Box 4.1). The dorsal vascular

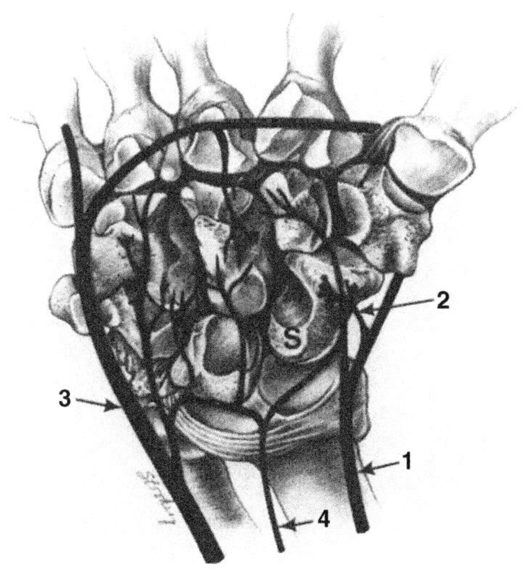

FIG. 4.1 Schematic drawing of the palmar external blood supply of the scaphoid. (*S*, scaphoid; *1*, radial artery; *2*, volar scaphoid branches; *3*, ulnar artery; *4*, anterior division of the anterior interosseous artery.) (From Gelberman RH, Menon J. The vascularity of the scaphoid bone. *J Hand Surg (Am)*. 1980;5(5):508; with permission.)

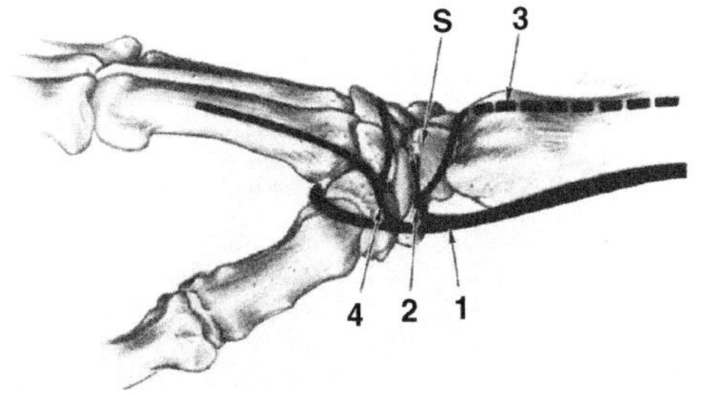

FIG. 4.2 Schematic drawing of the dorsal blood supply of the scaphoid. (*S*, scaphoid; *1*, radial artery; *2*, dorsal scaphoid branch; *3*, dorsal division of the anterior interosseous artery; *4*, intercarpal artery.) (From Gelberman RH, Menon J. The vascularity of the scaphoid bone. *J Hand Surg (Am)*. 1980;5(5):509; with permission.)

supply to the scaphoid accounts for 70%–80% of the internal vascularity of the bone, all in the proximal region.[7] On the dorsum of the scaphoid, there is an oblique ridge that lies between the articular surfaces for the radius and for the trapezium and trapezoid. The major dorsal vessels to the scaphoid enter the scaphoid through small foramina located on this dorsal ridge. The dorsal ridge is in the region of the scaphoid waist, and the entering vessels are often referred to as the dorsal ridge vessels.

The origin of the dorsal ridge vessels is from the radial artery. In most (70%) studied specimens, the dorsal ridge vessels originate directly from the radial artery; in others (23%), the dorsal ridge vessels are from a separate branch of the radial artery, the intercarpal artery. In the remaining 7%, both arteries supply the dorsal ridge vessels (as described below).

The intercarpal artery arises from the radial artery at the level of the intercarpal joint of the wrist. The intercarpal artery immediately divides into two branches. One branch runs transverse to the dorsum of the wrist to contribute to the dorsal intercarpal arch and anastomose with a branch from the ulnar artery. The other branch runs vertically and distally over the index metacarpal.

Approximately 5 mm proximal to the origin of the intercarpal vessel at the level of the styloid process of the radius, another vessel is given off that runs over the radiocarpal ligament to enter the scaphoid through its waist along the dorsal ridge. In 70% of studied specimens, this dorsal vessel arises directly from the radial artery. In 23%, the dorsal branch has its origin from the common stem of the intercarpal artery. In 7%, the scaphoid receives its dorsal blood supply directly from the branches of both the intercarpal artery and the radial artery proper. There are consistent major communications between the dorsal scaphoid branch of the radial artery and the dorsal branch of the anterior interosseous artery. No vessels enter the proximal dorsal region of the scaphoid through the dorsal scapholunate ligament, and no vessels enter through the dorsal cartilaginous areas.

The palmar vascular supply to the scaphoid accounts for 20%–30% of the internal vascularity of the bone, all in the region of the distal pole (Figs. 4.1–4.4). At the level of the radioscaphoid joint, the radial artery gives off the superficial palmar branch. Just distal to the origin of the superficial palmar branch, several smaller branches course obliquely and distally over the palmar aspect of the scaphoid to enter through the region of the scaphoid tubercle. These branches, the volar (palmar) scaphoid branches, divide into several smaller branches just prior to penetrating the bone. In 75% of studies specimens, these arteries arise directly from the radial artery. In the remainder, they arise from the superficial palmar branch of the radial artery. Anastomoses are usually present between the palmar division of the anterior interosseous artery and the palmar scaphoid branch of the radial artery when the latter arises from the superficial palmar branch of the radial artery. There are no apparent communicating branches from the ulnar artery to the palmar branches of the radial artery supplying the scaphoid. There are usually several very small vessels that run over the palmar scapholunate ligament, but these do

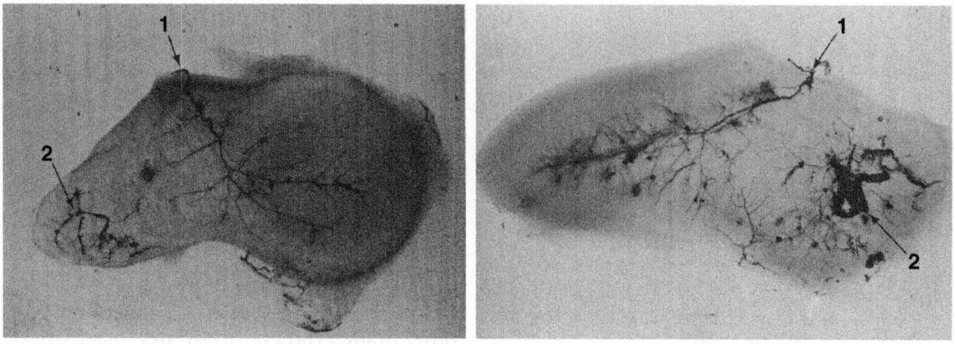

FIG. 4.3 **(A and B)** Photographs of cleared specimen showing the internal vascularity of the scaphoid (*1*, dorsal scaphoid branch of the radial artery [dorsal ridge vessel]); *2*, palmar scaphoid branch). (From Gelberman RH, Menon J. The vascularity of the scaphoid bone. *J Hand Surg (Am)*. 1980;5(5):511; with permission.)

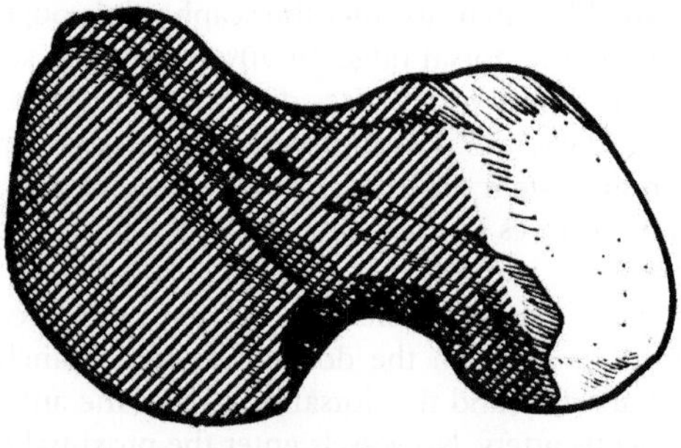

FIG. 4.4 The proximal 70%–80% of the scaphoid is supplied by the dorsal vessels (shaded area). The distal 20%–30% is supplied by the volar branches of the radial artery (white area). (From Gelberman RH, Menon J. The vascularity of the scaphoid bone. *J Hand Surg (Am)*. 1980;5(5):512; with permission.)

BOX 4.1
Extraosseous Vascularity of the Scaphoid

Origin of the dorsal ridge vessels that supply the proximal 70%–80% of the scaphoid:
Directly from radial artery proper (70%)
Intercarpal artery (23%)
Both (7%)
Origin of the palmar scaphoid branches that supply the distal 20%–30% of the scaphoid:
Directly from the radial artery proper (75%)
Superficial palmar branch (25%)

Data from Gelberman RH, Menon J. The vascularity of the scaphoid bone. *J Hand Surg (Am)*. 1980;5(5):508–513.

not penetrate the bone and do not contribute to the vascularity of the scaphoid in that region. The palmar cartilaginous areas of the scaphoid are devoid of any vascular structures. This palmar vascular supply is clinically important in isolated fractures of the scaphoid tubercle.

Internal Vascularity

In 79% of studied specimens, one to two dorsal vessels enter the scaphoid through foramina located on the dorsal ridge at the level of the waist. In 7%, the vessels entered proximally, and in 14% the vessels entered just distal to the waist. In most specimens, the dorsal vessels divided into two to three branches soon after entering in the scaphoid. These intraosseous vessels run volarly and proximally, in a retrograde fashion, dividing into smaller branches supplying the proximal pole as far as the proximal subchondral region. These vessels that entered dorsally supply 70%–80% of the proximal scaphoid (Fig. 4.3).

Clinical Correlations

The scaphoid is the most frequently injured bone in the carpus, and the long healing rates required for fractures are well established.[1-4,6-12,19-31] Additionally, development of osteonecrosis is common and is the second in incidence only to that of the femoral head, occurring in 13%–40% of scaphoid fractures.[6,7,9,10,12,19] Patients with fractures of the proximal one-third of the scaphoid have the highest incidence of nonunion and osteonecrosis, which has been reported to occur in 14%–100% of patients, whereas approximately 30%–50% of patients with fractures of the middle one-third develop nonunion or osteonecrosis.[6,9,10,12,19] If the fracture is in the most proximal one-fifth of the scaphoid, almost all fractures will develop nonunion or osteonecrosis. Although wide ranges of reported incidence of delayed union, nonunion, or osteonecrosis do exist, fracture location and displacement have been implicated in these problems.[7,11,19,22,30] Overall, the healing times for fractures of the scaphoid become progressively longer as the fracture location becomes more proximal. Healing time for tuberosity fractures ranges from about 4 to 6 weeks. For occult or stable fractures, healing times usually range from 6 to 8 weeks. For distal third and waist fractures, fractures healing times range from 10 to 12 weeks. From proximal pole or comminuted fractures, healing times range from 12 to 20 weeks, with occurrence of nonunion, the most common of all groups.[6,7,19]

These healing times, nonunion rates, and occurrence of osteonecrosis all correlate with the vascular anatomy, where the retrograde flow of the intraosseous vessels would be at more risk as the fracture becomes more proximal. The proximal portion is the farthest reaching of the terminal portions of the intraosseous vessels. Recent MRI studies have demonstrated loss of blood flow proximal to the fracture, suggesting that disruption of the intraosseous vessels at the fracture site would contribute to slow fracture healing rates.[25,26] In fractures in the tubercle or distal one-third, nonunion is rare. This correlates well to relatively good supply of the distal one-third. Independent of fracture location, nonunion and osteonecrosis have been reported to occur in as many as 50% of patients with fractures displaced greater than 1 mm.[6] This would correlate with a higher incidence of vascular disruption with greater fracture displacement.

RECOMMENDATIONS

- Inform patients of potential long healing times for fractures of the waist or proximal pole because of the unique and relatively limited blood supply to the scaphoid.
- Note to patients that the more proximal the fracture, the more potential for longer healing times because of progressively limited vascularity of the proximal pole and potential for disruption of these proximal vessels.
- When fractures occur in the distal scaphoid or tubercle, inform patients of the relatively timely healing expected good outcome for these fractures.
- During operative approach to the proximal or dorsal scaphoid, protect the vascular leash that attaches to the midscaphoid (which contains the dorsal ridge vessels).

CONCLUSIONS

1. The dorsal vascularity, comprising the dorsal ridge vessels, supplies 70%–80% of the vascular supply to the central and proximal portions of the scaphoid. This dorsal supply originates from the radial artery and enters the dorsal scaphoid in the midportion.
2. These dorsal vessels supply the scaphoid vascularity in the region of the waist and proximal pole, through retrograde vessels that extend to the proximal pole.
3. Fractures in the waist and proximal scaphoid depend on the dorsal vascular supply for adequate and timely healing.
4. The palmar vascularity supplies the distal 20%–30% of the scaphoid. In isolated fractures of the tubercle, the palmar vascularity will supply the distal portion of the scaphoid. Because of the greater vascularity of the distal pole, fractures of the distal scaphoid and tubercle usually heal in a timely fashion without sequela.

REFERENCES

1. Obletz BE, Halbstein BM. Non-union of fractures of the carpal navicular. *J Bone Joint Surg*. 1938;20:424–428.
2. Cave EF. The carpus with reference to fractured navicular bone. *Arch Surg*. 1940;40:54–76.
3. Russe O. Fracture of the carpal navicular: diagnosis, non-operative treatment, and operative treatment. *J Bone Joint Surg Am*. 1960;42:759–768.
4. Mazet Jr R, et al. Fractures of the carpal navicular, analysis of 91 cases and review of the literature. *J Bone Joint Surg Am*. 1963;45:82–112.
5. Vidal MA, Linscheid RL, Amadio PC, et al. Preisser's disease. *Ann Chir Main Memb Super*. 1991;10:227–235.
6. Cooney WP, Dobyns JH, Linscheid RL. Fractures of the scaphoid: a rational approach to management. *Clin Orthop*. 1980;149:90–97.
7. Gelberman RH, Wolock BS, Siegel DB. Current concepts review: fractures and nonunion of the carpal scaphoid. *J Bone Joint Surg*. 1989;71A:1560–1565.
8. Stewart MM. Fractures of the carpal navicular: a report of 436 cases. *J Bone Joint Surg*. 1954;36A:998–1006.
9. Wagner C. Fractures of the carpal navicular. *J Bone Joint Surg*. 1952;34A:774–784.
10. Herbert TJ. *The Fractured Scaphoid*. St. Louis: Quality Medical Publishing; 1990.
11. Cooney WP, Linscheid RTL, Dobyns JH. Fractures and dislocation of the wrist. In: Rockwood CA, Green DP, Buchholz RW, Heckman J, eds. *Rockwood and Greens Fractures in Adults*. Philadelphia: Lippincott-Raven; 1996:745–867.
12. Gaebler C. Fractures and dislocations of the carpus. In: Bucholz RW, Heckman JD, Court-Brown CM, eds. *Rockwood and Green's Fractures in Adults*. Philadelphia: Lippincott Williams and Wilkins; 2006:857–908.
13. Travaglini FG. Arterial circulation of the carpal bones. *Bull Hosp Joint Dis N Y*. 1959;20:424–428.
14. Barber H. The intraosseous arterial anatomy of the adult human carpus. *Orthopaedics*. 1972;5:1–19.

15. Gelberman RH, Menon J. The vascularity of the scaphoid bone. *J Hand Surg Am*. 1980;5:508–513.
16. Grettve S. Arterial anatomy of the carpal bones. *Acta Anat*. 1955;25:331–335.
17. Taleisnik J, Kelly PJ. Extraosseous and intraosseous blood supply of the scaphoid bone. *J Bone Joint Surg Am*. 1966;48:1125–1137.
18. Botte MJ, Mortensen WW, Gelberman RH, et al. Internal vascularity of the scaphoid in cadavers after insertion of the Herbert screw. *J Hand Surg*. 1988;13A:216–222.
19. Freedman DM, Botte MJ, Gelberman RH. Vascularity of the carpus. *Clin Orthop*. 2001;383:47–59.
20. Grewal R, Suh N, MacDermid JC. The missed scaphoid fractures—outcomes of delayed cast treatment. *J Wrist Surg*. 2015;4:27883.
21. Watanabe K. Analysis of carpal malalignment caused by scaphoid nonunion and evaluation of corrective bone graft on carpal alignment. *J H Hand Surg*. 2011;36A:10–16.
22. Kakar S, Shin AY. Ununited fracture of the proximal pole of the scaphoid with avascular necrosis. *J Hand Surg*. 2011;36A:1522–1524.
23. Dias JJ, Singh HP. Displaced fracture of the waist of the scaphoid. *J Bone Joint Surg Br*. 2011;93B. 1433–9, 2–11.
24. Song K, von Schroeder HP. Delays and poor management of scaphoid fractures: factors contributing to nonunion. *J Hand Surg*. 2011;36A:1471–1474.
25. Dawson JS, Martel A, Davis TRC. Scaphoid blood flow and acute fracture healing: a dynamic MRI study with enhancement with gadolinium. *J Bone Joint Surg BR*. 2001;83:B809–B814.
26. Megerle K, Worg H, Christopoulos G, et al. Gadolinium-enhanced preoperative MRI scans as a prognostic parameter in scaphoid nonunion. *J Hand Surg Eur Vol*. 2011; 36E:23–28.
27. Hannemann PFW, Gottens KWA, van Wely BJ, et al. The clinical and radiological outcome of pulsed electromagnetic field treatment for acute scaphoid fractures: a randomized double-blind placebo-controlled multicentre trial. *J Bone Joint Surg Br*. 2012;94-B: 1403–1408.
28. Malerich MM, Catalano III LW, Weidner ZD, et al. Distal scaphoid resection for degenerative arthritis secondary to scaphoid nonunion: a 20-year experience. *J Hand Surg Am*. 2014;39:1669–1676.
29. Mathoulin C, Brunelli F. Further experience with the index metacarpal vascularized bone graft. *J Hand Surg Br*. 1998;23B:311–317.
30. Kulkarni RW, Wollstein R, Tayar R, et al. Patterns of healing of scaphoid fractures: the importance of vascularity. *J Bone Joint Surg Br*. 1999;81-B:85–90.
31. Fernandez DL, Martin CJ. Gonzalez del Pino. Scaphoid Malunion: the significance of rotational malalignment. *J Hand Surg Br*. 1998;23B:771–775.

CHAPTER 5

Dynamic Imaging and Kinematics of the Scaphoid

MARIEKE G.A. DE ROO, MD • GEERT J. STREEKSTRA, IR, PHD • SIMON D. STRACKEE, MD, PHD

KEY POINTS

- Dynamic 3D CT imaging or 3D MRI allows quantitative analysis of dynamic in vivo carpal kinematics.
- The current available data acquired with dynamic 3D imaging modalities are very difficult to compare.
- We made suggestions for standardization of dynamic imaging and image analysis methods, aiming at reproducible dynamic imaging that facilitates comparison between patients groups.

PANEL 1
Case Scenario

A 28-year-old man visited the emergency department after a fall on his outstretched hand. Radiographs demonstrated a scaphoid waist fracture (Fig. 5.1A). On the CT a 1-mm palmar translation of the distal fragment was visible (Fig. 5.1B–C). Should we classify this scaphoid fracture as a stable or unstable fracture?

IMPORTANCE OF THE PROBLEM

Scaphoid fractures are considered "unstable" when they are more than 1 mm displaced, which is the most important diagnostic measurement associated with nonunion.[1–6] It is well reported that the nonunion rates are considerably higher when a fracture is more than 1 mm displaced, with up to a 55% chance of malunion or nonunion, in comparison with an 90%–95% overall rate of union in scaphoid fractures.[1,2] The interpretation to which scaphoid fractures are unstable differs among surgeons.[8,9] As stated by authors previously, the assumption that "nondisplaced" fractures are "stable," and "displaced" fractures are "unstable," should be considered with care.[10,11]

Whether displaced fractures demonstrate an unstable motion pattern during wrist motion remains to be analyzed extensively. Because static imaging modalities cannot evaluate instability of the scaphoid fragments during normal wrist motion,[12–14] some studies used arthroscopy to evaluate fracture instability, finding fracture comminution as a predictor for instability.[10] However, it is unknown if the traction that is applied during arthroscopy influences fracture stability.[10,11] As for nonoperative diagnostic modalities, dynamic imaging of the wrist, such as fluoroscopy and dynamic three-dimensional (3D) computed tomography (CT) imaging, could be essential to identify true in vivo instability between the scaphoid fragments.[9] However, fluoroscopic imaging cannot be analyzed quantitatively because it is a two-dimensional (2D) technique with the risk of overprojection of the surrounding carpals; therefore dynamic 3D imaging is the optimal method to determine fracture instability.

Recent advancements in the field of dynamic imaging may provide opportunities to evaluate fracture instability patterns and assess the effect of a scaphoid fracture on carpal kinematics. Because dynamic imaging is relatively new, there is no consensus about the best way to conduct this type of analysis. The results generated by the multiple approaches are difficult to compare; we evaluated the imaging techniques used to describe interfragmentary motion of a scaphoid fracture or a scaphoid nonunion.

MAIN QUESTION

With what kind of dynamic imaging methods or semi-dynamic imaging methods is the kinematical pattern of scaphoid fracture or scaphoid nonunion analyzed, and can we compare the motion parameters of those measurement methods?

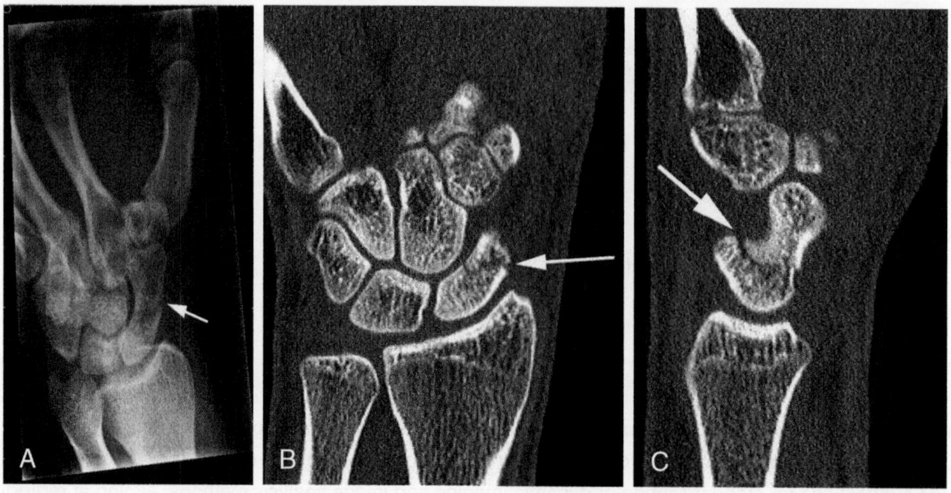

FIG. 5.1 **(A)** The radiograph demonstrates a scaphoid waist fracture. **(B)** Coronal CT scan. **(C)** Sagittal CT scan, 1 mm palmar translation of the distal fragment. The arrow indicates the fracture line.

Current Opinion

After some years of 3D research of scaphoid fractures and nonunions, the interest starts to shift toward dynamically scanning scaphoid fractures, with the aim to evaluate fracture instability and the effect on carpal alignment.

Finding the Evidence

We conducted an online literature search in Medline and Embase and a manual search of the reference lists for relevant articles. All reports with some type of dynamic imaging of scaphoid fractures were eligible for inclusion. Because we expected the data available to be small, we included articles analyzing scaphoid fractures, scaphoid nonunions, and cadaver studies. Inclusion criteria were as follows:

1. Original full-length articles focusing on dynamic imaging of the scaphoid fractures, scaphoid nonunions, or (human) cadaver studies
2. Availability of a full-text copy of a manuscript online or paper version

Exclusion criteria were as follows:

1. Reports focusing only on 3D reconstructions of the scaphoid with the wrist in a single position
2. Nonoriginal full-length articles
3. Articles not in English, French, or German language

Literature Search, Study Selection, and Data Extraction

We used Medical Subject Headings (MeSH) (=scaphoid bone; fractures; imaging, three-dimensional OR four-dimensional CT) and free search terms in the title and abstract with truncation (Table 5.1). We retrieved all titles and abstracts for eligibility assessment. EndNote X7 (Thomas Reuter, London, United Kingdom) was used to remove duplicates and assess titles and abstracts. If eligibility criteria were met, articles were obtained and reviewed. After final selection, we analyzed the following aspects that could be important for reproducible dynamic imaging:

1. What imaging technique is used?
2. Is a guided motion pattern used to replicate a specific motion?
3. What is the definition of the neutral position of the wrist?
4. How is global wrist motion defined?
5. Are the positions of the wrist in which the data are acquired described?
6. Are the measurements performed on 2D or 3D images of the carpal bones?
7. What coordinate system is used to express motion of the carpals?
8. How is the fracture location measured and described?
9. Are the kinematics of the scaphoid fragments analyzed separately?
10. Is the analysis technique validated?

Quality of the Evidence

All articles provided a relatively low quality of evidence. All articles were included.

Level III:

Case-controlled study: 1

TABLE 5.1
Online databases: MEDLINE (through Pubmed) and EMBASE (through Ovid)

	Search strategy	Records identified
Medline	("Scaphoid Bone"[Mesh] OR scaphoid*[tiab] OR Hand Navicular Bone*[tiab]) AND ("Fractures, Bone"[Mesh:NoExp] OR "Fractures, Ununited"[Mesh] OR "Fractures, Malunited" OR fracture*[tiab] OR nonunion*[tiab] OR non-union*[tiab] OR malunion*[tiab] OR mal-union*[tiab] OR malunited*[tiab] OR ununited*[tiab] OR delayed*[tiab] OR chronic*[tiab] OR recalcitrant*[tiab]) AND ("Imaging, Three-Dimensional"[Mesh:NoExp] OR "Four-Dimensional Computed Tomography"[Mesh] OR "Image Processing, Computer-Assisted"[Mes:NoExp] OR "Image Interpretation, Computer Assisted"[Mesh:NoExp] OR three-dimension*[tiab] OR four-dimension*[tiab] OR 3-dimension[tiab] OR 4-dimension[tiab] OR 3dimension*[tiab] OR 4dimension*[tiab] OR 3D[tiab] OR 4D[tiab] OR 3-d[tiab] OR 4-d[tiab] OR dynamic imag*[tiab] OR dynamic*[tiab] OR in-vivo[tiab] OR kinematic*[tiab] OR biomechanic*[tiab])	245
Embase	(scaphoid bone/or (scaphoid*).ti,ab,kw.) and (fracture nonunion/or scaphoid fracture/or fracture/or (fractur* or injur* or nonuni* or non-uni* or ununi* or un-uni* or maluni* or mal-uni*).ti,ab,kw.) and (three dimensional imaging/ or (three-dimension* or four-dimension* or 3-dimension* or 4-dimension* or 3-d* or 4-d* or 3d* or 4d* 3-D imag* or 3D imag* or 4-D imag* or 4D imag*or dynamic imag* or in-vivo* or kinematic*).ti,ab,kw.)	203
Total identified		448
	Duplicates removed	100
	Screening title + abstract	348
	Included for full text analysis	12
Included after full text analysis		9

Level IV:
- Case-controlled study with methodological limitations: 2
- Case series: 1

Level V:
- Cadaver study: 5

FINDINGS

Five cadaver studies were included; one study evaluated acute scaphoid fractures; and three studies observed motion patterns of scaphoid nonunions (Table 5.2).

What Imaging Technique Is Used?

Most studies evaluated stepwise motion patterns. The cadaver study of Werner et al. measured the dynamic motion patterns of the scaphoid fragments, lunate, and third metacarpal, using electromagnetic sensors to express the motion of the carpals.[13] Kaneshiro et al. implanted markers in the scaphoid and radius and used a dynamic biplane radiography system to register continuous motion of every 5 degrees of forearm rotation.[17] Eventually the statistical analysis was performed at 30 and 60 degrees of pronation, neutral, and 30 and 60 degrees of supination. The remaining studies used a stepwise motion pattern analysis, with a variety of carpal motion analysis methods, ranging from carpal markers,[18–20] a markerless bone registration technique,[14] a volume-based registration technique,[21] a "bony landmarks method,"[22] and a "cortical method."[23]

Is a Guided Motion Pattern Used to Replicate a Specific Motion?

A guided motion pattern is created through performing motion of the wrist with a device that imposes motion in a fixed plane. Only Tehranzadeh et al. did not use a guided motion pattern[23]; all other investigators performed motion in a set plane.

What Is the Definition of the Neutral Position of the Wrist?

Five studies defined the neutral position of the wrist as the alignment of the third metacarpal with

TABLE 5.2
Characteristics of Included Studies

Study	N	Type of Imaging	DYNAMIC?	Motion Axes	GUIDED MOTION?
ACUTE SCAPHOID FRACTURES					
Feipel[22]	13	3D CT	No	RU, FE	Yes
SCAPHOID NONUNIONS					
Tehranzadeh[23]	30	Radiographs	No	FE	No
Leventhal 2008[14]	6	3D CT	No	RU, FE, RE, FU, RF, UE	Yes
Moritomo[21]	13	3D CT and 3D MRI	No	RU, FE	Yes
CADAVER STUDY					
Smith[18]	5	Radiographs	No	RU, FE	Yes
Kaneshiro[17]	4	Radiographs	Yes	Pronation and supination	Yes
McAdams[20]	10	3D CT	No	Pronation and supination	Yes
Ivancic[19]	8	Optotrak	No	FE	Yes
Werner[13]	11	3D CT	Yes	RU, FE, DT	Yes

DT, dart-throwing motion; *FE*, flexion-extension motion; *FU*, flexion and ulnar deviation; *MRI*, magnetic resonance imaging; *RE*, radial deviation and extension; *RF*, radial deviation and flexion; *RU*, radioulnar deviation; *UE*, ulnar deviation and extension.

the dorsal surface of the forearm.[14,17,19,21,22] Two studies did not specify their definition of a neutral position,[13,20] one study described the amount of tendon load applied,[18] and one study positioned the wrist in a lateral position with an angle of 30–40 degrees to the tabletop with the elbow raised with padding.[23]

How Is Global Wrist Motion Defined?

Six of the nine studies did not specify how they determined global wrist motion.[17–20,22,23] Two studies expressed the global wrist motion as the motion of the capitate[14,21] and one study used the motion of the third metacarpal.[13]

Are the Positions of the Wrist in Which the Data Are Acquired Described?

Four studies described the angle of the wrist in which they analyzed the interfragmentary motion of the scaphoid[13,14,17,22] (Table 5.3).

Are the Measurements Performed on the 2D or 3D Images of the Carpal Bones?

All the measurement methods to estimate interfragmentary motion differed, from measurements from 2D images, used in the studies of McAdams,[20] Tehranzadeh,[23] and Feipel,[22] to all different types of 3D analysis by Ivancic,[19] Smith,[18] Leventhal,[14] Kaneshiro,[17] Moritomo,[17] and Werner.[13]

What Coordinate System Is Used to Express Motion of the Carpals?

Five studies used all different types of radial coordinate systems. Moritomo et al. used the coordinate system according to the International Society of Biomechanics (http://www.isbweb.org/standards/wrist.html).[21] Leventhal et al. preferred the coordinate system advised by Coburn et al.[14,24] Feipel et al. projected the coordinate system on the radial styloid process.[22] Two studies based on the radial coordinate system placed markers on the radial bone.[17,18] Ivancic et al. used a coordinate system projected on the most proximal point of the proximal scaphoid fragment.[19] Three studies did not use a coordinate system to express motion.[13,20,23]

How Is the Fracture Location Determined?

Two studies determined if the location of the fracture was proximal or distal to the scaphoid apex.[13,21] In the cadaver experiments the fracture was manually created, but only the study of Werner et al. investigated the precise location of the fracture afterward.[13] The other studies did not specify which classification system they used to describe the location of the fracture.[17–20]

Are the Kinematics of the Scaphoid Fragments Analyzed Separately?

The study of Feipel et al. did not analyze the motion patterns of the distal and proximal scaphoid fragment separately.[22] All other studies analyzed both fragments,

TABLE 5.3
The Characteristics of the Positioning of the Wrist in Which the Measurements of the Study Are Performed, in Degrees

	POSITIONING OF THE WRIST (DEGREES)									
Study	**F**	**E**	**R**	**U**	**U&E**	**R&F**	**R&E**	**U&F**	**Supination**	**Pronation**
ACUTE SCAPHOID FRACTURES										
Feipel[22]	45	45	15	30	–	–	–	–	–	–
SCAPHOID NONUNIONS										
Tehranzadeh[23]	Not described		–	–	–	–	–	–	–	–
Leventhal[14]	40	40	10	30	30U,40E	10R,40F	10R,40E	30U,40F	–	–
Moritomo[21]	Not described				–	–	–	–	–	–
CADAVER STUDY										
Smith[18]	Not described				–	–	–	–	–	–
Kaneshiro[17]	–	–	–	–	–	–	–	–	30, 60	30, 60
McAdams[20]	Not described				–	–	–	–	–	–
Ivancic[19]	Not described				–	–	–	–	–	–
Werner[13]	50	30	10	20	–	–	10R,30E	10U,30F	–	–

E, extension; *F*, flexion; *R*, radial deviation; *R&E*, radial deviation and extension; *R&F*, radial deviation and flexion; *U*, ulnar deviation; *U&E*, ulnar deviation and extension; *U&F*, ulnar deviation and flexion; –, not the motion pattern evaluated in the study.

describing motion between the distal fragment relative to the proximal fragment or relative to the position of the radius.

Is the Analysis Technique Validated?

Six studies validated their analysis technique.[13,14,17–19,21] One study performed some experiments to determine the accuracy of the measurement methods used, but did not specify the exact methods used.[22] The remaining two studies did not validate their analysis technique.[20,23]

RECOMMENDATIONS

In this study we did not investigate the effect of a treatment or intervention; therefore the GRADE system to score overall quality of the evidence could not be applied. To answer our research question, if we can compare the motion parameters of the scaphoid fragments with the measurement methods used; we evaluated several aspects important for dynamic imaging. The rationale behind these aspects is provided in a list below:

- **The imaging technique used**
  Quasi-dynamic imaging of the carpals with 3D images of the wrist in multiple positions provides an accurate but static motion pattern. Abrupt dynamic changes in the carpal alignment cannot be detected with static imaging modalities (25, 26). Ideally a dynamic imaging technique should be used for assessing pathological wrist kinematics.
- **Why a guided motion pattern?**
  Performing motion in a specific fixed plane provides an accurate and reproducible motion pattern. If the hand is allowed to move freely, the wrist can move through slightly different motion planes, with, for example, radioulnar deviation occurring, creating different outcomes.[25] It will be difficult to compare data if such bias is present.
- **Positioning of the wrist**
  To compare study outcomes, the measured interfragmentary motion should be related to the actual wrist position. To determine the wrist position, the position of the capitate has shown to be more accurate then external measurement methods.[26]
- **2D or 3D measurements of the carpal bones**
  Measurements should be performed on 3D images, not on 2D, because it allows for measurement of three degrees of freedom only.[27] As motion occurs in three translational parameters and three rotational parameters (i.e., six degrees of freedom), carpal motion can only be accurately described with 3D measurement methods. The fracture location should be determined on 3D images because it is a 3D problem.[9]

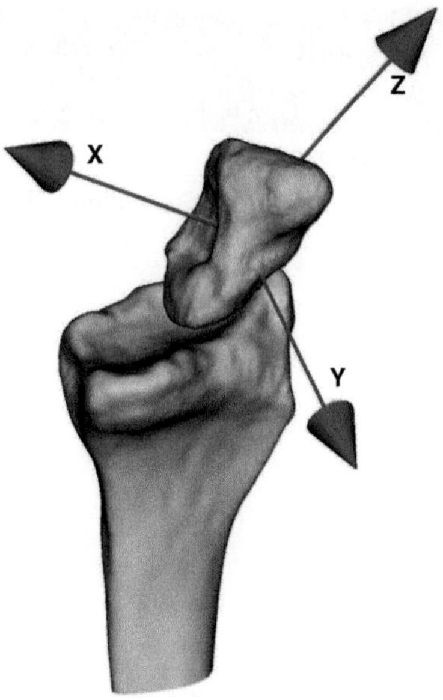

FIG. 5.2 Coordinate system of the scaphoid.

- **Why a coordinate system?**
To express motion in vivo, motion parameters of the individual carpal bones relative to an anatomically based coordinate system are needed (Fig. 5.2).[27]
- **Analysis of the scaphoid fragments**
Interfragmentary motion can be accurately described in three rotational and three translational parameters of the distal fragment relative to the proximal fragment.[27] When only distances are measured from single points opposite on the fragments, rotation of the fragment can occur, whereas the measured distance stays the same.
- **Validation of the technique**
It is important to validate the analysis technique; because the measured rotations and translations can be so small, results could be accounted to motion blurring, image acquisition, and image analysis.

CONCLUSION

Dynamic imaging of joints is a new and promising trend, creating opportunities to evaluate normal and pathologic wrist kinematics. We evaluated the current data available acquired with dynamic or stepwise imaging modalities. We found that the measurement methods and analysis techniques used to gather the available data was so diverse; we could not compare motion parameters found for interfragmentary motion of the scaphoid fragments. This can also be due to failed reporting of specific methods used. We evaluated what we consider to be important aspects of dynamic imaging to create awareness of the difficulties in performing dynamic imaging research. Therefore, we made suggestions for standardization of dynamic imaging and image analysis methods, aiming at future reproducible dynamic imaging that facilitates comparison between patient groups.

PANEL 2
Authors' Preferred Technique

DYNAMIC 3D CT PROTOCOL

- Validate the dynamic 3D CT technique used.
- Scan both wrists, use the uninjured wrist as a reference; because anatomic differences of ligament insertions are known (but are relatively small), this provides the best reference for the normal motion pattern of the patient.[7]
- Identify fracture location on 3D CT, with the contralateral uninjured scaphoid as a reference.
- Let the patient perform a guided active motion pattern of the wrist.
- Express global wrist motion as the rotation of the capitate with respect to the radius[15] because nonnegligible differences (3–5 degrees of rotation) between the capitate and third metacarpal are described.[16]
- Use a clearly defined radial coordinate system, with landmarks according to the International Society of Biomechanics (http://www.isbweb.org/standards/wrist.html).
- Interfragmentary motion should be described as the motion of the distal fragment relative to the proximal fragment in three translational and three rotational parameters.

PANEL 3
Pearls and Pitfalls of Dynamic Imaging

PEARLS

- Dynamic 3D CT or 3D MRI imaging provides the opportunity to quantitatively analyze dynamic in vivo carpal kinematics.
- When dynamic 3D CT is accurately performed, quantitative analysis of fracture instability is possible.

PITFALLS

- No validation of the analysis technique.
- A nondefined wrist angle in which the measurements are performed.
- The use of a nonguided motion pattern.

REFERENCES

1. Buijze GA, Ochtman L, Ring D. Management of scaphoid nonunion. *J Hand Surg Am*. 2012;37(5):1095–1100. quiz 1101.
2. Swart E, Strauch RJ. Diagnosis of scaphoid fracture displacement. *J Hand Surg Am*. 2013;38(4):784–787. quiz 787.
3. Eddeland A, Eiken O, Hellgren E, Ohlsson NM. Fractures of the scaphoid. *Scand J Plast Reconstr Surg*. 1975;9(3): 234–239.
4. Szabo RM, Manske D. Displaced fractures of the scaphoid. *Clin Orthop Relat Res*. 1988;(230):30–38.
5. Bhat M, McCarthy M, Davis TR, Oni JA, Dawson S. MRI and plain radiography in the assessment of displaced fractures of the waist of the carpal scaphoid. *J Bone Joint Surg Br*. 2004;86(5):705–713.
6. Langhoff O, Andersen JL. Consequences of late immobilization of scaphoid fractures. *J Hand Surg Br*. 1988;13(1):77–79.
7. Viegas SF, Yamaguchi S, Boyd NL, Patterson RM. The dorsal ligaments of the wrist: anatomy, mechanical properties, and function. *J Hand Surg Am*. 1999;24(3):456–468.
8. Steinmann SP, Adams JE. Scaphoid fractures and nonunions: diagnosis and treatment. *J Orthopaedic Science*. 2006;11(4):424–431.
9. Ten Berg PW, Drijkoningen T, Strackee SD, Buijze GA. Classifications of acute scaphoid fractures: a systematic literature Review. *J Wrist Surg*. 2016;5(2):152–159.
10. Buijze GA, Jorgsholm P, Thomsen NO, Bjorkman A, Besjakov J, Ring D. Factors associated with arthroscopically determined scaphoid fracture displacement and instability. *J Hand Surg Am*. 2012;37(7):1405–1410.
11. Buijze GA, Jorgsholm P, Thomsen NO, Bjorkman A, Besjakov J, Ring D. Diagnostic performance of radiographs and computed tomography for displacement and instability of acute scaphoid waist fractures. *J Bone Joint Surg Am*. 2012;94(21):1967–1974.
12. Oka K, Moritomo H, Murase T, Goto A, Sugamoto K, Yoshikawa H. Patterns of carpal deformity in scaphoid nonunion: a 3-dimensional and quantitative analysis. *J Hand Surg Am*. 2005;30(6):1136–1144.
13. Werner FW, St-Amand H, Moritomo H, Sutton LG, Short WH. The effect of scaphoid fracture site on scaphoid instability patterns. *J Wrist Surg*. 2016;5(1):47–51.
14. Leventhal EL, Wolfe SW, Moore DC, Akelman E, Weiss AP, Crisco JJ. Interfragmentary motion in patients with scaphoid nonunion. *J Hand Surg Am*. 2008;33(7):1108–1115.
15. de Lange A, Kauer JM, Huiskes R. Kinematic behavior of the human wrist joint: a roentgen-stereophotogrammetric analysis. *J Orthopaedic Research*. 1985;3(1):56–64.
16. Citteur JM, Ritt MJ, Bos KE. Carpal boss: destabilization of the third carpometacarpal joint after a wedge excision. *J Hand Surg Br*. 1998;23(1):76–78.
17. Kaneshiro SA, Failla JM, Tashman S. Scaphoid fracture displacement with forearm rotation in a short-arm thumb spica cast. *J Hand Surg Am*. 1999;24(5):984–991.
18. Smith DK, Cooney 3rd WP, An KN, Linscheid RL, Chao EY. The effects of simulated unstable scaphoid fractures on carpal motion. *J Hand Surg Am*. 1989;14(2 Pt 1): 283–291.
19. Ivancic PC, Save AV, Carlson EJ, Dodds SD. Scaphoid interfragmentary motions due to simulated transverse fracture and volar wedge osteotomy. *Clin Biomechanics (Bristol, Avon)*. 2014;29(2):189–195.
20. McAdams TR, Spisak S, Beaulieu CF, Ladd AL. The effect of pronation and supination on the minimally displaced scaphoid fracture. *Clin Orthop Relat Res*. 2003;(411): 255–259.
21. Moritomo H, Murase T, Oka K, Tanaka H, Yoshikawa H, Sugamoto K. Relationship between the fracture location and the kinematic pattern in scaphoid nonunion. *J Hand Surg Am*. 2008;33(9):1459–1468.
22. Feipel V, Dourdoufis M, Salvia P, Rooze M. The use of medical imaging-based kinematic analysis in the evaluation of wrist function and outcome. *Hand Clin*. 2003;19(3):401–409. viii.
23. Tehranzadeh J, Davenport J, Pais MJ. Scaphoid fracture: evaluation with flexion-extension tomography. *Radiology*. 1990;176(1):167–170.
24. Coburn J, Crisco JJ. Interpolating three-dimensional kinematic data using quaternion splines and hermite curves. *J Biomechanical Engineering*. 2005;127(2):311–317.
25. Shores JT, Demehri S, Chhabra A. Kinematic "4 dimensional" CT imaging in the assessment of wrist Biomechanics before and after surgical repair. *Eplasty*. 2013;13. e9.
26. Wolfe SW, Neu C, Crisco JJ. In vivo scaphoid, lunate, and capitate kinematics in flexion and in extension. *J Hand Surg Am*. 2000;25(5):860–869.
27. Foumani M, Strackee SD, Jonges R, et al. In-vivo three-dimensional carpal bone kinematics during flexion-extension and radio-ulnar deviation of the wrist: dynamic motion versus step-wise static wrist positions. *J Biomech*. 2009;42(16):2664–2671.

CHAPTER 6

Predictors of Scaphoid Fractures

ANDREW D. DUCKWORTH, BSC(HONS), MBCHB, MSC, FRCSED(TR&ORTH), PHD

KEY POINTS

- Between 5% and 20% of patients who present to the emergency department (ED) with a suspected fracture of the scaphoid are eventually diagnosed with a true fracture.
- The diagnosis of true scaphoid fractures among suspected scaphoid fractures continues to be a quandary as no single or combination of clinical signs has been documented to be adequately sensitive or specific.
- The most sophisticated imaging modalities have reported false-positive and false-negative rates because the rate of true fractures among suspected fractures is low and there is currently no agreed consensus reference standard for diagnosing a true fracture.
- Clinical predictions rules can incorporate demographic and clinical predictors of a true acute fracture of the scaphoid, aiming to increase the prevalence and pretest probability of true fractures among suspected fractures, and thus the various imaging modalities available will provide more useful and accurate data to help inform management.
- Surgeons and patients need to be accepting that the best we can do without an agreed reference standard is to define and refine the probability of a sustaining a true fracture of the scaphoid.

PANEL 1
Case Scenario

A 24-year-old woman presents to the emergency department complaining of left wrist pain following a simple fall onto the outstretched hand. She is tender in the region of the anatomic snuff box and over the scaphoid tubercle. There is a reduced range of movement at the wrist and thumb with associated radial sided wrist pain. Standard four-view scaphoid radiographs reveal no obvious bony injury to the scaphoid or the rest of the carpus or wrist. In such a patient, what is the probability of an occult scaphoid fracture and how is it best managed?

IMPORTANCE OF THE PROBLEM

The suspected fracture of the scaphoid continues to be a problematic and costly clinical scenario despite the improvements in knowledge and radiological imaging. When investigating and managing suspected fractures of the scaphoid, a clear knowledge of the epidemiology and etiology is invaluable. It is important to consider that the population affected is predominantly young and active, where a prompt diagnosis and avoidance of unnecessary immobilization is beneficial. The treating surgeon needs to balance the use of immobilization and restriction of day-to-day activities, against the potential risk of nonunion and arthrosis that can occur after undiagnosed and/or untreated fractures of the scaphoid.[1–3]

The suspected scaphoid fracture is defined by a patient with radial-sided wrist pain and tenderness following trauma, e.g., fall from standing height onto the outstretched hand, with up to 90% recalling a hyperextension injury. Standard four-view scaphoid radiographs are routinely performed (Fig. 6.1A–D). Despite this, literature quotes that up to 30%–40% of scaphoid fractures are not identified on primary clinical assessment and standard four-view radiographs.[4–12] Patients who consequently are confirmed as having a scaphoid fracture on repeat clinical assessment and radiologic imaging, which is commonly performed at 10–14 days postinjury, are defined as having an occult fracture of the scaphoid.[5,10,13–17]

The mind-set and drive of research in this area over recent years has been to determine the optimal "gold standard" radiologic test to diagnose all fractures early so that none are missed and that an early definitive diagnosis is made, with an aim of reducing unnecessary immobilization and the requirement for further clinical assessments.[14,18–24] However, despite strong advocates

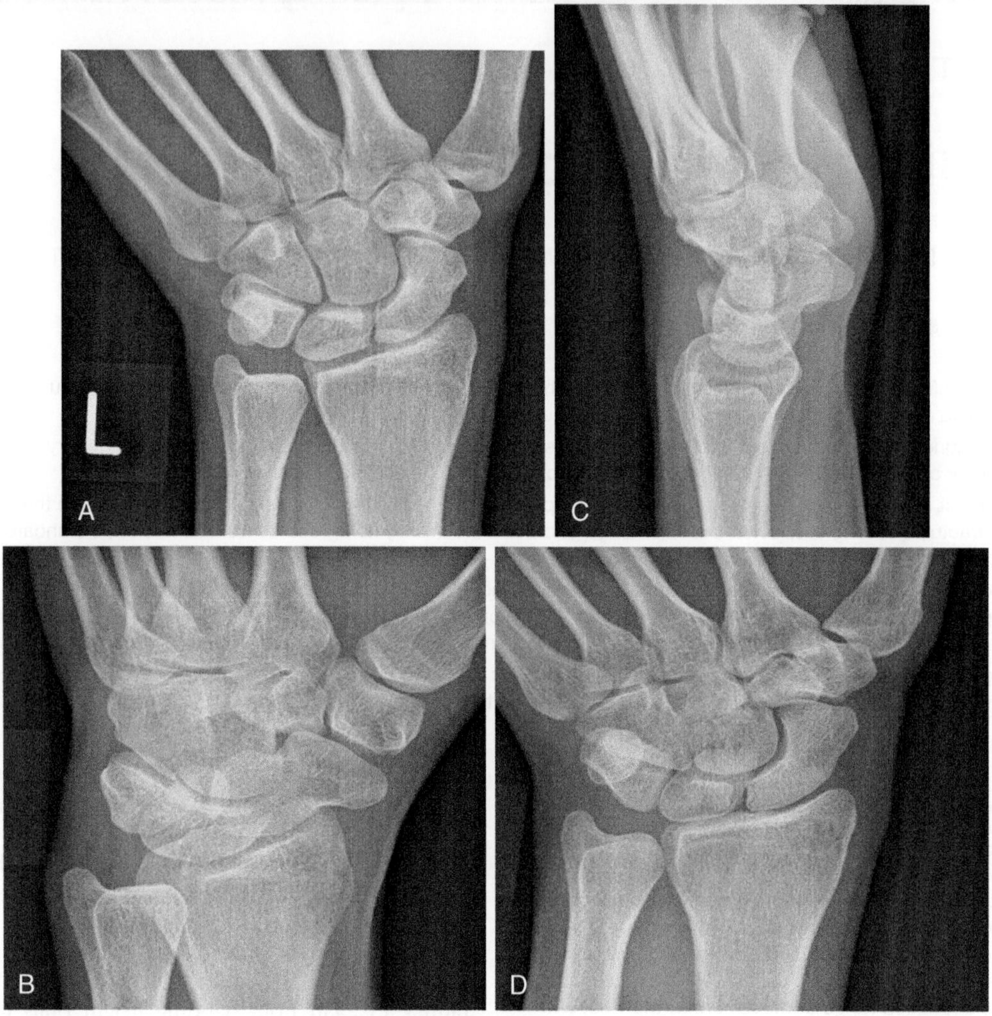

FIG. 6.1 The standard four scaphoid radiograph series. **(A)** Posteroanterior (PA), **(B)** Semi-pronated oblique, **(C)** Lateral, **(D)** PA with ulnar deviation

for the numerous secondary imaging modalities, a clear solution to the conundrum has not emerged.

Two critical issues need to be contemplated when considering the clinical and radiologic diagnostic tests used in the assessment of the suspected scaphoid fractures.[25,26] The first issue relates to the low prevalence of true fractures among suspected fractures. The data suggest that between 5% and 20% of patients who present with a suspected fracture of the scaphoid are eventually diagnosed with a true fracture.[6,24,25,27–30] This scenario notably lowers the probability that a positive clinical or radiologic test will correspond with a true fracture of the scaphoid as false-positive results are nearly as common as true-positive results (Table 6.1).[6,24–30] Because false positives and false negatives are quoted at 5%–10% for diagnostic tests, given the low prevalence of true fractures among the patients assessed for the fractures, the PPVs according to Bayes' theorem will be low even when the test has high sensitivity and specificity (Fig. 6.2).[25,31] The second issue is the absence of a consensus reference standard for confirming a true fracture,[31,32] which means that an alternative method for calculating diagnostic performance characteristics (latent class analysis) is needed.[33,34] The most commonly used reference standard in the literature is the absence of a fracture on radiographs at 6 weeks postinjury,[10,25,28,35,36] although this has recently been refuted in one study because of the low agreement between observers.[37]

TABLE 6.1
Contingency Table of Commonly Used Statistical Terms and Diagnostic Performance Characteristics in the Literature Investigating Clinical Tests and Imaging Used for the Suspected Scaphoid Fracture

Terminology	Explanation
Sensitivity	The ability of clinical test or imaging to correctly identify a patient with a true scaphoid fracture.
Specificity	The ability of clinical test or imaging to correctly identify a patient with no fracture.
False-positive rate	Equivalent to the type I error and is equal to 1 − specificity.
False-negative rate	Equivalent to the type II error and is equal to 1 − sensitivity.
Positive predictive value (PPV)	The proportion of actual true scaphoid fractures in relation to the number of positive clinical tests or imaging. PPV is directly proportional to the prevalence of true scaphoid fractures and can be adjusted after the test.
Negative predictive value	The proportion of actual patients with no scaphoid fracture in relation to the number of negative clinical tests or imaging.
Likelihood Ratio	Utilizes the sensitivity and specificity to ascertain the effect of a clinical test or imaging being associated with a true scaphoid fracture. The likelihood ratio is calculated for both positive (+) and negative (−) clinical tests or imaging.
Incidence	The rate of new true scaphoid fractures in a population over a given time.
Prevalence	The proportion of patients with a true scaphoid fracture in a defined population.
Pretest probability	Probability of the presence of a true scaphoid fracture before a clinical test or imaging.
Posttest probability	Probability of the presence of a true scaphoid fracture after a clinical test or imaging.

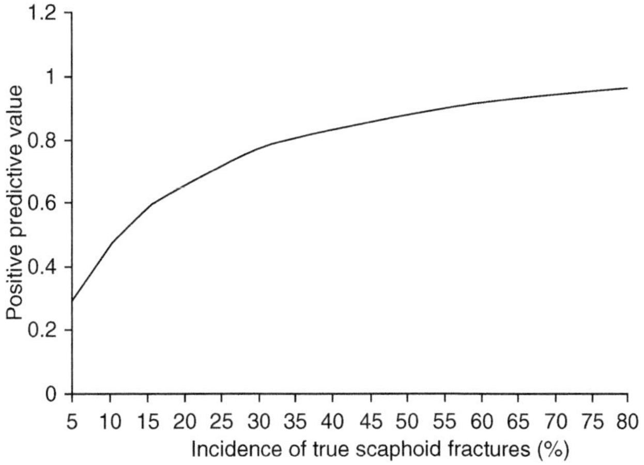

FIG. 6.2 The effect seen between fracture prevalence and the positive predictive value of diagnostic tests. (From Duckworth AD, Ring D, McQueen MM. Assessment of the suspected fracture of the scaphoid. *J Bone Joint Surg Br*. 2011;93(6):714; with permission.)

The consequence of the low prevalence of a true fracture and the distinct lack of a consensus reference standard for diagnosing a fracture is that, despite advances in imaging, there will probably be an unavoidable very low probability of missing a true fracture among the numerous suspected fractures of the scaphoid that present. Given the growing evidence that the various imaging modalities may not be the answer, an option is to increase the pretest probability of a patient having a true fracture prior to ordering such advanced imaging. This could be done by implementing clinical prediction rules incorporating predictors of fracture so to indicate when advanced imaging may be beneficial.

MAIN QUESTION

In adult patients, what are the demographic and clinical predictors for the presence of a true scaphoid fracture? (Table 6.2)

Current Opinion

Current practice suggests that diagnosis of scaphoid fractures is through a combination of clinical history, examination, and radiographic assessment. No single sign, or even when the signs are combined, has been found to be sufficiently sensitive and specific[38–40] (see Chapter 7). As a consequence of oversensitive clinical signs and the lack of a consensus gold standard for imaging the suspected scaphoid fracture, a large number of patients with a suspected fracture undergo unnecessary mobilization and persistent imaging,[7,10,11,38,39,41–43] which can result in stiffness and high costs to both the healthcare system and the patient.[18,20,21,44]

National guidelines of some professional associations, as well as research advocates, are optimistic on the use of MRI. The Royal College of Radiologists (United Kingdom) suggests that current evidence demonstrate equivocal diagnostic performance characteristics for bone scintigraphy, CT, and MRI for suspected fractures.[45] In contrast, the American College of Radiology (ACR) advocates radiographs and MRI.[46] Despite strong diagnostic performance characterizes for MRI as the secondary imaging modality for suspected fractures, in low prevalence situations such as this, the positive predictive value (PPV) has been shown to be only 88% and the literature has documented the potential for false-positive MRI scans.[47] In a prospective cohort study comparing CT and MRI for diagnosing true fractures among suspected fractures, both had comparable diagnostic performance characteristics with the PPV for CT 76% and 54% for MRI.[48] This study raises the issue of whether small unicortical lines on CT or bone edema on MRI are a true fracture (Fig. 6.3), with the rate of scaphoid bone bruising on MRI leading to occult fracture noted to be 2% in one study.[49]

An international survey of 105 hospitals worldwide documented a high rate of inconsistency with regard to the imaging protocol for suspected scaphoid fractures, with only 22% noted to have a fixed protocol.[50] This is consistent with two recent surveys performed in the United Kingdom that reported a high rate of variability in both the use of repeat radiographs and the indication and mode of secondary imaging.[51,52] A potential solution to these issues and variation in practice would be employing clinical prediction rules that are known to effectively guide patient management throughout all areas of medicine.[53,54] Clinical prediction rules for suspected scaphoid fractures would incorporate a combination of demographic and clinical risk factors that could potentially increase the prevalence of true fractures among suspected fractures.[25,26] This would mean utilizing advanced secondary imaging modalities such as MRI in higher risk patients, which would likely improve the diagnostic performance characteristics currently reported.

Finding the Evidence

- Cochrane Search: Scaphoid Fracture
- Pubmed (Medline): "Suspected Scaphoid Fracture" [Mesh] OR "Predictors Scaphoid Fracture" OR "Scaphoid Fracture Epidemiology"
- Bibliography of eligible articles
- Articles that were not in English were excluded from the review

Quality of the Evidence

Level III:

Prospective or retrospective comparative studies: 3

Level IV:

Case series: 8

FINDINGS

The incidence of scaphoid fractures is conflicting in the literature, ranging from 1.5 to 121 fractures per

TABLE 6.2
Demographic and Clinical Predictors for the Presence of a True Scaphoid Fracture

Population	Adults ≥16 years of Age or Older With a Suspected Fracture of the Scaphoid
Intervention	Not applicable
Comparison	Demographic and clinical risk factors including age, gender, mechanism of injury, comorbidities, clinical symptoms and signs
Outcomes	True confirmed fracture of the scaphoid on radiologic imaging
Study designs	Metaanalyses, systematic reviews, randomized controlled trials, cohort studies, case series

100,000 persons/year.[20,27,30,55–59] The wide disparity is possibly due to analysis of predominantly retrospective data, investigation of exact patient populations, e.g., military, along with the limitation of large national databases to differentiate between a true and suspected fracture of the scaphoid.[20,27,30,55–58] In a prospective study from a single center with a defined captive adult population an annual incidence of 29 per 100,000 per year was reported for true radiographically confirmed acute scaphoid fractures.[59] This literature is consistent with data from Scandinavia reporting annual incidences ranging from 26 to 39 per 100,000 persons/year.[30,56] The quoted mean age of adult patients with a true scaphoid fractures ranges from 25 to 35 years. Males are noted to be significantly younger at the time of injury compared with their female counterparts, most closely fitting a type B fracture distribution curve (Fig. 6.4).[20,27,30,55–59] A male gender predominance is consistently reported throughout the literature, with a male to female ratio of ~2.5:1.[20,27,30,55–59] Two studies have also reported male gender as a predictor or a true fracture of the scaphoid.[24,34]

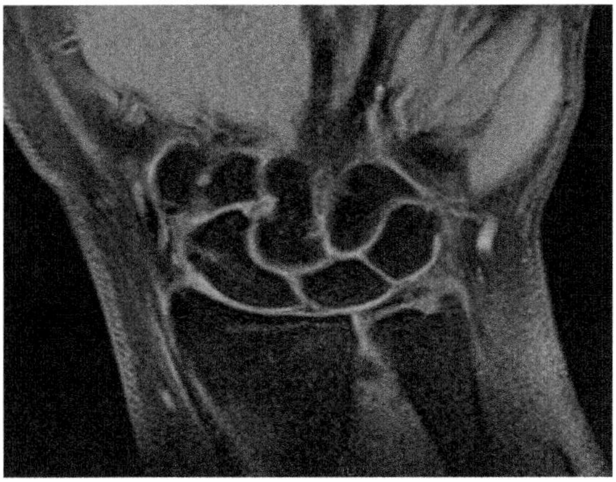

FIG. 6.3 MRI demonstrating bone marrow edema and curvilinear sagittal band of low signal in keeping with microtrabecular damage/bone edema.

With regard to mechanism of injury, true scaphoid fractures commonly follow a fall on to the outstretched hand or during sports.[24,30,58,59] Two studies have found that sports injuries are associated with a true fracture.[24,34] Sports associated with an increased risk of fracture include football, cycling, basketball, and skateboarding, although this is dependent on the study source.[58,59] True scaphoid fractures are also being increasingly reported following punching or assault-related injuries.[60,61] An epidemiologic study from Edinburgh noted that females frequently sustained a fracture following a low energy fall from standing height, whereas males were more likely to sustain their fracture after a high-energy mechanism such as sports or a motor vehicle accident.[59] This is consistent with the younger age at which a true scaphoid fracture occurs in males.

Two prospective cohort studies have identified demographic and clinical predictors of a true fracture and suggest the use of potential clinical prediction

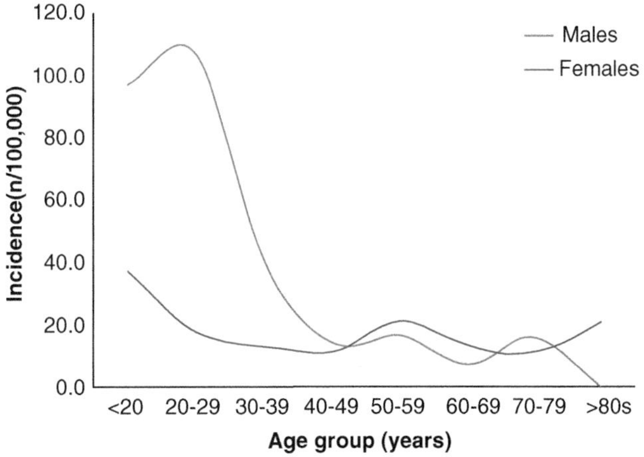

FIG. 6.4 A type B fracture distribution curve for acute true fractures of the scaphoid that presented in Edinburgh over a 1-year period. (From Wohlauer MV, Sauaia A, Moore EE, et al. Acute kidney injury and post-trauma multiple organ failure: the canary in the coal mine. *J Trauma Acute Care Surg*. 2012;72(2):373–378; with permission.)

rules for the assessment of suspected scaphoid fractures. Rhemrev and colleagues performed a prospective cohort study with an aim to develop a clinical prediction rule to determine predictors of fracture.[29] On multivariate analysis, they found in 78 patients with a suspected scaphoid fracture that a reduction in extension of <50%, supination strength of ≤10% and the presence of a previous scaphoid fracture were independently predictive of a true scaphoid fracture.[29] A potential limitation of the study is that the clinical tests are not routinely performed in day-to-day clinical practice, making the general uptake less likely. However, this study does clearly establish the potential of a clinical prediction rule to improve the assessment of suspected scaphoid fractures.

In our recent prospective study from Edinburgh and Boston, we performed a prospective cohort analysis of 223 patients with a clinically suspected fracture or radiographically confirmed scaphoid fracture (n = 62).[34] This study used radiologic imaging at 6 weeks postinjury as the reference standard. The study found that predictors for a true scaphoid fracture were male gender, sports injury, anatomical snuff box (ASB) pain on ulnar deviation of the wrist (negative predictive value, 100%), and pain on thumb-index finger pinch at presentation. Predictors at the 2-week review were scaphoid tubercle tenderness. These demographic and clinical signs were incorporated to develop clinical prediction rules that could guide the assessment of these patients. This study demonstrated that clinical prediction rules have a substantial and meaningful influence on the probability of a suspected scaphoid fracture.

Considerations for Future Research

It is improbable that a consensus reference standard will ever be agreed. Advanced and more sophisticated imaging currently has identified a higher number of abnormalities that are inconsistently interpreted. Therefore, to progress there needs to be an appreciation that we are really dealing with probabilities rather than certainties with regard to the assessment of suspected scaphoid fractures. The aim would then be to reach optional negative and PPVs and reaching agreed and acceptable thresholds. With the preimaging probability of a fracture (i.e., prevalence of true scaphoid fractures among suspected fractures) inherently related to the PPV of diagnostic tests, future research should aim to develop the attempts to produce clinical prediction rules that incorporate demographic and clinical factors predictive of a true fracture. This will better identify patients in whom advanced imaging will have acceptable diagnostic performance characteristics.

RECOMMENDATIONS

In adult patients with a suspected fracture of the scaphoid but normal scaphoid radiographs, the evidence regarding predictors of a true fracture suggests the following:

- 5%–20% of patients who present to the ED with a suspected fracture of the scaphoid are eventually diagnosed with a true fracture (overall quality: moderate).
- Male gender, sports injuries, and a previous scaphoid fracture are risk factors for a true acute fracture of the scaphoid (overall quality: moderate).
- Clinical signs suggestive of a true fracture are ASB pain on ulnar deviation of the wrist (presentation), pain on thumb-index finger pinch (presentation), and scaphoid tubercle tenderness (2 weeks) (overall quality: moderate).
- Clinical prediction rules incorporating demographic and clinical predictors of a true scaphoid fracture have the potential to increase the pretest probability of a fracture (overall quality: moderate).

CONCLUSION

Although there is currently limited data, prospective cohort studies have identified a combination of demographic and clinical predictors associated with a true acute fracture of the scaphoid. Combining and implementing these factors through clinical prediction rules could increase the prevalence of true fractures among suspected fractures and lead to the utilization of advanced imaging in high-risk patients. If the preimaging probability of a true fracture is ≥40%, bone scintigraphy, CT, or MRI will likely have better diagnostic performance characteristics and thus will provide superior accurate information to guide management in this predominantly young and active patient population.[25,26]

Finally, with regard to the general mindset, it is important to consider an analogy to the acceptance of the documented risks and complications associated with joint replacement surgery, e.g., risk of infection less than 1%. This would suggest that a change in the mind-set is likely required when considering the suspected scaphoid fracture where patients, doctors, and society are willing to accept a likely less than 1% probability of missing a true fracture.

PANEL 2
Author's Preferred Technique

For such a young female patient with a low-energy injury and a suspected occult scaphoid fracture but negative four-view scaphoid radiographs, the pretest probability of a fracture is low (5%–20% according to the literature but possibly less), so we would reassess the patient after 2 weeks of immobilization in a wrist splint. Clinical assessment would be performed at this stage by a specialist once the injury was more comfortable. Repeat four-view scaphoid radiographs would also be performed. If the clinical symptoms and signs had resolved and the radiographs were normal, the patient would be discharged with advice.

If symptoms/signs persist and the probability of a fracture was high, e.g., male and high-energy injury, an informed discussion would be carried out with the patient. For those higher risk cases, advanced imaging (routinely MRI) would be performed to exclude a fracture and thus avoid prolonged immobilization in a predominantly young and active population. For the small number of low-risk cases, the patient would continue with the splint for a further 4 weeks at most. Patients would then be reviewed at the 6-week mark and a repeat and hopefully final clinical assessment including radiographs would be carried out.

In our center, we are currently auditing a new pathway that is based on previous work we have done on developing clinical prediction rules. An example of such a clinical prediction rule is found in Fig. 6.5A–C. This formalizes the pathway described above, but is more robustly based on clinical data. Although such clinical prediction rules are still in development, it is clear that they can have a substantial and meaningful influence on the probability of a suspected fracture of the scaphoid.

PANEL 3
Pearls and Pitfalls

PEARLS

- Demographic and clinical risk factors for a true acute fracture of the scaphoid are evident in the literature.
- Advanced imaging for all suspected scaphoid fractures is not likely the answer given the documented false-positive and false-negative rates associated with the low prevalence of true fractures among suspected fractures.
- Clinical prediction rules incorporating demographic and clinical predictors should aid in the assessment of the suspected fracture by increasing the pretest probability of a fracture, thus improving the various imaging modalities available.

PITFALLS

- Although demographic risk factors have been identified, the evidence is currently limited.
- Despite these predictors, epidemiologic data would still suggest that a third of true scaphoid fractures occur in women and over 40% following a low-energy fall.
- Although clinical signs have been incorporated within clinical prediction rules, the specificity of all signs in isolation remains low.

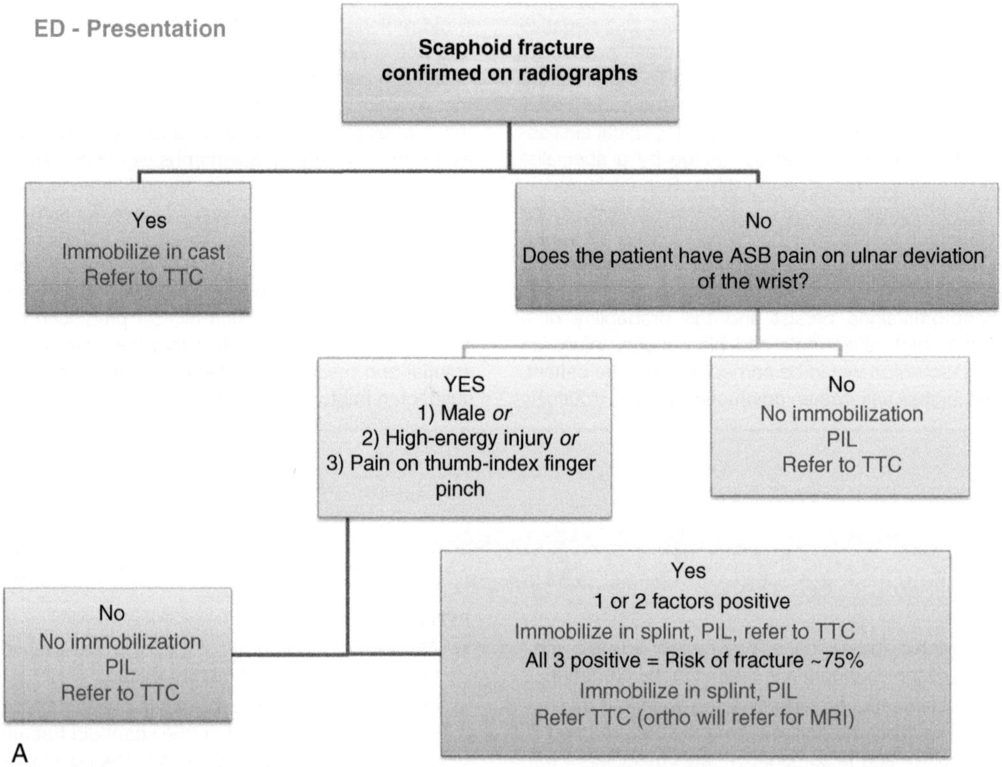

FIG. 6.5 A management algorithm for suspected fractures of the scaphoid based on data and a clinical prediction rule developed by Duckworth et al. **(A)** Presentation, **(B)** 2-week review, and **(C)** 6-week review algorithms. *ED*, emergency department; *PIL*, patient information leaflet; *TTC*, trauma triage clinic. (Adapted from Duckworth AD, Buijze GA, Moran MJ, et al. *J Bone Joint Surg Br*. 2012;94(7):961–968; with permission.)

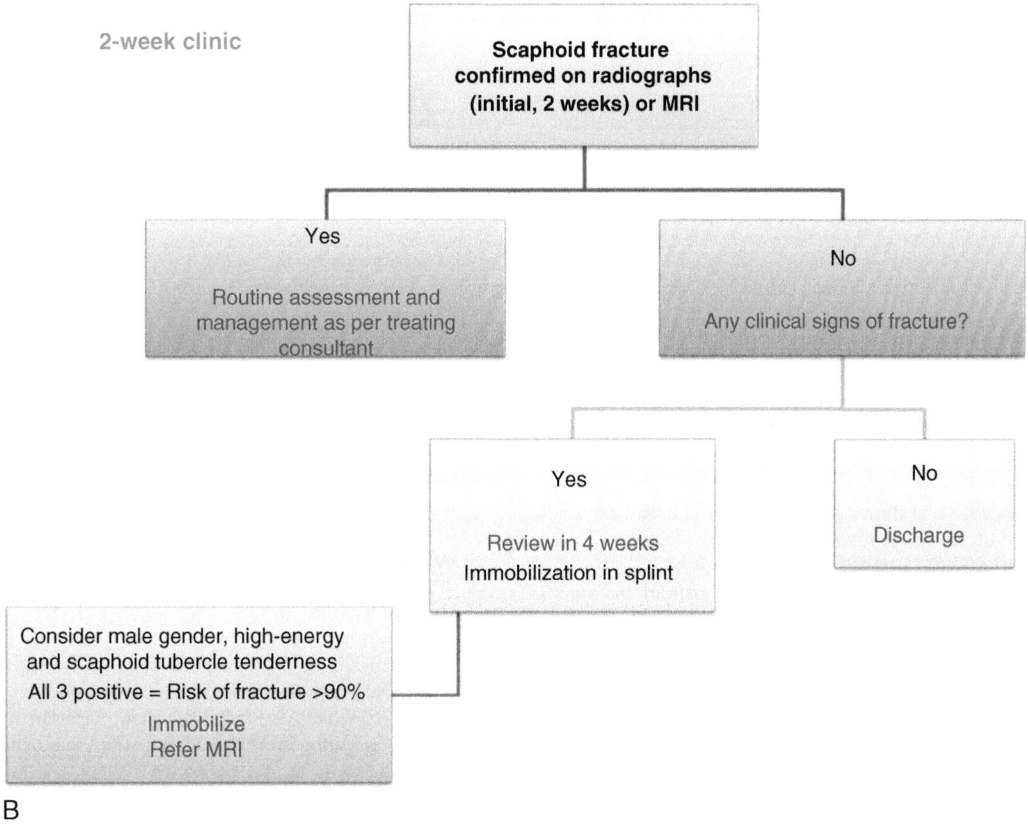
2-week clinic
Scaphoid fracture confirmed on radiographs (initial, 2 weeks) or MRI
Yes
Routine assessment and management as per treating consultant
No
Any clinical signs of fracture?
Yes
Review in 4 weeks
Immobilization in splint
No
Discharge
Consider male gender, high-energy and scaphoid tubercle tenderness
All 3 positive = Risk of fracture >90%
Immobilize
Refer MRI
B

FIG. 6.5, cont'd

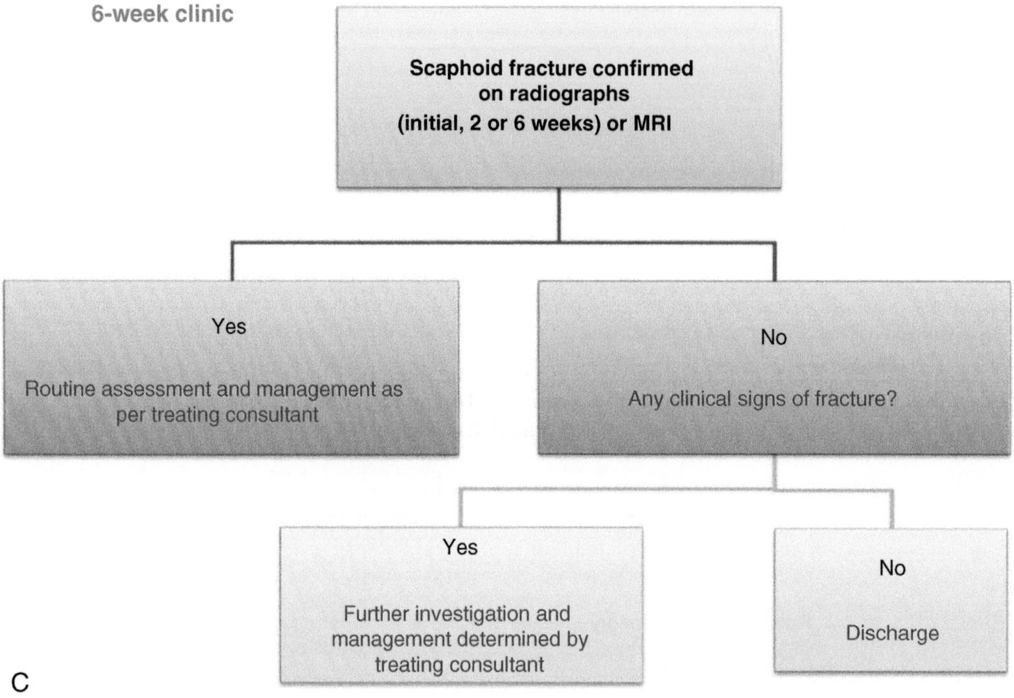

FIG. 6.5, cont'd

REFERENCES

1. Cooney WP. Failure of treatment of ununited fractures of the carpal scaphoid. *J Bone Joint Surg Am.* 1984;66(7):1145–1146.
2. Ruby LK, Stinson J, Belsky MR. The natural history of scaphoid non-union. A review of fifty-five cases. *J Bone Joint Surg Am.* 1985;67(3):428–432.
3. Kawamura K, Chung KC. Treatment of scaphoid fractures and nonunions. *J Hand Surg Am.* 2008;33(6):988–997.
4. Gaebler C, McQueen MM. Carpus fractures and dislocations. In: Bucholz RW, Court-Brown CM, Heckman JD, Tornetta P, eds. *Rockwood and Green's Fractures in Adults.* 7th ed. Philadelphia: Lippincott Williams & Wilkins; 2010:781–828.
5. Ring D, Jupiter JB, Herndon JH. Acute fractures of the scaphoid. *J Am Acad Orthop Surg.* 2000;8(4):225–231.
6. Kozin SH. Incidence, mechanism, and natural history of scaphoid fractures. *Hand Clin.* 2001;17(4):515–524.
7. Barton NJ. Twenty questions about scaphoid fractures. *J Hand Surg Br.* 1992;17(3):289–310.
8. Waizenegger M, Barton NJ, Davis TR, Wastie ML. Clinical signs in scaphoid fractures. *J Hand Surg Br.* 1994;19(6):743–747.
9. Gaebler C, Kukla C, Breitenseher MJ, Mrkonjic L, Kainberger F, Vecsei V. Limited diagnostic value of macroradiography in suspected scaphoid fractures. *Acta Orthop Scand.* 1998;69(4):401–403.
10. Gabler C, Kukla C, Breitenseher MJ, Trattnig S, Vecsei V. Diagnosis of occult scaphoid fractures and other wrist injuries. Are repeated clinical examinations and plain radiographs still state of the art? *Langenbecks Arch Surg.* 2001;386(2):150–154.
11. Unay K, Gokcen B, Ozkan K, Poyanli O, Eceviz E. Examination tests predictive of bone injury in patients with clinically suspected occult scaphoid fracture. *Injury.* 2009;40(12):1265–1268.
12. Brooks S, Wluka AE, Stuckey S, Cicuttini F. The management of scaphoid fractures. *J Sci Med Sport.* 2005;8(2):181–189.
13. Annamalai G, Raby N. Scaphoid and pronator fat stripes are unreliable soft tissue signs in the detection of radiographically occult fractures. *Clin Radiol.* 2003;58(10):798–800.
14. Fusetti C, Poletti PA, Pradel PH, et al. Diagnosis of occult scaphoid fracture with high-spatial-resolution sonography: a prospective blind study. *J Trauma.* 2005;59(3):677–681.
15. Breitenseher MJ, Metz VM, Gilula LA, et al. Radiographically occult scaphoid fractures: value of MR imaging in detection. *Radiology.* 1997;203(1):245–250.
16. Kusano N, Churei Y, Shiraishi E, Kusano T. Diagnosis of occult carpal scaphoid fracture: a comparison of magnetic resonance imaging and computed tomography techniques. *Tech Hand Up Extrem Surg.* 2002;6(3):119–123.

17. Memarsadeghi M, Breitenseher MJ, Schaefer-Prokop C, et al. Occult scaphoid fractures: comparison of multidetector CT and MR imaging-initial experience. *Radiology*. 2006;240(1):169–176.
18. Tiel-van Buul MM, Broekhuizen TH, van Beek EJ, Bossuyt PM. Choosing a strategy for the diagnostic management of suspected scaphoid fracture: a cost-effectiveness analysis. *J Nucl Med*. 1995;36(1):45–48.
19. McQueen MM, Gelbke MK, Wakefield A, Will EM, Gaebler C. Percutaneous screw fixation versus conservative treatment for fractures of the waist of the scaphoid: a prospective randomised study. *J Bone Joint Surg Br*. 2008;90(1):66–71.
20. van der Molen AB, Groothoff JW, Visser GJ, Robinson PH, Eisma WH. Time off work due to scaphoid fractures and other carpal injuries in The Netherlands in the period 1990 to 1993. *J Hand Surg Br*. 1999;24(2):193–198.
21. Dorsay TA, Major NM, Helms CA. Cost-effectiveness of immediate MR imaging versus traditional follow-up for revealing radiographically occult scaphoid fractures. *AJR Am J Roentgenol*. 2001;177(6):1257–1263.
22. Hansen TB, Petersen RB, Barckman J, Uhre P, Larsen K. Cost-effectiveness of MRI in managing suspected scaphoid fractures. *J Hand Surg Eur Vol*. 2009;34.
23. Gooding A, Coates M, Rothwell A. Cost analysis of traditional follow-up protocol versus MRI for radiographically occult scaphoid fractures: a pilot study for the Accident Compensation Corporation. *N Z Med J*. 2004;117(1201):U1049.
24. Jenkins PJ, Slade K, Huntley JS, Robinson CM. A comparative analysis of the accuracy, diagnostic uncertainty and cost of imaging modalities in suspected scaphoid fractures. *Injury*. 2008;39(7):768–774.
25. Ring D, Lozano-Calderon S. Imaging for suspected scaphoid fracture. *J Hand Surg Am*. 2008;33(6):954–957.
26. Duckworth AD, Ring D, McQueen MM. Assessment of the suspected fracture of the scaphoid. *J Bone Joint Surg Br*. 2011;93(6):713–719.
27. Hove LM. Epidemiology of scaphoid fractures in Bergen, Norway. *Scand J Plast Reconstr Surg Hand Surg*. 1999;33(4):423–426.
28. Adey L, Souer JS, Lozano-Calderon S, Palmer W, Lee SG, Ring D. Computed tomography of suspected scaphoid fractures. *J Hand Surg Am*. 2007;32(1):61–66.
29. Rhemrev SJ, Beeres FJ, van Leerdam RH, Hogervorst M, Ring D. Clinical prediction rule for suspected scaphoid fractures A Prospective Cohort Study. *Injury*. 2010;41.
30. Larsen CF, Brondum V, Skov O. Epidemiology of scaphoid fractures in Odense, Denmark. *Acta Orthop Scand*. 1992;63(2):216–218.
31. Altman DG, Bland JM. Diagnostic tests 2: predictive values. *BMJ*. 1994;309(6947):102.
32. Altman DG, Bland JM. Diagnostic tests. 1: sensitivity and specificity. *BMJ*. 1994;308(6943):1552.
33. Buijze GA, Mallee WH, Beeres FJ, Hanson TE, Johnson WO, Ring D. Diagnostic performance tests for suspected scaphoid fractures differ with conventional and latent class analysis. *Clin Orthop Relat Res*. 2011;469(12):3400–3407.
34. Duckworth AD, Buijze GA, Moran M, et al. Predictors of fracture following suspected injury to the scaphoid. *J Bone Joint Surg Br*. 2012;94(7):961–968.
35. Munk B, Frokjaer J, Larsen CF, et al. Diagnosis of scaphoid fractures. A prospective multicenter study of 1,052 patients with 160 fractures. *Acta Orthop Scand*. 1995;66(4):359–360.
36. Yin ZG, Zhang JB, Kan SL, Wang XG. Diagnosing suspected scaphoid fractures: a systematic review and meta-analysis. *Clin Orthop Relat Res*. 2010;468(3):723–734.
37. Mallee WH, Mellema JJ, Guitton TG, Goslings JC, Ring D, Doornberg JN. 6-week radiographs unsuitable for diagnosis of suspected scaphoid fractures. *Arch Orthop Trauma Surg*. 2016;136(6):771–778.
38. Parvizi J, Wayman J, Kelly P, Moran CG. Combining the clinical signs improves diagnosis of scaphoid fractures. A prospective study with follow-up. *J Hand Surg Br*. 1998;23(3):324–327.
39. Powell JM, Lloyd GJ, Rintoul RF. New clinical test for fracture of the scaphoid. *Can J Surg*. 1988;31(4):237–238.
40. Duckworth AD, Ring D. Carpus fractures and dislocations. In: Court-Brown CM, Heckman JD, McQueen MM, Ricci III WMTP, eds. *Rockwood and Green's Fractures in Adults*. 8th ed. Philadelphia, PA: Lippincott Williams & Wilkins; 2014:991–1056.
41. Freeland P. Scaphoid tubercle tenderness: a better indicator of scaphoid fractures? *Arch Emerg Med*. 1989;6(1):46–50.
42. Grover R. Clinical assessment of scaphoid injuries and the detection of fractures. *J Hand Surg Br*. 1996;21(3):341–343.
43. Esberger DA. What value the scaphoid compression test? *J Hand Surg Br*. 1994;19(6):748–749.
44. Skirven T, Trope J. Complications of immobilization. *Hand Clin*. 1994;10(1):53–61.
45. Royal College of Radiologists. *Making the Best Use of a Department of Clinical Radiology; Guidelines for Doctors*. 5th ed. London, UK: Royal College of Radiologists; 2003.
46. American College of Radiology (ACR). Expert Panel on Musculoskeletal Imaging, ACR Appropriateness Criteria. In: Reston VA, ed. *Acute Hand and Wrist Trauma*. 1st ed. American College of Radiology; 2001:1–7.
47. de Zwart AD, Beeres FJ, Ring D, et al. MRI as a reference standard for suspected scaphoid fractures. *Br J Radiol*. 2012;85(1016):1098–1101.
48. Mallee W, Doornberg JN, Ring D, van Dijk CN, Maas M, Goslings JC. Comparison of CT and MRI for diagnosis of suspected scaphoid fractures. *J Bone Joint Surg Am*. 2011;93(1):20–28.
49. Thavarajah D, Syed T, Shah Y, Wetherill M. Does scaphoid bone bruising lead to occult fracture? A prospective study of 50 patients. *Injury*. 2011;42(11):1303–1306.
50. Groves AM, Kayani I, Syed R, et al. An international survey of hospital practice in the imaging of acute scaphoid trauma. *Am J Roentgenol*. 2006;187(6):1453–1456.

51. Brookes-Fazakerley SD, Kumar AJ, Oakley J. Survey of the initial management and imaging protocols for occult scaphoid fractures in UK hospitals. *Skeletal Radiol.* 2009;38(11):1045–1048.
52. Smith JE, House RH, Gallagher J, Phillips A. The management of suspected scaphoid fractures in English hospitals: a national survey. *Eur J Emerg Med.* 2016;23(3):190–193.
53. Reilly BM, Evans AT. Translating clinical research into clinical practice: impact of using prediction rules to make decisions. *Ann Intern Med.* 2006;144(3):201–209.
54. Llewelyn H. Assessing properly the usefulness of clinical prediction rules and tests. *BMJ.* 2012;344:e1238.
55. Yardley MH. Upper limb fractures: contrasting patterns in Transkei and England. *Injury.* 1984;15(5):322–323.
56. Jonsson BY, Siggeirsdottir K, Mogensen B, Sigvaldason H, Sigursson G. Fracture rate in a population-based sample of men in Reykjavik. *Acta Orthop Scand.* 2004;75(2): 195–200.
57. Wolf JM, Dawson L, Mountcastle SB, Owens BD. The incidence of scaphoid fracture in a military population. *Injury.* 2009;40(12):1316–1319.
58. Van Tassel DC, Owens BD, Wolf JM. Incidence estimates and demographics of scaphoid fracture in the U.S. population. *J Hand Surg Am.* 2010;35(8):1242–1245.
59. Duckworth AD, Jenkins PJ, Aitken SA, Clement ND, Court-Brown CM, McQueen MM. Scaphoid fracture epidemiology. *J Trauma Acute Care Surg.* 2012;72(2):E41–E45.
60. Sutton PA, Clifford O, Davis TR. A new mechanism of injury for scaphoid fractures: 'test your strength' punch-bag machines. *J Hand Surg Eur Vol.* 2010;35(5):419–420.
61. Horii E, Nakamura R, Watanabe K, Tsunoda K. Scaphoid fracture as a "puncher's fracture". *J Orthop Trauma.* 1994;8(2):107–110.

CHAPTER 7

Diagnostic Work-up for Suspected Scaphoid Fractures

WOUTER H. MALLEE, MD • MAARTEN J. DE VOS, MD, PHD

KEY POINTS

- Fear of missing scaphoid fractures results in unnecessary overtreatment.
- Magnetic resonance imaging (MRI) and computed tomography (CT) are able to establish a definitive diagnosis.
- MRI and CT are more expensive diagnostic tools than radiography, but with the right timing, they could lead to lower costs.
- Societal costs benefit from immediate MRI or CT.

IMPORTANCE OF THE PROBLEM

Delayed diagnosis of a true scaphoid fracture in clinically suspected scaphoid fractures increases the risk of persistent wrist problems and nonunion.[2,3] Its blood supply is fragile and can be interrupted when fractured. Early treatment results in satisfactory results.[4]

Trauma mechanism and physical examination in the emergency department (ED) can point toward a suspected scaphoid fracture. If radiographs of the wrist and scaphoid appear normal, 20% of the patients will still have a scaphoid fracture.[5] With the risks of delayed treatment and occult fracture rate in mind, defensive management is usually started.[6] Usually, temporary cast immobilization is prescribed until further examination or imaging is performed. The fear of undertreatment, therefore, results in overtreating 80% of patients with normal radiographs.

Numerous studies have been done to determine the diagnostic accuracy of imaging modalities such as magnetic resonance imaging (MRI), computed tomography (CT), and bone scintigraphy (BS) in detecting occult scaphoid fractures.[7–13] The variety in techniques consequently results in a variation in diagnostic work-up as showed in national and international surveys.[14–16] This is due to the availability of the scanning tools per hospital, differences in costs per technique, and the lack of a consensus reference standard.

At 1- to 2-week follow-up, repeat radiographs can detect the occult fracture; however, the diagnostic accuracy is questionable. Additional imaging is often needed for definitive diagnosis.

PANEL 1
Case Scenario

A 27-year-old man visited the emergency department with complaints of his right wrist after a fall on the outstretched hand during a tennis match. He has tenderness of the anatomic snuffbox and pain around the scaphoid with ulnar deviation. Radiographs in four views show no fracture (Fig. 7.1). You are considering your diagnostic work-up for this suspected scaphoid fracture. What is your best practice: immobilization and repeat radiography in 10–14 days or additional imaging as soon as possible?

Cost-effectiveness

Advanced imaging techniques used to be costly diagnostic tools; however, in present days, these prices have dropped significantly in most countries. Most imaging techniques, especially CT, are becoming more available in the EDs, which provides the physician with better options for immediate diagnosis and thereby adequate treatment. In suspected scaphoid fractures, unnecessary cast treatment is one of the main issues due to its effect on loss of productivity of the patient. By improving the diagnostic work-up, both healthcare and societal costs could drop significantly.

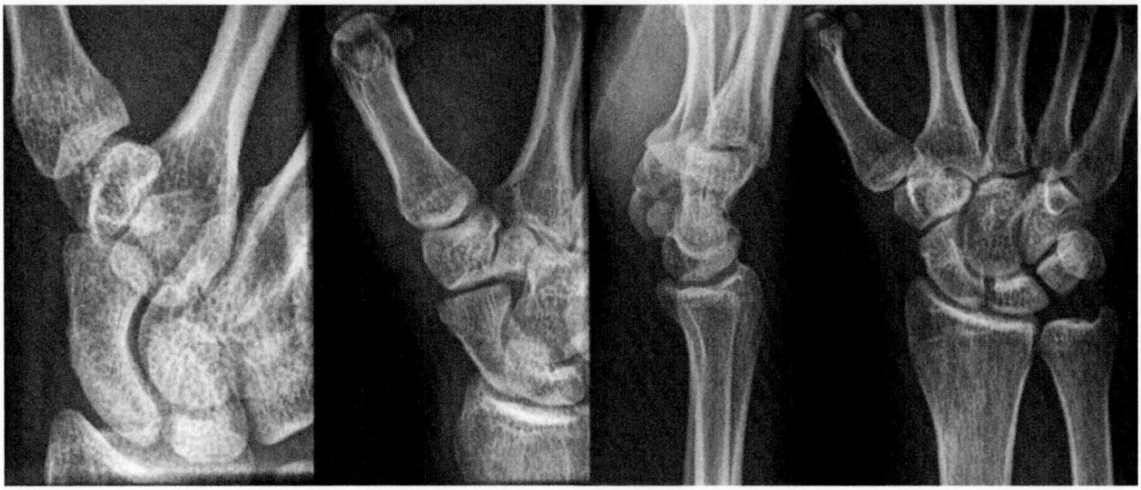

FIG. 7.1 Initial radiographs in four views.

MAIN QUESTIONS

What is the best and most cost-effective diagnostic work-up for clinically suspected scaphoid fractures with normal radiographs?

Current Opinion

There is a wide variety in diagnostic management for suspected scaphoid fractures. Repeating radiographs is often performed after 1–2 weeks of cast immobilization.

Finding the Evidence

The literature search was done in the following libraries:

- Cochrane Database of Systematic Reviews
- Cochrane Register of Diagnostic Test Accuracy Studies
- NHS Economic Evaluation Database
- Pubmed

  Diagnostic accuracy studies:
- Search extracted studies till 2012
- The Cochrane libraries were searched using the term: Scaphoid
- The NHS database was searched using the term: Scaphoid
- Pubmed (Medline) was searched using: "Scaphoid Bone" [Mesh] OR scaphoid fracture*[tiab] OR scaphoid bone Fracture*[tiab] OR scaphoid[tiab] AND "diagnos* OR Computed Tomography OR Magnetic Resonance Imaging OR Bone Scintigraphy OR Diagnos*
- Only systematic reviews and prospective cohort studies were included. This chapter is based on a recent Cochrane Review for Diagnostic Test Accuracy[5]

  Cost-effectiveness studies:
- Search extracted studies from 2000 to 2016
- Additional search terms used: "cost-effectiveness" OR "costs"

Quality of Evidence

Diagnostic accuracy studies

1A = Systematic review of prospective cohort studies/direct comparison studies
1B = Prospective cohort studies/direct comparison studies
2A = Systematic review cohort studies
2B = Cohort study/low-quality randomized controlled trial

Economic and decision analysis

I = Reasonable costs and alternatives used in a study with values obtained from many studies—the study used multiway sensitivity analysis
II = Reasonable costs and alternatives used in a study with values obtained from limited studies—the study used multiway sensitivity analysis
III = Analysis based on a limited section of alternatives and costs or poor estimates of costs
IV = No sensitivity analysis performed
V = Expert opinion

Quality of evidence for diagnostic accuracy studies

Level 1A: 1[5]

Quality of evidence for cost-effectiveness studies

Level 1B: 3[17–19]
Level 2B: 1[20]
Economic and decision analysis level II: 1[21]
Economic and decision analysis level IV: 3[22–24]

CT

Study	TP	FP	FN	TN	Sensitivity (95% CI)	Specificity (95% CI)
De Zwart 2012	14	1	6	138	0.70 [0.46, 0.88]	0.99 [0.96, 1.00]
Ilica 2011	14	0	2	39	0.88 [0.62, 0.98]	1.00 [0.91, 1.00]
Mallee 2011	4	1	2	27	0.67 [0.22, 0.96]	0.96 [0.82, 1.00]
Memarsadeghi 2006	8	0	3	18	0.73 [0.39, 0.94]	1.00 [0.81, 1.00]

MRI

Study	TP	FP	FN	TN	Sensitivity (95% CI)	Specificity (95% CI)
Beeres 2008	16	0	4	80	0.80 [0.56, 0.94]	1.00 [0.95, 1.00]
Breitenseher 1997	14	0	0	28	1.00 [0.77, 1.00]	1.00 [0.88, 1.00]
Mallee 2011	4	3	2	25	0.67 [0.22, 0.96]	0.89 [0.72, 0.98]
Memarsadeghi 2006	11	0	0	18	1.00 [0.72, 1.00]	1.00 [0.81, 1.00]
Tiel-van Buul 1996	5	0	2	9	0.71 [0.29, 0.96]	1.00 [0.66, 1.00]

BS

Study	TP	FP	FN	TN	Sensitivity (95% CI)	Specificity (95% CI)
Beeres 2008	20	8	0	72	1.00 [0.83, 1.00]	0.90 [0.81, 0.96]
De Zwart 2012	19	9	1	130	0.95 [0.75, 1.00]	0.94 [0.88, 0.97]
Nielsen 1983	11	43	0	47	1.00 [0.72, 1.00]	0.52 [0.41, 0.63]
O'Carroll 1982	6	5	0	19	1.00 [0.54, 1.00]	0.79 [0.58, 0.93]
Stordahl 1984	9	0	0	19	1.00 [0.66, 1.00]	1.00 [0.82, 1.00]
Tiel-van Buul 1993	21	14	0	90	1.00 [0.84, 1.00]	0.87 [0.78, 0.92]

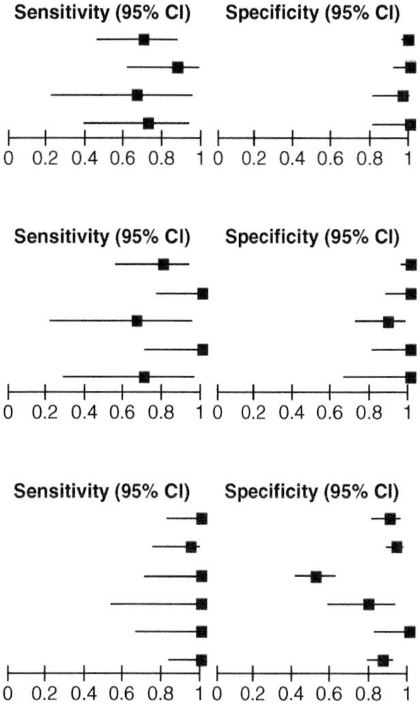

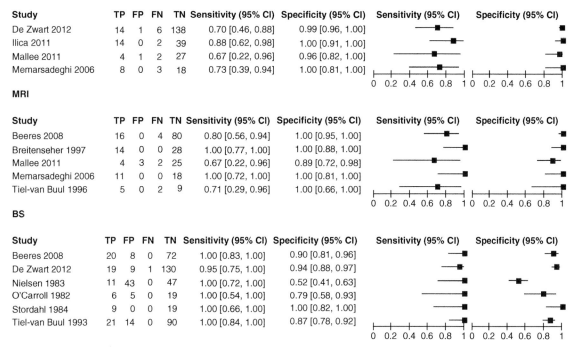

FIG. 7.2 Forrest plots for diagnostic accuracies of computed tomography (CT), magnetic resonance imaging (MRI), and bone scintigraphy (BS). *TP* True positives; *FP* False Positives; *FN* False Negatives; *TN* True Negatives (From Mallee WH, Wang J, Poolman RW, et al. Computed tomography versus magnetic resonance imaging versus bone scintigraphy for clinically suspected scaphoid fractures in patients with negative plain radiographs. *Cochrane Database Syst Rev*. 2015;6:13; with permission.)

FINDINGS

Diagnostic Accuracy

The systematic review shows the results of 11 prospective studies.[7–13,25–28] They reported diagnostic accuracy data for CT (4 studies; 277 patients), MRI (5 studies; 221 patients), and BS (6 studies; 543 patients). They included both comparison and noncomparison studies. Fig. 7.2 presents the diagnostic performance characteristics of the imaging modalities. For overall diagnostic accuracy, CT showed a summary sensitivity and specificity of 0.72 (0.36–0.92) and 0.99 (0.71–1.00), respectively. For MRI, summary sensitivity and specificity was 0.88 (0.64–0.97) and 1.00 (0.38–1.00), respectively. For BS, this was 0.99 (0.69–1.00) and 0.86 (0.73–0.94). BS showed a significant higher diagnostic accuracy compared with CT and MRI ($P<.01$); this is based on a higher sensitivity rate. CT and MRI showed comparable diagnostic accuracies ($P=.17$).

Only one study directly compared CT and BS and did not report a significant higher sensitivity; however, CT showed a significant higher specificity over BS.[11] One study directly compared MRI and BS and did not report a significant difference in correct predictions.[8]

The median prevalence of missed fractures was 20%. Given this prevalence, it is interesting to evaluate the effect of these diagnostic accuracies in a large cohort of 1000 patients (200 occult scaphoid fractures). These data are presented in Table 7.1. It is clear to extract that MRI would result in the lowest rate of over- and undertreatment.

The overall quality of the included studies was moderate to high.

Cost-effectiveness

The literature review found eight eligible studies, evaluating the costs applicable to incorporating advanced imaging techniques in suspected scaphoid fractures.[17–24] Most studies compared MRI with conventional protocols that mainly consist of 2 weeks of cast immobilization and repeat radiography. Because data were scarce and methodology was too diverse, pooling of data could not be performed.

TABLE 7.1
Effect of Diagnostic Accuracy on a Cohort of 1000 Patients With 200 Scaphoid Fractures

	Number of Missed Fractures	Number of Overtreated Patients
CT	56	8
MRI	24	0
BS	2	112

BS, bone scintigraphy, *CT*, computed tomography, *MRI*, magnetic resonance imaging.

Using MRI in the diagnostic work-up was the subject of all included studies. CT was subject in two studies.[21,22] Most studies looked at immediate scanning or within 3 days after injury compared with follow-up radiography and cast immobilization for 10–14 days. Immediate MRI or CT was the most cost-effective approach in three studies.[18,21,23] Costs were comparable in four studies,[19,20,22,24] and only one study reported slightly higher costs for MRI; however this was due to known high costs per MRI in Australia.[17]

All studies stress the effect of early diagnosis by immediate MRI and CT on societal costs. It is also emphasized that CT and MRI have the ability to detect other injuries such as carpal or distal radius fractures and ligamentous injury. Benefit is thereby expected in treatment of other occult injuries as well.

RECOMMENDATIONS

In patients with a clinically suspected scaphoid fracture and normal initial radiographs:

- Comparable diagnostic accuracy results are presented for MRI, CT, and BS. Direct comparisons showed no differences, and pooled estimates showed a higher sensitivity for BS over CT and MRI (overall quality: moderate to high).
- In large cohorts, BS still results in a considerable amount of overtreatment (overall quality: high).
- Immediate CT or MRI is comparable or beneficial over 10–14 days of cast immobilization and follow-up in terms of direct hospital costs (overall quality: moderate).
- Immediate CT or MRI is of great benefit for societal costs (overall quality: moderate).
- Incorporating CT or MRI in the diagnostic work-up results in detection of other occult injuries besides scaphoid fractures (overall quality: low).

CONCLUSIONS

In patients with a clinically suspected scaphoid fracture and normal radiographs, the best and most cost-effective diagnostic work-up is to perform immediate MRI; CT is a comparable alternative. This management will not increase direct hospital costs, can decrease the societal costs, and assures early diagnosis and adequate treatment.

A remaining issue in diagnosis of scaphoid fractures is the lack of an adequate reference standard. The most used reference standard is repeated radiography after 6 weeks; however, this test is known to have only slight interobserver agreement and limited specificity.[29]

A valuable additive to current literature is to raise the a priori chance of a true scaphoid fracture among suspected fractures. Improvement in clinical evaluation is one of the aspects that could lead to better diagnostic performance of MRI or CT and thereby even lower rates of over- and undertreatment.

PANEL 2
Author's Preferred Technique

In this case, we prefer to perform MRI in the acute setting when a patient presents with a clinically suspected scaphoid fracture and normal radiographs. A comparable alternative is CT (Fig. 7.3). A scaphoid fracture was detected on both scans. This will establish an early and definitive diagnosis and thereby adequate treatment without the risk for unnecessary immobilization and loss in productivity. If scans are negative, pressure bandage without further follow-up is sufficient.

PANEL 3
Pearls and Pitfalls

PEARLS

- With CT scanning in the acute setting, other fractures in the carpus and/or distal radius can be frequently found. CT scanning in the longitudinal axis of the scaphoid might result in an improved visualization of the scaphoid to distinguish vascular channels from minor fractures.[1]
- With MRI in the acute setting, other fractures and ligamentous injuries in the wrist can be frequently found.
- Immediate scanning protocols have been shown to be cost-effective.

PITFALLS

- Performing BS is both a time-consuming and an invasive diagnostic tool and is therefore not recommended.

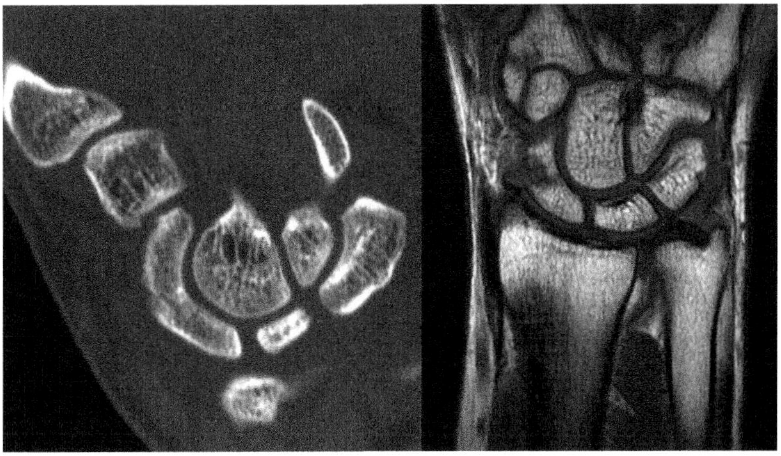

FIG. 7.3 CT and MRI scans of an occult scaphoid waist fracture

REFERENCES

1. Mallee WH, Doornberg JN, Ring D, et al. Computed tomography for suspected scaphoid fractures: comparison of reformations in the plane of the wrist versus the long axis of the scaphoid. *Hand (N Y)*. 2014;9(1):117–121.
2. Merrell GA, Wolfe Sw Fau - Slade 3rd JF, Slade 3rd JF. Treatment of scaphoid nonunions: quantitative meta-analysis of the literature. *J Hand Surg Am*. 2002. 0363–5023 (Print).
3. Gelberman Rh, Gross MS. The vascularity of the wrist. Identification of arterial patterns at risk. *Clin Orthop Relat Res*. 1986. 0009–921X (Print).
4. Dias JJ, Wildin CJ, Bhowal B, Thompson JR. Should acute scaphoid fractures be fixed? A randomized controlled trial. *J Bone Joint Surg Am*. 2005;87(10):2160–2168.
5. Mallee WH, Wang J, Poolman RW, et al. Computed tomography versus magnetic resonance imaging versus bone scintigraphy for clinically suspected scaphoid fractures in patients with negative plain radiographs. *Cochrane Database Syst Rev*. 2015;(6):CD010023.
6. Reigstad O, Grimsgaard C, Thorkildsen R, Rokkum M. Scaphoid non-unions, where do they come from? The epidemiology and initial presentation of 270 scaphoid non-unions. *Hand Surg*. 2012. 1793–6535 (Electronic).
7. Mallee W, Doornberg JN, Ring D, van Dijk CN, Maas M, Goslings JC. Comparison of CT and MRI for diagnosis of suspected scaphoid fractures. *J Bone Joint Surg Am*. 2011;93(1):20–28.
8. Beeres FJ, Rhemrev SJ, den Hollander P, et al. Early magnetic resonance imaging compared with bone scintigraphy in suspected scaphoid fractures. *J Bone Joint Surg Br*. 2008;90(9):1205–1209.
9. Breitenseher MJ, Metz VM, Gilula LA, et al. Radiographically occult scaphoid fractures: value of MR imaging in detection. *Radiology*. 1997;203(1):245–250.
10. Memarsadeghi M, Breitenseher MJ, Schaefer-Prokop C, et al. Occult scaphoid fractures: comparison of multidetector CT and MR imaging–initial experience. *Radiology*. 2006;240(1):169–176.
11. de Zwart A, Rhemrev SJ, Kingma LM, Kingma Lm Fau - Meylaerts SAG, et al. Early CT compared with bone scintigraphy in suspected schapoid fractures. *Clin Nucl Med*. 2010. 1536–0229 (Electronic).
12. Ilica AT, Ozyurek S, Kose O, Durusu M. Diagnostic accuracy of multidetector computed tomography for patients with suspected scaphoid fractures and negative radiographic examinations. *Jpn J Radiol*. 2011. 1867–108X (Electronic).
13. Tiel-van Buul MM, Roolker W, Verbeeten BW, Broekhuizen AH. Magnetic resonance imaging versus bone scintigraphy in suspected scaphoid fracture. *Eur J Nucl Med*. 1996;23(8):971–975.
14. Mallee WH, Veltman ES, Doornberg JN, Blankevoort L, van Dijk CN, Goslings JC. [Variations in management of suspected scaphoid fractures]. *Ned Tijdschrift Voor Geneeskunde*. 2012;156(28):A4514.
15. Groves AM, Kayani I, Syed R, et al. An international survey of hospital practice in the imaging of acute scaphoid trauma. *AJR Am J Roentgenol*. 2006;187(6):1453–1456.
16. Brookes-Fazakerley SD, Kumar Aj, Oakley J. Survey of the initial management and imaging protocols for occult scaphoid fractures in UK hospitals. *Skeletal Radiol*. 2009. 1432–2161 (Electronic).
17. Brooks S, Cicuttini FM, Lim S, Taylor D, Stuckey S, Wluka AE. Cost effectiveness of adding magnetic resonance imaging to the usual management of suspected scaphoid fractures. *Br J Sports Med*. 2005. 1473–0480 (Electronic).
18. Patel NK, Davies N, Mirza Z, Watson M. Cost and clinical effectiveness of MRI in occult scaphoid fractures: a randomised controlled trial. *Emerg Med J*. 2013. 1472–0213 (Electronic).

19. Gooding A, Coates M, Rothwell A. Cost analysis of traditional follow-up protocol versus MRI for radiographically occult scaphoid fractures: a pilot study for the Accident Compensation Corporation. *N. Z Med J.* 2004. 1175-8716 (Electronic).
20. Kelson T, Davidson R, Baker T. Early MRI versus conventional management in the detection of occult scaphoid fractures: what does it really cost? A rural pilot study. *J Med Radiat Sci.* 2016. 2051-3909 (Electronic).
21. Yin ZG, Zhang JB, Gong KT. Cost-effectiveness of diagnostic strategies for suspected scaphoid fractures. *J Orthop Trauma.* 2015. 1531-2291 (Electronic).
22. Karl JW, Swart E, Strauch RJ. Diagnosis of occult scaphoid fractures: a cost-effectiveness analysis. *J Bone Joint Surg Am.* 2015. 1535-1386 (Electronic).
23. Saxena P, McDonald R, Gull S, Hyder N. Diagnostic scanning for suspected scaphoid fractures: an economic evaluation based on cost-minimisation models. *Injury.* 2003. 0020-1383 (Print).
24. Dorsay TA, Major NM, Helms CA. Cost-effectiveness of immediate MR imaging versus traditional follow-up for revealing radiographically occult scaphoid fractures. *AJR Am J Roentgenol.* 2001. 0361-803X (Print).
25. Nielsen Pt, Hedeboe J, Thommesen P. Bone scintigraphy in the evaluation of fracture of the carpal scaphoid bone. *Acta Orthop Scand.* 1983. 0001-6470 (Print).
26. O'Carroll Pf, Doyle J, Duffy G. Radiography and scintigraphy in the diagnosis of carpal scaphoid fractures. *Ir J Med Sci.* 1982. 0021-1265 (Print).
27. Stordahl A, Schjoth A, Woxholt G, Fjermeros H. Bone scanning of fractures of the scaphoid. *J Hand Surgery Edinb Scotl.* 1984;9(2):189–190.
28. Tiel-van Buul MM, Broekhuizen AH, Bakker AJ, Bos KE, van Royen EA. Radiography and scintigraphy of suspected scaphoid fracture. A long-term study in 160 patients. *J Bone Joint Surg Br.* 1993. 0301-620X (Print).
29. Mallee WH, Mellema JJ, Guitton TG, et al. 6-week radiographs unsuitable for diagnosis of suspected scaphoid fractures. *Arch Orthop Trauma Surg.* 2016;136(6):771–778.

Classification Systems of Scaphoid Fractures

TESSA DRIJKONINGEN, MD • PAUL W. TEN BERG, MD •
SIMON D. STRACKEE, MD, PHD • GEERT A. BUIJZE, MD, PHD

KEY POINTS

- Acute scaphoid fractures know many different classifications based on (1) fracture location, (2) fracture plane orientation, and (3) fracture stability/displacement.
- The most popular classifications include the Herbert, Mayo, and Russe classifications, although none of them are completely reliable.
- The choice of applied classification system is based on preference of the surgeon.

PANEL 1
Typical scaphoid fracture case

CASE
An 18-year-old man visited the emergency department after a fall from his skateboard on the outstretched hand with complaints of right wrist pain. A series of scaphoid radiographs and a CT scan showed a nondisplaced fracture approximately at the distal third of the scaphoid. Because of the availability of many heterogeneous classification systems based on subjective radiographic interpretations, you are undetermined whether this fracture should be classified as a distal pole/distal third fracture or a distal waist fracture. Recent technologic advances in imaging enables analyzing scaphoid fracture lines in full 3D space, providing clearly defined anatomic landmarks, including the scapho-trapezio-trapezoid joint, scapho-capitate joint, and scapholunate joint, which might be useful for clinicians to use as more objective cutoff (Fig. 8.1). How can this scaphoid fracture best be classified, and how will that influence your management?

IMPORTANCE OF PROBLEM

There is great heterogeneity and controversy among surgeons worldwide in classifying scaphoid fractures. Dr. Étienne Destot first documented scaphoid fractures in 1905 following the discovery of radiography.[1] Later in 1939, Cravener clarified contributing factors of scaphoid nonunion and classified scaphoid fractures taking age and location into account.[2] "In discussing carpal scaphoid fractures, we must first arrive on a common ground. Is the fracture through the tuberosity, the waist, or the body? If it is through the tuberosity we can practically neglect it, for it will heal. If it is through the body will not easily."

The most commonly used classifications include the Herbert, Mayo, and Russe classifications (Figs. 8.2, 8.3, and 8.4), but more systems are known in literature presenting considerable controversies.[3–5] Treatment of acute scaphoid fractures is often based on how they are classified. Most surgeons do not use a specific classification but describe morphology of the fracture (e.g., a nondisplaced distal third fracture), which is dependent on the angle of a radiograph. Some surgeons consider all scaphoid fractures unstable, irrespective of displacement, when a fracture line is readily identified on radiographs[6] or shows bicortical involvement.[7] Consequently, those surgeons[6,7] believe that all these fractures have an indication for surgery, which may lead to overtreatment.

More than 70 years later, there is still no consensus mainly because of the number of different scaphoid fracture classifications available in the literature, each trying to improve prognosis and treatment selection. Scaphoid fractures should be characterized in a reliable and reproducible way that facilitates comparison among different groups or among similar groups treated differently.[8,9] The aim of this chapter is to clarify different concepts and classifications of acute scaphoid fractures and their popularity. As reported incidence

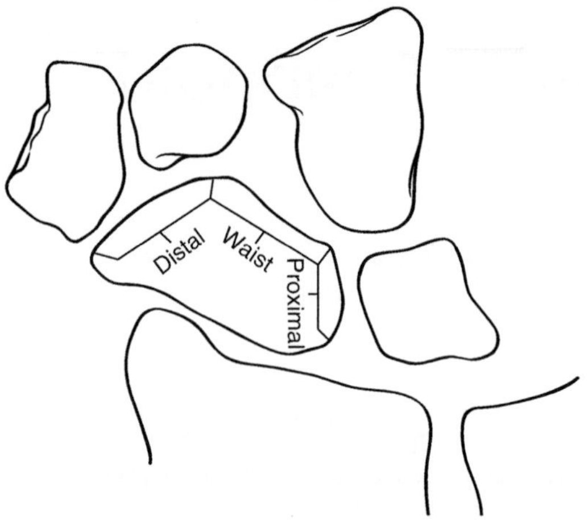

FIG. 8.1 The Simplified Scaphoid Fracture Classification by Drijkoningen and Buijze based on scapho-trapezio-trapezoid joint, scaphocapitate joint, and scapholunate joint anatomy on posteroanterior radiographs.

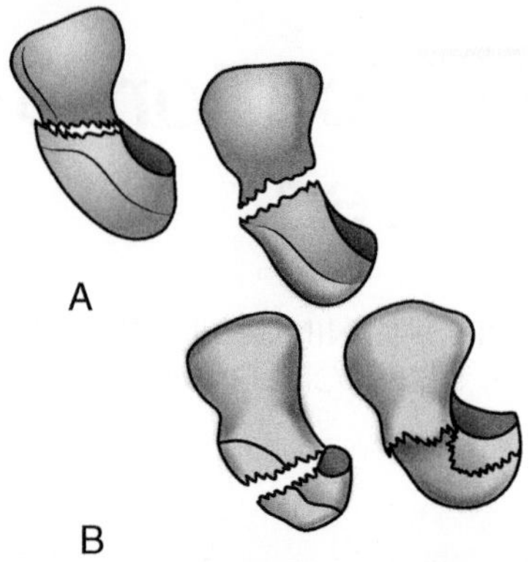

FIG. 8.3 Herbert divided acute scaphoid fractures into **(A)** acute stable and **(B)** unstable. Stable acute fractures included fractures of the tubercle and incomplete unicortical "crack" fractures. A type B2 is an acute unstable complete fracture of the waist.

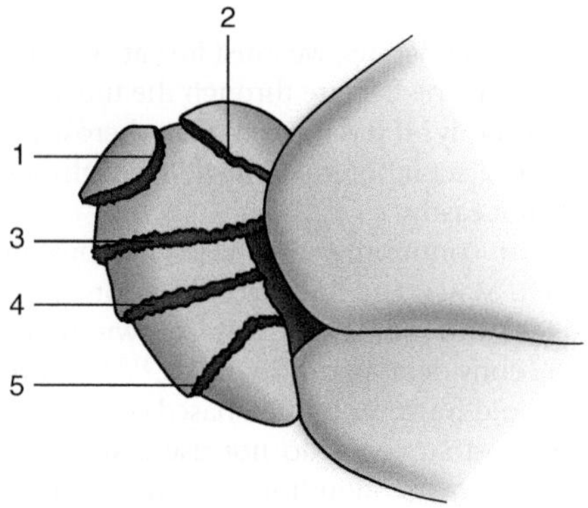

FIG. 8.2 Cooney divided scaphoid fractures into fractures of the (1) distal tubercle, (2) distal intraarticular surface, (3) distal third, (4) waist, and (5) proximal pole.

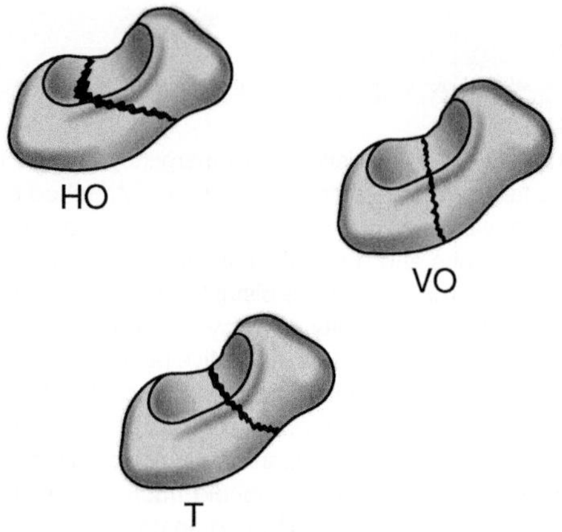

FIG. 8.4 Russe separated fractures based on fracture plane orientation into transverse (T), horizontal oblique (HO), and vertical oblique (VO) fractures.

rates of different fracture types vary considerably in literature, our second aim is clarifying incidence rates based on the original reports.

MAIN QUESTION

How are scaphoid fractures preferably classified, and according to these classifications, which fractures are most common?

Current Opinion

Based on surgeon's preference, currently the most popular classifications are the Herbert (fracture displacement), Russe (fracture plane orientation) and Mayo (fracture location) classification. Transverse fractures through the body of the scaphoid seem to be most often detected.

Finding Evidence

- Medical literature from 1950 to 2016
- Pubmed: ("Scaphoid Bone"[Mesh] OR scaphoid fracture [tiab] OR scaphoid bone fracture_[tiab] OR scaphoid[tiab]) AND ("classification" [Subheading] OR class_)

- Inclusion criteria:
  1. Original description of novel classifications of acute scaphoid fractures in an adult population (>18 years)
  2. Availability of a (translated) full-text copy of a manuscript online or paper version
  3. All types of articles, including clinical, biomechanic, cadaver, and imaging studies
- Exclusion criteria:
  1. (Original) description of an already existing classification of acute scaphoid fractures
  2. (Original) description of wrist pathologies other than acute scaphoid fractures
  3. Languages other than English, French, or German
- Classification systems were considered clinically relevant only when applicable to clinical practice. A threshold of >10 times cited in the database of Web of Science (WoS) was used
- Google Scholar was the additional database to record the number of citations as second measure for popularity of classifications

Quality of the Evidence

No guidelines have yet been developed to assess the quality of these articles classifying acute scaphoid fractures, so for this chapter, no distinction was made between study design or image modalities used.
Level I: Systematic reviews: 2
Level III: Retrospective studies: 10
Level IV: Case series: 3

FINDINGS

Three hundred eight potential eligible articles can be found in literature using the inclusion criteria named above which finally lead to a total of 13 different classification systems found based on the following:

1. Fracture location
2. Fracture plane orientation
3. Fracture stability and displacement

Classifications Based on Fracture Location (Table 8.1)

Bohler et al.[10] described 873 conservatively treated fractures between 1925 and 1952. Tuberosity fractures showed 100% healing rate; all other fractures showed a 97% healing rate. Proximal fractures were immobilized for 10–12 weeks, and middle and distal fractures for 6–8 weeks. Cooney et al.[4] (Mayo) (Fig. 8.2) and Schernberg et al.[11] also distinguished fractures by location, and Prosser et al.[12] classified solely distal fractures. Osteoarthritis might develop in the scapho-trapezio-trapezoid joint because of malunion after compression fractures (type II). The AO foundation introduced a general fracture classification system.[13] Standardizing research and communication among surgeons, the Orthopaedic Trauma Association (OTA) adopted this system, known as the AO/OTA system.[8]

Classifications Based on Fracture Plane Orientation (Table 8.2)

Bohler et al.[10] also distinguished fractures based on fracture planes, resembling Pauwels classification[15] of femoral neck fractures. Horizontal oblique fractures might show compressive forces across fracture sites, resulting in a tendency to heal. Transverse fractures might have both compressive and shear forces, resulting in an average tendency to heal. Vertical oblique fractures were considered to be caused by shearing forces, considering them unstable with consequently a higher risk of nonunion. Russe[5] described a similar system (Fig. 8.3), which receives more attention, probably because of international publications and presentations. Compson[14] distinguished 80 fractures based on dorsal alignment of fracture planes. He reconstructed fracture outlines on transparent solid three-dimensional scaphoid models by looking at multiple standard radiological views. He classified fractures as being transverse fractures when continued through the "surgical waist," oblique fractures when through the dorsal sulcus, and a separate group of proximal pole fractures.

Classifications Based on Displacement and/or Instability (Table 8.3)

McLaughlin and Parkes[16] classified fractures by stability, ranging from incomplete fractures with intact shell of cartilage and bone to undisplaced/stable fractures and displaced/unstable fractures. Cooney et al.[4] (Mayo) also classified fractures by stability (Table 8.4). Based on biomechanical experiments, Weber[17] described nondisplaced fractures without disruption of ligamentous attachments, angulated fractures with dorsal intercarpal ligamentous disruption due to increasing injury forces, and displaced fractures with complete disruption of ligamentous attachments. Angulation may decrease surface contact, which lead to an increased risk of nonunion. Herbert and Fisher[3] proposed a classification intending to identify fractures most likely needing screw fixation caused by instability (Fig. 8.3). All complete bicortical fractures (except for tubercle fractures) were considered unstable. According to Garcia-Elias and Lluch,[18] proximal scaphoid fractures are stable when located proximal to the scapholunate

TABLE 8.1
Classification of Acute Scaphoid Fractures Based on Fracture Location

Author Cited (#)[a]	Cases (#)	Classification	Rate (%)
Böhler (I)[b,10] 38; 67	873	1 Tuberosity	16
		2-a Proximal third	10
		2-b Border, middle/proximal third	7
		2-c Middle third	55
		2-d Middle third: wedge chipped out	4
		2-e Distal third	9
Cooney (I) (Mayo)[4] 110; 330	45	1 Tuberosity	16
		2 Distal articular surface	16
		3 Distal one-third	16
		4 Waist, middle one-third	67
		5 Proximal pole	18
Schernberg[c,11] 16; 37	325	I Proximal pole	4
		II, III, IV Waist	82
		V Distal pole	8
		VI-a, b, c Distal tubercle	6
Prosser[12] 13; 29	37	I Tuberosity	54
		II (A, B, C) Distal intraarticular	41, 0, 5
		III Osteochondral fracture	0
AO/OTA[8] N/A[d]	–	72-A1 Proximal pole, noncommunited	
		72-A2 Waist, noncommunited	
		72-A3 Distal pole, noncommunited	
		72-B2 Waist, communited	

OTA, Orthopaedic Trauma Association.
[a]Number of citations in World of Science; Google Scholar.
[b]German article.
[c]French article.
[d]Not applicable, since the article comprised fracture classification systems of the entire musculoskeletal system.

TABLE 8.2
Classification of Acute Scaphoid Fractures Based on Fracture Plane Orientation

Author Cited (#)[a]	Cases (#)	Classification	Rate (%)
Böhler (I)[b,10] 38; 67	734	HO—Horizontal oblique	47
		T—Transverse	50
		VO—Vertical oblique	3
Russe[5] 277; 501	220	HO—Horizontal oblique	35
		T—Transverse	60
		VO—Vertical oblique	5
Compson[14] 41; 69	80	1 Transverse waist (surgical waist)	30
		2 Oblique waist (dorsal sulcus)	36
		3 Proximal pole	34

[a]Number of citations in World of Science; Google Scholar.
[b]German article.

TABLE 8.3
Classification of Acute Scaphoid Fractures Based on Displacement/Instability

Author Cited (#)[a]	Cases (#)	Classification	Rate (%)
McLaughlin[16]	–	A Incomplete	x
37; 70		B Undisplaced and stable	x
		C Displaced and unstable	x
Cooney (II)	45	1 Nondisplaced/stable	71
(Mayo)[4]		2 Displaced/unstable	29
110; 330			
Weber[17]	36	1 Nondisplaced	53
35; 127		2 Angulated	17
		3 Displaced	30
Herbert[3]	200/431	A1 Stable, tubercle	x
331; 739		A2 Stable, incomplete waist	x
Modified		B1 Unstable, distal oblique	19[b]
Herbert 1996		B2 Unstable, complete waist	60[b]
139; 268		B3 Unstable, proximal pole	21[b]
		B4 Unstable fracture dislocation	x
		B5 Communited fractures	x
Garcia-Elias[18]	–	1 Stable, proximal to SL ligament	x
27; 53		2 Unstable, distal to SL ligament	x

SL, scapholunate.
[a]Omitted in the modified Herbert classification.
[b]Based on 82 B1, B2, and B3 fractures reported in the article of 1996.

TABLE 8.4
Mayo Classification (Instability of Acute Scaphoid Fractures and Their Characteristics)

Stable Fractures	Unstable Fractures
Displacement less than 1 mm	Displacement more than 1 mm
Normal intercarpal alignment	Dorsal intercalated segmental instability alignment
Capitate-lunate angle 0–15 degrees	Capitate-lunate angle > 15 degrees
Scaphoid-lunate angle 30–60 degrees	Scaphoid-lunate angle > 60 degrees
Lateral intrascaphoid angle less than 35 degrees	Lateral intrascaphoid angle more than 35 degrees
Distal fractures	Comminuted fractures
	Perilunate fractures

From Cooney WP, Dobyns JH, Linscheid RL. Fractures of the scaphoid: a rational approach to management. *Clin Orthop Relat Res*. 1980;(149):90–97; with permission.

ligaments, forming the important link between the lunate and the distal scaphoid, but are unstable when located distal to these structures.

RECOMMENDATION

In patients with an acute scaphoid fracture of the scaphoid, evidence suggests the following:

- Based on citations of the World of Science and Google Scholar, the Herbert (1984) classification was the most popular classification with respectively 331 and 739 citations, Russe followed with 277 and 501 citations, and the third most popular classification was Cooney with the Mayo classification with 110 and 330 citations (overall quality: moderate).
- When dividing acute scaphoid classifications in fracture location, fracture plane orientation, and fracture displacement or instability:
  - Incidence based on fracture location shows that waist fractures occur most often with percentages ranging from 66% to 82%[4,10,11] (overall quality: moderate).
  - Based on fracture plane orientation, most fractures are transverse, ranging from 36% to 60%, followed by horizontal oblique fractures ranging from 30% to 47%[5,10,15] (overall quality: low).
  - Considering fracture stability, most fractures are described as stable and/or nondisplaced (53% and 71%)[4,17] (overall quality: low).

CONCLUSION

All classification systems were based on plain radiography. Scaphoid classifications can roughly be divided based on fracture location, fracture plane orientation, and fracture displacement or instability. The most clinically used classifications include the Herbert, Mayo, and Russe classifications, which, respectively, consider unstable, proximal, and vertical fractures to be at risk of nonunion development. Because of the many different fracture descriptions as described in literature, there is a need for an unambiguous classification system with well-defined cutoff points based on more reliable imaging techniques, facilitating comparison among different patient groups or similar patient groups treated differently.

PANEL 2
Authors' Preferred Technique

In clinical practice, the Herbert, Russe, and Mayo classifications are most frequently used to classify acute scaphoid fractures, but cannot reliably predict outcome or prognosis.[3–5] Most original articles describing a classification used radiography as the sole method of assessing union, which has limited reliability compared with the use of CT.[19–21] Moreover, clear radiographic definitions of union were often lacking. For example, the original article of the Herbert classification assessed union on a scale ranging from sound union, to apparent union, doubtful union, and nonunion, without providing further details. Consequently, none of the described classification systems can reliably predict the outcome in terms of fracture union.

In addition, the various fracture subgroups lack well-defined criteria, and their identification on radiographs has limited reproducibility as well.[9,22–24] For example, the step-offs to identify displacement were often not defined and cannot reliably be detected on radiographs.[25] Definitions proposed for displacement ranges from nondisplaced to minimally, moderately, and severely displaced fractures.[26] In particular, it is often unclear when displacement is considered minimal.[27] Displacement and instability are often used interchangeably, which is incorrect, as these characteristics have different meaning. Displaced fractures may be stable, whereas unstable fractures may have a nondisplaced appearance as observed on standard imaging.

Individual predictors for troublesome healing have been studied previously in clinical series,[6,28–30] irrespective to fracture classification systems, which seem to have more clinical relevance. The following characteristics were found to be associated with troublesome healing: proximal fractures,[30] displacement,[29] comminution,[30] and time from injury to treatment.[31,32] These predictors have a continuous nature and they are often dichotomized with arbitrary cutoff points. Because of the lack of consensus, the clinical application of these predictors is also limited.

To be able to reach consensus on interpretation of the latter fracture characteristics, more reliable imaging modalities should be applied in clinical research using well-defined criteria. Two- or three-dimensional CT may improve assessment of fracture displacement, compared with standard radiographs.[29] In addition, motion-imaging modalities of the wrist, e.g., fluoroscopy or dynamic three-dimensional CT, may be useful in detecting interfragmentary motion, i.e., true instability, which cannot reliably be detected on static imaging, in contrast to displacement. Improving the way instability and displacement are detected may lead to better identification of the troublesome acute scaphoid fractures requiring more aggressive treatment. In follow-up, ideally union should be determined using a CT, by assessing at least the presence of crossing trabeculae.[33]

PANEL 2
Authors' Preferred Technique—Cont'd

Based on the controversial and ambiguous classifications systems as described earlier, the authors used 3D CT fracture mapping analysis in 51 patients aiming for a simplified classification system with well-defined anatomic cutoff points on a posteroanterior radiograph (unpublished work). It showed that the vast majority of fractures can be classified on posteroanterior radiographs as follows:

1. Proximal pole fractures (proximal to the distal scapholunate interval)
2. A range of waist fractures (involving the scaphocapitate interval)
3. Distal tubercle fractures (involving the scapho-trapezio-trapezoid interval) (Fig. 8.1)

Displacement is best diagnosed using additional CT imaging in the longitudinal plane of the scaphoid. Stability can only be diagnosed using dynamic imaging (e.g., fluoroscopy, dynamic three-dimensional CT, or arthroscopy).

In the case of the 18-year-old male subject, we prefer to use the simplified anatomic classification system described above to classify the fracture as a nondisplaced (distal) waist fracture because the fracture line extends to the scaphocapitate joint (not the scapho-trapezio-trapezoid joint) as interpreted on 2D CT. Hence, the decision for this type of treatment is best based on shared-decision making. Surgery yields to a shorter immobilization period and allows early return to work but has a higher risk of complications.[34–39]

PANEL 3
Pearls and Pitfalls

PEARLS

- A reliable scaphoid fracture classification should enable guiding decision-making and estimating prognosis and risk for complication.
- A reliable scaphoid fracture classification may enhance clinical investigation about the optimal treatment for acute scaphoid fractures on which there is currently no consensus.
- Proximal location, displacement, and delayed treatment seem to be predictors of higher risk for scaphoid nonunion, irrespective to classification system.
- The authors' newly proposed simplified anatomic classification is validated by 3D imaging, but can still be used straightforwardly in posteroanterior radiographs. Based on 3D mapping analysis, it distinguishes the three main fracture types as (1) proximal pole fractures (proximal to the distal scapholunate interval), (2) waist fractures (involving the scaphocapitate interval), and (3) distal tubercle fractures (involving the scapho-trapezio-trapezoid interval).

PITFALLS

- The existing classification systems are all based on the 2D radiographic interpretation of scaphoid characteristics, which have limited reproducibility.
- None of the existing systems can reliably predict the outcome of acute scaphoid fractures in terms of fracture consolidation. Therefore, the clinical relevance of dividing scaphoid fractures into the various subgroups as proposed in literature is currently unknown. Moreover, no consensus exists on the radiologic criteria defining consolidation of the fracture.

REFERENCES

1. Peltier LF. The classic. Injuries of the wrist. A radiological study. By Etienne Destot. 1926. *Clin Orthop Relat Res.* 1986;202:3–11.
2. Cravener EK, McElroy DG. Fractures of the carpal (navicular) scaphoid. *Am J Surg.* 1939;44(1):8.
3. Herbert TJ, Fisher WE. Management of the fractured scaphoid using a new bone screw. *J Bone Joint Surg Br.* 1984;66(1):114–123.
4. Cooney WP, Dobyns JH, Linscheid RL. Fractures of the scaphoid: a rational approach to management. *Clin Orthop Relat Res.* 1980;149:90–97.
5. Russe O. Fracture of the carpal navicular. Diagnosis, nonoperative treatment, and operative treatment. *J Bone Joint Surg Am.* 1960;42-A:759–768.
6. Steinmann SP, Adams JE. Scaphoid fractures and nonunions: diagnosis and treatment. *J Orthop Sci.* 2006;11(4): 424–431.
7. Herbert TJ. *The Fractured Scaphoid.* 1st ed. St. Louis, MO: Quality Medical Publishing; 1990.
8. Marsh JL, Slongo TF, Agel J, et al. Fracture and dislocation classification compendium – 2007: Orthopaedic Trauma Association classification, database and outcomes committee. *J Orthop Trauma.* 2007;21(suppl 10):S1–S133.
9. Desai VV, Davis TR, Barton NJ. The prognostic value and reproducibility of the radiological features of the fractured scaphoid. *J Hand Surg Br.* 1999;24(5):586–590.
10. Bohler L, Trojan E, Jahna H. Treatment of 734 cases of fresh fracture of the scaphoid bone of the hand [in German]. *Wiederherstellungschir Traumatol.* 1954;2:86–111.

11. Schernberg F, Elzein F, Gérard Y. Anatomo-radiological study of fractures of the carpal scaphoid bone. Problems of abnormal callus [in French]. *Rev Chir Orthop Repar Appar Mot.* 1984;70(suppl 2):55–63.
12. Prosser AJ, Brenkel IJ, Irvine GB. Articular fractures of the distal scaphoid. *J Hand Surg Br.* 1988;13(1):87–91.
13. Mu¨ller ME, Allgöwer M, Willenegger H. *Technik der operative Frakturenbehandlung.* 1st ed. Berlin: Springer; 1963.
14. Compson JP. The anatomy of acute scaphoid fractures: a threedimensional analysis of patterns. *J Bone Joint Surg Br.* 1998;80(2):218–224.
15. Pauwels F. *Der schenkelhalsbruch ein mechanisches problem: Grundlagen des Haeilungsvorganges Prognose und kausale Therapie.* Stuttgart: Ferdinand Enke Verlag; 1935.
16. McLaughlin HL, Parkes II JC. Fracture of the carpal navicular (scaphoid) bone: gradations in therapy based upon pathology. *J Trauma.* 1969;9(4):311–319.
17. Weber ER. Biomechanical implications of scaphoid waist fractures. *Clin Orthop Relat Res.* 1980;149:83–89.
18. Garcia-Elias M, Lluch A. Partial excision of scaphoid: is it ever indicated?. *Hand Clin.* 2001;17(4):687–695. x.
19. Hannemann PF, Brouwers L, van der Zee D, Stadler A, Gottgens KW, Weijers R. Multiplanar reconstruction computed tomography for diagnosis of scaphoid waist fracture union: a prospective cohort analysis of accuracy and precision. *Skeletal Radiol.* 2013;42(10):1377–1382.
20. Buijze GA, Guitton TG, van Dijk CN, Ring D. Science of Variation Group. Training improves interobserver reliability for the diagnosis of scaphoid fracture displacement. *Clin Orthop Relat Res.* 2012;470(7):2029–2034.
21. Dias JJ, Taylor M, Thompson J, Brenkel IJ, Gregg PJ. Radiographic signs of union of scaphoid fractures. An analysis of inter-observer agreement and reproducibility. *J Bone Joint Surg Br.* 1988;70(2):299–301.
22. Lozano-Calderón S, Blazar P, Zurakowski D, Lee SG, Ring D. Diagnosis of scaphoid fracture displacement with radiography and computed tomography. *J Bone Joint Surg Am.* 2006;88(12):2695–2703.
23. Bhat M, McCarthy M, Davis TR, Oni JA, Dawson S. MRI and plain radiography in the assessment of displaced fractures of the waist of the carpal scaphoid. *J Bone Joint Surg Br.* 2004;86(5):705–713.
24. Temple CL, Ross DC, Bennett JD, Garvin GJ, King GJ, Faber KJ. Comparison of sagittal computed tomography and plain film radiography in a scaphoid fracture model. *J Hand Surg Am.* 2005;30(3):534–542.
25. Lozano-Calderón S, Blazar P, Zurakowski D, Lee SG, Ring D. Diagnosis of scaphoid fracture displacement with radiography and computed tomography. *J Bone Joint Surg Am.* 2006;88(12):2695–2703.
26. Swart E, Strauch RJ. Diagnosis of scaphoid fracture displacement. *J Hand Surg Am.* 2013;38(4):784–787. quiz 787.
27. Swart E, Strauch RJ. Diagnosis of scaphoid fracture displacement. *J Hand Surg Am.* 2013;38(4):784–787. quiz 787. http://dx.doi.org/10.1016/j.jhsa.2012.10.025.
28. Moritomo H. Radiographic clues for determining carpal instability and treatment protocol for scaphoid fractures. *J Orthop Sci.* 2014;19(3):379–383.
29. Buijze GA, Jørgsholm P, Thomsen NO, Bjorkman A, Besjakov J, Ring D. Diagnostic performance of radiographs and computed tomography for displacement and instability of acute scaphoid waist fractures. *J Bone Joint Surg Am.* 2012;94(21):1967–1974.
30. Moritomo H, Murase T, Oka K, Tanaka H, Yoshikawa H, Sugamoto K. Relationship between the fracture location and the kinematic pattern in scaphoid nonunion. *J Hand Surg Am.* 2008;33(9):1459–1468.
31. Ramamurthy C, Cutler L, Nuttall D, Simison AJ, Trail IA, Stanley JK. The factors affecting outcome after non-vascular bone grafting and internal fixation for nonunion of the scaphoid. *J Bone Joint Surg Br.* 2007;89(5):627–632.
32. Langhoff O, Andersen JL. Consequences of late immobilization of scaphoid fractures. *J Hand Surg Br.* 1988;13(1):77–79.
33. Ferguson DO, Shanbhag V, Hedley H, Reichert I, Lipscombe S, Davis TR. Scaphoid fracture non-union: a systematic review of surgical treatment using bone graft. *J Hand Surg Eur Vol.* 2016;41(5):492–500.
34. Adolfsson L, Lindau T, Arner M. Acutrak screw fixation versus cast immobilisation for undisplaced scaphoid waist fractures. *J Hand Surg Br.* 2001;26(3):192–195.
35. Arora R, Gschwentner M, Krappinger D, Lutz M, Blauth M, Gabl M. Fixation of nondisplaced scaphoid fractures: making treatment cost effective. Prospective controlled trial. *Arch Orthop Trauma Surg.* 2007;127(1):39–46.
36. McQueen MM, Gelbke MK, Wakefield A, Will EM, Gaebler C. Percutaneous screw fixation versus conservative treatment for fractures of the waist of the scaphoid: a prospective randomised study. *J Bone Joint Surg Br.* 2008;90(1):66–71.
37. Vinnars B, Pietreanu M, Bodestedt A, Ekenstam FA, Gerdin B. Nonoperative compared with operative treatment of acute scaphoid fractures. A randomized clinical trial. *J Bone Joint Surg Am.* 2008;90(6):1176–1185.
38. Saedén B, Törnkvist H, Ponzer S. HöglundM. Fracture of the carpal scaphoid. A prospective, randomised 12-year follow-up comparing operative and conservative treatment. *J Bone Joint Surg Br.* 2001;83(2):230–234.
39. Bond CD, Shin AY, McBride MT, Dao KD. Percutaneous screw fixation or cast immobilization for nondisplaced scaphoid fractures. *J Bone Joint Surg Am.* 2001;83-A(4):483–488.

FURTHER READING

1. Luria S, Schwarcz Y, Wollstein R, Emelife P, Zinger G, Peleg E. 3- dimensional analysis of scaphoid fracture angle morphology. *J Hand Surg Am.* 2015;40(3):508–514.

CHAPTER 9

Three-Dimensional Imaging of Scaphoid Fractures

SHAI LURIA, MD • YONATAN SCHWARCZ, MD

KEY POINTS

- The majority of scaphoid fractures are horizontal oblique and not transverse.
- Acute displaced fractures have extension and supination of the proximal fragment (a "proximal extension" deformity). In fracture nonunion distal to the dorsal apex of the scaphoid ridge (and not in acute fractures), there is additional dorsal translation of the distal fragment.
- There are two types of displaced fracture nonunions, proximal or distal to the dorsal apex of the ridge of the scaphoid. Distal "mobile" fractures have increased deformity and interfragmentary motion, more bone loss, and larger dorsal osteophytes than proximal "stable" fractures.
- A volar-distal approach to screw placement can only accommodate a central screw in the proximal fragment. Central screw positioning throughout the length of the scaphoid may be possible through a distal-transtrapezial or proximal-dorsal approach.
- Three-dimensional (3D) imaging techniques for preoperative planning, including optimal surgical approach, screw direction, graft size, and the need for osteophyte resection, are good clinical aids, although they have not yet been clinically proven to improve outcome in scaphoid fractures.
- Intraoperative 3D imaging may enable the correction of malreduction during the procedure, although the use of current imaging modalities is still limited by technical factors.

IMPORTANCE OF THE PROBLEM

The treatment of scaphoid fractures is challenging because of the complexity of wrist and scaphoid anatomy, kinematics, and fracture morphology. Understanding and classification of these injuries have been based on two-dimensional (2D) images,[1-3] even when examining CT and MRI scans.[4-7] The notion of fracture instability governs decision-making, but there is limited evidence to support commonly used criteria.[8] Although extensively debated, the treatment of these fractures is still controversial[9] and can include long periods of immobilization and high rates of complications.[10] In contrast to common fracture surgical techniques, the scaphoid fracture is in fact currently treated with disregard to its morphology.[8,11,12]

Three-dimensional (3D) imaging is changing our understanding of wrist and scaphoid physiology and pathology. It is used extensively by surgeons not only to better understand the patient's pathology[13,14] but also to enable measurement of fracture characteristics, which are less accurately assessed in two dimensions.[15,16] 3D imaging is thus likely to change the way we treat these injuries.

MAIN QUESTIONS

- How has 3D imaging changed our knowledge of scaphoid fractures?
- Can 3D imaging improve the treatment of scaphoid fractures?

PANEL 1
Case Scenario

A 20-year-old healthy man falls on his outstretched left hand during a soccer match. He goes to the emergency room complaining of wrist pain and swelling. Radiographs reveal a displaced scaphoid waist fracture (Herbert type B2) (Fig. 9.1). A CT scan shows extension of the proximal fragment (Fig. 9.2). You are considering open reduction and screw fixation of the fracture. Can preoperative 3D imaging help you understand the fracture more accurately, preplan the procedure, and perform percutaneous reduction and fixation instead? Would intraoperative 3D imaging help analyze the reduction achieved?

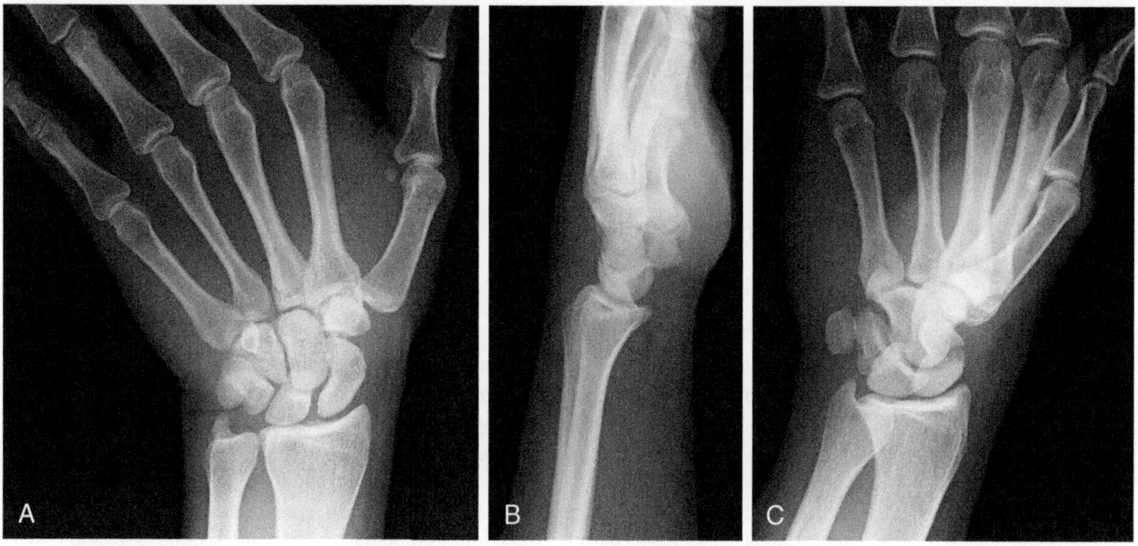

FIG. 9.1 **(A)** posteroanterior, **(B)** lateral, and **(C)** oblique radiographs of a displaced waist fracture (Herbert type B2) of the scaphoid.

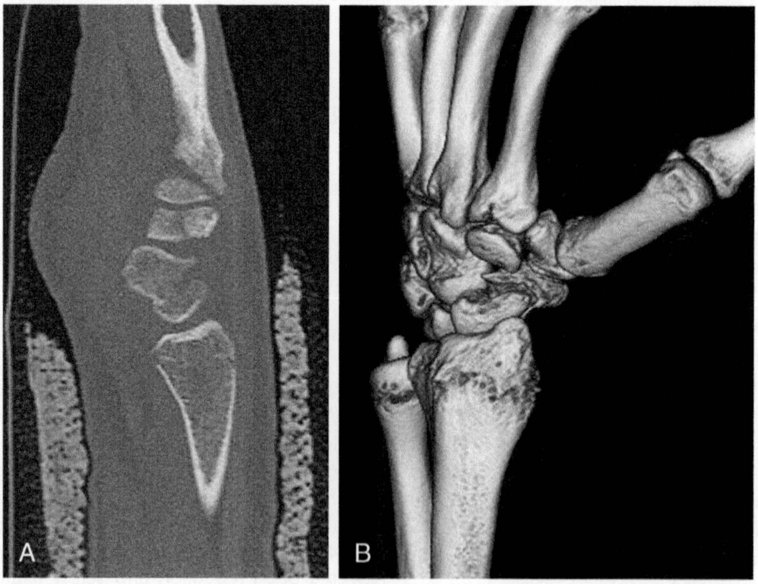

FIG. 9.2 **(A)** Sagittal reconstruction and **(B)** 3D reconstruction of a wrist CT scan of a displaced waist fracture. Note the "proximal fragment extension" deformity of the fracture.

Current Opinion

Scaphoid fractures are treated according to their degree of instability. Instability is currently defined according to fracture characteristics using two-dimensional measures such as the degree of displacement, measures of carpal instability, or fracture angle. The evidence supporting the choice of these criteria and the ability to evaluate them using radiographs is limited.

Finding the Evidence

- Cochrane search: Scaphoid Fracture
- Pubmed (Medline):
  1. ((scaphoid bone[MeSH Terms]) AND bone fracture[MeSH Terms]) AND 3d imaging[MeSH Terms]
  2. (3d imagings[MeSH Terms]) AND orthopedic [MeSH Terms]
  3. (((((((CT[Title]) OR imaging[Title]) OR computed tomography[Title]) OR MRI[Title]) OR scintigraphy[Title]) OR dimensional[Title]) OR 3d[Title]) AND scaphoid[Title]
- Bibliography of eligible articles
- Articles that were not in English were excluded

Quality of the evidence

Diagnostic Level II: 2
Diagnostic Level IV: 27

FINDINGS

Three-dimensional imaging of scaphoid fractures using computed tomography (CT) has been reported since 1985,[17] followed by reports of carpal bone surface reconstruction.[14] Reconstruction was said to be "a tool to communicate the spatial information of the complex bony structure to nonradiologists."[14] 3D wrist models can be used to generate an orthogonal reference system and compare the injured wrist to the contralateral one.[18] These models have been used to study different aspects of scaphoid fractures, including displacement patterns and the kinematics of fractures and fracture nonunion, and to calculate the scaphoid long axis; compute the fracture angle, orientation, and bone loss; design preferred surgical approaches for optimal screw placement; and detect malreduction intraoperatively.

Fracture displacement patterns have been examined in several case series using 3D models. The displacement of fracture nonunions was quantified finding the proximal fragment extended, radially deviated, and supinated relative to the distal fragment.[18–20] In acute fractures, the displacement of the fragments in relation to the distal radius as a reference was recently described.[16] When comparing the CT scans of 57 patients with nondisplaced and 23 with displaced fractures with a control group of 27 patients with no wrist pathology, a similar displacement was found between the fragments as described for fracture nonunions. Relative to the reference system (the distal radius joint surface), only the proximal fragment was displaced, i.e., it was found to be supinated, extended, and volarly translated. The so-called "humpback" deformity, which characterizes the perceived flexion of the distal fragment, emerged actually as a "proximal (fragment) extension" deformity of the acute fracture.[16]

Using 3D imaging, two displacement patterns of fracture nonunion or malunion, termed the volar and dorsal types, were first identified in 22 patients and measured using two-dimensional measures.[19] In 5 of these 22 cases, the fracture offset could be seen in the scans but not in the radiographs.[19] In another study of 11 patients with nonunion, these patterns were defined according to their location proximal or distal to the dorsal apex of the scaphoid ridge (the dorsal ulnar edge of the scaphoid where the dorsal intercarpal ligament and the dorsal part of the dorsal scapholunate interosseous ligament are attached).[21] The volar pattern was associated with more transverse and distal fracture lines; the dorsal pattern was associated with more horizontal and proximal fracture lines.[19,21,22] In a study comparing radiographic and CT scan parameters, these patterns could not be differentiated on the radiographs of 8 of 43 fractures (19%) despite the use of appropriate radiographs and the proximal fragment ratio (ratio of proximal fragment length to scaphoid length on radiographs).[22]

More advanced 3D models of fracture nonunion enabled 3D measures. They revealed that the displacement in both previously described patterns was dorsal, but to a more significant extent, with fractures distal to the dorsal apex of the scaphoid ridge.[23] In 20 fracture nonunions distal to the apex, the proximal scaphoid extended and supinated with the lunate and the distal scaphoid and capitate translated dorsally. In four fractures proximal to the apex, the scaphoid extended and slightly pronated and the distal scaphoid and capitate translated dorsally but less than the more distal fractures.[23] The effect of the fracture patterns on wrist kinematics was presented in an in vivo 3D motion analysis study of 13 patients.[24] The patterns were then reclassified into mobile (distal) or stable (proximal) types.[24] In seven cases of the mobile type, the fracture was distal to the dorsal apex of the ridge and showed a "book opening" motion with flexion and extension of the wrist. In six cases of the stable type, the fracture was proximal to the apex with little deformity and interfragmentary motion.[24] The differential motion of the fracture fragments was reported in another study of six patients with fracture nonunion using a markerless CT scan registration technique. Carpal bone motion, with wrist flexion and extension, with or without a scaphoid fracture, showed a 38% decrease in extension of the proximal fragment coupled with the lunate compared with the healthy wrist.[25] There was no difference in the distal fragment motion in fractured versus healthy wrists.[25]

In a study of the angle and direction of inclination of acute fractures, the scaphoid long axis was used as a reference. In contrast to the two-dimensional radiographic perception of most fractures as transverse waist fractures,[3,26] all waist and proximal fractures were found to be horizontal oblique with an angle of 56 degrees for 86 acute waist fractures and 48 degrees for 25 acute proximal fractures. This was significantly different from a 90-degree transverse fracture.[15]

Two studies measured bone loss and the graft size needed for treatment of fracture nonunions using 2D (and not 3D) measurements of selected slices of CT and MRI scans.[5,18] Using a 3D CT model and 3D measures, the bone defect could be better quantified.[27] The defect in 24 fracture nonunions was compared as a function of the fracture position distal or proximal to the dorsal apex of the scaphoid ridge, using the contralateral scaphoid as a template. In the 20 distal fractures, the defect had a wedge shape facing the volar side and accounted for 9% of the scaphoid volume. In the four proximal fractures, the defect had a flat, crescent configuration and consisted of 1% of the scaphoid volume.[27] Dorsal callus formation was evaluated in one study comparing nonunions with contralateral scaphoids.[20] Virtual reduction of the fractures demonstrated that without dorsal appositional callus resection, adequate reduction might not be possible.[20] A study of 28 patients with fracture nonunion found that osteophyte volume and bone loss volume were positively correlated to each other and increased with time.[28]

To accurately examine scaphoid morphology, fracture characteristics, and fracture fixation alternatives using 3D models, the long axis of the scaphoid has been characterized in several ways.[15,29] In one study, by examining different available implants placed on this long axis in a 3D model, the authors found that a longer screw could be placed using a volar-distal approach.[30] This has to do with the shape of the scaphoid, as well as the conical or differential size of the leading and trailing ends of the screws.

Several attempts have been made using CT-generated 3D models to delineate a safe zone to evaluate possible screw positions, which would not protrude into the joint.[29,31–33] In terms of the safe zone, one study found that computing the maximum screw length and using a volar-distal approach would allow central placement in the central one-third of the scaphoid of 10 cadaver specimens. The optimal starting point was on the dorsal and radial side of the scaphoid tubercle.[29] One study examined the possibility of placing a screw in the central third of the entire length of the scaphoid but found this to be impossible.[31] The authors showed that a screw placed from a distal approach along the distal central third would need to be placed through the scaphotrapezial joint (transtrapezial approach).[31]

Placing a long axis screw, which is common practice, disregards the fracture morphology and has been questioned.[34] 3D analysis of horizontal oblique fractures of 10 dry bone specimens indicated that a perpendicular screw took up a smaller area of the fracture surface, which is an advantage for fracture apposition and healing.[35]

The use of a 3D model to preoperatively plan surgical repair of waist fracture nonunions was examined in a case series of seven patients.[36] The authors simulated and calculated the reduction of the fragments, as well as the size of the bone defect and possible positioning of the screw. Epoxy resin models were created from the computer model, including the position of the screw, and were used as guides during the actual procedure. The authors reported good clinical results, although they could only state that the hard models aided in surgical orientation.

3D imaging intraoperatively was examined in one study.[37] The authors compared two imaging modalities and examined the quality of fracture reduction, wire position, and possible extrusion, after preliminary reduction and fixation. The modalities were found to be useful in the diagnosis of malreduction in 2 of 25 cases. Adequate analysis of the position of the wire was limited by artifacts and dependency on the technician's skills.

RECOMMENDATIONS

- New approaches to fracture fixation should be assessed to address the actual configuration of most scaphoid fractures, which are horizontal oblique. The current long axis or central screw approach results in fixation that is at a significant angle to the fracture and may not be the optimal approach (overall quality: moderate).
- The proximal fragment should be flexed and pronated to achieve reduction (overall quality: moderate). Fracture reduction is possible using a single K-wire placed in the proximal fragment, with no manipulation of the distal fragment.

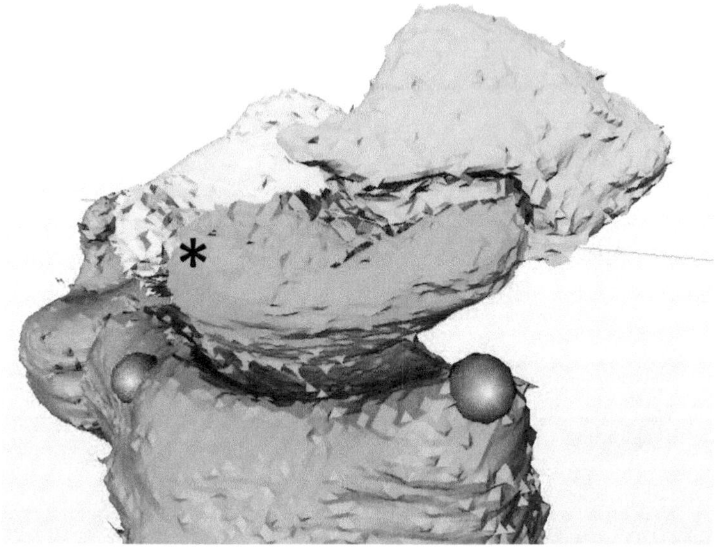

FIG. 9.3 3D analysis of the fracture reveals a horizontal oblique fracture distal to the dorsal apex of the scaphoid ridge (*) viewed from a radiodorsal direction. *Brown sphere* markers on the distal radius rim enable the creation of a reference system to which the directions can be measured. The *thin green line* depicts the projection of the volar-dorsal axis on the fracture plane. The lunate is marked in yellow, the distal radius and ulna in turquoise, and the scaphoid in light blue and green.

- 3D imaging may aid in the preplanning of fracture and fracture nonunion operative treatment (overall quality: low).
- 3D intraoperative imaging may reveal malreduction of the fracture prior to definitive fixation (overall quality: low).

CONCLUSION

3D imaging models show that most acute scaphoid fractures are horizontal oblique and, when displaced, have displacement only of the proximal fragment. In fracture nonunion, there is additional dorsal translation of the distal fragment. Two patterns have been found to exist in fracture nonunion as a function of their location proximal or distal to the dorsal apex of the scaphoid ridge. 3D imaging shows that a central screw can be positioned throughout the length of the scaphoid in a distal-transtrapezial or proximal-dorsal approach. These techniques can thus contribute to the preoperative planning of surgery, as well as the intraoperative analysis of malreduction. However, their advantages still need to be clinically proven and simplified for their widespread utilization.

PANEL 2
Author's Preferred Technique

3D analysis of the CT scan of an acute scaphoid fracture (Panel 1) reveals a horizontal oblique fracture with no comminution, distal to the dorsal apex of the scaphoid ridge (Fig. 9.3). Measured between the fracture plane and the longitudinal axis of the scaphoid, the fracture angle was 38 degrees and was inclined in a dorsal-ulnar direction (Fig. 9.4). The fracture was treated percutaneously, by reducing the proximal fragment using the Kirschner-wire "joystick" technique (Fig. 9.5). This wire or an additional wire may be inserted into the lunate to facilitate reduction indirectly. Percutaneous fixation was achieved through a dorsal proximal approach (Fig. 9.6).

The apex of the dorsal ridge is located at the dorsal ulnar edge of the scaphoid where the dorsal intercarpal ligament and the dorsal part of the dorsal scapholunate interosseous ligament are attached.

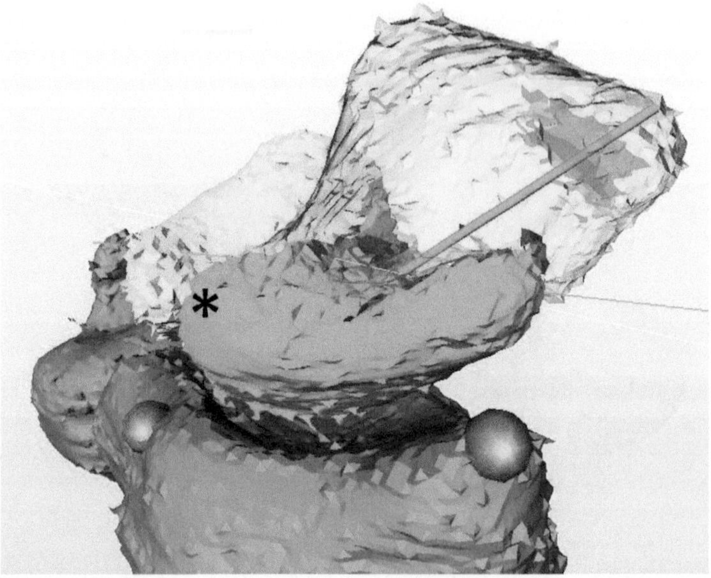

FIG. 9.4 After virtual reduction of the scaphoid fracture, viewed from a radiodorsal direction. The fracture angle is 38 degrees, measured between the fracture plane and the longitudinal axis of the scaphoid (*bold green line*). The longitudinal axis was calculated using the statistical procedure of principal component analysis. Considering a volarly directed inclination as a fracture inclination of 0 degree and a dorsally directed inclination (horizontal oblique) as an inclination of 180 degrees, the fracture in this case is inclined 224 degrees in a dorsal and ulnar direction. * - dorsal apex of the scaphoid ridge.

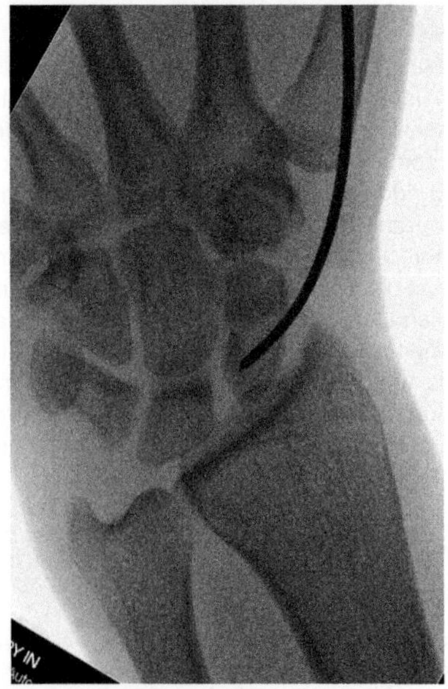

FIG. 9.5 Percutaneous reduction of the proximal fragment using the Kirschner-wire "joystick" technique.

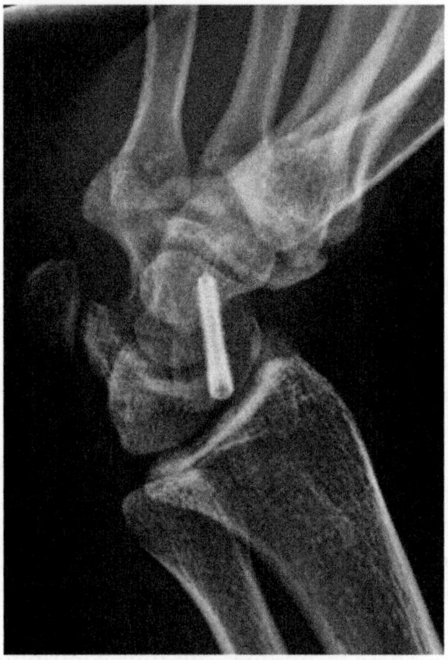

FIG. 9.6 Postoperative oblique radiograph of the fracture after reduction and fixation with a dorsal-proximal approach.

PANEL 3
Pearls and Pitfalls

PEARLS

- In acute scaphoid fractures, concurrent flexion of the extended lunate with the proximal scaphoid may aid in fracture reduction.
- Central screw placement is possible through a transtrapezial or dorsal-proximal approach. In the volar-distal approach, the screw is central only proximally.

PITFALLS

- Failure to resect the dorsal osteophyte in fracture nonunions may result in failure of fracture reduction or dorsal impingement.

REFERENCES

1. Compson JP. The anatomy of acute scaphoid fractures: a three-dimensional analysis of patterns. *J Bone Joint Surg Br*. 1998;80(2):218–224.
2. Herbert TJ, Fisher WE. Management of the fractured scaphoid using a new bone screw. *J Bone Joint Surg Br Vol*. 1984;66-B:114–123.
3. Russe O. Fracture of the carpal navicular: diagnosis, non-operative treatment, and operative treatment. *The J Bone Joint Surg*. 1960;42(5):759–768.
4. Bain GI, Bennett JD, MacDermid JC, Slethaug GP, Richards RS, Roth JH. Measurement of the scaphoid humpback deformity using longitudinal computed tomography: intra- and interobserver variability using various measurement techniques. *J Hand Surg Am*. 1998;23(1):76–81.
5. Topper SM. Magnetic resonance imaging of the humpback scaphoid: the technique and a mathematical performance evaluation. *Am J Orthoped*. 1999;28(11):639–643.
6. Sanders WE. Evaluation of the humpback scaphoid by computed tomography in the longitudinal axial plane of the scaphoid. *J Hand Surg Am*. 1988;13(2):182–187.
7. Ring D, Patterson JD, Levitz S, Wang C, Jupiter JB. Both scanning plane and observer affect measurements of scaphoid deformity. *J Hand Surg Am*. 2005;30(4):696–701.
8. LS K. Fractures of the carpal bones. In: Scott W, Wolfe RNH, Pederson William C, Kozin Scott H, Cohen Mark S, eds. *Green's Operative Hand Surgery*. 7th ed. vol. 1. Philadelphia, PA: Elsevier; 2016:588–652.
9. Dias JJ, Wildin CJ, Bhowal B, Thompson JR. Should acute scaphoid fractures be fixed? A randomized controlled trial. *J Bone Joint Surg*. 2005;87(10):2160–2168.
10. Pinder RM, Brkljac M, Rix L, Muir L, Brewster M. Treatment of scaphoid nonunion: a systematic review of the existing evidence. *J Hand Surg Am*. 2015;40(9):1797–1805. e1793.
11. McCallister WV, Knight J, Kaliappan R, Trumble TE. Central placement of the screw in simulated fractures of the scaphoid waist: a biomechanical study. *J Bone Joint Sur*. 2003;85-A(1):72–77.
12. Trumble TE, Gilbert M, Murray LW, Smith J, Rafijah G, McCallister WV. Displaced scaphoid fractures treated with open reduction and internal fixation with a cannulated screw. *J Bone Joint Surgery*. 2000;82(5):633–641.
13. Nakamura R, Horii E, Tanaka Y, Imaeda T, Hayakawa N. Three-dimensional CT imaging for wrist disorders. *J Hand Surg Br*. 1989;14(1):53–58.
14. Biondetti PR, Vannier MW, Gilula LA, Knapp RH. Three-dimensional surface reconstruction of the carpal bones from CT scans: transaxial versus coronal technique. *Comput Med Imaging Graph*. 1988;12(1):67–73.
15. Luria S, Schwarcz Y, Wollstein R, Emelife P, Zinger G, Peleg E. 3-dimensional analysis of scaphoid fracture angle morphology. *J Hand Surg Am*. 2015;40(3):508–514.
16. Schwarcz Y, Schwarcz Y, Peleg E, Joskowicz L, Wollstein R, Luria S. Three-dimensional analysis of acute scaphoid fracture displacement: proximal extension deformity of the scaphoid. *J Bone Joint Surg*. 2017;99(2):141–149.
17. Weeks PM, Vannier MW, Stevens WG, Gayou D, Gilula LA. Three-dimensional imaging of the wrist. *J Hand Surg Am*. 1985;10(1):32–39.
18. Belsole RJ, Hilbelink DR, Llewellyn JA, Dale M, Greene TL, Rayhack JM. Computed analyses of the pathomechanics of scaphoid waist nonunions. *J Hand Surg Am*. 1991;16(5):899–906.
19. Nakamura R, Imaeda T, Horii E, Miura T, Hayakawa N. Analysis of scaphoid fracture displacement by three-dimensional computed tomography. *J Hand Surg Am*. 1991;16(3):485–492.
20. Schweizer A, Furnstahl P, Nagy L. Three-dimensional computed tomographic analysis of 11 scaphoid waist nonunions. *J Hand Surg Am*. 2012;37(6):1151–1158.
21. Moritomo H, Viegas SF, Elder KW, et al. Scaphoid nonunions: a 3-dimensional analysis of patterns of deformity. *J Hand Surg Am*. 2000;25(3):520–528.
22. Inagaki H, Nakamura R, Horii E, Nakao E, Tatebe M. Differences in radiographic findings between scaphoid fracture patterns. *Hand Surg*. 2004;9(2):197–202.
23. Oka K, Moritomo H, Murase T, Goto A, Sugamoto K, Yoshikawa H. Patterns of carpal deformity in scaphoid nonunion: a 3-dimensional and quantitative analysis. *J Hand Surg Am*. 2005;30(6):1136–1144.
24. Moritomo H, Murase T, Oka K, Tanaka H, Yoshikawa H, Sugamoto K. Relationship between the fracture location and the kinematic pattern in scaphoid nonunion. *J Hand Surg Am*. 2008;33(9):1459–1468.
25. Leventhal EL, Wolfe SW, Moore DC, Akelman E, Weiss AP, Crisco JJ. Interfragmentary motion in patients with scaphoid nonunion. *J Hand Surg Am*. 2008;33(7):1108–1115.
26. Brondum V, Larsen CF, Skov O. Fracture of the carpal scaphoid: frequency and distribution in a well-defined population. *Eur J Radiol*. 1992;15(2):118–122.

27. Oka K, Murase T, Moritomo H, Goto A, Sugamoto K, Yoshikawa H. Patterns of bone defect in scaphoid nonunion: a 3-dimensional and quantitative analysis. *J Hand Surg Am*. 2005;30(2):359–365.
28. Ten Berg PW, Dobbe JG, Horbach SE, Gerards RM, Strackee SD, Streekstra GJ. Analysis of deformity in scaphoid non-unions using two- and three-dimensional imaging. *J Hand Surg Eur Vol*. 2016;41(7):719–726.
29. Leventhal EL, Wolfe SW, Walsh EF, Crisco JJ. A computational approach to the "optimal" screw axis location and orientation in the scaphoid bone. *J Hand Surg Am*. 2009;34(4):677–684.
30. Meermans G, Verstreken F. Influence of screw design, sex, and approach in scaphoid fracture fixation. *Clin Orthopaedics Related Res*. 2012;470(6):1673–1681.
31. Guo Y, Tian GL, Chen S, Tapia C. Establishing a central zone in scaphoid surgery: a computational approach. *Int Orthopaed*. 2014;38(1):95–99.
32. Levitz S, Ring D. Retrograde (volar) scaphoid screw insertion-a quantitative computed tomographic analysis. *J Hand Surg Am*. 2005;30(3):543–548.
33. Jung WS, Jung JH, Chung US, Lee KH. Spatial measurement for safe placement of screws within the scaphoid using three-dimensional analysis. *J Plast Surg Hand Surg*. 2011;45(1):40–44.
34. Luria S, Hoch S, Liebergall M, Mosheiff R, Peleg E. Optimal fixation of acute scaphoid fractures: finite element analysis. *J Hand Surg Am*. 2010;35(8):1246–1250.
35. Hart A, Mansuri A, Harvey EJ, Martineau PA. Central versus eccentric internal fixation of acute scaphoid fractures. *J Hand Surg Am*. 2013;38(1):66–71.
36. Murase T, Moritomo H, Goto A, Sugamoto K, Yoshikawa H. Does three-dimensional computer simulation improve results of scaphoid nonunion surgery? *Clin Orthopaedics Related Res*. 2005;(434):143–150.
37. Luria S, Safran O, Zinger G, Mosheiff R, Liebergall M. Intraoperative 3-dimensional imaging of scaphoid fracture reduction and fixation. *Orthop Traumatol Surg Res OTSR*. 2015;101(3):353–357.

CHAPTER 10

Diagnosis of Displaced Scaphoid Fractures

KANAI GARALA, BSC (HONS), MB CHB (HONS), MRCS, DIPMEDED • HARVINDER SINGH, MBBS, MS (ORTH), FRCS (ORTH), PHD • JOSEPH DIAS, MBBS, FRCS (ORTH), MD

KEY POINTS

- Displacement of scaphoid fractures can be described by the gap, step, angle, and rotation between the fracture fragments.
- Although a displaced scaphoid is commonly defined as one with a gap or translation of 1 mm or more, there is poor evidence for this.
- Radiographs of good quality and with sufficient views are a poor imaging modality to assess scaphoid fracture displacement but serve as a screening tool.
- High-resolution CT imaging with multiplanar reconstruction is currently the best modality to investigate displacement in scaphoid fractures.

PANEL 1
Case Scenario

A 25-year-old man was ice-skating and fell onto his outstretched right hand. He presented to the emergency department where radiographs showed a displaced scaphoid waist fracture (Fig. 10.1). What is the best imaging modality to identify more clearly the degree and nature of displacement?

IMPORTANCE OF THE PROBLEM

The incidence of displacement in scaphoid fracture is around 10%–20%.[1-3] Displaced scaphoid fractures have a greater rate of malunion and nonunion, leading to persistent pain, poor grip strength, osteoarthritis, and scaphoid nonunion advanced collapse.[3,4] The impact and costs to the patient and healthcare providers to manage scaphoid nonunion are significant. As most scaphoid fractures occur in young patients with most of their working lives ahead of them, it is imperative to identify displacement and intervene appropriately to prevent morbidity.[5]

What Is the Definition of Displacement?

The scaphoid has a complicated three-dimensional structure and is in close proximity to other carpal bones. This can make it difficult to clearly identify displacement. There are four separate types of displacements that could be present in scaphoid fractures and they are not mutually exclusive. The gap, translation, angulation, and rotation between fragments should be identified and assessed if displacement is suspected.[6]

Translation, gap, and angulation are the most studied types of displacement. Although any displacement changes the anatomy of the scaphoid, it is generally considered that 1 mm or greater translation or gap is clinically relevant.[2,6-8] However, there has been no scientific assessment to arrive at this cutoff value and therefore a 1-mm translation is not an evidence-based measurement of displacement, but an anecdotal one. Fractures with translation of more than 1 mm between scaphoid fracture fragments, in any direction but usually at the radial or dorsal cortex, are described as displaced. A fracture with a gap of more than 1 mm in the sagittal or coronal plane is also considered to be displaced.[6]

Fractures with an intrascaphoid angle of more than 35 degrees,[6,9] when viewing from the lateral aspect of the scaphoid, are described as displaced using the Mayo classification.[10] Once again, the scientific backing for this number is limited with a key paper only having three patients assessed.[9] However, we know that angulated scaphoid fractures are associated with poorer outcomes.[10-12]

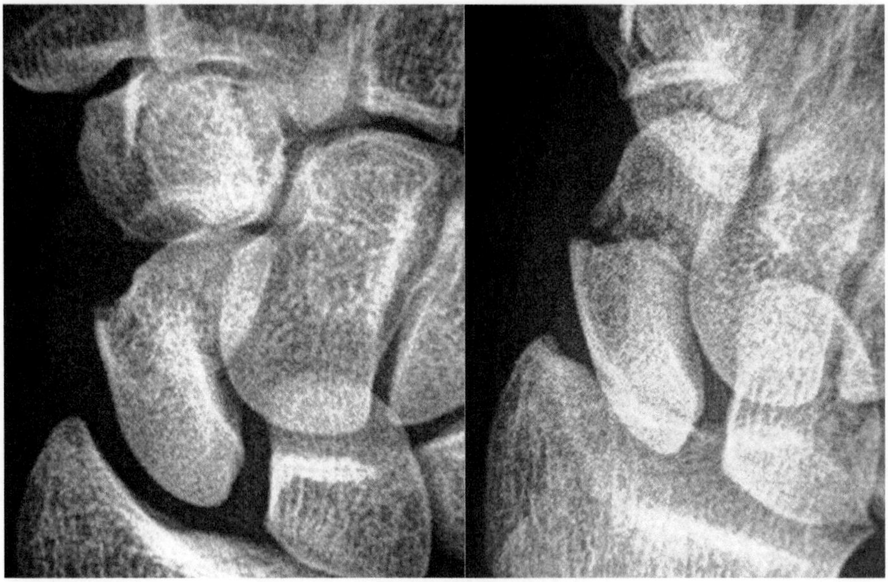

FIG. 10.1 A displaced scaphoid fracture.

With regard to rotation, there is limited evidence to determine a value to quote which can satisfactorily describe this displacement. Therefore a recommendation for this type of displacement cannot be made. One study described that, in 36% of scaphoid fractures, the distal fragment pronates on the proximal fragment.[13] A recent study has explored the native intraosseous rotation of uninjured scaphoids, and perhaps this will instigate more research to explore the role of rotation in scaphoid fractures.[14]

MAIN QUESTION

What is the best method to diagnose displacement in patients who have a fractured scaphoid?

In population, intervention, comparator, and outcomes of interest (PICO) format—*For all patients with displaced scaphoid waist fractures, what is the accuracy of diagnosing displacement using plain radiographs versus more complex imaging methodology, namely computed tomography (CT), magnetic resonance imaging (MRI), or ultrasound?*

Current Opinion

Although radiographs of good quality and with sufficient views are a useful screening tool for scaphoid fractures, the imaging modalities used most frequently to further assess displacement in scaphoid fractures are CT and MRI imaging. MRI is widely considered the gold standard to assess whether the scaphoid is fractured. What is not clear is whether MRI or CT should be preferred to assess displacement of scaphoid fractures.

Finding the Evidence

We provide below a list of Pubmed search algorithms used to construct this chapter:

For radiographs: [scaphoid OR [navicular AND [carpus OR hand OR wrist]]] AND [fracture NOT [TUBEROSITY OR PROXIMAL POLE]] + [[displacement OR displaced OR unstable] NOT [undisplaced OR stable]] + [gap OR step OR angle OR rotation OR swelling] AND [[radiograph OR X-ray OR X-ray] AND [pa OR posterior-anterior OR lateral OR oblique OR zitter OR angled OR [ulna AND [deviated OR deviation]]]] + [measure OR diagnose OR assess OR assessment OR analysis OR identify OR detect]

For CT: [scaphoid OR [navicular AND [carpus OR hand OR wrist]]] AND [fracture NOT [TUBEROSITY OR PROXIMAL POLE]] + [[displacement OR displaced OR unstable] NOT [undisplaced OR stable]] + [gap OR step OR angle OR rotation OR swelling] AND [[CT OR computed tomography OR CAT scan] AND [axial OR coronal OR sagittal]] + [measure OR diagnose OR assess OR assessment OR analysis OR identify OR detect]

For MRI: [scaphoid OR [navicular AND [carpus OR hand OR wrist]]] AND [fracture NOT [TUBEROSITY OR PROXIMAL POLE]] + [[displacement OR displaced OR unstable] NOT [undisplaced OR stable]] + [gap OR

TABLE 10.1
Diagnostic Performance Characteristics for Detecting Scaphoid Fracture Displacement

Author	Imaging Modality	Sensitivity	Specificity	PPV	NPV	Accuracy
Lozano-Calderón[16]	Radiographs	75	72	10	97	64
	CT	72	80	13	98	80
	CT + radiographs	80	73	16	99	73
Bhat[18]	Radiographs	33–47	78–97	27–86	77–83	70–78
Buijze[15]	Radiographs	45	95	53	94	70
	CT	77	86	39	97	82
Temple[17]	Radiographs	52	84	76	63	68
	CT (sagittal view only)	49	89	81	63	69

PPV, positive predictive value; *NPV*, negative predictive value
Sensitivity: true positives/(true positives + false negatives)
Specificity: true negatives/(true negatives + false positives)
PPV: (sensitivity – prevalence)/[(sensitivity – prevalence) + (1 – specificity) – (1 – prevalence)]
NPV: [specificity – (1 – prevalence)]/[(1 – sensitivity) – (prevalence + specificity) – (1 – prevalence)]

step OR angle OR rotation OR swelling] AND [[MRI OR magnetic resonance imaging OR MR] AND [coronal OR sagittal]] + [measure OR diagnose OR assess OR assessment OR analysis OR identify OR detect]

For ultrasonography: [scaphoid OR [navicular AND [carpus OR hand OR wrist]]] AND [fracture NOT [TUBEROSITY OR PROXIMAL POLE]] + [[displacement OR displaced OR unstable] NOT [undisplaced OR stable]] + [gap OR step OR angle OR rotation OR swelling] AND [US OR ultrasound OR sonography] + [measure OR diagnose OR assess OR assessment OR analysis OR identify OR detect]

For operative assessment: [scaphoid OR [navicular AND [carpus OR hand OR wrist]]] AND [fracture NOT [TUBEROSITY OR PROXIMAL POLE]] + [[displacement OR displaced OR unstable] NOT [undisplaced OR stable]] + [gap OR step OR angle OR rotation OR swelling] AND [surgery OR endoscopy OR intraoperative OR intra-operative OR intra operative OR arthroscopy OR arthroscopic] + [measure OR diagnose OR assess OR assessment OR analysis OR identify OR detect]

Quality of Evidence

Overall no randomized controlled trials, systematic reviews, or metaanalyses were found, which specifically answered the headline question. The vast majority of high-level studies on scaphoid fracture imaging are dedicated to discussing imaging of occult scaphoid fractures. However, we found 13 studies of some relevance to imaging in displaced scaphoid fractures. The evidence in relation to these is as follows:

Level III: 5 studies
Level IV: 8 studies

FINDINGS

Evidence From Level III Studies

Thirteen studies were selected for inclusion in the review. Of these, five papers were comparative studies.[15–19] Three have compared the accuracy of detecting scaphoid fracture displacement between CT imaging and plain radiographs,[15–17] whereas one has compared MRI and plain radiography.[18] The sensitivities, specificities, positive predictive values, and negative predictive values for the studies can be found in Table 10.1. The final comparative study examines the role of training to improve detection of displacement in scaphoid fractures.[19]

Lozano-Calderón et al. compared CT with radiography to assess scaphoid fracture displacement.[16] 30 scaphoid fractures were used in the study of which 10 were displaced and 20 were undisplaced. Because there were many physicians assessing the imaging for the project, no raw numbers for detection of displacement were given. The authors found that CT imaging improved intraobserver and interobserver reliability of diagnosing scaphoid fracture displacement. This was significantly better than radiography alone. On CT scans, angular displacement of the fracture had the greatest interobserver reliability, followed by fracture gapping of more than 1 mm. With regard to radiographs, tilting of the lunate and a fracture gap of more than 1 mm had the highest interobserver reliability. When CT and radiographs were used together, interobserver reliability for angular displacement and fracture gapping improved further. The combination of imaging modalities led to an improved sensitivity and positive predictive value than when CT was used in isolation.

The caveat with this study was that displacement was never directly confirmed by arthroscopy.

Buijze et al. also compared the diagnostic performance characteristics of CT and radiographs when attempting to diagnose displacement in scaphoid fractures.[15] Of 44 scaphoid fractures, 22 were displaced and 22 were undisplaced. Radiography identified 11 of the 22 displaced fractures, whereas CT diagnosed 20 of 22 displaced fractures. This study used arthroscopy as the reference standard to confirm displacement intraoperatively. The authors stated that CT was a better imaging modality to identify fracture displacement. However, this study was subject to selection bias as radiographically displaced fractures were overrepresented.

Bhat et al. compared radiography and MRI in a total of 50 patients; 9 of 50 fractures were displaced.[18] MRI was used as the reference standard for displacement. Lateral intrascaphoid angles (LISAs) and height to length (H/L) ratios were assessed. The authors found it difficult to assess these measurements on MRI because the borders of the proximal and distal articular surfaces of the scaphoid were difficult to locate. Nevertheless, only three of the nine fractures, which were displaced on MRI, were identified as displaced on radiography.

Temple et al. compared plain radiographs with CTs in scaphoid fractures created in cadavers.[17] Thrity-three cadaveric wrists were divided into three equal groups: no fracture, undisplaced fracture, and displaced (>1 mm) fracture. The scaphoid fractures were stabilized with glue. The authors compared sensitivities and specificities between radiographs and CT in the sagittal plane for detecting displaced scaphoid fractures. Radiographic sensitivity and specificity were 52% and 84% (PPV 76%, NPV 63%), respectively, whereas the sensitivity and specificity of CT in the sagittal plane were 49% and 89% (PPV 81%, NPV 63%). The sensitivity was reduced for diagnosing displacement with CT because the authors only used sagittal reconstructions and therefore found it difficult to detect coronal displacement.

The final Level III study examined the effect of training on the interobserver reliability for the diagnosis of scaphoid fracture displacement.[19] This randomized trial assessed 64 surgeons' ability to detect displacement with both CT and radiographs of fractured scaphoids. Twenty fractures were assessed of which half were displaced. The sensitivity and specificity for detecting displacement in the nontraining group was 83% and 85%, respectively. In the trained group, this improved to 87% sensitivity and 86% specificity. There was a significant improvement in interobserver reliability with training.

There have been no studies comparing the accuracy between using CT and MRI to assess displacement in scaphoid fractures.

Evidence From Level IV Studies

There were 10 Level IV studies, which involved radiologic diagnosis of displacement in scaphoid fractures. A study in 25 patients using three-dimensional CT to assess displacement noted two types of translation or offset of the distal scaphoid fragment, volar and dorsal.[13] The volar type was associated with humpback deformities and axial rotation. Axial rotation specifically was found in 9 of 25 fractures in axial top views. The authors recommended that CT was the best radiologic assessment for displacement. The best views were the coronal and sagittal CT reconstructions.

Further studies comment on specific measures for displacement. The LISA and dorsal cortical angle (DCA) are quantitative measures of the humpback deformity in a scaphoid. The H/L ratio can also be measured. Sanders et al. describe an intrascaphoid angle of more than 35 degrees to be a displaced fracture.[9] However, this study only had three scaphoids for assessment. Nevertheless, this measurement has become accepted as the de facto assessment for angular displacement. Bain et al. used CT to measure the scaphoid humpback deformity in 37 scaphoids.[20] They noted that a DCA of greater than 160 degrees was abnormal. However, the authors found that there was poor intraobserver reliability when assessing LISA, moderate when assessing DCA, but excellent intraobserver reliability when assessing H/L ratio. Another study only recommended using H/L on CT because of the poor interobserver reliability when assessing DCA and LISA.[21] Berg et al. compared H/L of normal scaphoids to those of scaphoid fractures, which progress to nonunion.[22] A mean H/L of 0.61 (sagittal view) and 0.42 (coronal view) was found in nonunion cases compared with H/L of 0.65 (sagittal view) and 0.48 (coronal view) in normal scaphoids.

Buijze et al., as an addition to their arthroscopically determined scaphoid fracture displacement study, noted that radiographic comminution on CT was associated with operatively determined displacement.[23] This paper also explored the importance of differentiating between stability and displacement. They described instability as the potential for a fracture to displace. 38 scaphoid fractures were considered unstable, meaning that the fragments could be easily moved out of position arthroscopically; 27 scaphoid fractures were diagnosed as displaced on CT; 11 were thought to be undisplaced by CT imaging, but intraoperatively they were unstable. This paper was unique in that it broaches the topic of the undisplaced but unstable fracture, which has not been discussed in the literature previously.

The quantitative measurements of scaphoid displacement assessed on CT are difficult to measure on radiographs. A study in 36 patients examined several radiographic carpal alignment indices in wrists with scaphoid fractures.[24] The authors found that scapholunate and radiolunate angles had the highest reliability with respective intraclass correlation coefficients of 0.745 and 0.726 and may be used to assess scaphoid fracture displacement. However, no sensitivities or specificities were provided in the paper. Inagaki et al. explored the role of different radiographic views on assessing two types of displaced fractures, volar and dorsal displacement.[25] Oblique radiographs demonstrated volar displacement in 28 of 37 (76%) volar displaced fractures and dorsal displacement in 10 of 18 (56%) dorsal displaced fractures. The authors used CT as their reference standard to define displacement.

Recommended Sequences for Radiography, CT, and MRI

It is recommended that four projections are taken for radiography of the scaphoid. These are the posterior-anterior projection, lateral projection, oblique projections, and posterior-anterior projection in ulnar deviation of the wrist (elongated scaphoid projection). The oblique views should be performed in 45 degrees semipronated position to assess the scaphoid adjacent to the lunate and in 45 degrees semisupinated position to assess the proximal pole.[26]

For CT scans, it is recommended to take high-resolution images using 0.5-mm slices.[27] The scan should be viewed in bone windows and the entire scaphoid should be captured. With modern CT, multiplanar reconstruction is possible after data acquisition. Coronal and sagittal reconstructions in the plane of the longitudinal axis of the scaphoid are best to appreciate any fracture characteristics.[28]

For MRI, it is recommended that flux densities of 1.5 or 3.0 T and a gradient field strength of more than 15 mT/m are needed to investigate scaphoid fractures.[29,30] Slice thickness of 1.5 mm in an interleaved technique are required to not miss minimally displaced fractures. The aim of the sequences is to detect bone marrow edema. This makes MRI perfect for identifying undisplaced fractures, but more difficult to clearly define bony displacement. STIR (short tau inversion recovery) and TSE (turbo spin echo) sequences with T2 weighting are the recommended MRI protocols as both sequences highlight the bone marrow edema. The use of contrast medium aids assessment of nearby ligamentous structures such as the scapholunate ligament.

RECOMMENDATION

Displacement of scaphoid fractures is best assessed by a high-quality CT scan with bone windows and multiplanar reconstructions in the sagittal and coronal planes along the longitudinal axis of the scaphoid (overall quality: moderate).

PANEL 2
Author's Preferred Technique

In this case scenario, a CT scan was made to identify more clearly the degree and nature of displacement before operative intervention (Fig. 10.2). Based on the assessment of angulation, gap and translation treatment strategy was selected. The patient had internal fixation of the fracture using a headless compression screw after an open reduction (Fig. 10.3). The standard to investigate displacement of scaphoid fractures is high-resolution spiral CT of the wrist. With modern CT and reconstruction software, it is possible to manipulate the images in multiple planes and formulate a reconstruction of the bone. CT provides the necessary images for preoperative planning to occur. This allows the surgeon to select the best approach to fix the displaced scaphoid. The vast majority of published data on imaging in scaphoid fractures investigate occult fractures using MRI.[31] We do not believe that MRI is the best investigation for displaced fractures because the soft tissue edema seen will cloud the exact morphology of the fracture plane; however, a comparative study to assess the accuracy of MRI versus CT for diagnosing displacement of a scaphoid fracture has not been performed. We recommend good-quality radiography with sufficient views as an adequate initial investigation for displaced scaphoid fractures. However, to characterize the exact nature of displacement and adequately measure it, we recommend high-resolution CT.

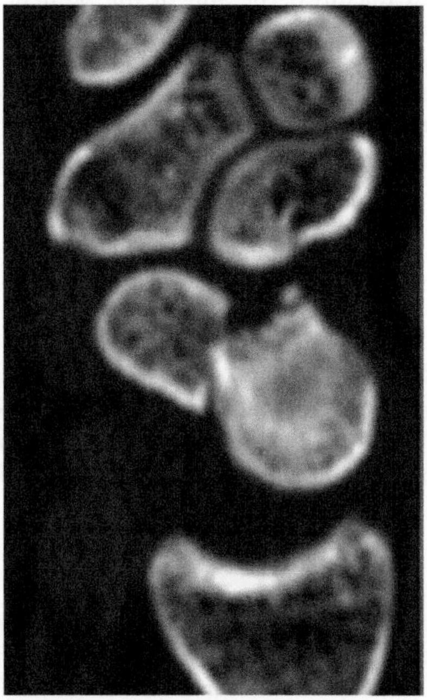

FIG. 10.2 Computerized tomography demonstrating the same scaphoid fracture from Fig. 10.1.

PANEL 3
Pearls and Pitfalls

PEARLS

1. Displacement of scaphoid fracture can be translation, gap, angulation, and rotation.
   a. Translation is measured as the maximum displacement of corresponding cortices in the coronal or sagittal planes.
   b. Gap is measured as the maximal distance between two corresponding fracture fragments.
   c. If either of these measures are 1 mm or more, then the fracture is considered displaced (or severely displaced if 2 mm or more).
2. Consider a high-resolution CT scan with postprocessing multiplanar reconstruction of the scaphoid in patients with appearance of displacement on any of the radiographic views of the scaphoid.
3. Height to length ratio has a higher interobserver reliability when measuring angular displacement.
   a. Angulation can be directly measured by the intrascaphoid angle, but because of poor interobserver reliability, the authors recommend indirect measurement of the angulation by calculating the height to length ratio.
4. Displaced fractures have a higher risk of nonunion.

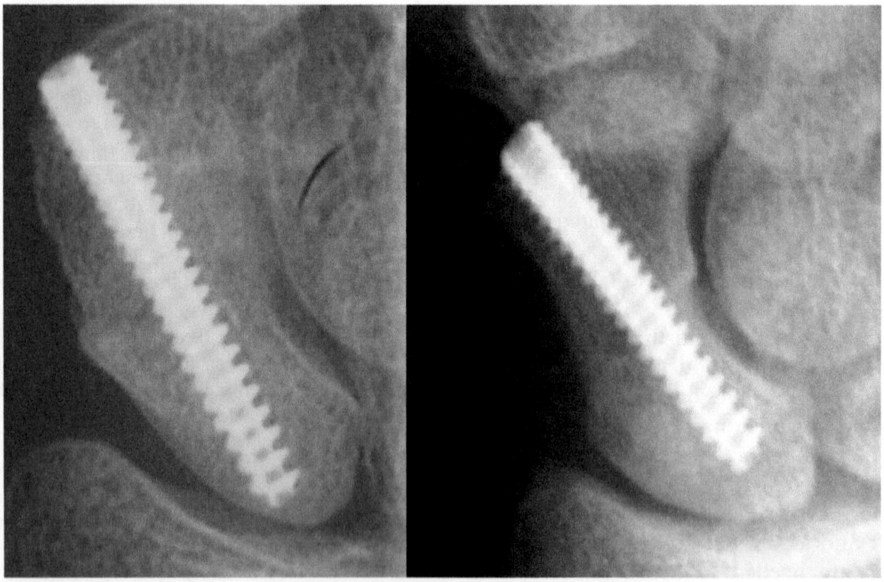

FIG. 10.3 Radiographs after open reduction and internal fixation.

PANEL 3
Pearls and Pitfalls—cont'd

PITFALLS

1. Even good-quality radiographs with sufficient views may miss revealing fracture displacement or its extent.
2. Correction of displacement during surgery can be technically challenging.
3. Displacement may be worsened during fixation if the screw is not perpendicular to the fracture plane or eccentrically positioned.

CONCLUSIONS

There is no universally agreed consensus in the literature regarding two key elements of the diagnosis of displacement in scaphoid fractures. Firstly, the best imaging modality to detect scaphoid fracture displacement is unclear because there are no high-level studies comparing MRI and CT. Secondly, there is no clear definition of displacement with regard to the measure of displacement on CT; some authors use 1 mm and others use 2 mm as a cutoff. The authors recommend high-resolution CT to delineate the fracture morphology and a gap or translation of 1 mm as a cutoff.

REFERENCES

1. Clay N, Dias J, Costigan P, et al. Need the thumb be immobilised in scaphoid fractures? A randomised prospective trial. *Bone Joint J*. 1991;73(5):828–832.
2. Cooney W, Dobyns JH, Linscheid RL. Fractures of the scaphoid: a rational approach to management. *Clin Orthop Relat Res*. 1980;149:90–97.
3. Thorleifsson R, Karlsson J, Sigurjonsson K. Fractures of the scaphoid bone A follow-up study. *Arch Orthop Trauma Surg*. 1984;103(2):96–99.
4. Szabo RM, Manske D. Displaced fractures of the scaphoid. *Clin Orthop Relat Res*. 1988;230:30–38.
5. Garala K, Taub N, Dias J. The epidemiology of fractures of the scaphoid. *Bone Joint J*. 2016;98(5):654–659.
6. Dias J, Singh H. Displaced fracture of the waist of the scaphoid. *J Bone Joint Surg Br*. 2011;93(11):1433–1439.
7. Buijze G, Goslings J, Rhemrev S, et al. Cast immobilization with and without immobilization of the thumb for nondisplaced and minimally displaced scaphoid waist fractures: a multicenter, randomized, controlled trial. *J Hand Surg*. 2014;39(4):621–627.
8. Eddeland A, Eiken O, Hellgren E, Ohlsson N-M. Fractures of the scaphoid. *Scand J Plastic Reconstruct Surg*. 1975;9(3):234–239.
9. Sanders WE. Evaluation of the humpback scaphoid by computed tomography in the longitudinal axial plane of the scaphoid. *J Hand Surg*. 1988;13(2):182–187.
10. Cooney 3rd W. Scaphoid fractures: current treatments and techniques. *Instr Course Lect*. 2002;52:197–208.
11. Amadio PC, Berquist TH, Smith DK, et al. Scaphoid malunion. *J Hand Surg*. 1989;14(4):679–687.
12. Burgess RC. The effect of a simulated scaphoid malunion on wrist motion. *J Hand Surg*. 1987;12(5):774–776.
13. Nakamura R, Imaeda T, Horii E, et al. Analysis of scaphoid fracture displacement by three-dimensional computed tomography. *J Hand Surg*. 1991;16(3):485–492.
14. Schmidle G, Rieger M, Klauser AS, et al. Intraosseous rotation of the scaphoid: assessment by using a 3D CT model—an anatomic study. *Eur Radiol*. 2014;24(6):1357–1365.
15. Buijze GA, Jørgsholm P, Thomsen NO, et al. Diagnostic performance of radiographs and computed tomography for displacement and instability of acute scaphoid waist fractures. *J Bone Joint Surg Am*. 2012;94(21):1967–1974.
16. Lozano-Calderón S, Blazar P, Zurakowski D, et al. Diagnosis of scaphoid fracture displacement with radiography and computed tomography. *J Bone Joint Surg Am*. 2006;88(12):2695–2703.
17. Temple CL, Ross DC, Bennett JD, et al. Comparison of sagittal computed tomography and plain film radiography in a scaphoid fracture model. *The J Hand Surg*. 2005;30(3):534–542.
18. Bhat M, McCarthy M, Davis T, et al. MRI and plain radiography in the assessment of displaced fractures of the waist of the carpal scaphoid. *Bone Joint J*. 2004;86(5):705–713.
19. Buijze GA, Guitton TG, van Dijk CN, Ring D. Training improves interobserver reliability for the diagnosis of scaphoid fracture displacement. *Clin Orthop Relat Res*. 2012;470(7):2029–2034.
20. Bain GI, Bennett JD, MacDermid JC, et al. Measurement of the scaphoid humpback deformity using longitudinal computed tomography: intra-and interobserver variability using various measurement techniques. *The J Hand Surg*. 1998;23(1):76–81.
21. Ring D, Patterson JD, Levitz S, et al. Both scanning plane and observer affect measurements of scaphoid deformity. *The J Hand Surg*. 2005;30(4):696–701.
22. ten Berg PW, Dobbe JG, Strackee SD, Streekstra GJ. Quantifying Scaphoid malalignment based upon height-to-length ratios obtained by 3-dimensional computed tomography. *J Hand Surg*. 2015;40(1):67–73.
23. Buijze GA, Jørgsholm P, Thomsen NO, et al. Factors associated with arthroscopically determined scaphoid fracture displacement and instability. *J Hand Surg*. 2012;37(7):1405–1410.
24. Roh YH, Noh JH, Lee BK, et al. Reliability and validity of carpal alignment measurements in evaluating deformities of scaphoid fractures. *Arch Orthop Trauma Surg*. 2014;134(6):887–893.
25. Inagaki H, Nakamura R, Horii E, et al. Differences in radiographic findings between scaphoid fracture patterns. *Hand Surg*. 2004;9(02):197–202.
26. Compson J, Waterman J, Heatley F. The radiological anatomy of the scaphoid Part 2: radiology. *J Hand Surg Br Eur Vol*. 1997;22(1):8–15.

27. Coblenz G, Christopoulos G, Fröhner S, et al. [Scaphoid fracture and nonunion: current status of radiological diagnostics]. *Der Radiol.* 2006;46(8):664. 666–676.
28. Mallee WH, Doornberg JN, Ring D, et al. Computed tomography for suspected scaphoid fractures: comparison of reformations in the plane of the wrist versus the long axis of the scaphoid. *Hand.* 2014;9(1):117–121.
29. Ring D, Lozano-Calderón S. Imaging for suspeced scaphoid fracture. *J Hand Surg.* 2008;33(6):954–957.
30. Yin Z, Zhang J, Kan S, Wang X. Diagnostic accuracy of imaging modalities for suspected scaphoid fractures. *J Bone Joint Surg Br.* 2012;94(8):1077–1085.
31. Mallee WH, Wang J, Poolman RW, et al. Computed tomography versus magnetic resonance imaging versus bone scintigraphy for clinically suspected scaphoid fractures in patients with negative plain radiographs. *Cochrane Libr.* 2012.

CHAPTER 11

Scaphoid Fracture Instability

PETER JØRGSHOLM, MD, PHD • ANDERS BJÖRKMAN, MD, PHD •
GEERT A. BUIJZE, MD, PHD • JAN-RAGNAR HAUGSTVEDT, MD, PHD

KEY POINTS

1. No imaging method can accurately predict scaphoid fracture stability.
2. Stability in a scaphoid fracture can be assessed by open or arthroscopic approach.
3. Fracture comminution has a strong correlation to instability.
4. Fracture displacement on radiographs or CT nearly always indicates instability.
5. CT scans have higher sensitivity than radiographs in diagnosing comminution and displacement.
6. An unstable scaphoid fracture has longer time to union when treated conservatively.

PANEL 1
Case Scenario

An 18-year-old right-handed male toolmaker crashed on his mountain bike. Following the injury he visited the emergency room complaining of radial-sided pain in his left wrist pain. According to the treating doctor and the radiologist, no sign of fracture was seen on initial X-rays (Fig. 11.1). He was treated with a dorsal splint and planned for orthopedic follow-up, but he never received any appointment and removed his splint after 2 weeks. Because of persistent pain, he was referred to a hand surgeon by his general practitioner 3 weeks following the initial injury.

Fluoroscan showed a scaphoid waist fracture and CT revealed a translunate arc injury (Box 11.1): a comminuted transverse scaphoid waist fracture, a volar chip fracture in the lunate, and a transverse fracture in the triquetrum (Fig. 11.2).

How can you determine whether this fracture is unstable?

How would this influence your decision for the most appropriate treatment?

IMPORTANCE OF THE PROBLEM

Stability of the fractured scaphoid as related to the prognosis for union has been debated because Herbert brought up his classification of scaphoid fractures: type A, acute stable fractures, and type B, acute unstable fractures[2] (Table 11.1). This evaluation was mainly assessed on four-view wrist radiographs and partly by open surgical evaluation.

Since then sophisticated radiologic modalities (CT) and minimally invasive surgery (arthroscopy) have gained increased popularity and made it possible to correlate these two investigations.

MAIN QUESTION

How can instability of a scaphoid fracture be diagnosed and how does it affect management?

Current Opinion

Grossly displaced scaphoid fractures are considered unstable and require reduction and internal fixation. However, current opinion varies among hand and orthopedic surgeons on when a scaphoid fracture is stable and could be treated conservatively.

Finding the Evidence

- **Cochrane Database:** "scaphoid fracture" 1; "scaphoid fracture instability" 0
- **Pubmed (systematic reviews):** "scaphoid fracture" 19; "scaphoid fracture instability" 1
- **Pubmed:** "scaphoid fracture" 2623; "scaphoid fracture instability" 265
- Articles that were not in English, French, or German were excluded.

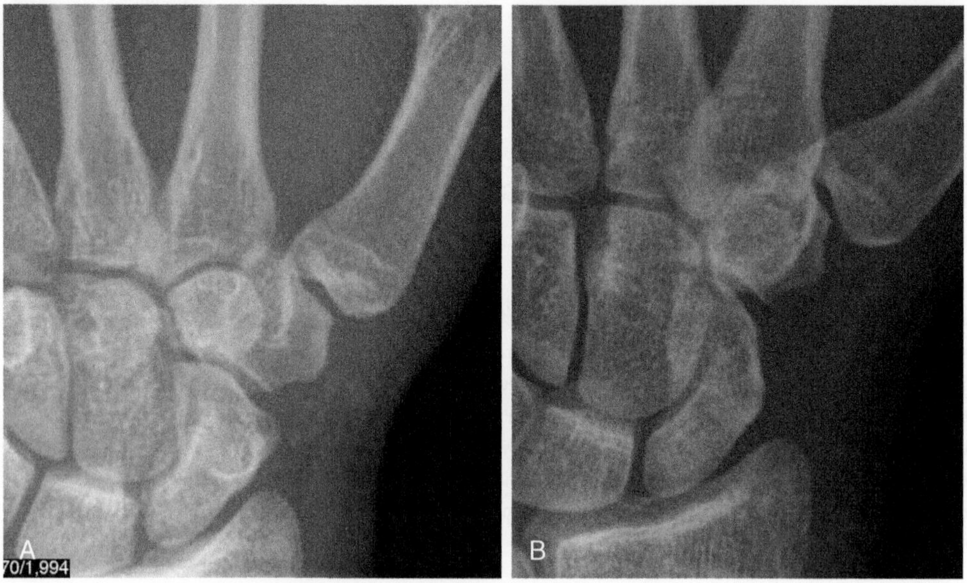

FIG. 11.1 Posterior anterior radiographs of left wrist. Six initial views all evaluated normal. **(A)** Plain Posterior anterior view. **(B)** Stecher's view (clenched fist and ulnar deviation).

BOX 11.1
Translunate Arc Injury

Biomechanically, combined scaphoid injuries have been explained as part of lesser or greater arc injuries. Lesser arc injuries are mainly ligament injuries and dislocations around the lunate, and greater arc injuries are mainly transcarpal fracture dislocations. As many variants of these injuries exist, and not all are explained by the lesser and greater arc theory, Bain and coworkers have proposed that translunate and inferior arc injuries should be added.[1]

Quality of the Evidence

Level III:
- Prospective diagnostic studies: 2

Level IV:
- Case series: 3

Level V:
- Expert opinion: 1

FINDINGS

CT is superior in assessing fracture displacement,[3,4] and it has been shown that displacement, angulation, and comminution significantly increase the time to union (CT verified) and are related to higher risks of nonunion.[5] The attributable risk of nonunion will approximately double for each half a millimeter the translation is increased (Fig. 11.3), reaching a clinically critical level with >1 mm of displacement. Displacement, angulation, and comminution "were independently significant in increasing the time required to achieve union and were shown to have an overall additive effect."[5]

In a prospective study comparing CT and arthroscopy, Buijze et al.[6] showed that radiographically displaced scaphoid waist fractures are almost always unstable (90%), but unstable fractures are not always radiographically displaced (54%). In another study on very much the same cohort, it was shown that fracture comminution was strongly correlated with fracture instability when assessed arthroscopically (Fig. 11.4).[7]

The incidence of displaced scaphoid fractures varies in different studies probably because of inconsistent definition of displacement and whether plain radiographs, CT, or MRI scans are used for diagnosis. Using radiographs the incidence varies from 5% to 25%,[8] using CT it is reported to be 19%,[5] and using MRI it is reported to be 17%.[9]

The incidence of comminuted scaphoid fracture is sparsely described. One partly retrospectively study on 80 scaphoid fractures with meticulous review of radiographs[10] had 9% comminuted fractures—all in the waist area—and using CT the incidence of comminution has been reported to be 13%.[5]

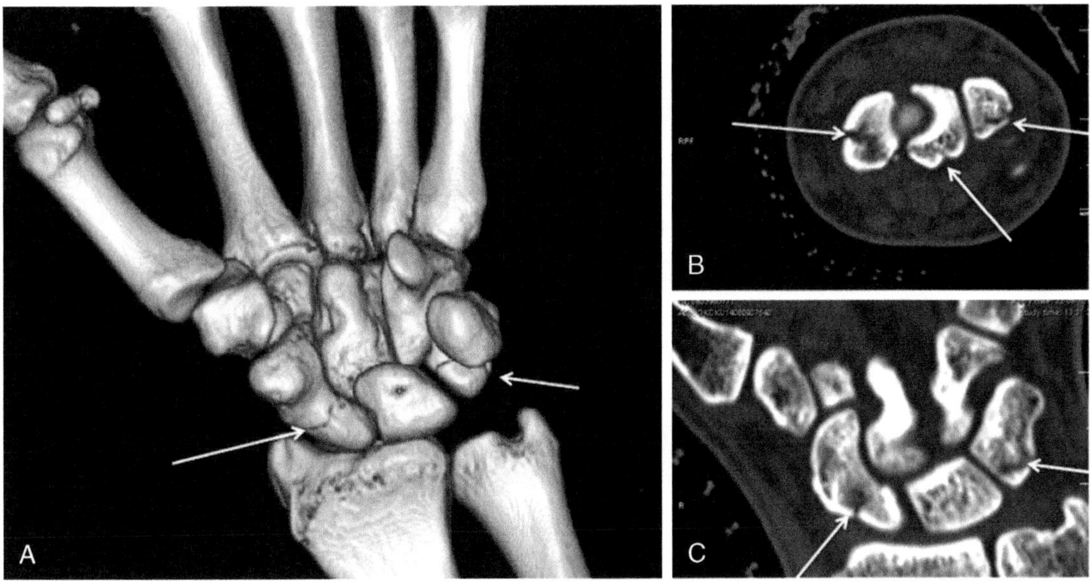

FIG. 11.2 A translunate arc injury. **(A)** Three-dimensional CT with the scaphoid and triquetral fractures (arrows) visible. **(B)** Transectional view showing all three fractures (arrows) (scaphoid, lunate, and triquetral fractures). **(C)** Coronal view showing scaphoid and triquetral fractures (arrows).

TABLE 11.1
Scaphoid Fracture: Herbert Classification

A	Acute, stable	**A1**	Tubercle
		A2	Nondisplaced crack in the waist
B	Acute, unstable	**B1**	Oblique, distal third
		B2	Displaced or mobile, waist
		B3	Proximal pole
		B4	Fracture dislocation
		B5	Comminuted

Adapted from Herbert TJ, Fisher WE. Management of the fractured scaphoid using a new bone screw. *J Bone Joint Surg Br*. 1984; 66(1):119; with permission.

The overall union rate for conservatively treated scaphoid fractures as evaluated by CT scans is found to be 95%.[5] Translation or fracture gap >1 mm or volar angulation >15 degrees is often used as a criterion for displacement and the diagnosis is best made by CT with reconstruction in the long axis of the scaphoid. Displacement is correlated to higher nonunion rate, and longer time to union and instability is often found in displaced fractures. Comminution is correlated to longer time to union and most often instability is found in comminuted fractures.

It is attempting to assume that stability of the fracture as seen by arthroscopy influences the time to union and ultimately nonunion in combination with all other factors (fracture location, adjacent ligament injury, concomitant fractures, time delay from injury, smoking, medication, age, etc.).

Reduction and internal fixation of displaced scaphoid fractures whether done open or arthroscopically has a high union rate but can be a technical challenge.[11-12]

Special attention is needed in case of combined scaphoid injuries. Scaphoid fractures in combination with other carpal fractures have been considered rare[13] and are mainly described as part of greater arc injuries or perilunate fracture dislocations,[14] most often involving high-energy trauma.[15] Studies with MRI have shown that the occurrence of more than one carpal fractures at the same time is not uncommon.[16] Furthermore, several variants of simultaneous carpal fractures without dislocation have been reported.[17-18] Herzberg has suggested a new classification of combined carpal injuries without dislocation and has proposed to call them perilunate injuries, not dislocated (PLIND)[19]; furthermore, he argues that these injuries initially could have been dislocated and spontaneously reduced

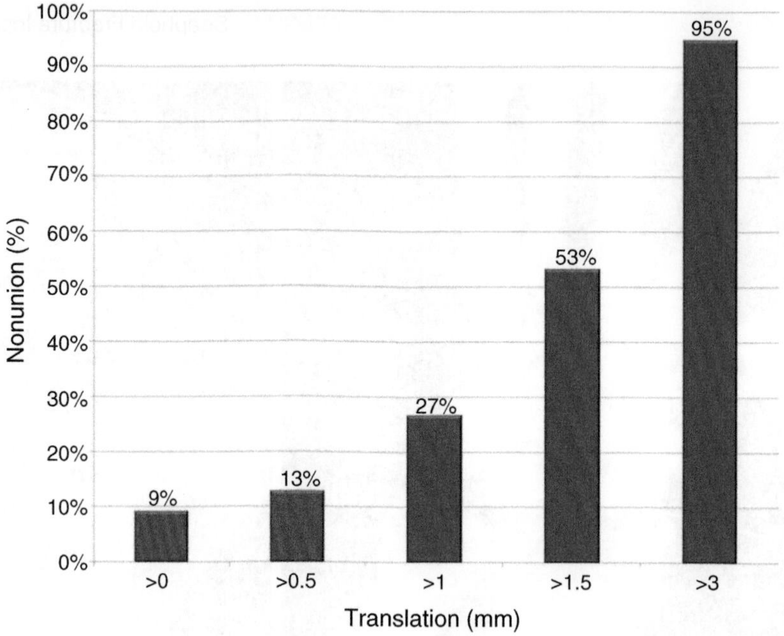

FIG. 11.3 Relationship between risk of nonunion (%) and fracture displacement (mm) in conservatively treated scaphoid fractures. Nonunion as seen by CT scan. (From Grewal R, Suh N, Macdermid JC. Use of computed tomography to predict union and time to union in acute scaphoid fractures treated nonoperatively. *J Hand Surg Am*. 2013;38(5):876; with permission.)

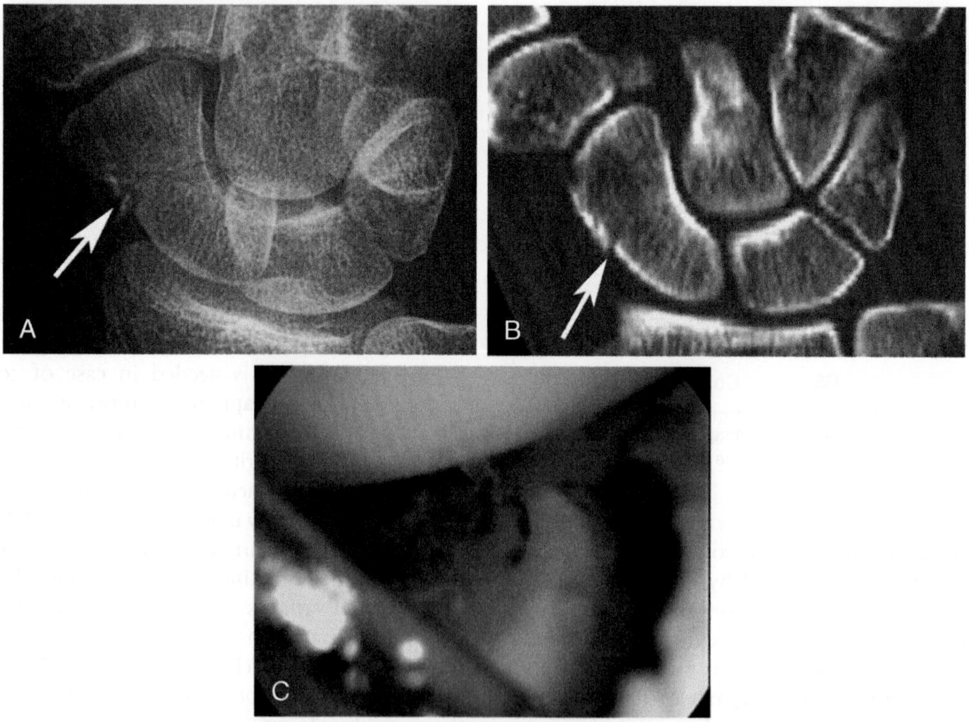

FIG. 11.4 **(A)** Radiographically comminuted (arrow) and **(B)** minimally displaced fracture (arrow) on CT. **(C)** Arthroscopically unstable. ((**A** and **B**) From Buijze GA, Jørgsholm P, Thomsen NO, et al. Factors associated with arthroscopically determined scaphoid fracture displacement and instability. *J Hand Surg Am*. 2012;37(7):1407; with permission.)

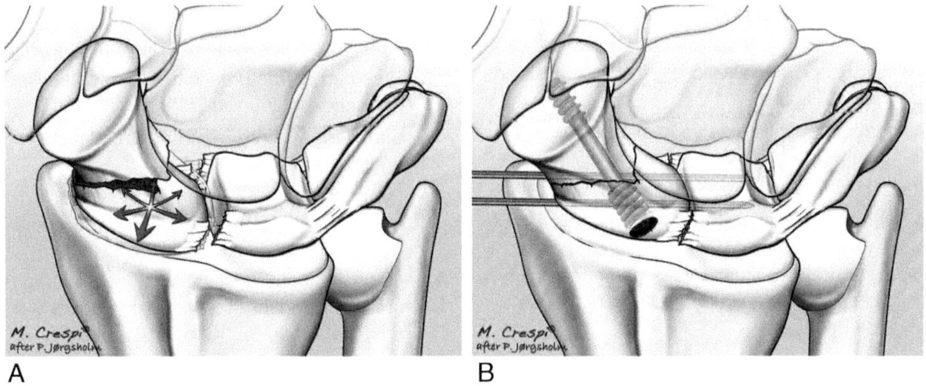

FIG. 11.5 **(A)** The combined unstable scaphoid waist fracture and complete scapholunate (SL) ligament rupture result in a "floating" (arrows) proximal scaphoid fracture fragment with minimal vascular supply. **(B)** Arthroscopy-assisted screw fixation of the scaphoid fracture and temporary percutaneous K-wire fixation of the SL joint. (Courtesy of P. Jørgsholm, MD, PhD, Kerteminde, Denmark.)

themselves. As instability is a prevalent issue, they often require reduction and internal fixation of fractures with temporary pinning of ligament injuries, which gives good union rates and reasonable results.[15,19] An example of a highly unstable PLIND injury is the combination of an unstable scaphoid fracture and a complete scapholunate (SL) ligament rupture, leading to a floating proximal scaphoid fragment (Fig. 11.5A).

Recommendation

In patients with intraarticular scaphoid fracture, CT is recommended to assess the fracture location and whether comminution or >1 mm displacement or >15 degrees angulation is evident (overall quality: moderate).

When a comminuted and/or displaced scaphoid fracture is found, the fracture is likely to be unstable and correlated with longer time to union and with a higher risk of nonunion, and the evidence suggests that open or arthroscopic-assisted reduction and internal fixation with cannulated screw provides good to excellent rates of union (overall quality: moderate).

When a proximal pole fracture is found, moderate instability is anticipated, and the evidence suggests that open or arthroscopic-assisted reduction and internal fixation with cannulated screw provides good to excellent rates of union (overall quality: moderate).

In case of severe instability as seen in transscaphoid perilunate fracture dislocations, a high risk of nonunion is expected when treated conservatively, and the evidence suggests that open or arthroscopic internal fixation with cannulated screw and temporary pinning of ligament injuries provide high rates of union (overall quality: low).

CONCLUSION

An unstable scaphoid fracture is ultimately diagnosed by arthroscopic or open surgical findings as no gold standard for noninvasive assessment exists. On the other hand, by using CT scans, one will get a rather good estimation of fracture stability: fracture comminution, >1 mm displacement, and >15 degrees humpback angulation are correlated to instability. Proximal pole fractures are surprisingly stable but have a tendency to open like a book. Unstable fractures have higher nonunion rates—most will unite by conservative treatment, but time to union may be significantly longer.

Most scaphoid fractures are nondisplaced and stable (approximately 75%) and can be successfully treated conservatively in a below-elbow cast with high rates of union at 6 weeks.

PANEL 2
Case Scenario Continued

COMBINED SCAPHOID FRACTURE (LUNATE ARC INJURY) CONTINUED:
A comminuted fracture in the scaphoid was observed and instability therefore likely. An arthroscopy was offered to estimate fracture stability and revealed an unstable scaphoid and lunate volar chip fracture (too small for osteosynthesis) and a stable triquetrum fracture. The scaphoid fracture was stabilized with an antegrade cannulated screw and the lunate and triquetrum fractures were treated conservatively with a thumb-spica below-elbow cast. The fractures were united as seen by CT at 9 weeks and cast treatment discontinued. The patient was able to return to part-time work at 12 weeks.

PANEL 3
Authors' Preferred Technique

1. Radiographs: Posterior anterior, lateral, and Stecher's projection (Fig. 11.5).
2. Dynamic fluoroscopic examination by treating physician (see paragraph 1, Panel 4).
3. Negative radiographs: MRI as soon as possible.
4. Positive radiographs and/or MRI: CT scan with 3D reconstruction.
5. In case of displacement more than 1 mm of diastasis or step-off, angulation more than 15 degrees, comminution present or proximal pole or perilunate injury arthroscopic-assisted reduction and percutaneous screw fixation (ARIF).
6. Proximal pole fractures (ARIF).
7. Transscaphoid perilunate dislocations (ARIF).
8. Pure carpal fractures with stable osteosynthesis do not need any immobilization.
9. Simultaneous intercarpal ligament lesions pinned and casted for 6–8 weeks.
10. Minimally and nondisplaced distal and waist fractures are treated in a below-elbow cast for 6 weeks.
11. Once 50% of the scaphoid shows evidence of union on CT discontinuation of cast treatment. If less than 50% united, repeat CT at 10 weeks.

PANEL 4
Pearls and Pitfalls

PEARLS

1. Fluoroscopic dynamic investigation of scaphoid fractures will give additional information on fractures' morphology and stability if CT is not available. Clenched fist and wrist rotation is particularly useful to visualize a fracture line similar to the technique in Stecher's view (Fig. 11.6).
2. Dorsal approach either with arthroscopy-assisted surgery, percutaneous K-wire placement, and screw insertion under fluoroscopic guidance alternatively by a miniarthrotomy makes correct screw placement more feasible. During maximum volar wrist flexion the K-wire is inserted as volar as possible and close to the SL ligament. Aiming K-wire toward thumb base facilitate central K-wire placement. A vertical traction device could be used for this and would even be helpful during reduction if necessary (Fig. 11.7).

PITFALLS:

1. Some waist fractures (one-fourth) have a complete scapholunate ligament injury[20] and are highly unstable with a floating proximal scaphoid fragment and often need K-wire fixation and/or cast treatment (Fig. 11.5).
2. Coronal fractures are unstable in a sliding manner and are difficult to reduce even openly. Twin small headless screw inserted dorsally perpendicular to the fracture line can stabilize such fractures (Fig. 11.8).

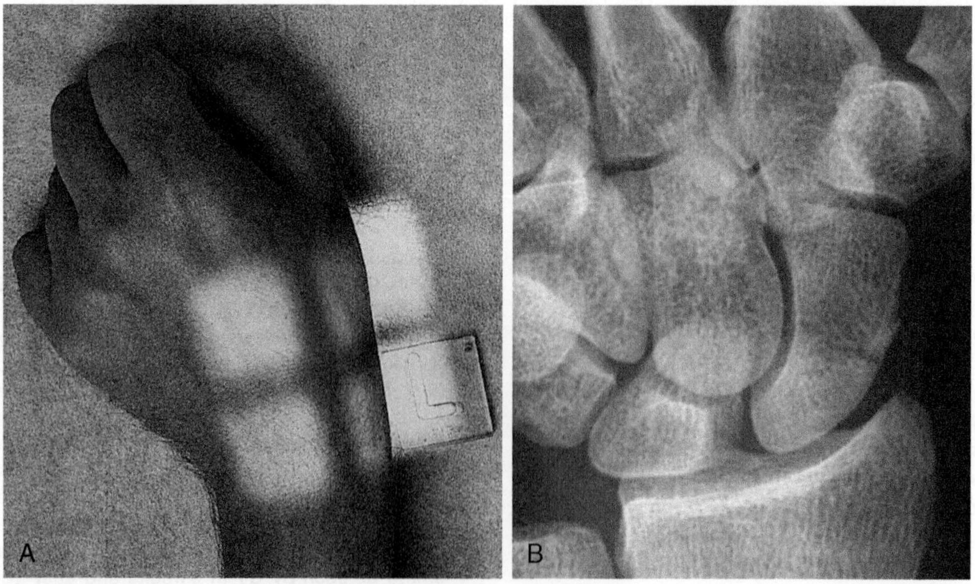

FIG. 11.6 Stecher's view: clenched fist and maximum ulnar deviation extend the scaphoid for paralleling X-ray beam to fracture plane and minimize a superimposing of the scaphoid. (A) Posterior anterior projection of ulnar deviated clenched fist. (B) The scaphoid extended and no superimposed carpal bones and fracture plane parallel to X-ray beam.

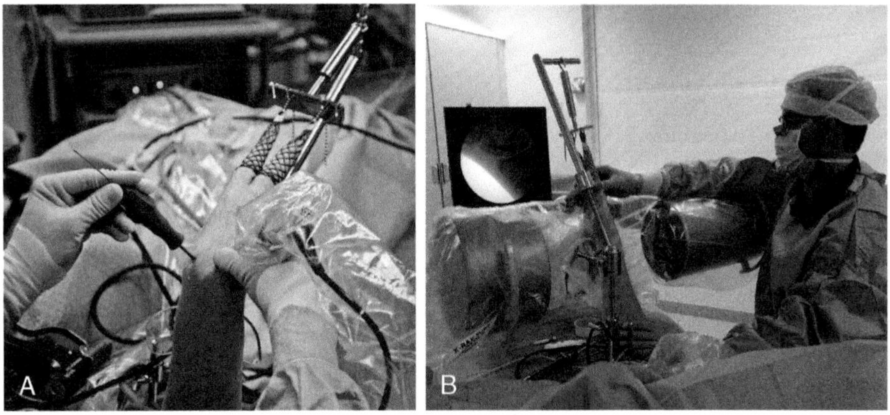

FIG. 11.7 Intraoperative settings for arthroscopy-assisted screw fixation of scaphoid fractures. **(A)** Wrist traction tower with the wrist in flexion to facilitate the dorsal insertion of the cannulated screw into the scaphoid. **(B)** Image intensifier designed for hand and wrist surgery used to check the placement of the screw. (From Jörgsholm, P. Scaphoid Fractures – epidemiology, diagnosis and treatment. Hand Surgery Research Group. Doctoral Dissertation Series; 2015:6 Lund University, Sweden; with permission.)

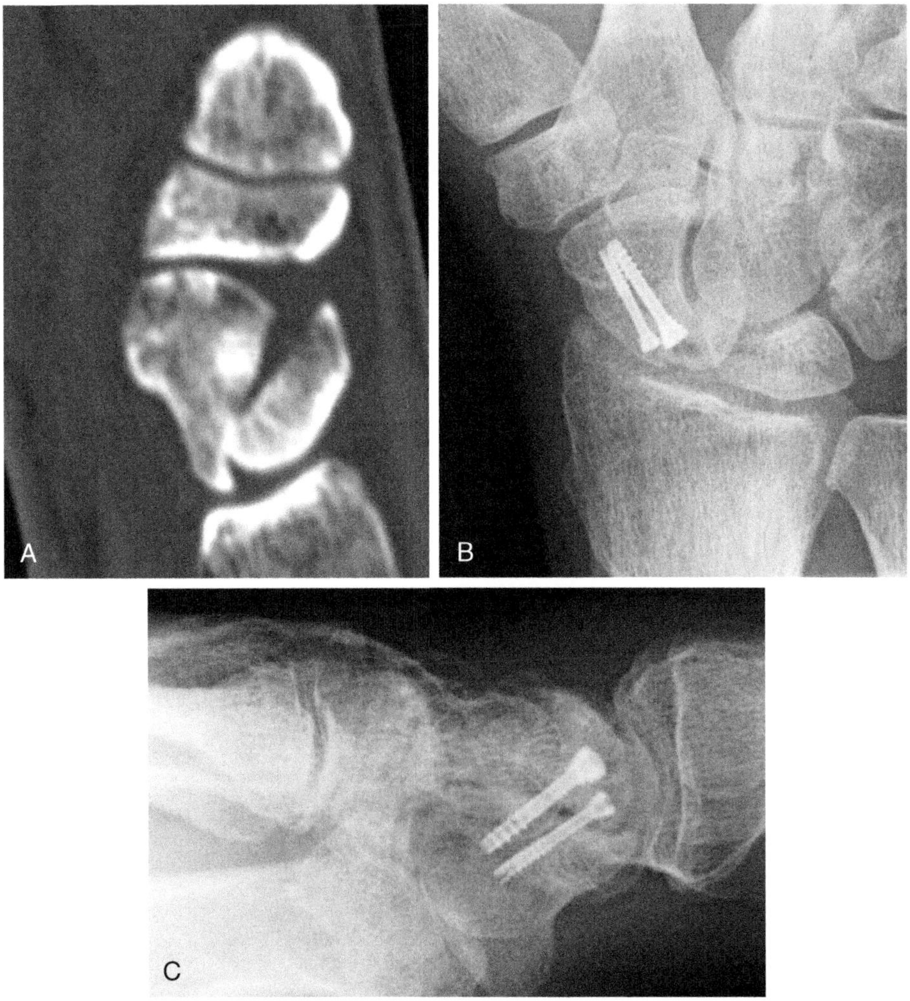

FIG. 11.8 Highly unstable coronal scaphoid fracture not recognized on initial radiographs. **(A)** Sagittal CT scan. Twin cannulated screws perpendicular to fracture plane. **(B)** PA view. **(C)** Lateral view.

REFERENCES

1. Bain GI, Pallapati S, Eng K. Translunate perilunate injuries-a spectrum of this uncommon injury. *J Wrist Surg.* 2013;2(1):63–68.
2. Herbert TJ, Fisher WE. Management of the fractured scaphoid using a new bone screw. *J Bone Joint Surg Br.* 1984;66(1):114–123.
3. Nakamura R, Imaeda T, Horii E, Miura T, Hayakawa N. Analysis of scaphoid fracture displacement by three-dimensional computed tomography. *J Hand Surg Am.* 1991;16(3):485–492.
4. Buijze GA, Wijffels MM, Guitton TG, Grewal R, van Dijk CN, Ring D. Interobserver reliability of computed tomography to diagnose scaphoid waist fracture union. *J Hand Surg Am.* 2012;37(2):250–254.
5. Grewal R, Suh N, Macdermid JC. Use of computed tomography to predict union and time to union in acute scaphoid fractures treated nonoperatively. *J Hand Surg Am.* 2013;38(5):872–877.
6. Buijze GA, Jørgsholm P, Thomsen NO, Björkman A, Besjakov J, Ring D. Diagnostic performance of radiographs and computed tomography for displacement and instability of acute scaphoid waist fractures. *J Bone Joint Surg Am.* 2012;94(21):1967–1974.
7. Buijze GA, Jørgsholm P, Thomsen NO, Björkman A, Besjakov J, Ring D. Factors associated with arthroscopically determined scaphoid fracture displacement and instability. *J Hand Surg Am.* 2012;37(7):1405–1410.
8. Singh HP, Taub N, Dias JJ. Management of displaced fractures of the waist of the scaphoid: meta-analyses of comparative studies. *Injury.* 2012;43(6):933–939.
9. Bhat M, McCarthy M, Davis TR, Oni JA, Dawson S. MRI and plain radiography in the assessment of displaced fractures of the waist of the carpal scaphoid. *J Bone Joint Surg Br.* 2004;86(5):705–713.
10. Compson JP. The anatomy of acute scaphoid fractures: a three-dimensional analysis of patterns. *J Bone Joint Surg Br.* 1998;80(2):218–224.
11. Trumble TE, Gilbert M, Murray LW, Smith J, Rafijah G, McCallister WV. Displaced scaphoid fractures treated with open reduction and internal fixation with a cannulated screw. *J Bone Joint Surg Am.* 2000;82(5):633–641.
12. Slade JF1, Lozano-Calderón S, Merrell G, Ring D. Arthroscopic-assisted percutaneous reduction and screw fixation of displaced scaphoid fractures. *J Hand Surg Eur Vol.* 2008;33(3): 350–354. http://dx.doi.org/10.1177/1753193408090121.
13. Apergis E, Darmanis S, Kastanis G, Papanikolaou A. Does the term scaphocapitate syndrome need to be revised? A report of 6 cases. *J Hand Surg Br.* 2001;26(5):441–445.
14. Mayfield JK, Johnson RP, Kilcoyne RK. Carpal dislocations: pathomechanics and progressive perilunar instability. *J Hand Surg Am.* 1980;5(3):226–241.
15. Herzberg G, Comtet JJ, Linscheid RL, Amadio PC, Cooney WP, Stalder J. Perilunate dislocations and fracture-dislocations: a multicenter study. *J Hand Surg Am.* 1993;18(5):768–779.
16. Jørgsholm P, Thomsen NO, Besjakov J, Abrahamsson SO, Bjorkman A. The benefit of magnetic resonance imaging for patients with posttraumatic radial wrist tenderness. *J Hand Surg Am.* 2013;38(1):29–33.
17. Robison JE, Kaye JJ. Simultaneous fractures of the capitate and hamate in the coronal plane: case report. *J Hand Surg Am.* 2005;30(6):1153–1155.
18. Buijze GA, Mudgal CS. Nondisplaced fractures of the proximal carpal row: case report. *J Hand Surg Am.* 2011;36(8):1310–1312.
19. Herzberg G. Perilunate injuries, not dislocated (PLIND). *J Wrist Surg.* 2013;2(4):337–345.
20. Jørgsholm P, Thomsen NO, Björkman A, Besjakov J, Abrahamsson SO. The incidence of intrinsic and extrinsic ligament injuries in scaphoid waist fractures. *J Hand Surg Am.* 2010;35(3):368–374.

CHAPTER 12

Surgical Versus Conservative Treatment for Nondisplaced Scaphoid Waist Fractures

BASTIAAN N.P. DE BOER, BSC • JOB N. DOORNBERG, MD, PHD • WOUTER H. MALLEE, MD • GEERT A. BUIJZE, MD, PHD

KEY POINTS

- Surgical and conservative treatments show no significant differences in long-term patient-based self-reported disability scores.
- Surgical treatment provides earlier return to work compared with conservative treatment; however, this applies to manual laborers only.
- Union rates are reproducibly high and complication rates consistently low for both treatment methods.
- Risks and short-term benefits of surgery should be carefully weighted in clinical decision-making.

PANEL 1
Case Scenario

A 36-year-old male entrepreneur visited the emergency department with complaints of moderate right wrist pain after a fall on his outstretched right dominant hand during a bike crash. Radiographs and CT show a minimally displaced scaphoid waist fracture (Fig. 12.1). On discussing the options of surgical and conservative treatment, the patient discloses that he is not eager to undergo surgery but would like to return to his desk-based labor as soon as possible. How can you best counsel the patient and manage his fracture considering his preferences?

IMPORTANCE OF THE PROBLEM

Surgical and conservative treatments for nondisplaced or minimally displaced scaphoid waist fractures are both reliable options with good comparable functional outcomes. In the past decades, there has been an increasing trend toward surgical treatment, but the question—is this evidence based? Time to return to work and sports are generally considered to be much shorter with surgical treatment. As many patients with scaphoid fractures are young and active, this may be important in decision-making.

MAIN QUESTION

When is operative treatment preferred over conservative treatment in nondisplaced or minimally displaced scaphoid waist fractures?

Current Opinion

There is no treatment superior for nondisplaced or minimally displaced scaphoid fractures. Different patients have different priorities regarding preferred treatment, which reflect pros and cons of both (e.g., risk of surgical complications vs. shorter time to return to work). There is controversy whether conservative or surgical treatment is favorable for an individual patient.[1] An ongoing tendency toward surgical treatment is observed, which can be partially explained by development in advanced surgical fixation technology. Surgical interventions for nondisplaced or minimally displaced scaphoid fractures have developed toward percutaneous (minimally invasive) fixation, usually performed with a headless cannulated compression screw. However, cast immobilization has

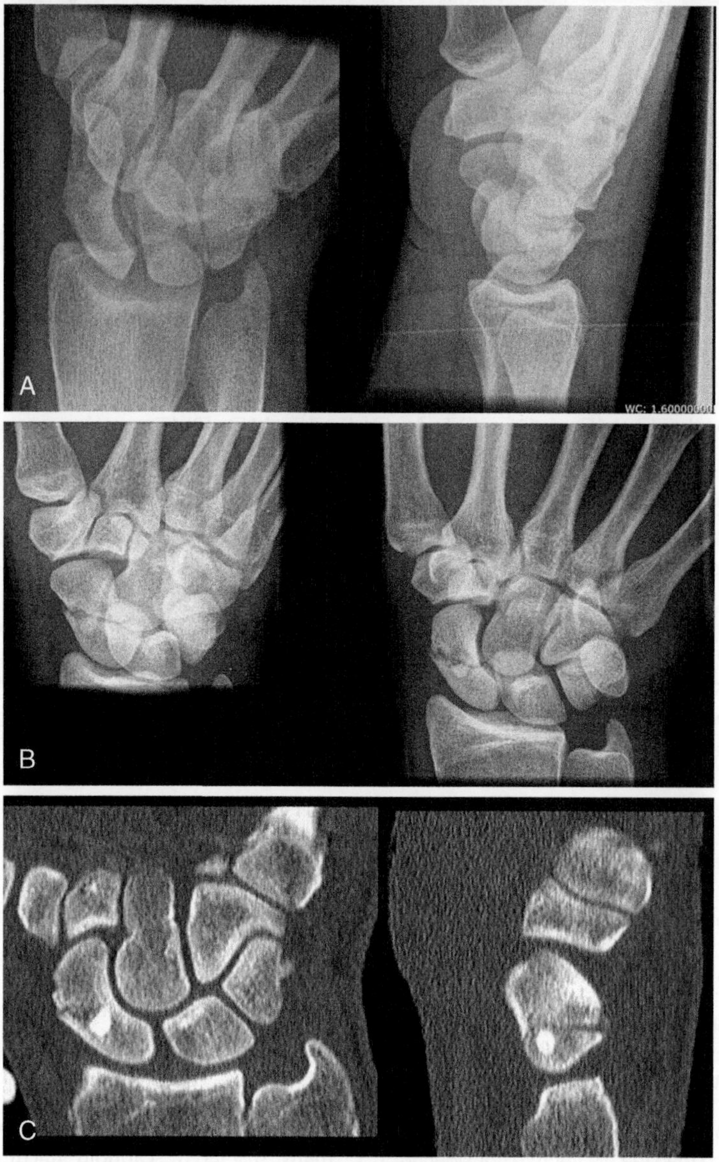

FIG. 12.1 **(A and B)** Radiographs and **(C)** CT show a minimally displaced scaphoid waist fracture.

also advanced toward less disabling treatment options—from above-elbow casting toward below-elbow casting with or without immobilization of the thumb, all displaying reproducibly high rates of union (90–100%).[2] To date there is limited evidence to support this tendency toward surgical treatment as we have previously reported.[1]

Finding the Evidence

- A systematic search was performed with the following terms: scaphoid* and fracture* and random*. Databases included the Cochrane Bone, Joint and Muscle Trauma Group Specialised Register, the Cochrane Central Register of Controlled Trials (CENTRAL), MEDLINE, EMBASE, CINAHL, and reference lists of articles.
- Bibliography of eligible articles.
- Articles that were not in English, French, or German were excluded.
- The search through the above databases was performed by a trained Cochrane librarian.

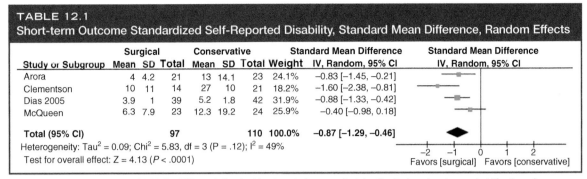

TABLE 12.1
Short-term Outcome Standardized Self-Reported Disability, Standard Mean Difference, Random Effects

Study or Subgroup	Surgical Mean	Surgical SD	Surgical Total	Conservative Mean	Conservative SD	Conservative Total	Weight	Standard Mean Difference IV, Random, 95% CI
Arora	4	4.2	21	13	14.1	23	24.1%	−0.83 [−1.45, −0.21]
Clementson	10	11	14	27	10	21	18.2%	−1.60 [−2.38, −0.81]
Dias 2005	3.9	1	39	5.2	1.8	42	31.9%	−0.88 [−1.33, −0.42]
McQueen	6.3	7.9	23	12.3	19.2	24	25.9%	−0.40 [−0.98, 0.18]
Total (95% CI)			**97**			**110**	**100.0%**	**−0.87 [−1.29, −0.46]**

Heterogeneity: $Tau^2 = 0.09$; $Chi^2 = 5.83$, df = 3 (P = .12); $I^2 = 49\%$
Test for overall effect: Z = 4.13 ($P < .0001$)

Standard Mean Difference IV, Random, 95% CI

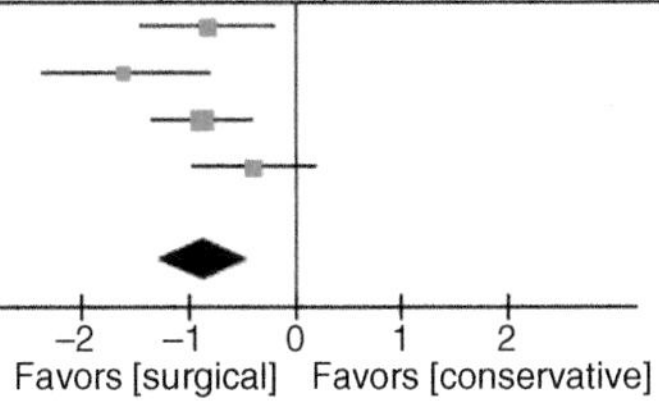

From de Boer BNP, Doornberg JN, Mallee WH, et al. Surgical treatment of non- and minimally-displaced acute scaphoid fractures favours over-conservative treatment but only in the short term: an updated meta-analysis. *J ISAKOS: Joint Disorders & Orthop Sports Med.* 2016;1(6):329–337; with permission.

Quality of the Evidence

Level I:

- Randomized controlled trials: 9

FINDINGS

This chapter only included randomized controlled trials and is an update of a previously published review concerning outcomes in surgical and conservative treatment for minimally and nondisplaced scaphoid waist fractures.[1] We compared two different groups of interventions. Surgical interventions encompass all open reduction and internal fixation or percutaneous (minimally invasive) fixation techniques. In general, fixation was performed with a headless cannulated compression screw.[3] Conservative intervention may include any form of cast immobilization, above- or below-elbow, with or without immobilization of the thumb.

Outcome Description

Functional outcome was based on validated—and/or standardized—function scores in both short- and long-term, including the Disabilities of the Arm, Shoulder and Hand (DASH) score, the Patient-Rated Wrist Evaluation (PWRE), the Patient Evaluation Measure (PEM), and the Modified Green and O'Brien score.[3–6]

Negative (adverse) outcomes included infection, malunion, nonunion, and avascular necrosis. Nonunion was defined as an absence of trabecular fracture healing at more than 6 months postinjury, with radiographic evidence. Outcomes between 16 weeks and 2 years were considered as short-term and outcomes over 2 years were considered as long-term.

Other outcome measures of this review were patient satisfaction, wrist pain, range of wrist motion, grip strength, time to union, time to return to work, resuming of previous activity, and financial costs. Pain was measured on a scale from 0 to 4 (with 0 as best and 4 as worst). Patient satisfaction was measured on a five-point scale.

Results on Functional Outcome

Of seven studies that reported on standardized functional outcomes, two studies reported long-term functional outcome (median follow-up of 7.8 and 10.2 years).[7,8] Three studies reported short-term functional outcome (median follow-up of 24 weeks and 1 year). One study reported both the short- and the long-term (median follow-up of 26 weeks and 6 years).[9] Short-term data showed significant difference in functional outcome, suggesting that surgical treatment was slightly favorable over conservative treatment in the short-term (Table 12.1).

The data of the functional outcome on the long-term revealed no significant difference (Table 12.2).

Secondary Outcomes

The rate of infection was reported in seven studies.[7,10–15] Five of seven analyzed studies reported no infections.[7,11,13–15] In the remaining studies, one infection occurred in the surgical intervention group[10,12]: two cases of superficial wound infection were both successfully treated with oral antibiotics (Table 12.3).

Seven studies reported on malunion as an outcome measure.[7,10–15] In two studies there were five cases of malunion.[10,11] All five cases occurred in the conservative intervention group. This difference, however, was not statistically significant (Table 12.4).

Nonunion was reported in six studies.[7,10,12–15] No significant difference between surgical and conservative treatments on the rate of nonunion was revealed (Table 12.5).

TABLE 12.2
Long-term Outcome Standardized Self-Reported Disability, Standard Mean Difference, Random Effects

	Surgical			Conservative				Standard Mean Difference
Study or Subgroup	Mean	SD	Total	Mean	SD	Total	Weight	IV, Random, 95% CI
Clementson	0	4.5	14	1	1.6	21	24.1%	−0.32 [−1.00, 0.36]
Dias 2008	10.3	1.7	35	9.9	2	36	37.6%	0.21 [−0.25, 0.68]
Vinnars 2008	4.5	1	40	5	1.5	35	38.3%	−0.39 [−0.85, 0.06]
Total (95% CI)			**89**			**92**	**100.0%**	**−0.15 [−0.55, 0.26]**

Heterogeneity: Tau^2 = 0.06; Chi^2 = 3.63, df = 2 (P = .16); I^2 = 45%
Test for overall effect: Z = 0.71 (P = .48)

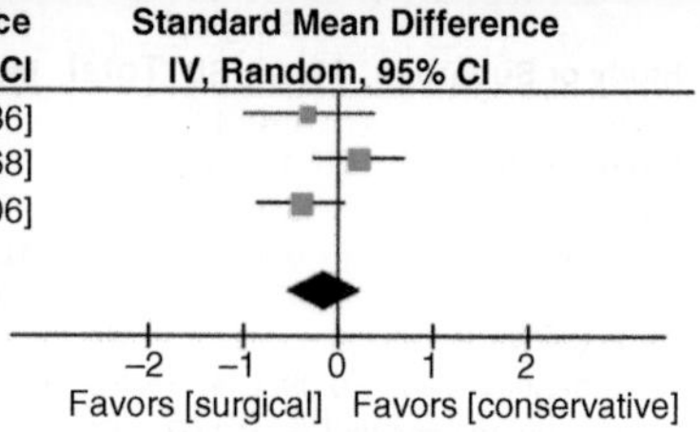

From de Boer BNP, Doornberg JN, Mallee WH, et al. Surgical treatment of non- and minimally-displaced acute scaphoid fractures favours over-conservative treatment but only in the short term: an updated meta-analysis. *J ISAKOS: Joint Disorders & Orthop Sports Med.* 2016;1(6):329–337; with permission.

TABLE 12.3
Rate of Infection, Risk Ratio, Random Effects

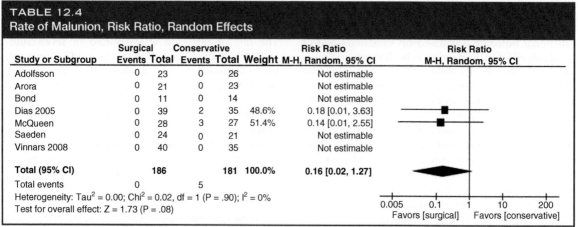

	Surgical		Conservative			Risk Ratio
Study or Subgroup	Events	Total	Events	Total	Weight	M-H, Random, 95% CI
Adolfsson	0	23	0	26		Not estimable
Arora	1	21	0	23	50.4%	3.27 [0.14, 76.21]
Bond	0	11	0	14		Not estimable
Dias 2005	1	39	0	42	49.6%	3.23 [0.14, 76.90]
McQueen	0	28	0	27		Not estimable
Saeden	0	24	0	21		Not estimable
Vinnars 2008	0	40	0	35		Not estimable
Total (95% CI)		**186**		**188**	**100.0%**	**3.25 [0.35, 30.34]**
Total events	2		0			

Heterogeneity: Tau^2 = 0.00; Chi^2 = 0.00, df = 1 (P = .99); I^2 = 0%
Test for overall effect: Z = 1.03 (P = .30)

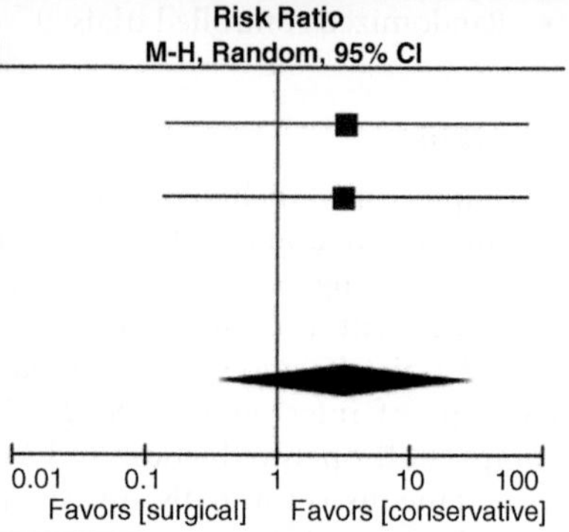

From de Boer BNP, Doornberg JN, Mallee WH, et al. Surgical treatment of non- and minimally-displaced acute scaphoid fractures favours over-conservative treatment but only in the short term: an updated meta-analysis. *J ISAKOS: Joint Disorders & Orthop Sports Med.* 2016;1(6):329–337; with permission.

TABLE 12.4
Rate of Malunion, Risk Ratio, Random Effects

	Surgical		Conservative			Risk Ratio
Study or Subgroup	Events	Total	Events	Total	Weight	M-H, Random, 95% CI
Adolfsson	0	23	0	26		Not estimable
Arora	0	21	0	23		Not estimable
Bond	0	11	0	14		Not estimable
Dias 2005	0	39	2	35	48.6%	0.18 [0.01, 3.63]
McQueen	0	28	3	27	51.4%	0.14 [0.01, 2.55]
Saeden	0	24	0	21		Not estimable
Vinnars 2008	0	40	0	35		Not estimable
Total (95% CI)		**186**		**181**	**100.0%**	**0.16 [0.02, 1.27]**
Total events	0		5			

Heterogeneity: Tau^2 = 0.00; Chi^2 = 0.02, df = 1 (P = .90); I^2 = 0%
Test for overall effect: Z = 1.73 (P = .08)

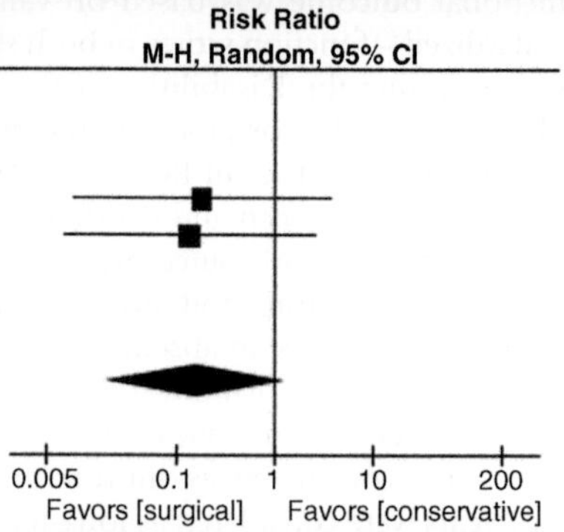

From de Boer BNP, Doornberg JN, Mallee WH, et al. Surgical treatment of non- and minimally-displaced acute scaphoid fractures favours over-conservative treatment but only in the short term: an updated meta-analysis. *J ISAKOS: Joint Disorders & Orthop Sports Med.* 2016;1(6):329–337; with permission.

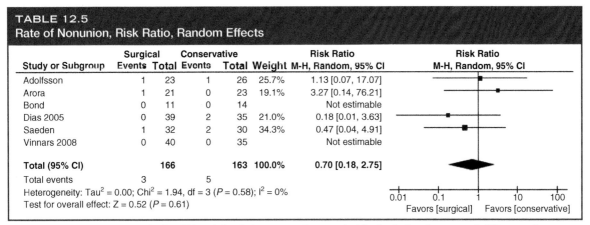

TABLE 12.5
Rate of Nonunion, Risk Ratio, Random Effects

Study or Subgroup	Surgical Events	Surgical Total	Conservative Events	Conservative Total	Weight	Risk Ratio M-H, Random, 95% CI
Adolfsson	1	23	1	26	25.7%	1.13 [0.07, 17.07]
Arora	1	21	0	23	19.1%	3.27 [0.14, 76.21]
Bond	0	11	0	14		Not estimable
Dias 2005	0	39	2	35	21.0%	0.18 [0.01, 3.63]
Saeden	1	32	2	30	34.3%	0.47 [0.04, 4.91]
Vinnars 2008	0	40	0	35		Not estimable
Total (95% CI)		**166**		**163**	**100.0%**	**0.70 [0.18, 2.75]**
Total events	3		5			

Heterogeneity: $Tau^2 = 0.00$; $Chi^2 = 1.94$, $df = 3$ ($P = 0.58$); $I^2 = 0\%$
Test for overall effect: $Z = 0.52$ ($P = 0.61$)

Risk Ratio M-H, Random, 95% CI

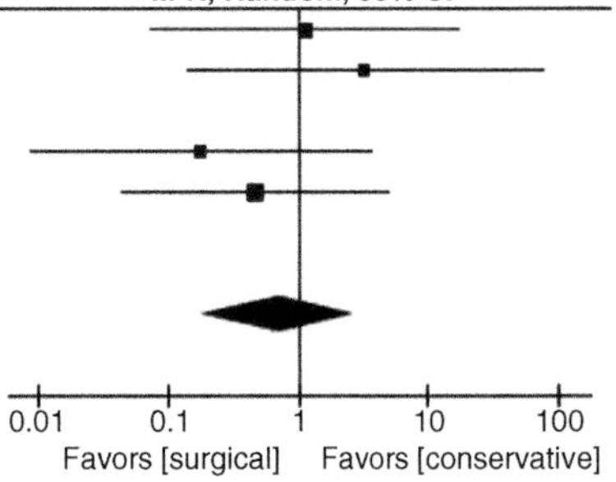

From de Boer BNP, Doornberg JN, Mallee WH, et al. Surgical treatment of non- and minimally-displaced acute scaphoid fractures favours over-conservative treatment but only in the short term: an updated meta-analysis. *J ISAKOS: Joint Disorders & Orthop Sports Med.* 2016;1(6):329–337; with permission.

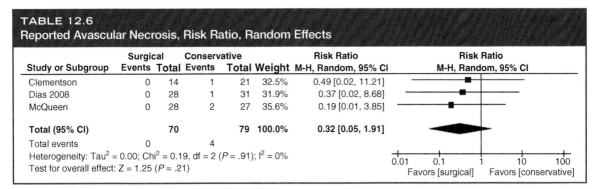

TABLE 12.6
Reported Avascular Necrosis, Risk Ratio, Random Effects

Study or Subgroup	Surgical Events	Surgical Total	Conservative Events	Conservative Total	Weight	Risk Ratio M-H, Random, 95% CI
Clementson	0	14	1	21	32.5%	0.49 [0.02, 11.21]
Dias 2008	0	28	1	31	31.9%	0.37 [0.02, 8.68]
McQueen	0	28	2	27	35.6%	0.19 [0.01, 3.85]
Total (95% CI)		**70**		**79**	**100.0%**	**0.32 [0.05, 1.91]**
Total events	0		4			

Heterogeneity: $Tau^2 = 0.00$; $Chi^2 = 0.19$, $df = 2$ ($P = .91$); $I^2 = 0\%$
Test for overall effect: $Z = 1.25$ ($P = .21$)

Risk Ratio M-H, Random, 95% CI

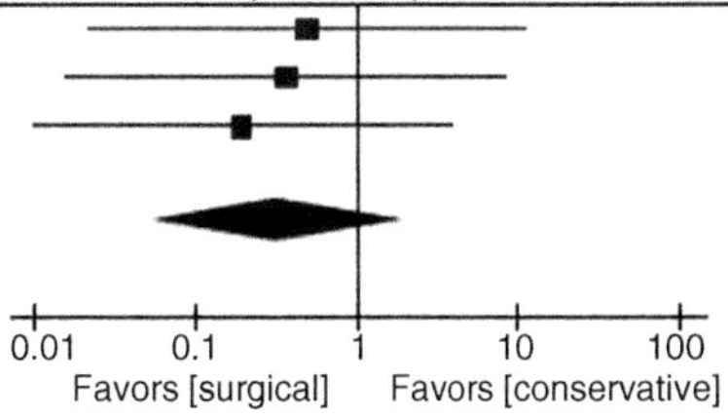

From de Boer BNP, Doornberg JN, Mallee WH, et al. Surgical treatment of non- and minimally-displaced acute scaphoid fractures favours over-conservative treatment but only in the short term: an updated meta-analysis. *J ISAKOS: Joint Disorders & Orthop Sports Med.* 2016;1(6):329–337; with permission.

In three studies, avascular necrosis was assessed.[8,9,11] No events of avascular necrosis were reported in the surgical intervention group, and avascular necrosis was reported in 4 of 79 patients in the conservative intervention group. This difference was not significant (Table 12.6).

In Favor of Conservative Treatment

One study[10] reported wrist pain; it showed a significant difference in favor of conservative treatment, $P<.0001$; the standard mean difference was 2.06 (range, 1.06–3.07).

In Favor of Surgical Treatment

Patient satisfaction was assessed in one study.[13] In this study there was a significant difference in favor of surgical treatment, $P<.0001$. The standard mean difference was 2.06 (range, 1.06–3.07).

A significant difference in time to union was reported in three studies in favor of surgical treatment.[11–13] The standard mean difference was −4.80 (weeks) (range, −5.15 to −4.44).

Five studies reported a significant difference in time to return to work, in favor of surgical treatment.[11–13,15,16] The mean difference was −7.04 (weeks) (range, −7.57 to −6.50).

In grip strength there was also a significant difference in favor of surgical treatment, according to six studies.[7,10–13,15] The standard mean difference of the loss of grip strength was −2.59% (range, −4.24 to −0.94).

Equivalence Between Surgical and Conservative Treatment

Seven studies reported range of wrist motion.[7,9–13,15] They showed no significant difference and a strong heterogeneity among the data because of different techniques of measuring the grip strength.

Two studies reported financial costs and no significant difference was found.[12,16]

RECOMMENDATION

In patients with a nondisplaced or minimally displaced scaphoid waist fracture, the evidence suggests the following:

- Short-term patient-based functional outcome slightly favors surgical treatment, although this may not be considered a minimal clinical important difference (overall quality: high).
- Long-term patient-based functional outcomes are equivalent (overall quality: high).
- Union rates are reproducibly high and complication rates are consistently low for both treatment methods (overall quality: high).
- Return to work is significantly faster in surgical treatment; however, this applies to manual laborers only (overall quality: high).

CONCLUSION

Perhaps the most clinically relevant advantage of surgical treatment of nondisplaced or minimally displaced scaphoid fractures is a significant earlier return to work for manual workers, with a standard mean difference of 7 weeks. It may explain increased (short-term) satisfaction, as well as the slightly better short-term functional outcome, because long-term wrist (as well as thumb) immobilization equally results in more weeks of—transient—joint stiffness and disability after cast removal. An earlier return to work is an important factor for the absence of difference in costs—from a societal perspective—the costs of surgery are weighed out by a reduced loss of work productivity.

PANEL 2
Authors' Preferred Techniques

In follow-up of the case, we prefer a shared decision-making approach. Because the patient had a substantial preference for conservative treatment and performs desk-based labor, we opted for a below-elbow cast without immobilization of the thumb, enabling him to perform his main daily activities, such as typing and writing. Additionally, we offered an optional conversion to surgical treatment within 2 weeks if he would experience considerable loss of productivity due to the cast. After 10 weeks, the patient was no longer tender and a CT confirmed that just over half of the fracture was consolidated (partial union, Fig. 12.2). The cast was discontinued and the patient was followed-up until radiographic union was confirmed at 6 months (Fig. 12.3).

Conservative treatment is still considered the mainstay of treatment of nondisplaced and minimally displaced scaphoid waist fractures. However, to achieve a reliably high union rate, in our opinion, it is imperative to rule out displacement. In shared decision-making, the clinician and the patient can carefully consider the differences between conservative and operative treatments. Patients who are professionally dependent on the function of their wrist, such as (light) manual laborers, musicians, and athletes, may consider operative treatment. For those who are not professionally dependent on the function of their wrist, we would favor conservative treatment.

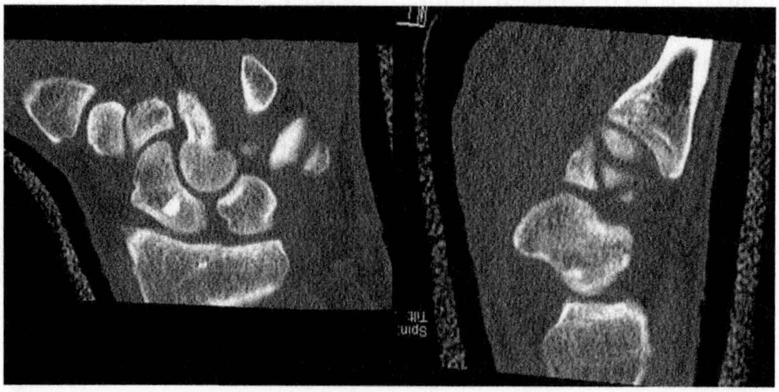

FIG. 12.2 A 10-week CT scan shows trabecular bridging just over half of the fracture site.

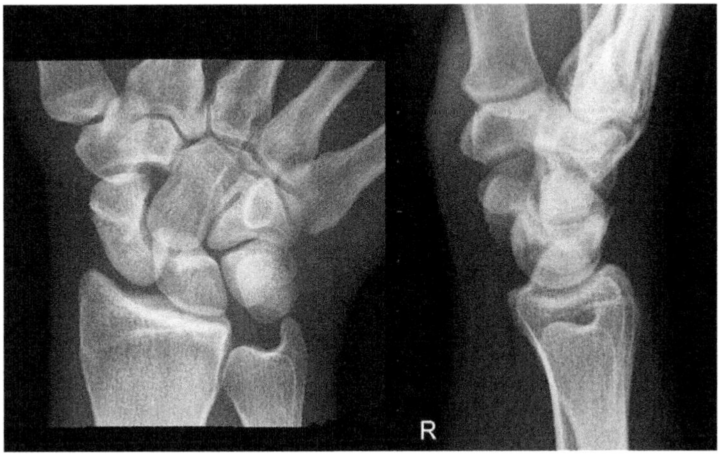

FIG. 12.3 Six-month radiographs confirm union.

PANEL 3
Pearls and Pitfalls

PEARLS

- All patients with nondisplaced and minimally displaced scaphoid waist fractures qualify for conservative treatment; surgical intervention may be performed in a select population with preference for early restoration of manual ability.
- The vast majority (>95%) of CT-scan confirmed nondisplaced and minimally displaced scaphoid waist fractures continue to union following conservative treatment, even if a follow-up CT scan at 6–12 weeks shows delayed union.
- Decision-making for either conservative or surgical treatment is preferably done by carefully weighing the optional benefits of surgical fixation and risks of surgery with each individual patient.

PITFALLS

- Displaced fractures may seem nondisplaced on radiographs only and have a poorer union rate with conservative treatment. In case of any doubt (anything more than a simple crack), CT is highly recommended.
- Surgical treatment of scaphoid fractures can be risky in the absence of adequate training or experience.

REFERENCES

1. Buijze GA, Doornberg JN, Ham JS, et al. Surgical compared with conservative treatment for acute nondisplaced or minimally displaced scaphoid fractures: a systematic review and meta-analysis of randomized controlled trials. *J Bone Joint Surg Am*. 2010;92(6):1534–1544. http://dx.doi.org/10.2106/JBJS.I.01214. [published Online First: 2010/06/03].
2. Buijze GA, Goslings JC, Rhemrev SJ, et al. Cast immobilization with and without immobilization of the thumb for nondisplaced and minimally displaced scaphoid waist fractures: a multicenter, randomized, controlled trial. *J Hand Surg Am*. 2014;39(4):621–627. http://dx.doi.org/10.1016/j.jhsa.2013.12.039.
3. Kwok IH, Leung F, Fau - Yuen G, Yuen G. Assessing results after distal radius fracture treatment: a comparison of objective and subjective tools. *Geriatr Orthop Surg Rehabil*. 2011. http://dx.doi.org/10.1177/2151458511422701. PMC3597314.
4. Gumesson C, Atroshi I, Ekdahl C. The disabilities of the arm, shoulder and hand (DASH) outcome questionnaire: longitudinal construct validity and measuring self-rated health change after surgery. *BMC Musculoskelet Disord*. 2003.
5. Bialocerkowski A. Patient rated wrist evaluation. *Aust J Physiother*. 2008;54(3):221. http://dx.doi.org/10.1016/s0004-9514(08)70035-7.
6. MacDermid JC. *The Patient-rated Wrist Evaluation (PRWE)© User Manual*. Hamilton: McMaster University; 2007.
7. Vinnars B, Pietreanu M, Bodestedt A, et al. Nonoperative compared with operative treatment of acute scaphoid fractures. A Randomized Clinical Trial. *The J Bone Joint Surgery Am Volume*. 2008;90(6):1176–1185. http://dx.doi.org/10.2106/JBJS.G.00673.
8. Dias J, Dhukaram V, Abhinav A, et al. Clinical and radiological outcome of cast immobilisation versus surgical treatment of acute scaphoid fractures at a mean follow-up of 93 months. *JBJS*. 2008. http://dx.doi.org/10.1302/0301-620X.90B7.

9. Clementson M, Jorgsholm P, Besjakov J, et al. Conservative treatment versus arthroscopic-assisted screw fixation of scaphoid waist fractures-a randomized trial with minimum 4-year follow-up. *J Hand Surg*. 2015. http://dx.doi.org/10.1016/j.jhsa.2015.03.007.
10. Dias JJ, Wildin CJ, Bhowal B, et al. Should acute scaphoid fractures be fixed A randomized controlled trial. *J Bone Joint Surg Am*. 2005.
11. McQueen M, Gelbke M, Wakefield A, et al. Percutaneous screw fixation versus conservative treatment for fractures of the waist of the scaphoid: a prospective randomised study. *J Bone Joint Surg Br*. 2007. http://dx.doi.org/10.1302/0301-620X.90B1.
12. Arora R, Gschwentner M, Krappinger D, et al. Fixation of nondisplaced scaphoid fractures: making treatment cost effective. Prospective controlled trial. *Arch Orthop Trauma Surg*. 2007;127(1):39–46. http://dx.doi.org/10.1007/s00402-006-0229-z.
13. Bond C, Shin A, McBride M, et al. Percutaneous screw fixation or cast immobilization for nondisplaced scaphoid fractures. *JBJS*. 2001;83-A(4).
14. Adolfsson L, Lindau T, Arner M. Acutrak screw fixation versus cast Immobiliastion for undisplaced scaphoid waist fractures. *J Hand Surgery*. 2001. British and European Volume.
15. Saeden B, Tornkvist H, Ponzer S, et al. Fracture of the carpal scaphoid. A prospective, randomised 12-year follow-up comparing operative and conservative treatment. *J Bone Joint Surg Br*. 2001;83.
16. Vinnars B, Ekenstam F, Gerdin B. Comparison of direct and indirect costs of internal fixation and cast treatment in acute scaphoid fractures: a randomized trial involving 52 patients. *Acta Orthop*. 2007;78(5):672–679. http://dx.doi.org/10.1080/17453670710014383.

CHAPTER 13

Conservative Treatment of Nondisplaced and Minimally Displaced Scaphoid Waist Fractures

JORIS P. COMMANDEUR, MD • STEVEN J. RHEMREV, MD, PHD • FRANK J.P. BEERES, MD, PHD

KEY POINTS

- The outcome of treating nondisplaced and minimally displaced waist scaphoid fractures with a below-elbow cast is similar to treatment with an above-elbow cast.
- The outcome of treating nondisplaced and minimally displaced waist scaphoid fractures in a cast without immobilization of the thumb is similar to a treatment with a scaphoid cast (including the thumb).
- Immobilization can be done in neutral position or in 20 degrees extension of the wrist, which is preferred over immobilization in 20 degrees flexion of the wrist.
- Traditional immobilization periods for nondisplaced and minimally displaced scaphoid waist fractures range between 6 and 12 weeks, but recent evidence suggests that 4–6 weeks of immobilization may be enough for most cases.

PANEL 1
Case Scenario

A 40-year-old healthy man (*Patient A*) and a 45-year-old man (*Patient B*) visit the emergency department with complaints of the right wrist after a cycling fall and a fall on the outstretched hand from standing height, respectively. Radiographs of both patients show a minimally (<1 mm) displaced waist fracture of the scaphoid (Figs. 13.1 and 13.2).

Patient A works as a window cleaner and *Patient B* does not perform manual labor. When deciding for a conservative treatment, exactly in what type of cast and for how long will you immobilize each patient?

IMPORTANCE OF THE PROBLEM

In contrast to the low nonunion rate (0%–1%) of fractures of the distal third of the scaphoid, the nonunion rate of nondisplaced and minimally displaced scaphoid fractures in the proximal and middle third is considerably higher. In his review, Beeres et al. describe a nonunion rate of 36% in proximal pole fractures.[1] Nonunion rates of 0%–10% in nondisplaced and minimally displaced waist fractures have been described after conservative treatment.[2,3] To confirm union of a scaphoid fracture, conventional radiographs and CT are often used.[4,5] However, there is no consensus for the use of a CT for the diagnosis of early union.[4–6]

Adequate treatment has to be started as soon as possible because delay negatively influences outcome.[1] While displaced (>1 mm) and proximal pole fractures are generally treated operatively, nondisplaced or minimally displaced fractures (<1 mm) are mainly treated conservatively in a cast.[1,7] There is debate about the joints that need to be immobilized. Moreover, the position of the wrist and the period of immobilization remain unclear. Some studies have been published showing that immobilization in a below-elbow cast does not contribute to a higher nonunion rate than immobilization in an above-elbow cast.[2] Furthermore, a cast without immobilization of the thumb does not contribute to a higher nonunion rate than a cast with immobilization of the thumb.[3] A position of the wrist in 20 degrees dorsal flexion during cast immobilization has been advocated.[8] In this position, it is hypothesized that the function of the musculus abductor pollicis longus and musculus abductor brevis are neutralized.[1] Finally, there is no consensus about the length of time of immobilization for nondisplaced and minimally displaced scaphoid fractures. In the literature, periods

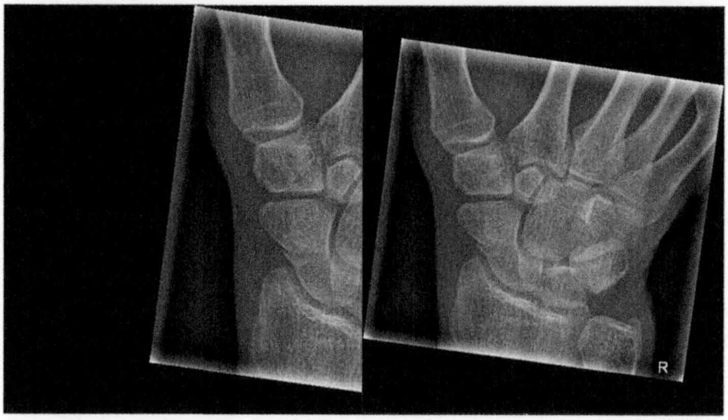

FIG. 13.1 Patient A, at presentation in the emergency department.

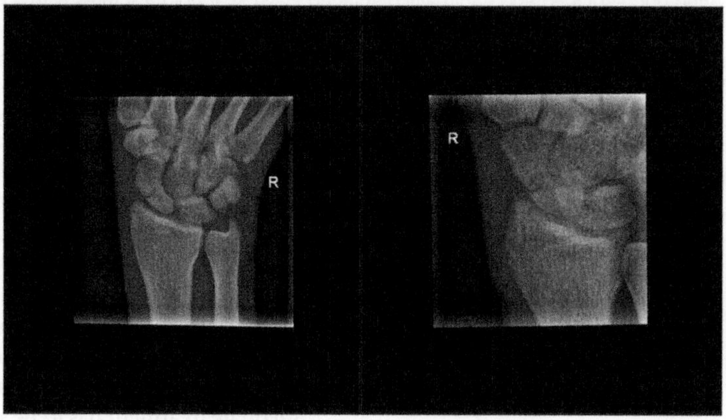

FIG. 13.2 Patient B, at presentation in the emergency department.

of immobilization commonly range between 6 and 12 weeks.[9]

MAIN QUESTION

What is the optimal conservative treatment for a nondisplaced or minimally displaced waist fracture?

Current Opinion

In contrast to displaced scaphoid fractures that are generally treated operatively, current opinion in the treatment of nondisplaced and minimally displaced scaphoid fractures is highly divergent in terms of type and length of immobilization.

Finding of Evidence

- Cochrane: Scaphoid Fracture
- Pubmed (Medline): ("Fractures, Bone"[Mesh] AND "Scaphoid Bone"[Mesh]) OR "Scaphoid Bone/injuries" [Mesh] OR ((scaphoid*[tiab] OR scafoid*[tiab] OR schapoid*[tiab] OR os scaph*[tiab] OR (os[ti] AND navicular*[ti]) OR os navicular*[tiab] OR navicular bone*[tiab]) AND (fractur*[tiab] OR injur*[tiab] OR trauma*[tiab] OR (broken*[tiab] AND ("bone" [tiab] OR bone'*[tiab] OR bones*[tiab])))) AND ("Casts, Surgical"[Mesh] OR conservativ*[tiab] OR nonoperative*[tiab] OR non-operative*[tiab] OR nonsurgical*[tiab] OR non-surgical*[tiab] OR immobiliz*[tiab] OR immobilis*[tiab] OR "cast"[tiab]ORcast'*[tiab]OR"casts"[tiab]ORcasts'* [tiab]OR"Braces"[Mesh]OR"brace"[tiab]ORbrace'* [tiab] OR braces*[tiab] OR bracing*[tiab] OR braced*[tiab] OR plaster of paris*[tiab] OR paris plaster*[tiab] OR paris bandage*[tiab] OR pressure dressing*[tiab] OR "Calcium Sulfate"[Mesh] OR "gypsite"[tiab] OR "gypsum"[tiab])) NOT (("Scaphoid Bone"[Mesh] OR scaphoid*[tiab] OR scafoid*[tiab] OR schapoid*[tiab] OR os scaph*[tiab]

OR (os[ti] AND navicular*[ti]) OR os navicular*[tiab] OR navicular bone*[tiab]) AND (non-displace*[tiab] OR non-dislocat*[tiab] OR nondisplace*[tiab] OR nondislocat*[tiab] OR minimally displace*[tiab] OR minimal displace*[tiab])

- Bibliography of eligible articles
- Publications prior to 1985 were excluded
- Case reports were excluded
- Articles that were not in English, German, French, and Dutch were excluded

Quality of Evidence

Below-elbow versus above-elbow cast

Level I:

Systematic reviews/etaanalyses: 2

Randomized trials: 2

Thumb or no-thumb cast

Level I:

Systematic reviews/metaanalyses: 2

Randomized trials: 2

Position of the wrist in the cast

Level I:

Systematic reviews/metaanalyses: 2

Randomized trials: 1

Removable cast

Level III:

Retrospective comparative studies: 1

Immobilization time

Level II:

Prospective cohort study: 1

Level III:

Retrospective comparative studies: 1

Pulsed electromagnetic field and pulsed low-intensity ultrasound therapy

Level I:

Randomized trials: 1

Level II:

Randomized trials with methodological limitations: 1

FINDINGS

Below-Versus Above-Elbow Cast

Historically, an above-elbow cast was advocated to reduce movement at the fracture site, which occurs during pronation and supination.[2,10] Nevertheless, according to two systematic reviews, this movement does not contribute to a higher nonunion rate.

These systematic reviews have been published considering a treatment with a cast (including thumb) above the elbow and a cast (including thumb) below the elbow. Doornberg et al. and Alshryda et al. describe the two randomized controlled trials published addressing this topic.[11,12] Alho et al. performed a randomized controlled trial with 99 patients, sustaining 100 fractures of the scaphoid, whereas Gellman et al. included 51 patients with this fracture. Both study results were pooled together, resulting in no statistically significant difference in the union and complication rate (RR = 1.02, 95% confidence interval [CI] = 0.05–19.23, $P = .99$).[13,14]

Thumb or No-Thumb Immobilization

The same two systematic reviews have focused on a treatment comparing a cast with or without thumb immobilization (both below-elbow casts).[11,12] Both authors describe the study of Clay et al. who found a similar nonunion rate in both groups: 14 of 143 patients in the thumb group and 15 of 148 patients in the no-thumb group (RR = 0.97, 95% CI = 0.48–1.93, $P = .92$).[2] A limitation of this study is the fact that patients sustaining scaphoid fractures of type A1, A2, B1, B2, B3, and B5, according to the Herbert classification, were included. A nonunion rate of 10% was found.

Therefore, Buijze et al. performed a randomized controlled trial, including only nondisplaced and minimal displaced fractures of the waist of the scaphoid. In this multicenter study, 62 patients were enrolled, 31 in both groups. Inadvertently seven patients with a fracture of the distal third of the scaphoid were included as well, four in the thumb group and three in the no-thumb group.[3]

After 10 weeks, using CT as a reference standard, there was a significant difference in the extent of union favoring the no-thumb group (85% vs. 70%). In this group, only one patient, who elected an operative treatment after 1 week sustained a nonunion. The union rate in both groups, excluding this patient, was 100%.

After 10 weeks of immobilization, one patient in the thumb group had persistent wrist pain and was immobilized for an additional 4 weeks. After 10 weeks, there were no significant differences between both groups for nonunion rate. After 6 months, there were no significant differences between both groups for wrist motion, grip strength, disabilities of the arm, shoulder and hand score, the Mayo Modified Wrist Score, and pain score. A subgroup analysis (excluding the patients who sustained a distal scaphoid fracture) also gave no significant differences, concerning the abovementioned parameters.

Position in the Cast

To date, one study has been performed evaluating the position of wrist immobilization (in a below-elbow cast without immobilization of the thumb). Hambidge et al. included 121 patients with a waist fracture or a distal pole fracture. 58 patients were treated in a 20-degree (palmar) flexion cast and 63 patients in a 20-degree (dorsal) extension cast. After 12 weeks, all casts were removed. Regarding the nonunion rate in the flexion (9%) and extension groups (13%), no significant difference was found on radiographs after 6 months. Moreover, there was no significant difference in secondary outcome measures (wrist flexion, grip strength, and level of pain) after 6 months. However, wrist extension was significantly lower in the flexion group with a mean difference of 12° ($P = < .01$),[8] although the authors have not corrected for multiple outcome testing.

Removable Cast

Terkelsen et al. published a retrospective study in 1988. They compared their new casting method, a removable below-elbow cast with immobilization of the thumb, used between 1981 and 1984 with their previous method, an above-elbow cast with immobilization of the thumb, used between 1978 and 1981. The patients in the first group were able to move the arm out of the cast. Weight bearing was not allowed. The nonunion rate in the removable cast was 3 of 44, and it was 7 of 48 in the above-elbow cast group, which does not contribute to a significant difference ($P = .25$). The number of patients needing physiotherapy and the number of patients complaining of inconvenience of the cast at rest was significantly lower in the removable cast group (both $P = .01$).[15] Although these results are in favor of a removable cast, this study has some inherent limitations due to its retrospective study design. Moreover, the information provided in this paper is very limited and should therefore be interpreted with care. Additionally, the overall nonunion rate of 11%, which was confirmed clinical and radiologic (by an X-ray of the scaphoid in two projections), is high.

Comparable studies that confirm the favorability of a removable cast have not been published.

Immobilization Time

Rhemrev et al. performed a retrospective study reviewing conservatively treated nondisplaced and minimally displaced scaphoid fracture over a 3-year period in a Level I trauma center. The patients were treated with a below-elbow cast with thumb immobilization for 6 weeks. In case of persistent clinical signs of a fracture after 6 weeks of immobilization, the casting period was extended consecutively every 2 weeks. In case of clinical and radiologic nonunion after 12 weeks, an operative treatment was advocated. 71 patients were included in this study, 58 patients (81.7%) demonstrated full consolidation after 6 weeks, 11 patients (15.5%) required an immobilization of 8–12 weeks, and 2 patients (2.8%) required an immobilization of more than 12 weeks.[16] Considering the retrospective design, this study has inherent limitations.

Geoghegan et al. performed a prospective nonrandomized study in 43 patients with nondisplaced scaphoid waist fractures who were treated in a below-elbow cast without immobilization of the thumb. After 4 weeks a CT scan was performed. This showed union in 26 cases; for the other patients cast immobilization was extended.[17] In the literature no prospective randomized controlled trial has been published comparing the immobilization time for nondisplaced or minimally displaced scaphoid fractures. In the majority of the trials performed with nondisplaced and minimally displaced scaphoid fractures, the immobilization time ranges between 6 and 12 weeks.[2–6,8,13,16,18–20]

Pulsed Electromagnetic Field and Pulsed Low-Intensity Ultrasound Therapy

Pulsed electromagnetic field therapy has been extensively studied by Hannemann et al. (see Chapter 23).[20] With regard to pulsed low-intensity ultrasound therapy, Mayr et al. performed a single-blind randomized controlled trial with patients sustaining scaphoid fractures type B1 or B2 (Herbert classification). 29 patients (30 fractures) were divided into two groups; all patients were treated with a below-elbow cast with immobilization of the thumb until radiologic consolidation occurred. The intervention group additionally underwent a pulsed low-intensity ultrasound treatment of 20 min daily. The consolidation was assessed by a CT scan every 2 weeks. The time until consolidation was 43.2 ± 10.9 days in the intervention group, compared with 62 ± 19.2 days in the placebo group, a significant difference ($P = .0055$). Limitations of this study include the small groups, lacking sample size calculation, a single-blinded design, and more importantly the imprecision and unreliability of the primary outcome time until consolidation, despite the fact that evaluation by a CT-scan was performed every 2 weeks.[21] No further publications considering both subjects have been found in the literature.

RECOMMENDATIONS

In patients with nondisplaced and minimal displaced scaphoid waist fractures, evidence suggests the following:

- There is no difference in nonunion and complication rates between patients treated with either a below- or above-elbow cast. Therefore a below-elbow cast is advocated for the conservative treatment of these fractures (overall quality: high).
- There is no difference in nonunion rate nor functional outcome between patients treated with a below-elbow cast with or without immobilization of the thumb (overall quality: high).
- The nonunion rate is not influenced by the position of the cast, either in 20 degrees palmar flexion or 20 degrees dorsal extension. However, there is a significant difference considering the wrist function after 6 months, in favor of the extension group compared with the flexion group (overall quality: high).
- There is not enough evidence to advocate a removable cast (overall quality: moderate).
- An immobilization time of 6 weeks is enough in the majority of cases. In case of a nonconsolidated fracture, 2 weeks repeatedly of additional immobilization may be advisable (overall quality: low to moderate).
- There is not enough evidence that pulsed low-intensity ultrasound accelerates the healing of acute nondisplaced and minimal displaced scaphoid fractures (overall quality: low).

CONCLUSION

To date, the best evidence-based treatment of a nondisplaced or minimally displaced fracture of the scaphoid waist is a cast immobilization in a below-elbow cast, without immobilization of the thumb in a neutral position for 6 weeks. In case of persistent signs of a fracture, a new cast should be applied for an additional 2 weeks, repeating until clinical union has been confirmed in up to 12 weeks. Currently, there is not enough evidence to treat these nondisplaced or minimally displaced fractures safely with a removable cast. Pulsed electromagnetic field bone stimulators do not accelerate bone healing. There is not enough evidence that pulsed low-intensity ultrasound accelerates the healing of scaphoid fractures.

PANEL 2
Authors' Preferred Treatment

The authors treat these fractures conservatively in a below-elbow cast, without immobilization of the thumb for a minimum 6 weeks. In case of persistent clinical signs of a fracture, the casting period will be prolonged per 2 weeks, until union has been reached after a maximum of 12 weeks of immobilization.

After 6 weeks of immobilization *Patient A* is clinically pain free, radiographically there are no signs of complications (Fig. 13.3). *Patient B* was treated in the same fashion. However, because of persistent clinical symptoms of a nonunited fracture and the absence of radiologic union, the casting period was extended for 2 weeks. This was repeated until clinical and radiologic union occurred after 12 weeks (Fig. 13.4).

PANEL 3
Pearls and Pitfalls

PEARLS

- Individualizing treatment based on clinical evaluation of consolidation reduces the average time of immobilization. This approaches limits the casting period to 6 weeks for >80% of patients.
- Using clinical evaluation of consolidation limits the use of CT scans to a small minority of patients in whom a doubtful union remains.
- Immobilization in a below-elbow cast, without immobilization of the thumb, for 6 weeks is a reliable treatment for nondisplaced and minimally displaced scaphoid waist fractures.

PITFALLS

- Nondisplaced and minimally displaced scaphoid waist fractures could be difficult to diagnose on radiographs. Therefore, often additional CT or MRI should be performed.
- Radiologic assessment of union has shown poor interreliability.
- It has not been scientifically established whether clinical consolidation accurately predicts radiographic union on the long-term.
- A delayed start of the treatment is a risk factor for nonunion.

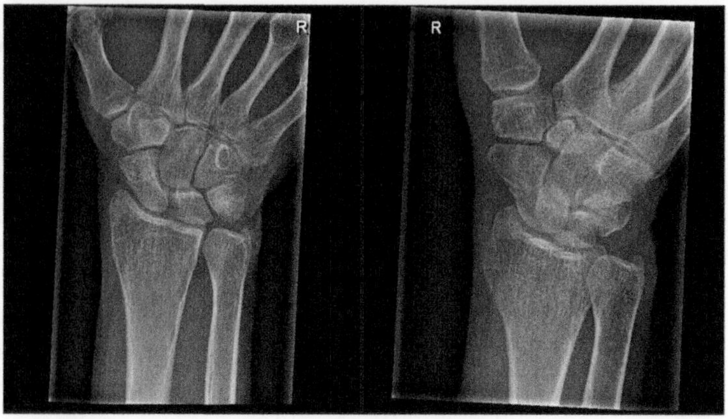

FIG. 13.3 Patient A, after 6 weeks of treatment.

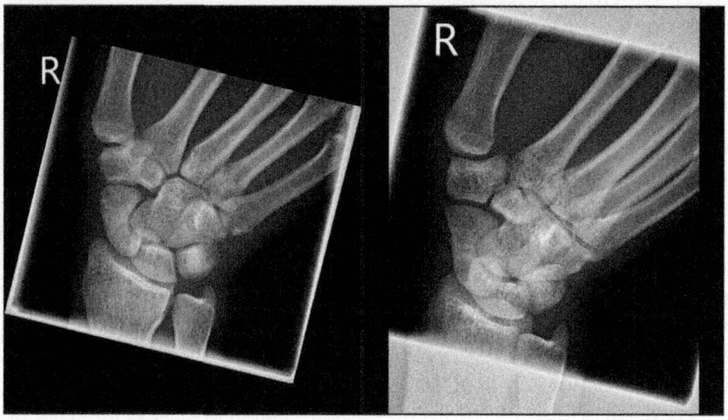

FIG. 13.4 Patient B, after 12 weeks of treatment.

REFERENCES

1. Beeres FJP, Rhemrev SJ, Hogervorst M, den Hollander P, Jukema GN. Scaphoid fractures: diagnostic and therapy. *Ned Tijdschr Voor Geneeskd.* 2007;13:742–747.
2. Clay NR, Dias JJ, Costigan PS, Barton NJ. Need the thumb be immobilized in scaphoid fractures? A randomized prospective trial. *J Bone Joint Surg Br.* 1991;73B: 828–832.
3. Buijze GA, Goslings JC, Rhemrev SJ, et al. CAST Trial Collaboration. Cast immobilization with and without immobilization of the thumb for nondisplaced and minimally displaced scaphoid waist fractures: a multicenter, randomized controlled trial. *J Hand Surg Am.* 2014;39: 621–627.
4. Hannemann PFW, Brouwers L, Dullaert K, van der Linden EX, Poeze M, Brink PRG. Determining scaphoid waist fracture union by conventional radiographic examination an analysis of reliability and validity. *Arch Orthop Trauma Surg.* 2015;135:291–296.
5. Hannemann PFW, Brouwers L, van der Zee D, et al. Multiplanar reconstruction computed tomography for diagnosis of scaphoid waist fracture union: a prospective cohort analysis of accuracy and precision. *Skeletal Radiol.* 2013;42:1377–1382.
6. Buijze GA, Wijffels MME, Guitton TG, Grewal R, van Dijk CN, Ring D. The Science of Variation Group. Interobserver reliability of computed tomography to diagnose scaphoid waist fracture union. *J Hand Surg.* 2012;37A:250–254.
7. Buijze GA, Doornberg JN, Ham JS, Ring D, Bhandari M, Poolman RW. Surgical compared with conservative treatment for acute nondisplaced or minimally displaced scaphoid fractures. *J Bone Joint Surg Am.* 2010;92:1534–1544.
8. Hambidge JE, Desai VV, Schranz PJ, Compson JP, Davis TRC, Barton NJ. Acute fractures of the scaphoid. *J Bone Joint Surg. Br.* 1999;81B:91–92.
9. Browner BD, Jupiter JB, Levine AM, Trafton PG, Green NE, Swiontkowski MF, eds. *Skeletal Trauma*. 3rd ed. Philadelphia: Elsevier Saunders; 2003:1271.

10. Kaneshiro SA, Failla JM, Tashman S. Scaphoid fracture displacement with forearm rotation in a short-arm thumb spica cast. *J Hand Surg*. 1999;24A:984–991.
11. Alshryda S, Shah A, Odak S, Al-Shryda J, Ilango B, Murali SR. Acute fractures of the scaphoid bone. systematic review and meta-analysis. *Surgeon*. 2012;10:218–229.
12. Doornberg JN, Buijze GA, Ham J, Ring D, Bhandari M, Poolman RW. Nonoperative treatment for acute scaphoid fractures: a systematic review and meta-analysis of randomized controlled trials. *J Trauma*. 2011;71:1073–1081.
13. Alho A, Kankaanpaa U. Management of fractures scaphoid bone: a prospective study of 100 fractures. *Acta Orthop Scand*. 1975;46:737–743.
14. Gellman H, Caputo RJ, Carter V, Aboulafia A, McKay M. Comparison of short and long thumb-spica casts for nondisplaced fractures of the carpal scaphoid. *J Bone Joint Surg*. 1989;71A:354–357.
15. Terkelsen CJ, Jepsen JM. Treatment of scaphoid fractures with a removable cast. *Acta Orthop Scand*. 1988;59:452–453.
16. Rhemrev SJ, van Leerdam RH, Ootes D, Beeres FJP, Meylaerts SAG. Non-operative treatment of non-displaced scaphoid fractures may be preferred. *Injury*. 2009;40:638–641.
17. Geoghegan JM, Woodruff MJ, Bhatia R, et al. Undisplaced scaphoid waist fractures: is 4 weeks' immobilization in a below-elbow cast sufficient if a week 4 CT-scan suggests fracture union? *J Hand Surg Eu*. 2009;34E:631–637.
18. Papaloizos MY, Fusetti C, Christen T, Nagy L, Wasserfallen JB. Minimally invasive fixation versus conservative treatment of undisplaced scaphoid fractures: a cost-effectiveness study. *J Hand Surg Br*. 2004;29B:116–119.
19. Vinnars B, FAf Ekenstam, Gerdin B. Comparison of direct and indirect costs of internal fixation and cast treatment in acute scaphoid fractures: a randomized trial involving 52 patients. *Acta Orthop*. 2007;78:672–679.
20. Hannemann PFW, van Wezenbeek MR, Kolkman KA, et al. CT-scan evaluated outcome of pulsed electromagnetic fields in the treatment of acute scaphoid fractures. A randomized, multicenter, double-blind, placebo-controlled trial. *Bone Joint J*. 2014;96B:1070–1076.
21. Mayr E, Rudzki MM, Rudzki M, Borchardt B, Häusser H, Rüter A. Does pulsed low-intensity ultrasound accelerate healing of scaphoid fractures? *Handchir Mikrochir Plast Chir*. 2000;32:115–122.

CHAPTER 14

Acute Management of Proximal Pole Scaphoid Fractures

ELIANA B. SALTZMAN, BA • SCHNEIDER K. RANCY, BA •
STEVE K. LEE, MD • SCOTT W. WOLFE, MD

KEY POINTS

- Proximal pole scaphoid fractures are the least common site of scaphoid fracture but are associated with a higher incidence of nonunion.
- Because of their inherent compromised vascularity and stability, proximal pole fractures are best managed surgically.
- Operative management of proximal pole fractures reduces time to union and length of cast immobilization.
- A dorsal "miniopen" antegrade approach is recommended for proximal pole fractures and is not associated with an increased risk of iatrogenic compromise of scaphoid vascularity.

PANEL 1
Case Scenario

A 37-year-old female communications agent presented to the emergency department with complaints of left wrist pain and swelling after falling on an outstretched wrist. An oblique radiograph 2 days postinjury demonstrates an oblique lucency, concerning for acute fracture (Fig. 14.1A–C). Axial and coronal computed tomography (CT) imaging 11 days postinjury confirm a nondisplaced proximal pole fracture extending to the scaphoid waist (Fig. 14.2A–C). As you outline the treatment options of fixation versus casting, your patient discloses that she is reluctant to undergo surgery, given the option of conservative treatment, and that she does not rely on her wrist for work. What risks and benefits do you outline for each treatment choice to make your recommendation?

IMPORTANCE OF THE PROBLEM

The proximal pole is the least frequently fractured site, with an incidence ranging from 6% to 20%, and yet is associated with the worst prognosis.[1] Proximal pole fractures not only result in a longer time to union, compared with distal or waist fractures,[2] but are also associated with a higher incidence of nonunion, ranging from 5% to 10% in nondisplaced fractures to 50% in displaced fractures.[2–4] Cadaveric and clinical studies have demonstrated that scaphoid nonunion can result in carpal collapse and posttraumatic arthritis.[5] The consequential pain, weakness, and diminished motion can confer significant functional impairment on this young patient population.

Displaced fractures can compromise the tenuous blood supply of the scaphoid, which is largely limited to the distal tubercle and the nonarticular dorsoradial ridge vessels that enter from the carpal arches in the dorsal wrist capsule.[6,7] Although there is some controversy on what constitutes stability, proximal pole fractures are often considered unstable because of separation from retrograde blood flow, the small size of the fracture fragment, and the large extension moment of the proximal row.[8–10] Herbert classified all proximal pole fractures as unstable and recommended surgical management in each case.[11]

Cast treatment of proximal pole fractures has been associated with a 90% union rate and a time to union ranging from 3 to 9 months.[2] Rettig and Raskin demonstrated that surgical open reduction and internal fixation resulted in a 100% union rate for proximal pole fractures at 9.5 weeks for nondisplaced fractures and 11 weeks for displaced fractures.[12] Given that these fractures most commonly occur in young healthy men, successful surgical intervention, if associated with minimal complication rate, would be a desirable intervention to reduce the risk of nonunion and rapidly restore productivity.

MAIN QUESTION

What is the preferred treatment for acute proximal pole fractures?

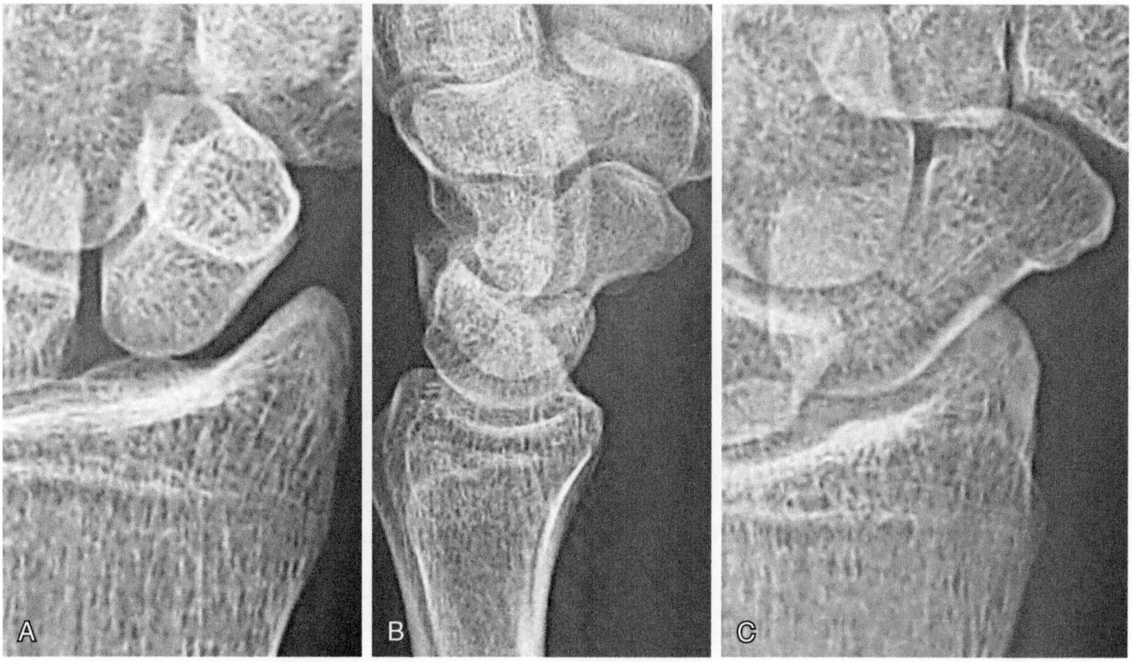

FIG. 14.1 Three radiographic views of the left wrist of a 37-year-old right-handed woman taken 2 days following a fall on an outstretched hand. **(A–C)** Posteroanterior, lateral, and oblique views. **(C)** An oblique lucent line in the proximal scaphoid suggestive of an acute fracture.

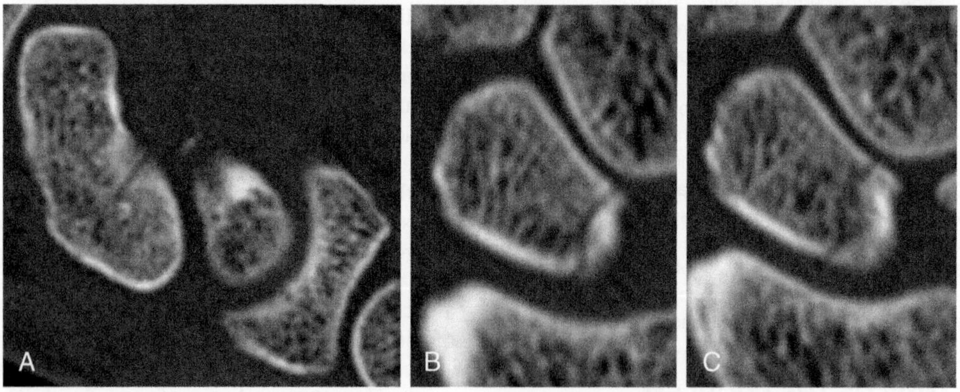

FIG. 14.2 CT scan of the left wrist acquired 11 days following injury. **(A)** A sagittal cut demonstrating a nondisplaced fracture through the proximal pole of the scaphoid, extending to the scaphoid waist. The fracture line also extends into the scapholunate, radioscaphoid, and scaphocapitate joints. **(B and C)** Sequential coronal cutes highlighting the fracture line extension into the scaphoid waist.

Current Opinion

Acute proximal pole fractures are best managed with surgical intervention because of the inherent vascular compromise and instability associated with this fracture pattern. Given the young patient population that typically sustains this injury, surgical fixation allows for earlier rehabilitation, reduced time of immobilization, reduced cost, and earlier return to work and activity.

Finding the Evidence

- Cochrane search: Scaphoid proximal pole

TABLE 14.1
Operative Treatment of Scaphoid Proximal Pole Fractures

Author	Year	n	n (%) Healed	n (%) Nonunion	Time to Union (Weeks)	n Complications (%)
Filan and Hebert[32]	1996	13	11 (85%)	2 (15%)		
Rettig and Raskin[12]	1999	17	17 (100%)	0 (0%)	10	0 (0%)
De Vos and Vandenberghe[33]	2003	8	6 (75%)	2 (25%)	11	2 (25%)
Slade and Gillon[34]	2008	65	65 (100%)	0 (0%)	6–8	1 (2%)
Brogan et al.[8]	2015	23	20 (87%)	3 (13%)	14	3 (13%)
Grewal et al.[35]	2016	4	4 (100%)	0 (0%)	14	0 (0%)
Total		130	123 (95%)	7 (5%)	9	6 (5%)

Complications: defined as other than nonunion, such as delayed union, revision surgery, AVN, carpal collapse, and/or arthritic progression.

- Pubmed (Medline): "scaphoid proximal pole," "scaphoid fracture," "acute scaphoid fracture," "acute scaphoid proximal pole fracture"
- Bibliography of eligible articles
- Articles that were not written in English, French, or German were excluded

Quality of the Evidence

- Level I:
  - Systematic reviews/metaanalyses: 6
  - Randomized trials: 3
- Level III:
  - Retrospective comparative studies: 4
- Level IV:
  - Case series: 13
- Level V:
  - Expert opinion: 5
  - Cadaveric/biomechanical studies: 3

FINDINGS

Although opinions on preferred treatment for acute proximal pole fractures differ, current prevailing dogma dictates that all acute proximal pole fractures require immediate operative fixation and rigid immobilization.[5,13-16] However, few studies report outcomes for surgical versus nonsurgical treatment of acute proximal pole fractures. As a result, there is insufficient "evidence" to perform a high-quality systematic review of the treatment of acute proximal pole fractures. Existing metaanalyses examine union rates, time to union, return to work time, and quantitative outcomes, such as range of motion and grip strength. However, these studies do not segregate data by fracture location or exclude proximal pole fractures from the analysis entirely.[15-21]

In their review of the "available evidence," Eastley and colleagues[16] identified 162 proximal pole fractures among a cohort of 1147 scaphoid fractures. Although the authors were limited by the criteria that each study utilized to define union, they found that 67 proximal poles were treated nonoperatively and 34% progressed to nonunion, whereas 95 were treated with surgical fixation and 2% progressed to nonunion. Cast-treated proximal pole fractures were determined to be at 7.5 times greater risk (95% confidence interval [CI], 4.9–11.5) for nonunion relative to acute distal or waist fractures, although fracture displacement and use of CT were inconsistently reported across studies.[16] Clay et al. similarly reported a 31% proximal pole nonunion rate with cast immobilization alone, but did not comment on the degree of fracture displacement, and union was assessed by radiographs alone.[22]

AUTHORS' METAANALYSIS

Seventeen studies detailing outcomes for surgical versus nonsurgical treatment of acute proximal pole fractures were identified for inclusion in our review (285 proximal pole fractures; range, 2-65).[2,8,12,22-35] Of these, six studies reported outcomes of operative treatment (130 proximal scaphoids; range, 4-65).[8,12,32-35] Four studies were case series and two were retrospective comparative studies. Union was achieved in 123 of 130 proximal poles (95%) at an average of 9 weeks (range, 9–14) [8,12,34,35] (Table 14.1).

TABLE 14.2
Nonoperative Treatment of Scaphoid Proximal Pole Fractures

Author	Year	n	n (%) Healed	n (%) Nonunion	Time to Union (Weeks)	n Complications (%)
Watson Jones[23]	1934	6	5 (83%)	1 (17%)	22	
London[24]	1961	9	5 (56%)	4 (44%)		
Margo and Seely[25]	1963	5	3 (60%)	2 (40%)		
Thorleifsson et al.[26]	1984	9	7 (78%)	9 (22%)	11	
Riester et al.[27]	1985	3	1 (33%)	2 (67%)	28	1 (33%)
Langhoff and Andersen[28]	1988	19	11 (58%)	8 (42%)	12	
Terkelsen and Jepsen[29]	1988	5	3 (60%)	2 (40%)		
Gellman et al.[30]	1989	5	4 (80%)	5 (20%)	12	2 (40%)
Clay et al.[22]	1991	12	8 (67%)	4 (33%)		
Düppe et al.[31]	1994	2	1 (50%)	1 (50%)		
Grewal et al.[2]	2013	28	24 (86%)	4 (14%)	8	
Grewal et al.[35]	2016	52	47 (90%)	5 (10%)	14	1 (2%)
Total		155	119 (77%)	36 (23%)	15	4 (3%)

Complications: defined as other than nonunion, such as AVN, carpal collapse, and/or arthritic progression.

Surgical technique varied and included fixation with noncannulated screws or cannulated headless compression screws using an open volar, open dorsal, or percutaneous approach.[8,12,32–34] In these studies, the dorsal approach was strongly advocated to improve fixation of the small proximal pole fragment and facilitate access to central screw placement.[12,34,36,37]

Twelve studies report treatment with cast immobilization in 155 proximal pole fractures.[2,22–31,34,35] There were two randomized trials, eight case series, and two retrospective comparative studies. Average length of casting was 15 weeks (range, 8–28). Patients were treated with a variety of casting techniques, including long-arm thumb spica and short-arm thumb spica, as well as different variations of wrist positioning. Although there is no reported difference in nonunion rate between long- and short-arm casting ($RR = 6.04$, 95% $CI = 0.30–119.88$, $P = .24$)[20] or differences related to wrist position, one prospective study demonstrated a shorter time to union with long-arm thumb spica casting for acute proximal pole fractures ($P < .05$).[30]

Union rate for cast treatment of proximal pole fractures averaged 119 of 155 (77%) (Table 14.2).[2,22–31,35] Time to union was longer for proximal pole fractures (113 days) versus distal (53 days) and waist fractures (65 days).[2] Additionally, fracture displacement was shown to be associated with a higher likelihood of nonunion (odds ratio, 3.4) and increased time to union (Pearson $r = 0.24$; $P < .001$).[2]

Refracture of the proximal pole after previous successful surgical treatment is a decidedly rare complication, with only five reported cases.[18,27,38] The most common pattern of refracture was a small displaced volar marginal shear fracture originating at the screw head.[38] In two of five cases, subsequent treatment was not reported. In the remaining three cases, secondary fracture was successfully treated with screw removal, debridement, grafting of the screw tract, and fragment fixation with miniscrews or wires.[18,38]

RECOMMENDATION

In adult patients with acute scaphoid proximal pole fractures, the available evidence supports the following:

- There is a higher risk for nonunion with cast treatment compared with internal fixation (overall quality: high).

- Time to union is greater with cast treatment than internal fixation (overall quality: low to moderate).
- A dorsal antegrade approach is recommended for proximal pole fractures to improve fixation of the small proximal pole fragment (overall quality: moderate).

CONCLUSION

Given the increased likelihood of nonunion and the prolonged time to union with cast treatment, immediate surgical fixation is strongly recommended as the treatment of choice for acute scaphoid proximal pole fracture.

PANEL 2
Authors' Preferred Technique, Pearls and Pitfalls

- In the case discussed, we opted for immediate surgical fixation in accordance with our standard treatment algorithm.
- High-resolution imaging is important for visualization and surgical planning of small proximal pole fractures. Contiguous and overlapping 0.625-mm thick computed tomographic scans in the long axis of the scaphoid (both coronal plane and sagittal plane long axes) are recommended. Images should be obtained in the "superman" position with the wrist overhead in the center of the unit.
- The authors recommend a miniopen approach rather than a percutaneous insertion method for cannulated screw placement to precisely identify screw insertion site and avoid soft tissue complications.[39]
- An oblique fracture plane may necessitate changes in screw trajectory, as central screw placement may be oblique to the fracture plane and may not maximize the compressive capabilities of the implant.
- When possible, pass the guide wire entirely through the palmar skin after confirmation and measurement of screw length. Apply a clamp to the distal end in case the wire breaks during drilling or screw placement.
- Fluoroscopic confirmation of guide wire and screw placement is essential to avoid breaching of the articular surface or screw head prominence (Fig. 14.3A–B).
- Remove any traction when tightening the screw to maximize fracture site compression.
- Choose a screw length 4–5 mm shorter than the guide wire to bury hardware on both ends.
- Computed tomography at 10–14 weeks postoperatively is essential to confirm healing prior to return to sports and activities, especially in small proximal pole fractures (Fig. 14.4A–D).
- Consider the use of smaller screws (1.7 mm) in cases where the proximal pole is very small.

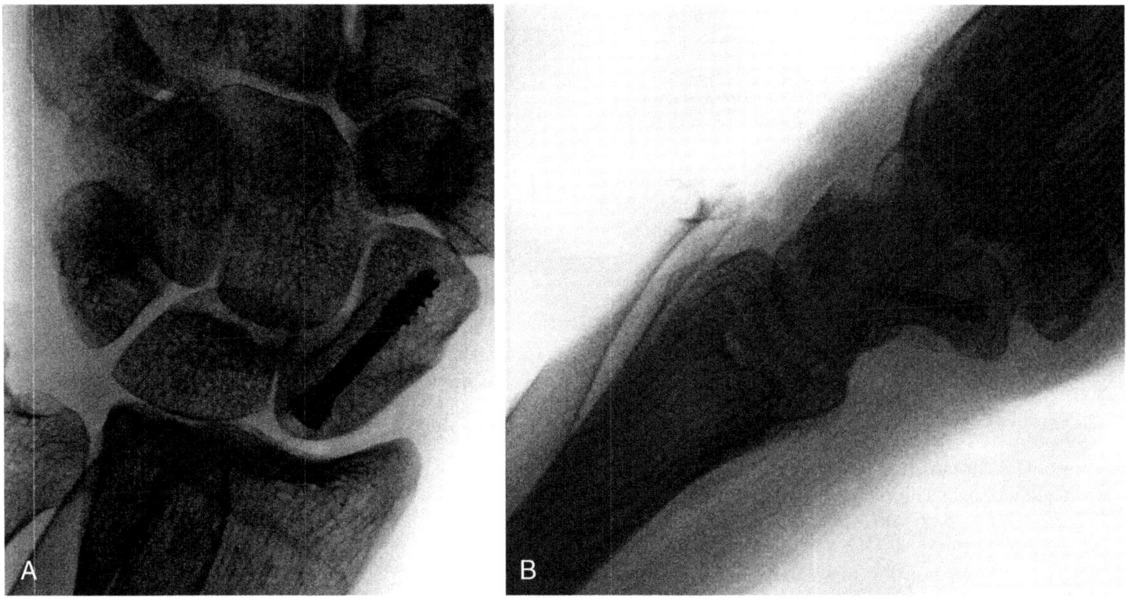

FIG. 14.3 **(A)** Intraoperative posteroanterior and **(B)** lateral fluoroscopy confirming hardware position following open reduction and internal fixation of a left scaphoid proximal pole fracture.

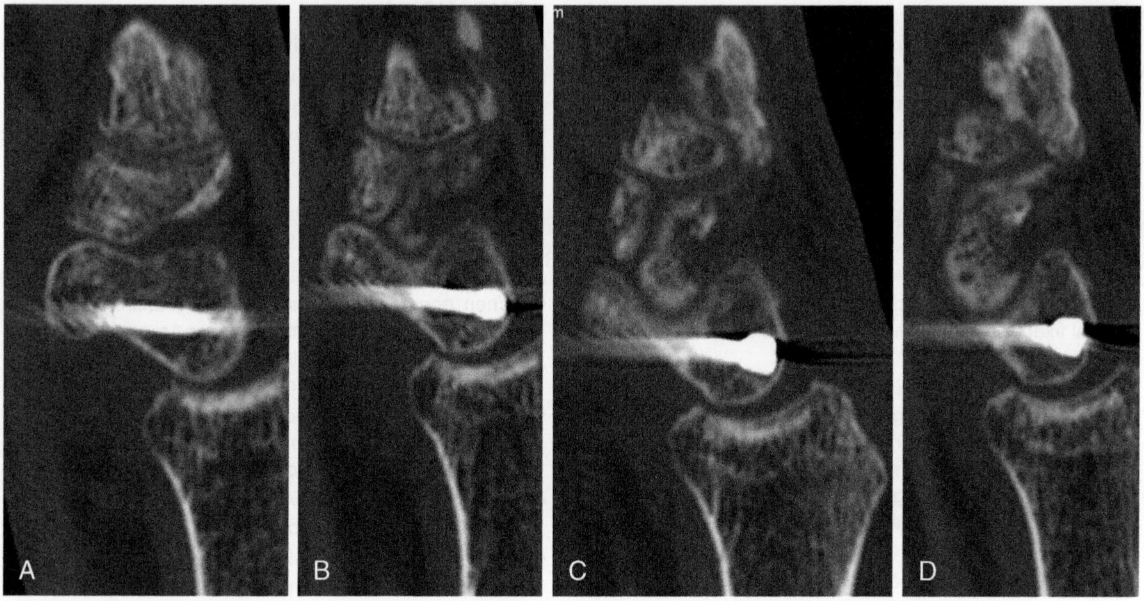

FIG. 14.4 (A–D) A CT scan of the left wrist without contrast 9.5 weeks postoperative demonstrating sequential radial to ulnar images of a healed nondisplaced fracture through the proximal pole of the scaphoid.

REFERENCES

1. Segalman KA, Graham TJ. Scaphoid proximal pole fractures and nonunions. *J Am Soc Surg Hand*. 2004;4:233–249.
2. Grewal R, Suh N, Macdermid JC. Use of computed tomography to predict union and time to union in acute scaphoid fractures treated nonoperatively. *J Hand Surg Am*. 2013;38(5):872–877.
3. Steinmann SP, Adams JE. Scaphoid fractures and nonunions: diagnosis and treatment. *J Orthop Sci*. 2006;11(4):424–431.
4. Gholson JJ, Bae DS, Zurakowski D, Waters PM. Scaphoid fractures in children and adolescents: contemporary injury pattern and factors influencing time to union. *J Bone Joint Surg Am*. 2011;93(13):12010–12019.
5. Ring D, Jupiter JB, Herndon JH. Acute fractures of the scaphoid. *J Am Acad Orthop Surg*. 2000;8(4):225–231.
6. Gelberman RH, Menon J. The vascularity of the scaphoid bone. *J Hand Surg*. 1980;5:508–513.
7. Taleisnik J, Kelly PJ. The extraosseous and intraosseous blood supply of the scaphoid bone. *J Bone Joint Surg*. 1996;48A:1125–1137.
8. Brogan DM, Moran SL, Shin AY. Outcomes of open reduction and internal fixation of acute proximal pole scaphoid fractures. *Hand (N Y)*. 2015;10(2):227–232.
9. Moritomo H, Murase T, Oka K, Tanaka H, Yoshikawa H, Sugamoto K. Relationship between the fracture location and the kinematic pattern in scaphoid nonunion. *J Hand Surg Am*. 2008;33(9):1459–1468.
10. Wolfe SW, Neu C, Crisco JJ. In vivo scaphoid, lunate, and capitate kinematics in flexion and in extension. *J Hand Surg Am*. 2000;25(5):860–869.
11. Herbert TJ, Fisher WE. Management of the fractured scaphoid using a new bone screw. *J Bone Joint Surg Br*. 1984;66(1):114–123.
12. Rettig ME, Raskin KB. Retrograde compression screw fixation of acute proximal pole scaphoid fractures. *J Hand Surg Am*. 1999;24(6):1206–1210.
13. Krimmer H. Management of acute fractures and nonunions of the proximal pole of the scaphoid. *J Hand Surg Br*. 2002;27(3):245–248.
14. Kawamura K, Chung KC. Treatment of scaphoid fractures and nonunions. *J Hand Surg Am*. 2008;33(6):988–997.
15. Alshryda S, Shah A, Odak S, Al-Shryda J, Ilango B, Murali SR. Acute fractures of the scaphoid bone: systematic review and meta-analysis. *Surgeon*. 2012;10(4):218–229.
16. Eastley N, Singh H, Dias JJ, Taub N. Union rates after proximal scaphoid fractures; meta-analyses and review of available evidence. *J Hand Surg Eur Vol*. 2013;38(8):888–897.
17. Yin ZG, Zhang JB, Kan SL, Wang P. Treatment of acute scaphoid fractures: systematic review and meta-analysis. *Clin Orthop Relat Res*. 2007;460:142–151.
18. Vinnars B, Pietreanu M, Bodestedt A, Ekenstam FA, Gerdin B. Nonoperative compared with operative treatment of acute scaphoid fractures. A randomized clinical trial. *J Bone Joint Surg Am*. 2008;90(6):1176–1185.

19. Buijze GA, Doornberg JN, Ham JS, Ring D, Bhandari M, Poolman RW. Surgical compared with conservative treatment for acute nondisplaced or minimally displaced scaphoid fractures: a systematic review and meta-analysis of randomized controlled trials. *J Bone Joint Surg Am*. 2010;92(6):1534–1544.
20. Doornberg JN, Buijze GA, Ham SJ, Ring D, Bhandari M, Poolman RW. Nonoperative treatment for acute scaphoid fractures: a systematic review and meta-analysis of randomized controlled trials. *J Trauma*. 2011;71(4): 1073–1081.
21. Symes TH, Stothard J. A systematic review of the treatment of acute fractures of the scaphoid. *J Hand Surg Eur Vol*. 2011;36(9):802–810.
22. Clay NR, Dias JJ, Costigan PS, Gregg PJ, Barton NJ. Need the thumb be immobilised in scaphoid fractures? A randomised prospective trial. *J Bone Joint Surg Br*. 1991;73:828–832.
23. Watson Jones R. Inadequate immobilization and nonunion of fractures. *Br Med J*. 1934;1:936–939.
24. London PS. The broken scaphoid bone: the case against pessimism. *J Bone Joint Surg Br*. 1961;43-B:237–244.
25. Margo MK, Seely JA. A statistical review of 100 cases of fracture of the carpal navicular bone. *Clin Orthop Relat Res*. 1963;31:102e105.
26. Thorleifsson R, Karlsson J, Sigurjonsson K. Fractures of the scaphoid bone. A follow-up study. *Arch Orthop Trauma Surg*. 1984;103:96–99.
27. Riester JN, Baker BE, Mosher JF, Lowe D. A review of scaphoid fracture healing in competitive athletes. *Am J Sports Med*. 1985;13(3):159–161.
28. Langhoff O, Andersen JL. Consequences of late immobilization of scaphoid fractures. *J Hand Surg Br*. 1988;13: 77–79.
29. Terkelsen CJ, Jepsen JM. Treatment of scaphoid fractures with a removable cast. *Acta Orthop Scand*. 1988;59: 452–453.
30. Gellman H, Caputo RJ, Carter V, Aboulafia A, McKay M. Comparison of short and long thumb-spica casts for nondisplaced fractures of the carpal scaphoid. *J Bone Joint Surg Am*. 1989;71:354–357.
31. Düppe H, Johnell O, Lundborg G, Karlsson M, Redlund-Johnell I. Long-term results of fracture of the scaphoid. A follow-up study of more than thirty years. *J Bone Joint Surg Am*. 1994;76:249–252.
32. Filan SL, Herbert TJ. Herbert screw fixation of scaphoid fractures. *J Bone Joint Surg Br*. 1996;78(4):519–529.
33. De Vos J, Vandenberghe D. Acute percutaneous scaphoid fixation using a non-cannulated Herbert screw. *Chir Main*. 2003;22(2):78–83.
34. Slade JF, Gillon T. Retrospective review of 234 scaphoid fractures and nonunions treated with arthroscopy for union and complications. *Scand J Surg*. 2008;97:280–289.
35. Grewal R, Lutz K, MacDermid JC, Suh N. Proximal pole scaphoid fractures: a computed tomographic assessment of outcomes. *J Hand Surg Am*. 2016;41(1):54–58.
36. Leventhal EL, Wolfe SW, Walsh EF, Crisco JJ. A computational approach to the "optimal" screw axis location and orientation in the scaphoid bone. *J Hand Surg Am*. 2009;34(4):677–684.
37. Martus JE, Bedi A, Jebson PJ. Cannulated variable pitch compression screw fixation of scaphoid fractures using a limited dorsal approach. *Tech Hand Up Extrem Surg*. 2005;9(4):202–206.
38. Rancy SK, Zelken JA, Lipman JD, Wolfe SW. Scaphoid proximal pole fracture following headless screw fixation. *J Wrist Surg*. 2016;5(1):71–76.
39. Weinberg AM, Pichler W, Grechenig S, Tesch NP, Heidari N, Grechenig W. The percutaneous antegrade scaphoid fracture fixation – safe method? *Injury*. 2009;40(6): 642–644.

CHAPTER 15

Distal Scaphoid Fractures

ANDERS BJÖRKMAN, MD, PHD • MARTIN CLEMENTSON, MD, PHD •
PETER JØRGSHOLM, MD, PHD • NIELS THOMSEN, MD, PHD

KEY POINTS

- Fractures in the distal third of the scaphoid are common.
- Fractures in the distal third of the scaphoid are the most common fracture type in young children.
- An avulsion of then radiovolar tip of the tuberosity with nonarticular or minimal articular involvement is the most common among distal fractures.
- A majority of distal scaphoid fractures unite if treated 4–8 weeks in a cast.

PANEL 1
Case Scenario

THE PATIENT
A 29-year-old man fell onto his right dominant hand during sports. Physical examination revealed tenderness in the anatomic snuffbox and on palpation on the scaphoid tubercle, as well as on longitudinal compression of the first metacarpal. Radiographs and CT showed a distal scaphoid fracture, type IIA according to Prosser (Fig. 15.1A–B). What is the most appropriate treatment for this patient?

IMPORTANCE OF THE PROBLEM AND CURRENT OPINION

The literature concerning scaphoid fractures has focused on diagnosis and treatment of fractures in the waist and proximal pole. Little attention has been paid to fractures in the distal third of the scaphoid, although they account for roughly 25% of all scaphoid fractures.[1,2] The distal third of the scaphoid is well vascularized and fractures in this part of the scaphoid are often nondisplaced or minimally displaced, which has led to the current opinion that fractures in the distal part of the scaphoid heal uneventful if treated in a cast for 6–8 weeks.[3] However, there are no randomized studies assessing different treatment regimes. Furthermore, available literature focuses on fracture union and provides no information on clinical or functional outcome.

Because of the frequency and diversity in fracture patterns, distal scaphoid fractures merit more attention than has been given so far.

MAIN QUESTION

What is the best treatment for a fracture in the distal third of the scaphoid when considering union rate and functional outcome?

Finding the Evidence

- Cochrane search: "scaphoid" AND "fracture" AND "distal" OR "tubercle"
- Pubmed: "scaphoid bone" or "scaphoid" AND "fracture" OR "nonunion" AND "distal" OR "tubercle"
- Only articles written in English were included

Quality of Evidence

Level II: Outcomes research[5]
Level IV: Case series[1,6–11]

ANATOMY

Cadaver studies on human specimens has shown that blood supply derives from the radial artery or its superficial palmar branch entering the scaphoid at the palmar, lateral aspect of the tubercle and from an intercarpal arch of the radial artery, which enters the scaphoid along its dorsal ridge.[12,13] Because of its direct blood supply, the distal scaphoid is well vascularized independent

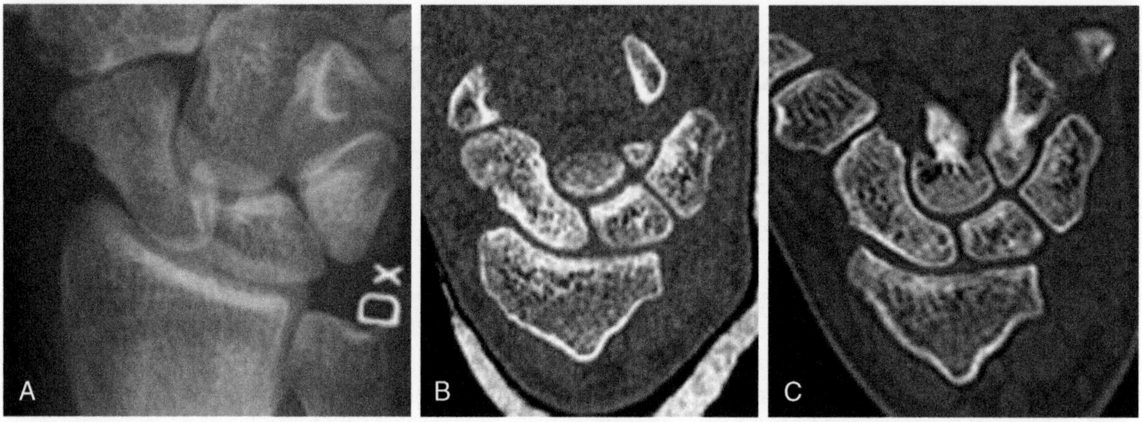

FIG. 15.1 Case scenario. A 29-year-old man who fell on his hand and sustained a Prosser type IIA injury. (A) Radiographs and (B) CT at the time of injury. (C) CT at a follow-up of 10 years after injury.

of which vascular branch is the main contributor of intraosseous blood supply.

The distal scaphoid has a biarticular surface, which articulates radiovolarly with the trapezium and ulnodorsally with the trapezoid. Ligaments of importance for function and stabilization of the distal scaphoid are the scapho-trapezio-trapezoid (STT) ligament, the scapho-capitate ligament, and the radioscaphocapitate ligament.

EPIDEMIOLOGY

In general, the majority of scaphoid fractures occur at the waist (64%–77%) followed by fractures in the distal part (21%–31%) and at the proximal pole (5%–10%).[1,2,14] In contrast, scaphoid fractures in children are reported to occur most frequently in the distal third (59%–87%), followed by waist fractures (12%–38%), and very rarely to affect the proximal pole (0%–3%).[8,15,16] Tubercle avulsion from the distal third is the single most common fracture site in children (33%–52%).[8,16] However, some reports have indicated a shift in the fracture pattern of children to resemble that in adults.[9,17] This has been attributed to a change in high-energy sporting activity early on in life.

FRACTURE BIOMECHANICS

Most patients with fractures in the distal third of the scaphoid report a fall on an outstretched hand. Several different mechanisms causing a distal fracture has been suggested such as avulsion of a radial fragment by the collateral ligament, capsular attachments, or the transverse carpal ligament[18,19] or fracture due to a direct blow to the palm.[6] A combination of compression and shearing force through the trapezium, resulting in a more extensive fracture of the articular surface, has also been suggested.[7]

CLASSIFICATION

The Mayo classification divides fractures in the distal third of the scaphoid into fractures of the tuberosity or intraarticular fractures of the STT joint.[20]

> Cooney and coworkers[20] developed a classification mainly based on fracture location where they divided the scaphoid into thirds. However, distal fractures were subdivided into fractures in the distal tubercle, distal intraarticular fractures, and distal fractures. They also acknowledged that location influences both tendency and time to healing.

Prosser et al. combined their own clinical experience with results from the literature and identified five different fracture types, involving the distal articular surface of the scaphoid(Fig. 15.2, type I–III).[7,21]

- Type I, is an avulsion of the radiovolar tip of the tuberosity with nonarticular or minimal articular involvement. It is the most common type accounting for more than 50% of all distal fractures.[7,8]
- Type II is an intraarticular fracture caused by a compressing or shearing force through the trapezium.[7] The fracture fragment can be radial (type IIA), ulnar (type IIB), or a combination (type IIC). Type IIA represents the second most common fracture type of the distal scaphoid.

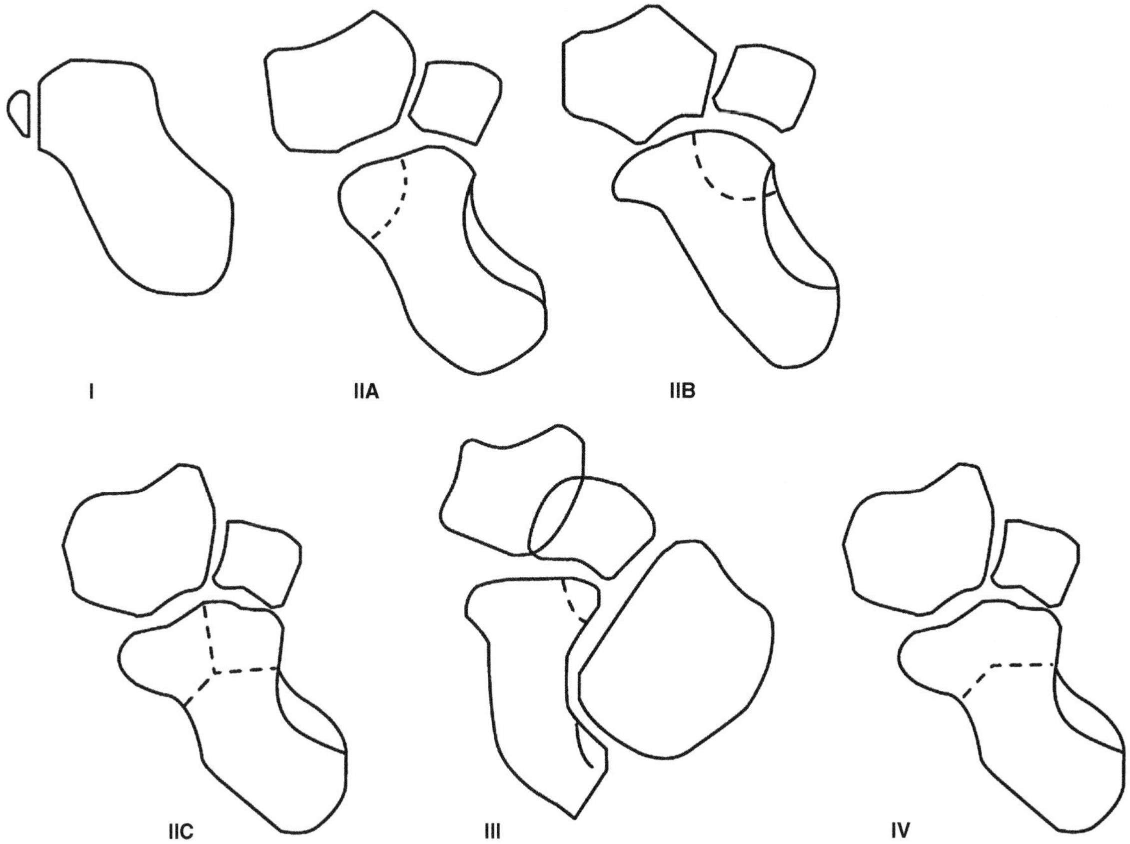

FIG. 15.2 Classification of distal scaphoid fractures according to Prosser et al., type I to III. Clementson et al.[4] added a type IV to make it possible to classify all distal scaphoid fractures.
Type I—extraarticular avulsion fracture
Type IIA—radial fragment
Type IIB—ulnar fragment
Type IIC—Y-fracture, combination of IIA and IIB
Type III—osteochondral fracture fragment of the capitate border of the distal articular surface
Type IV—extraarticular transverse distal fracture (Adapted from Prosser AJ, Brenkel IJ, Irvine GB. Articular fractures of the distal scaphoid. *J Hand Surg Br*. 1988;13(1):87; with permission.)

- Type III, which is rare, represents an osteochondral fracture fragment of the capitate border of the distal articular surface.[8] An accessory carpal bone, os centrale carpi,[22] can mimic the radiologic appearance of this fracture.

Clementson et al.[4] suggested including the transverse extraarticular fracture of the distal third of the scaphoid (synonymous with a Mayo type III fracture) as a type IV fracture (Fig. 15.2). This addition makes it possible to use the modified Prosser classification for all fractures in the distal third of the scaphoid.

IMAGING

Diagnosis and classification of distal scaphoid fractures are difficult on radiographs.[7] Although MRI is often preferred for the diagnosis of scaphoid fractures, CT with its higher spatial resolution and possibility for reconstruction of images in the long axis of the scaphoid is preferred for fracture classification. CT has also proven to be the investigation of choice for assessment of fracture union[23] and possibly also for evaluation of posttraumatic arthritis in the STT joint.[24]

TREATMENT

Fractures in the distal third of scaphoid represent a diverse group of fractures. They range from a distal small, extraarticular, avulsion of the radial palmar lip of the scaphoid tuberosity to more proximal fractures in the area of the watershed zone.[5,7]

There is a general agreement that fractures in the distal third of the scaphoid require shorter immobilization time compared with waist and proximal fractures, from 4 to 8 weeks,[1,3,5,25] and it has even been suggested that it is possible to treat avulsion/tubercle fractures in a removable splint.[26]

Some fractures in the distal scaphoid may benefit from operative treatment. However, in previous studies, there are no indications of evaluation for surgery in respect to fracture gap, dislocation, or step-off in the joint surface.

Nonunion

Delayed or nonunion of distal scaphoid fractures are extremely rare with few reports cases in the literature.[4,7,10,11,27,28] A common finding among nonunions is an inadequate initial treatment in a soft bandage or more commonly no treatment at all.[10,11] Nonunion in distal scaphoid fractures is often asymptomatic.[7,10] However, some nonunions give persisting symptoms that may necessitate operative treatment. Oron et al.[11] have reported that distal nonunions account for 4% of all scaphoid nonunions needing operative treatment.[11] The eight nonunions described by Oron et al. represented type IIC fractures in combination with dorsal intercalated segmental instability pattern, suggesting an associated and more extensive ligament injury.[11] One of these patients were relatively asymptomatic and did not want any treatment; seven patients were operated with cancellous bone grafting and internal fixation, five of which healed and two of which did not heal and were treated with excision of the distal pole.[11] In the case of a type I fracture that does not heal, a resection of the fracture fragment has been shown to relieve symptoms.[10]

Posttraumatic Arthritis

Distal scaphoid fractures may pose a risk for developing posttraumatic arthritis in the STT joint. However, in a 10-year follow-up of 41 distal fractures by Clementson et al.,[4] only seven patients (17%) showed radiologic signs of arthritis on CT. 5 of the 41 fractures were dislocated type II fractures, of which 2 had developed arthritis[4]. This rate of arthritis can be compared with studies with 10- to 12-year follow-up of conservatively treated scaphoid waist fractures, which have shown STT arthritis in 3%–25%.[29,30] The STT joint is the second most common site for degenerative changes in the wrist[31] and the arthritis is often asymptomatic.[32] In none of the seven patients in the study by Clementson et al.,[4] the arthritis had any clinical relevance and hence the risk for developing a symptomatic arthritis following a distal scaphoid fracture has to be considered as minor.

OUTCOME

Distal scaphoid fractures are generally considered benign and heal uneventfully, without any persisting symptoms.[1,8,15] In a 10-year follow-up of 41 distal fractures, patients had regained normal wrist range of motion, grip strength, and pinch strength compared with the uninjured side and had a mean DASH score of 2.[4]

RECOMMENDATION

In patients with a distal scaphoid fracture, evidence suggests the following:

- Cast immobilization provides excellent rates of union (overall quality: moderate).
- In case of nonunion, cancellous bone grafting and fracture fixation provide a high rate of union (overall quality: low).

CONCLUSION

Current evidence on treatment of distal scaphoid fractures relies on two level II and seven level IV studies. These studies suggest that distal scaphoid fractures should be treated with 4–8 weeks of cast immobilization. The duration of immobilization depends on the fracture type.

PANEL 2
Authors' Recommended Technique

Management according to the Prosser classification:

TYPE I

Type I is an extraarticular avulsion of the ligament attachment. The STT joint is stable and the fracture can be treated in a removable splint for 4 weeks.

TYPE IIA AND B

Type IIA is the more common type likely because the radial part of the STT ligament is the strongest. Given the stability of the STT ligament and because major parts of the articular surface are intact, these fractures can withstand axial load and thus can be treated in a short-arm cast for 4–6 weeks.

PANEL 2
Authors' Recommended Technique—cont'd

TYPE IIC

The fracture pattern with involvement of the entire articular surface in combination with less support from the ligaments around the STT joint suggests that this fracture type is more susceptive to axial load. Thus a short thumb spica cast for 6 weeks is appropriate.

TYPE III

In this fracture type the majority of the articulating surface is intact, but it may be accompanied by avulsion of the STT ligaments. Thus a short thumb spica cast for 4 weeks is appropriate.

TYPE IV

This fracture can be treated with the same principles as waist fractures with a short-arm cast for 6 weeks.

Fracture types II and IV with a gap or step-off of more than 1.5 mm should be considered for open reduction and internal fixation.

PANEL 3
Case Scenario Continued

Returning to the case scenario, the patient was treated in a short-arm cast for 4 weeks and then mobilized. At the 10-year follow-up, he did not experience any symptoms from his wrist, which showed a normal range of motion, grip strength, and pinch strength. CT (Fig. 15.1C) showed a healed fracture with a minimal step-off. There were no signs of STT arthritis.

REFERENCES

1. Leslie IJ, Dickson RA. The fractured carpal scaphoid. Natural history and factors influencing outcome. *J Bone Joint Surg Br*. 1981;63-B(2):225–230.
2. Brondum V, Larsen CF, Skov O. Fracture of the carpal scaphoid: frequency and distribution in a well-defined population. *Eur J Radiol*. 1992;15(2):118–122.
3. Lee S. Fractures of the carpal bones. In: Wolfe SW, Pederson W, Kozin SH, Cohen MS, eds. *Green's Operative Hand Surgery*. 7th ed. Philadelphia: Elsevier; 2017.
4. Clementson M, Thomsen N, Besjakov J, Jørgsholm P, Björkman A. Long-term outcomes after distal scaphoid fractures: a 10-year follow-up. *J Hand Surg Am*. 2017 Jul 18. [Epub ahead of print]. https://www.ncbi.nlm.nih.gov/pubmed/28733100
5. Morgan DA, Walters JW. A prospective study of 100 consecutive carpal scaphoid fractures. *Aust N Z J Surg*. 1984;54(3):233–241.
6. Cockshott WP. Distal avulsion fractures of the scaphoid. *Br J Radiol*. 1980;53(635):1037–1040.
7. Prosser AJ, Brenkel IJ, Irvine GB. Articular fractures of the distal scaphoid. *J Hand Surg Br*. 1988;13(1):87–91.
8. Vahvanen V, Westerlund M. Fracture of the carpal scaphoid in children. A clinical and roentgenological study of 108 cases. *Acta Orthop Scand*. 1980;51(6):909–913.
9. Gholson JJ, Bae DS, Zurakowski D, Waters PM. Scaphoid fractures in children and adolescents: contemporary injury patterns and factors influencing time to union. *J Bone Joint Surg Am*. 2011;93(13):1210–1219.
10. Mody BS, Belliappa PP, Dias JJ, Barton NJ. Nonunion of fractures of the scaphoid tuberosity. *J Bone Joint Surg Br*. 1993;75(3):423–425.
11. Oron A, Gupta A, Thirkannad S. Nonunion of the scaphoid distal pole. *Hand Surg*. 2013;18(1):35–39.
12. Gelberman RH, Menon J. The vascularity of the scaphoid bone. *J Hand Surg Am*. 1980;5(5):508–513.
13. Taleisnik J, Kelly PJ. The extraosseous and intraosseous blood supply of the scaphoid bone. *J Bone Joint Surg Am*. 1966;48(6):1125–1137.
14. Garala K, Taub NA, Dias JJ. The epidemiology of fractures of the scaphoid: impact of age, gender, deprivation and seasonality. *Bone Joint J*. 2016;98-B(5):654–659.
15. Ahmed I, Ashton F, Tay WK, Porter D. The pediatric fracture of the scaphoid in patients aged 13 years and under: an epidemiological study. *J Pediatr Orthop*. 2014;34(2):150–154.
16. Christodoulou AG, Colton CL. Scaphoid fractures in children. *J Pediatr Orthop*. 1986;6(1):37–39.
17. Stanciu C, Dumont A. Changing patterns of scaphoid fractures in adolescents. *Can J Surg*. 1994;37(3):214–216.
18. Mussbichler H. Injuries of the carpal scaphoid in children. *Acta Radiol*. 1961;56:361–368.
19. Fisk GR. Carpal instability and the fractured scaphoid. *Ann R Coll Surg Engl*. 1970;46(2):63–76.
20. Cooney WP, Dobyns JH, Linscheid RL. Fractures of the scaphoid: a rational approach to management. *Clin Orthop Relat Res*. 1980;(149):90–97.
21. Ten Berg PW, Drijkoningen T, Strackee SD, Buijze GA. Classifications of acute scaphoid fractures: a systematic literature review. *J Wrist Surg*. 2016;5(2):152–159.
22. Gerscovich EO, Greenspan A. Case report 598: os centrale carpi. *Skeletal Radiol*. 1990;19(2):143–145.
23. Buijze GA, Wijffels MM, Guitton TG, et al. Interobserver reliability of computed tomography to diagnose scaphoid waist fracture union. *J Hand Surg Am*. 2012;37(2):250–254.
24. Saltzherr MS, van Neck JW, Muradin GS, et al. Computed tomography for the detection of thumb base osteoarthritis: comparison with digital radiography. *Skeletal Radiol*. 2013;42(5):715–721.
25. Grewal R, Suh N, Macdermid JC. Use of computed tomography to predict union and time to union in acute scaphoid fractures treated nonoperatively. *J Hand Surg Am*. 2013;38(5):872–877.

26. Dias J. Nonoperative treatment of scaphoid fractures. In: Slutsky DJSJ, ed. *The Scaphoid*. New York: Thieme; 2011.
27. Wilson-MacDonald J. Delayed union of the distal scaphoid in a child. *J Hand Surg Am*. 1987;12(4):520–522.
28. Jonsson K. Nonunion of a fractured scaphoid tubercle. *J Hand Surg Am*. 1990;15(2):283–285.
29. Saeden B, Tornkvist H, Ponzer S, Hoglund M. Fracture of the carpal scaphoid. A prospective, randomised 12-year follow-up comparing operative and conservative treatment. *J Bone Joint Surg Br*. 2001;83(2):230–234.
30. Vinnars B, Pietreanu M, Bodestedt A, Ekenstam F, Gerdin B. Nonoperative compared with operative treatment of acute scaphoid fractures. A randomized clinical trial. *J Bone Joint Surg Am*. 2008;90(6):1176–1185.
31. Watson HK, Ballet FL. The SLAC wrist: scapholunate advanced collapse pattern of degenerative arthritis. *J Hand Surg Am*. 1984;9(3):358–365.
32. Wollstein R, Watson HK. Scaphotrapeziotrapezoid arthrodesis for arthritis. *Hand Clin*. 2005;21(4):539–543. vi.

CHAPTER 16

Percutaneous Scaphoid Fixation: Volar and Dorsal Techniques

NICHOLAS GODDARD, MB, FRCS

KEY POINTS

- Open fixation of acute, or complicated, scaphoid fractures results in a high rate of union, avoids potentially prolonged cast immobilization, but has a relatively high (approximately 30%) incidence of complications, especially wound/scar related.
- Percutaneous techniques convey all the advantages of open fixation but minimize the incidence of wound complications.
- Early percutaneous fixation may be offered as an alternative to cast immobilization.
- Volar and dorsal approaches result in similar outcomes.

PANEL 1
Case Scenario

CASE 1

A 21-year-old professional musician (keyboard and percussion) fell down while playing soccer. His initial radiographs showed no obvious scaphoid or distal radial fracture and accordingly his wrist was immobilized in a temporary backslab. Repeat radiographs at 10 days later were inconclusive, but an MRI scan confirmed the presence of a nondisplaced fracture through the waist of the scaphoid with associated bone edema involving the distal pole. Given his profession, he opted for percutaneous screw fixation. While preparing for surgery, you question the current best evidence: What is the optimal approach for a waist fracture: volar or dorsal?

IMPORTANCE OF THE PROBLEM

Fractures of the scaphoid lead to significant physical and economic morbidity. Early rigid fixation has recently been advocated to promote rapid functional recovery. Open reduction and internal fixation of the scaphoid is however technically demanding, damages the anterior radiocarpal ligaments, violates the scaphotrapezial joint, further endangers the already-compromised blood supply of the scaphoid, and not infrequently leads to troublesome hypertrophic scars. These problems may be overcome by percutaneous fixation.

MAIN QUESTION

What are the preferred methods and approaches of fixation for a nondisplaced or minimally displaced scaphoid fracture?

Current Opinion

Acute open reduction and rigid internal fixation of displaced or complicated scaphoid fractures is widely accepted as best practice, and we are indebted to Tim Herbert who introduced a reliable technique and suitable device, thus firmly establishing screw fixation of the scaphoid.[1,2]

The role of surgery for minimally displaced or nondisplaced fractures remains a subject of intense debate. It is, however, apparent that the greater majority of scaphoid fractures occur in young men who may be manual workers or may be involved in athletic activity. The avoidance of plaster immobilization in these patients would be very desirable. Early fixation would, therefore, provide the opportunity of early mobilization and earlier return to full function.

Finding the Evidence

- Cochrane search: Scaphoid Fracture
- Pubmed (Medline): (scaphoid fracture*[tiab]) AND ("minimally invasive surgical procedures" [Mesh] OR percutaneous [Subheading] OR volar* OR dorsal* OR minimally invasive)

- Bibliography of eligible articles
- Articles that were not in English, French, or German were excluded.

Quality of the Evidence

Level II:

Systematic reviews/metaanalyses: 1
Randomized trials with methodological limitations: 1
Prospective comparative studies: 1

Level III:

Retrospective comparative studies: 5

Level IV:

Case series: 11

FINDINGS

Although there are multiple studies comparing cast versus screw fixation, there are no studies comparing open versus percutaneous approaches for scaphoid fractures. Were metaanalysis, one RCT, and one prospective comparing volar with dorsal approaches; for acute fixation of waist fractures, the bulk of the literature is confined to either retrospective studies or case reports. Kang et al.[3] performed a metaanalysis of the available publications comparing dorsal and volar approaches for percutaneous fixation. They concluded that, although the dorsal approach allowed for better, more central screw positioning (which has been shown to result in possibly quicker union rates), there were no obvious advantages of one approach over another with regard to the incidence of nonunion, postoperative pain, grip strength, and overall functional outcome and range of motion with the exception of ulnar deviation, which was found to be significantly greater with the volar approach. Drac et al.[4]compared the volar percutaneous and limited dorsal approaches in a series of 76 patients with acute nondisplaced or minimally displaced type B2 fractures. In their study group there was a more rapid recovery with regard to the range of motion and grip strength in the volar fixation group, but by 1 year both groups were identical with regard to union rates, function, and range of motion by 12 months.

Historical Perspective

Satisfactory function following scaphoid fractures requires union in an anatomic position. This is facilitated, although not necessarily accelerated by stable fixation with a compression screw. Herbert and Fisher reported a far higher union rate for acutely stabilized scaphoid fractures. This was supported by the later work of Bunker[5] and of Wozasek and Moser.[6]

The open approach to scaphoid fracture fixation is technically demanding, damages the anterior radio carpal ligaments, violates the scaphotrapezial joint, further endangers the already compromised blood supply of the scaphoid, and not infrequently leads to troublesome hypertrophic scars.[2,7,8] In addition Garcia-Elias reported carpal instability after volar approaches to the scaphoid that damage the radiocapitate and radiolunate ligaments.[9]

A percutaneous technique minimizes operative trauma and preserves the blood supply of the scaphoid and the integrity of its surrounding ligaments. Percutaneous scaphoid fixation can be performed as a day case and allows for earlier mobilization, with fewer complications and has been shown to result in an increased speed of union with a very low rate of nonunion.[10]

Percutaneous screw fixation of the scaphoid was first reported by Streli in 1970[11] and subsequently adapted by Wozasek and Moser and later Ledoux.[6,12]

Scaphoid screw fixation has now been extensively evaluated both clinically and biomechanically, and the current selection of cannulated headless compression screws has facilitated the procedure.[13–16]

In 1996 we further modified and simplified the volar percutaneous technique using the cannulated Acutrak screw and extended the indications to stabilize minimally displaced or nondisplaced B1 or B2 acute scaphoid fractures.[17] In our pilot study we reported a union rate of 100% and our current experience continues to reflect this high rate of union. Encouraged by our early results we have now expanded the indications to include displaced fractures, delayed union, and some patterns of nonunions, where we would consider using supplementary percutaneous bone grafting.

Indications

There is still obviously a place for nonoperative (cast) treatment, which is undoubtedly safe, but with a known rate of nonunion and the associated inconvenience of plaster immobilization. In my opinion percutaneous fixation is now a justifiable alternative to cast immobilization and permits early rehabilitation with minimal risks and a high, if not guaranteed, rate of union.

The volar (distal to proximal) approach is applicable to all waist fractures and some proximal third fractures depending on the obliquity of the fracture line. Proximal pole fractures are best dealt with via a dorsal (proximal to distal) approach as described by Slade.[18] The direction of the fixation is obviously down to surgeon preference, but as a rule the trailing edge of the screw should be closest to the site of the fracture. For waist fractures the evidence suggests that the dorsal approach allowed for better, more central screw positioning (which has been shown to result in possibly quicker union rates[19]), and there were no obvious advantages of one approach over another with regard to the incidence of nonunion, postoperative pain, grip strength, overall functional outcome, and range of motion with the exception of ulnar deviation, which was found to be significantly greater with the volar approach.[3] Drac et al.[4] demonstrated that there was a more rapid recovery with regard to range of motion and grip strength in the volar fixation group, but by 1 year both groups were identical with regard to union rates, function, and range of motion by 12 months. One cautionary note, however, is that there have been reports of late fractures of the dorsal aspect of the proximal pole of the scaphoid following dorsal screw fixation.[20] This is thought to be the result of a potential stress riser at the pint of insertion of the screw. There have been no reports of a similar complication using the volar approach.

Having elected for percutaneous fixation, there is a distinct window of opportunity. Complex fracture dislocations require immediate intervention, but for other cases surgery can be postponed until the next suitable operating list and, in practice, can be delayed by up to 4 weeks without reducing the chance of ultimate fracture union. Beyond this stage, I would recommend supplementary measures such as cancellous bone grafting, which can be performed percutaneously, with or without arthroscopic assistance.

PANEL 2
Author's Preferred Technique

VOLAR APPROACH

Percutaneous scaphoid fixation using a cannulated headless compression screw can be performed under general or regional anesthesia. It is entirely feasible to perform the operation with the affected arm abducted on a hand table; we have found it easier to use a modification of the original technique described by Wozasek and Moser.[2,6]

For the volar technique the patient is placed supine on an operating table, the forearm and hand are prepared in a standard fashion and the rest of the upper limb and body covered with an extremity drape (Fig. 16.1A and B). I routinely infiltrate the proposed entry point of the guide wire with 2 ml 2% lignocaine with 1:200,000 adrenaline. The use of a tourniquet is optional.

The hand is suspended by the thumb alone in a single Chinese finger trap with no countertraction. This arrangement extends the scaphoid and ulnar deviates the wrist to improve access to the distal pole of the scaphoid. Importantly it permits free rotation of the hand throughout the operation, and the scaphoid remains in the center of the X-ray field throughout and facilitates arthroscopy if it is felt to be necessary to confirm the quality of the reduction[2] (Fig. 16.2).

The image intensifier C-arm is turned to a horizontal position and positioned so that the wrist is in the central axis. With the image intensifier in this position, it is then possible to screen the scaphoid continuously around the axis of the radial column. In most cases, there is no need for any additional measures to reduce the fracture. However, if it is felt that the position of the fracture is unacceptable then K wires can be inserted and used as joysticks to manipulate the fragments into position (see the section "Reduction Tips" below). The quality of the reduction can then be checked radiographically and if necessary arthroscopically without disturbing the overall setup. As with any closed fracture, fixation time spent in setting up and ensuring quality of the reduction is time well spent.

Having achieved an acceptable reduction the first, probably the most important step is to establish the entry point of the guide wire and hence ultimately the position of the screw. The ulnar deviation of the wrist allows the distal half of the scaphoid to slide out from under the radial styloid. The scaphoid tuberosity is easily palpable and is the key to the insertion point.

The entry point is then located using a 12G intravenous (IV) needle introduced on the anteroradial aspect of the wrist just radial and distal to the scaphoid tuberosity.[2] This serves as a trochar for the guide wire and proves to be invaluable as a direction aid so as to establish a central path along the scaphoid.[19] The needle is then insinuated into the scaphotrapezial joint, tilted into a more vertical position, and the position is checked under image intensifier. By gently levering on the trapezium, this maneuver brings the distal pole of the scaphoid more radial and thus ultimately facilitates screw insertion along a more central axis. It is then possible to screen the wrist by simply rotating the forearm in the X-ray beam and to line up the needle along the long axis of the scaphoid in all planes. The aim is to have the guide wire exiting the proximal pole just radial to the scapholunate junction.

I have found it helpful to have my thumb on the scaphoid tuberosity and index finger over Lister's tubercle and to aim the guide wire toward my index finger. This invariably gives the correct direction. Once I am happy with the entry point and the direction of the guide wire, I lightly tap the needle into the soft articular

Continued

PANEL 2
Author's Preferred Technique—cont'd

cartilage over the distal pole of the scaphoid so that the tip does not slip during the insertion of the guide wire. Any "fine-tuning" can be carried out at this point by rotating the IV cannula because the effect of the bevel can change the position of the ultimate entry point by up to 2 mm (Fig. 16.3).

The guide wire (0.045 in./1.1 mm) can then be passed down through the needle and drilled across the fracture continually checking the direction on the image intensifier and correcting as necessary, aiming for the radial aspect of the proximal pole. This requires an appreciation of the obliquity of the scaphoid in both anteroposterior and lateral planes. It is extremely important not to bend the guide wire, and any adjustments in direction should be made using the needle as a guide rather than attempting to alter the line of the guide wire alone (Fig. 16.4A and B).

The guide wire should be advanced to stop just short of the articular surface and should not breach it at this stage. The position, alignment, and length are checked once more. If the position is felt to be satisfactory, then a longitudinal incision of 0.5 cm is made at the entry point of the wire and deepened down to the distal pole of the scaphoid using a small hemostat and blunt dissection. This is a relatively safe zone with minimal risk to the adjacent neurovascular structures.[3]

The length of the screw is then determined using either the proprietary depth gauge or by advancing a second guide wire of the same length up the distal cortex of the scaphoid and subtracting the difference between the two. The correct screw size is 2 mm shorter than the measured length to ensure that the screw head is fully buried below the cartilage and the cortical surface. In practice, most screws in an adult male are 24–26 mm and 22–24 mm in females. The positioning guide wire is then advanced through the proximal pole of the scaphoid to exit on the dorsal aspect of the wrist. This is a precautionary measure to minimize the risk of inadvertent withdrawal of the wire during the reaming process and screw insertion and to facilitate the removal of the proximal portion if the wire were to break. In those rare cases where it is felt that there is a possibility of rotational instability, it is recommended that a second derotation wire be inserted parallel to the first prior to drilling and reaming. Such an instance would be encountered in early stabilization of a transscaphoid perilunate fracture dislocation, for example.

Having secured the guide wire, the 12G needle is then slid off and the cannulated drill is then passed over the wire using either a power drill or hand reamer stopping 1–2 mm short of the articular surface. My preference is to drill on power to minimize the risk of repeated bending of the guide wire, so reducing the chance of breakage. It is helpful to screen this process to ensure accurate drilling and especially to ensure that the guide wire has not been inadvertently bent (Fig 16.5).

The self-tapping screw is then advanced over the guide wire and the wire is removed. Compression can then be confirmed radiographically on the image intensifier (Fig 16.6).

The skin is closed using a single steristrip or suture, which is covered with a sterile compressive dressing. The tourniquet is released and the arm is elevated. Plaster immobilization is entirely optional and is not used in our unit when fixation appears stable.

DORSAL TECHNIQUE

The dorsal approach, as originally described by Slade,[18] is applicable to either midwaist fractures or, more appropriately, proximal pole fractures.

As with the volar approach, the surgery is carried out under image-intensifier (fluoroscopic) control. The patient is positioned supine with the arm on an arm table and the C-arm positioned horizontally (Fig 16.7).

The wrist is then examined to exclude any concomitant ligamentous injury or carpal instability. The hand is then visualized initially in a standard posteroanterior view and then flexed to almost 90°, superimposing the proximal and distal poles looking for the so-called "ring sign" confirming that one is then looking down the longitudinal axis of the scaphoid. The center of the "ring" now represents the central axis of the scaphoid (Fig. 16.8A and B).

A 12G cannula can then be used to identify the entry point in the center of the proximal pole and to orientate this along the central axis of the scaphoid, aiming distally to the scaphotrapezial joint. The cannula is lined up in the center of the pole, aiming distally. A guide wire is then drilled along the central axis of the scaphoid with the aim of exiting on the volar aspect of the wrist. The wrist *must* remain flexed at this time to avoid bending the guide wire. The wire is then withdrawn such that the proximal end of the wire remains in the proximal pole (Fig 16.9). The reduction is then confirmed and adjustments made if required. It is then possible to arthroscope the wrist at this stage to confirm the accuracy of the reduction.

Having confirmed the reduction, the wrist is then flexed once more and the wire is driven from a volar to a dorsal position to exit the dorsal aspect of the wrist. A small incision is then made to ensure that the extensor tendons are not impaled (Fig 16.10). The length of the screw is then established as with the volar approach, but the correct screw size is 4 mm shorter than the measured length to ensure that the screw head is fully buried below the articular cartilage and the cortical surface. A cannulated drill is then passed over the guide wire along the central axis of the scaphoid and the screw inserted in an antegrade fashion (Fig 16.11).

PANEL 2
Author's Preferred Technique—cont'd

COMBINED VOLAR/DORSAL APPROACH

Under some circumstances, it is possible to use a combined volar/dorsal approach; this can be used especially for small proximal pole fractures.

In a standard volar approach the aim is to insert as long a screw as possible down the central axis to speed up fracture union and to increase the biomechanical characteristics of the fixation. However, in a small proximal pole fragment, it is sometimes easier to fit this using a volar dorsal approach because the screw is relatively short.

The entry point under these circumstances on the volar aspect of the wrist is not quite so critical. The aim is to establish that the wire is centrally placed in the proximal pole fragment using a standard volar technique as described earlier. It is essential that the wire is exactly in the center of the proximal pole to maximize the strength of compression. The wrist is then flexed and the wire is driven through the dorsal aspect of the wrist, and standard fixation as per the Slade approach can then be effected. The important aspect of this method of fixation is that only a small screw (12–14mm) is required to achieve stable fixation.

POSTOPERATIVE CARE

The arm is elevated immediately postoperatively, and routine postanesthetic and neurovascular observations are recorded.

The patients are encouraged to begin active finger exercises prior to discharge. The patients are reviewed 10 days postoperatively to exclude sepsis and ensure that early mobilization is being carried out. The sutures are removed at this stage and carpal radiographs are taken to confirm that screw position is satisfactory. At this stage, patients are allowed to mobilize gently, but no heavy carrying or weight bearing activity is permitted.

We review the patient 4 weeks later and, further, radiographs are taken. Return to sedentary work is allowed as soon as the patient feels ready or when 75% of the contralateral range of movement is achieved. Manual work and athletic activity are deferred until there is radiographic evidence (either plain films or ideally CT scan) of fracture union. Patients are advised to wear a supportive splint for contact sports. There is usually no need to remove the screw at a later date.

REDUCTION TIPS

Under some circumstances, the fracture is unstable and a temporary second wire may become necessary to stabilize the fracture. Equally reduction can occasionally be difficult, especially when the fracture is mobile. Under these circumstances, certain reduction tips can be utilized. My favored technique is to use the IV cannula as a "joystick" in the distal pole. This is introduced into the chosen (ideal) entry point and advanced down to the fracture site. The cannula can then be used to manipulate the distal pole and line it up more accurately with the proximal pole, having achieved satisfactory alignment. An initial guide wire can then be inserted down the length of the scaphoid. Frequently, this is not in an ideal position and a more accurate guide wire can then be inserted prior to ultimate screw fixation.

Under certain circumstances, where the operation is being performed for delayed union, the fracture site can be a little stiff and a simple IV cannula is not really strong enough. Under these circumstances, a guide wire is introduced into the proximal pole and the cannulated drill is used as the "joystick." Finally, in later cases, where there is a potential humpback deformity with volar flexion of the scaphoid, two dorsal wires can be introduced and then used to manipulate the respective poles prior to insertion of the ultimate guide wire.

COMPLICATIONS

Fortunately, the percutaneous techniques are, in general, free of the complications previously reported using the traditional open approach. In my own experience the most frequent complication is of transient dysesthesia just distal to the scar. This is secondary to a neurapraxia of a sensory branch of the median nerve and usually resolves within 4–6 weeks. I have had no cases of infection in my personal series. The rate of nonunion in all reported series is low and can generally be attributed to technical errors in placement of the screw or confounding factors such as the patient being a smoker.

Most of the reported complications of percutaneous surgery can be attributed to technical errors, particularly leaving the screw too long protruding into the scaphotrapezial joint and possible resulting in premature degenerative changes. This can be avoided by appropriate screw selection and correct placement. In addition, there have been reports of guide wire breakage and screwdriver breakage.[21–23] Both are easily remedied and do not result in enduring harm to the patient nor jeopardize the final outcome.

I now have an experience of almost 600 percutaneous scaphoid fixations and remain encouraged by the high rate of fracture union (>98%) in the treatment of acute fractures. Indeed, my only failures to unite have been in those patients with proximal pole fractures that I have attempted to fix via the volar approach. All the acute waist fractures have united.

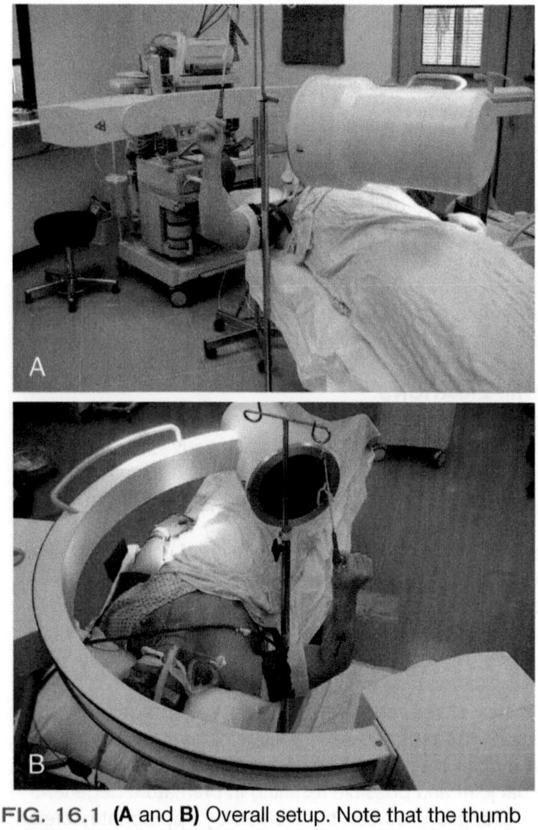

FIG. 16.1 **(A and B)** Overall setup. Note that the thumb is suspended by a single trap so placing the wrist in slight ulnar deviation and extension. The C-arm is brought in horizontally across the patient's upper body with the scaphoid at the center.

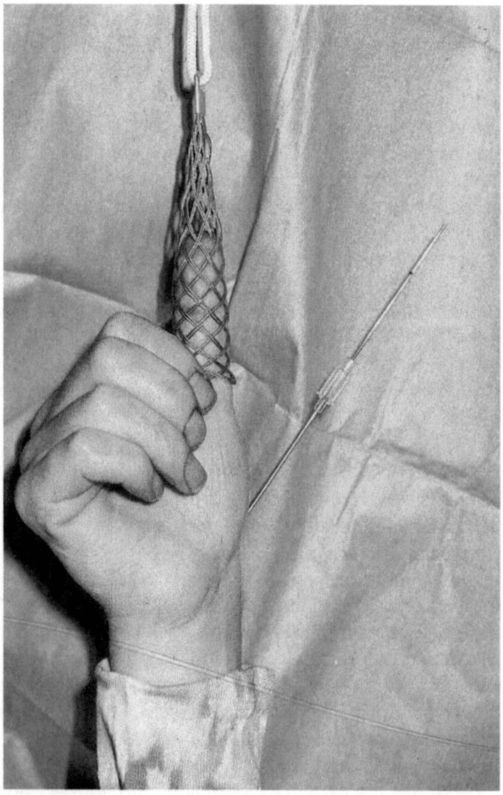

FIG. 16.2 Close-up of the entry point. Note that the entry point is more proximal and more volar than one might normally have assumed. It is helpful to use a 12 or 14G IV cannula as a trochar and aiming device, initially bringing it in virtually horizontally at the scaphotrapezial joint and then swinging it upward and anteriorly to line up the proposed direction of the guide wire aiming toward Lister's tubercle.

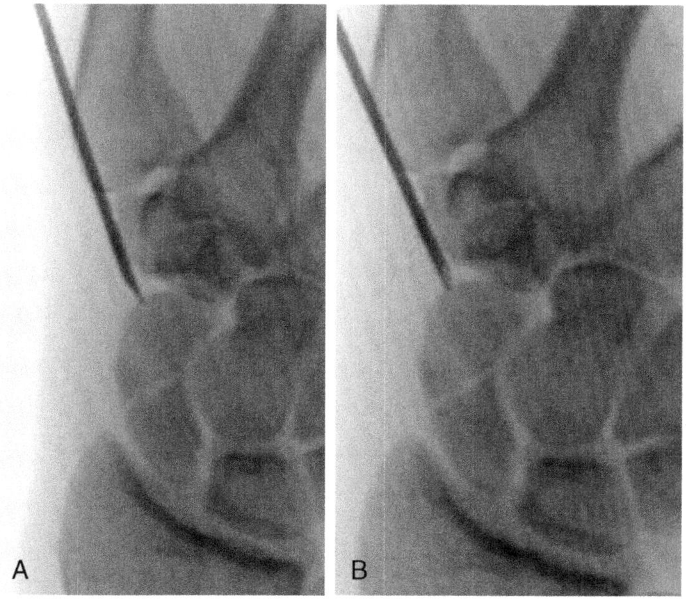

FIG. 16.3 (**A** and **B**) Fine-tuning by simple rotation of cannula so moving the entry point of the guide wire medially by 2 mm.

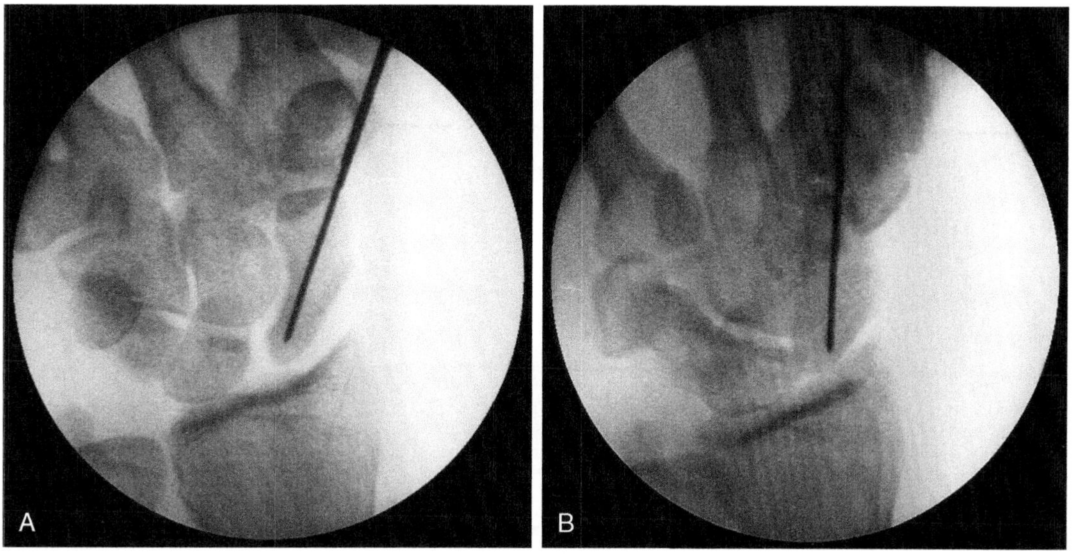

FIG. 16.4 **(A)** Anteroposterior position of the guide wire. Note the entry point at the lateral border of the scaphoid tuberosity and the 14G needle being used as an aiming device and trochar. The guide wire should be directed to the radial aspect of the scapholunate joint. **(B)** Lateral position of the guide wire. This position is just acceptable, but ideally could be a little more anterior. It is along the central axis of the bone.

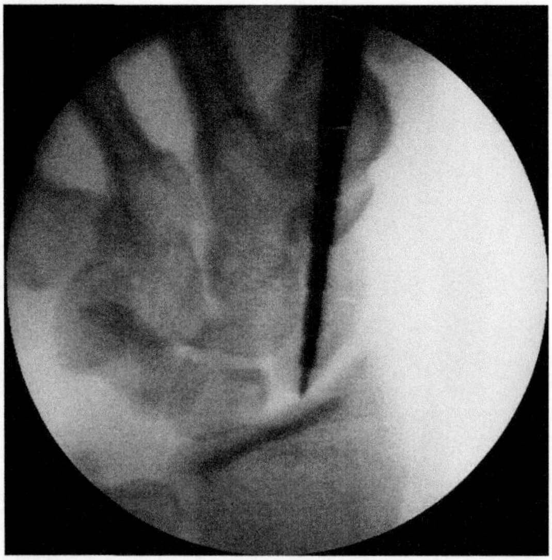

FIG. 16.5 After measuring the length of the screw, the guide wire is advanced through the articular surface to prevent inadvertent withdrawal while reaming and screw fixation. The chosen screw must be 2–4 mm shorter than the measured length. Note that the reamer has stopped 2–3 mm short of the proximal pole.

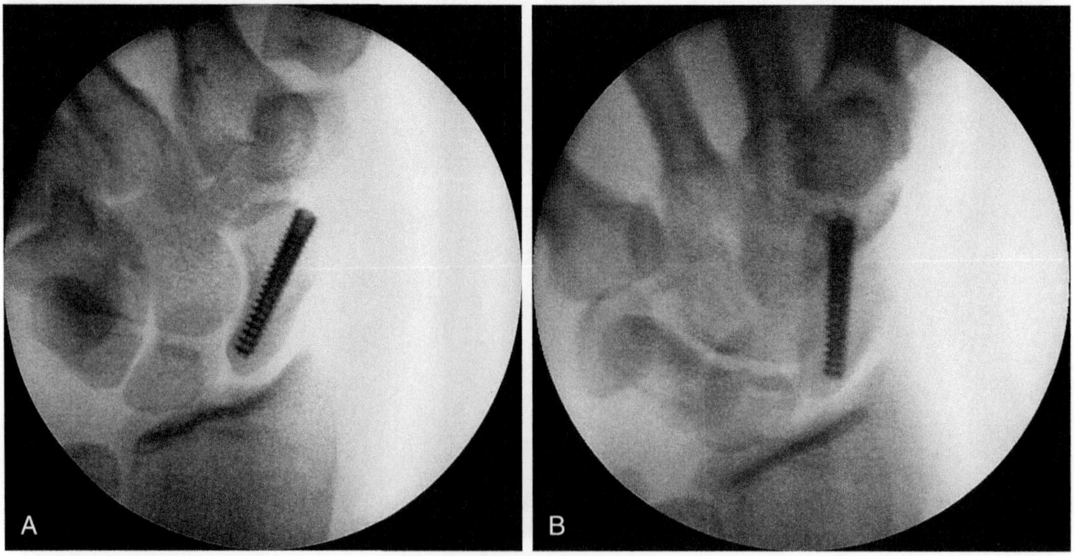

FIG. 16.6 (**A** and **B**) Final position of the screw. Note the position and alignment along the central axis and that both ends are buried beneath the articular surfaces.

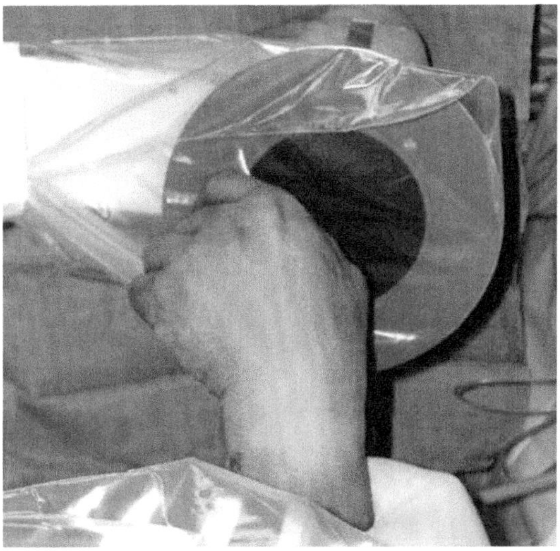

FIG. 16.7 Wrist pronated and flexed in the center of the mini C-arm.

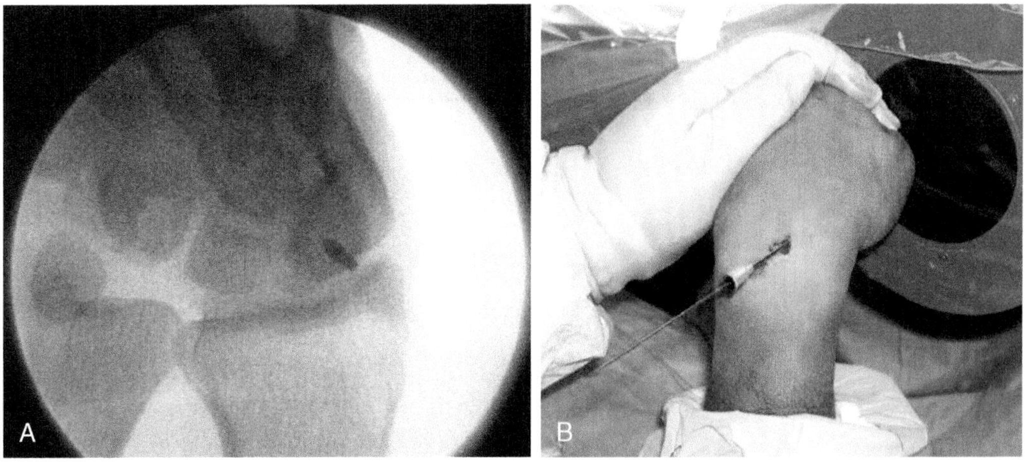

FIG. 16.8 **(A** and **B)** Wrist flexed and pronated with the scaphoid "ring" sign and entry point established in the center of the proximal pole.

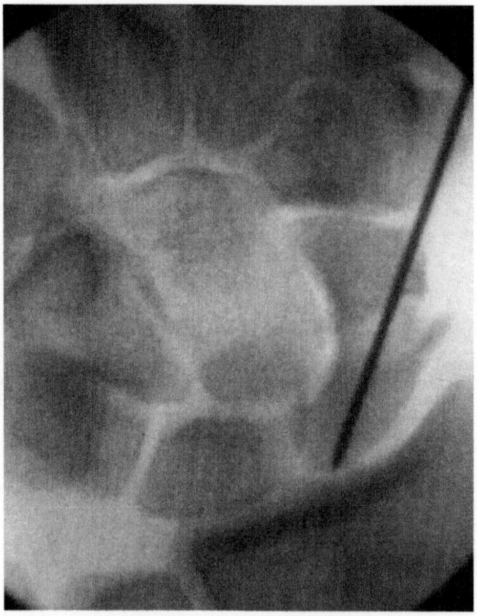

FIG. 16.9 Guide wire advanced through the volar aspect of the wrist, leaving the tip just in the proximal pole. The wrist can now be extended and reduction is confirmed. It is at this stage that an arthroscopy can be performed if required.

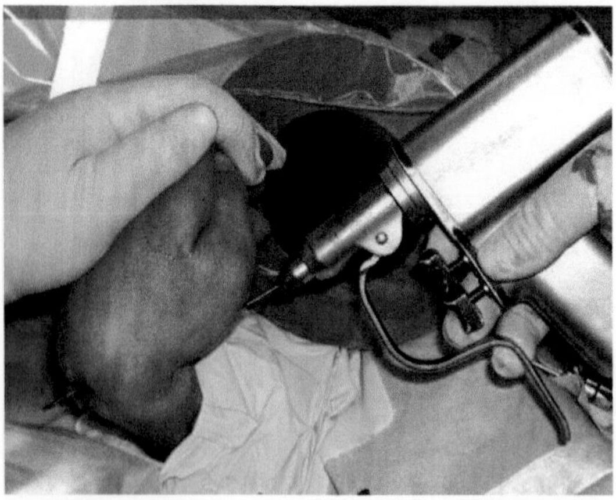

FIG. 16.10 Guide wire is then passed back through the dorsal aspect of the wrist and then the desired screw can be inserted.

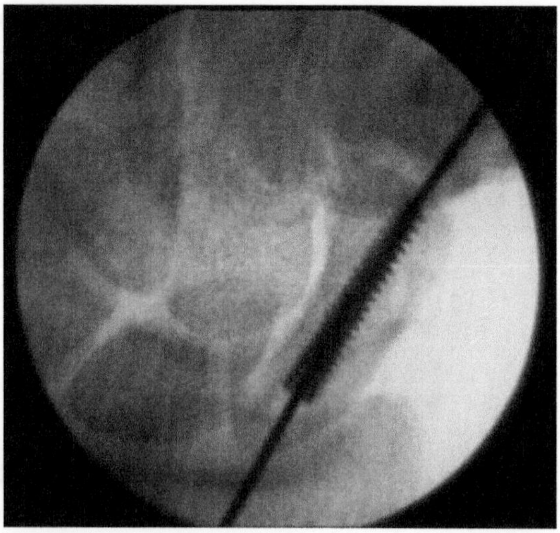

FIG. 16.11 Final positioning of screw from dorsal aspect of the wrist. Note that both ends are buried below the articular surfaces.

RECOMMENDATION

In patients with a nondisplaced or minimally displaced scaphoid waist fracture, evidence suggests the following:

- There is no difference between volar or dorsal approaches with regard to rates of union, overall function, and range of motion with the exception of ulnar deviation, which is better following a volar approach (overall quality: moderate).
- There is no difference in the rates of complications following volar and dorsal approaches, but there have been reports of late fractures of the proximal pole using the dorsal approach (overall quality: low).
- Surgeons should be familiar with both the dorsal and volar percutaneous approaches because not all acute scaphoid fractures can be dealt with completely with one approach (overall quality: very low).

CONCLUSION

The economic and social cost of plaster immobilization following scaphoid fractures must not be underestimated. This is particularly the case in young working men or those involved in athletic and sporting pursuits. Percutaneous fixation on the other hand allows early intervention with a minimally invasive day case procedure. This encourages early wrist and hand mobilization while minimizing the potential complications of open carpal surgery, especially scar hypersensitivity and hypertrophy. The current literature suggests that percutaneous fixation of acute scaphoid fractures has advantages over cast fixation.

PANEL 3
Pearls and Pitfalls

PEARLS

- Take time in positioning the patient to allow 360 degrees visualization of the scaphoid on the image intensifier.
- Establish the correct entry point, which should be just dorsal and radial to the tip of the scaphoid tuberosity.[3,19,24] Aim the guide wire to exit at the tip of the proximal pole at the scapholunate junction.
- Ensure that the guide wire is along the longest axis of the scaphoid and is as central as possible.
- Advance the guide wire to the 3/4 arthroscopic portal to minimize the risk of accidental withdrawal and to facilitate its removal in the event of breakage.
- Drill into the distal fragment even if using a self-drilling and self-tapping screw. This facilitates the screw "biting" as it is inserted and prevents "push-off" as the screw is advanced across the fracture site.
- Ensure that the screw is contained within the body of the scaphoid with both ends deep to the articular surface. The chosen screw must be 2–4 mm shorter than the measured length. Bear in mind that the average length of a male scaphoid is 28 mm (25.6–31.1 mm) and female 26.4 mm (23.7–28.4 mm).[3]
- Place the screw with the trailing edge closest to the fracture site. Thus distal pole fractures are best treated by volar placement, proximal pole fractures by proximal placement, and waist fractures by whichever the operator is most comfortable and familiar.

PITFALLS

- Malposition of the screw.
- Screw too long with protrusion into either radioscaphoid or scaphotrapezial joint (see above). Subtract 2 mm from the measured length for volar insertion and 4 mm for dorsal insertion.
- Breakage of the guide wire. This usually results when drilling by hand and is the effect of repeated bending of the wire during this maneuver. Drilling on power minimizes the risk.
- Screwdriver breakage. This usually results from failure to adequately predrill prior to screw implantation. Fortunately, the screwdriver is designed to break at a point where there is sufficient length for retrieval. I have found that straight arthroscopic grabbers are useful if this were to happen.

REFERENCES

1. Herbert TJ, Fisher WE. Management of the fractured scaphoid using a new bone screw. *J Bone Jt Surg Br.* 1984;66(0301-620X (Print)):114–123.
2. Filan SL, Herbert TJ. Herbert screw fixation of scaphoid fractures. *J Bone Jt Surg Br.* 1996;78(0301-620X (Print)): 519–529.
3. Kang K-B, Kim H-J, Park J-H, Shin Y-S. Comparison of dorsal and volar percutaneous approaches in acute scaphoid fractures: a meta-analysis. *PLoS One.* 2016;11(9):e0162779. http://dx.doi.org/10.1371/journal.pone.0162779.
4. Drac P, Cizmar I, Manak P, et al. Comparison of the results and complications of palmar and dorsal miniinvasive approaches in the surgery of scaphoid fractures. A prospective randomized study. *Biomed Pap Med Fac Univ Palacky Olomouc Czech Repub.* 2014;158(2):277–281. http://dx.doi.org/10.5507/bp.2012.060.
5. Bunker TD, McNamee PB, Scott TD. The Herbert screw for scaphoid fractures. A multicentre study. *J Bone Jt Surg Br.* 1987;69(0301-620X (Print)):631–634.
6. Wozasek GE, Moser KD. Percutaneous screw fixation for fractures of the scaphoid. *J Bone Jt Surg Br.* 1991;73(0301-620X):138–142.
7. Herbert TJ. Open volar repair of acute scaphoid fractures. *Hand Clin.* 2001;17(0749-0712):589–599. viii.
8. Dias JJ, Wildin CJ, Bhowal B, Thompson JR. Should acute scaphoid fractures be fixed? A randomized controlled trial. *J Bone Jt Surg Am.* 2005;87(0021-9355 (Print)):2160–2168.
9. Garcia-Elias M, Vall A, Salo JM, Lluch AL. Carpal alignment after different surgical approaches to the scaphoid: a comparative study. *J Hand Surg Am.* 1988;13(0363-5023 (Print)):604–612.
10. Adolfsson L, Lindau T, Arner M. Acutrak screw fixation versus cast immobilisation for undisplaced scaphoid waist fractures. *J Hand Surg Br.* 2001;26(3):192–195. http://dx.doi.org/10.1054/jhsb.2001.0558.
11. Streli R. [Percutaneous screwing of the navicular bone of the hand with a compression drill screw (a new method)]. *ZentralblChir.* 1970;95(0044-409X (Print)): 1060–1078.
12. Ledoux P, Chahidi N, Moermans JP, Kinnen L. [Percutaneous Herbert screw osteosynthesis of the scaphoid bone]. *Acta Orthop Belg.* 1995;61(0001-6462):43–47.
13. Shaw JA. A biomechanical comparison of scaphoid screws. *J Hand Surg [Am].* 1987;12(0363-5023 (Print)): 347–353.
14. Rankin G, Kuschner SH, Orlando C, McKellop H, Brien WW, Sherman R. A biomechanical evaluation of a cannulated compressive screw for use in fractures of the scaphoid. *J Hand Surg [Am].* 1991;16(0363-5023 (Print)): 1002–1010.
15. Kaulesar Sukul DM, Johannes EJ, Marti RK, Klopper PJ. Biomechanical measurements on scaphoid bone screws in an experimental model. *J Biomech.* 1990;23(0021-9290 (Print)):1115–1121.
16. Sagi AS. Scaphoid screws. *J Hand Surg [Am].* 1988;13 (0363-5023 (Print)):461–462.
17. Haddad FS, Goddard NJ. Acute percutaneous scaphoid fixation. A pilot study. *J Bone Jt Surg Br.* 1998;80(0301-620X): 95–99.
18. Slade III JF, Jaskwhich D. Percutaneous fixation of scaphoid fractures. *Hand Clin.* 2001;17(0749-0712):553–574.
19. McCallister WV, Knight J, Kaliappan R, Trumble TE. Central placement of the screw in simulated fractures of the scaphoid waist: a biomechanical study. *J Bone Jt Surg Am.* 2003;85-A(0021-9355):72–77.
20. Rancy SK, Zelken JA, Lipman JD, Wolfe SW. Scaphoid proximal pole fracture following headless screw fixation. *J Wrist Surg.* 2016;5(1):71–76. http://dx.doi.org/10.1055/s-0035-1565928.
21. Bushnell BD, McWilliams AD, Messer TM. Complications in dorsal percutaneous cannulated screw fixation of nondisplaced scaphoid waist fractures. *J Hand Surg Am.* 2007;32(0363-5023 (Print)):827–833.
22. McQueen MM, Gelbke MK, Wakefield A, Will EM, Gaebler C. Percutaneous screw fixation versus conservative treatment for fractures of the waist of the scaphoid: a prospective randomised study. *J Bone Jt Surg Br.* 2008;90(0301-620X (Print)):66–71.
23. Geurts G, Van Riet R, Meermans G, Verstreken F. Incidence of scaphotrapezial arthritis following volar percutaneous fixation of nondisplaced scaphoid waist fractures using a transtrapezial approach. *J Hand Surg Am.* 2011;36(11):1753–1758. http://dx.doi.org/10.1016/j.jhsa.2011.08.031.
24. Levitz S, Ring D. Retrograde (volar) scaphoid screw insertion-a quantitative computed tomographic analysis. *J Hand Surg Am.* 2005;30(0363-5023 (Print)):543–548.

FURTHER READING

1. Bond CD, Shin AY, McBride MT, Dao KD. Percutaneous screw fixation or cast immobilization for nondisplaced scaphoid fractures. *J Bone Jt Surg Am.* 2001;83-A(0021-9355):483–488.
2. Yip HS, Wu WC, Chang RY, So TY. Percutaneous cannulated screw fixation of acute scaphoid waist fracture. *J Hand Surg Br.* 2002;27(0266-7681):42–46.
3. Geissler WB, Adams JE, Bindra RR, Lanzinger WD, Slutsky DJ. Scaphoid fractures: what's hot, What's not. *J Bone Jt Surg.* February 2012;2012(61):169–181. http://dx.doi.org/10.2106/JBJS.942icl.
4. Neshkova IS, Jakubietz RG, Kuk D, Jakubietz MG, Meffert RH, Schmidt K. Percutaneous screw fixation of non- or minimally displaced scaphoid fractures. *Oper Orthop Traumatol.* 2015. http://dx.doi.org/10.1007/s00064-014-0325-0.
5. Davis EN, Chung KC, Kotsis SV, Lau FH, Vijan S. A cost/utility analysis of open reduction and internal fixation versus cast immobilization for acute nondisplaced mid-waist scaphoid fractures. *Plast Reconstr Surg.* 2006;117(1529-4242 (Electronic)):1223–1235.

6. Grewal R, King G. Percutaneous screw fixation led to faster recovery and return to work than immobilization for fractures of the waist of the scaphoid. *J Bone Jt Surg Am.* 2008;90(1535–1386 (Electronic)):1793.
7. Goddard N. Percutaneous scaphoid fixation: surgical technique volar approach with traction. *Atlas Hand Clin.* 2003;8:29–35.
8. Slade III JF, Gutow AP, Geissler WB. Percutaneous internal fixation of scaphoid fractures via an arthroscopically assisted dorsal approach. *J Bone Jt Surg Am.* 2002;84-A(suppl (0021–9355)):21–36.
9. Kamineni S, Lavy CB. Percutaneous fixation of scaphoid fractures. An anatomical study. *J Hand Surg Br.* 1999;24(0266–7681):85–88.
10. Leventhal EL, Wolfe SW, Walsh EF, Crisco JJ. A computational approach to the "optimal" screw axis location and orientation in the scaphoid bone. *J Hand Surg Am.* 2009;34(1531–6564 (Electronic)):677–684.
11. Heinzelmann AD, Archer G, Bindra RR. Anthropometry of the human scaphoid. *J Hand Surg Am.* 2007;32(0363–5023 (Print)):1005–1008.
12. Harding N. New wrist operation is key to my success. Daily Express. http://www.express.co.uk/life-style/health/124198/New-wrist-op-is-key-to-my-success; Published 2009.

CHAPTER 17

Optimal Screw Placement

GEERT MEERMANS, MD • MATTHIAS VANHEES, MD, PHD • FREDERIK VERSTREKEN, MD

KEY POINTS

- When treating a scaphoid fracture surgically, optimal screw position and length are essential to obtain solid fixation, allow early return to function, and minimize the risk of complications.
- Surgical treatment of scaphoid fractures can be technically demanding because of the shape of the scaphoid and its position in the carpus.
- Screws should be placed either centrally in the proximal and distal pole or perpendicular to the fracture plane.
- A standard volar approach results in more eccentric screw positioning at the distal pole compared with a modified volar or dorsal approach.
- The volar and dorsal approaches have similar outcomes regarding nonunion rate, function, grip strength, range of motion, postoperative complications, and pain.

PANEL 1
Case Scenario

A 31-year-old self-employed painter fell off his ladder at work and sustained a nondisplaced scaphoid waist fracture in his right-dominant wrist. Physical examination revealed pain at the anatomic snuffbox, restricted wrist movement, and decreased grip strength. He has no other associated injuries. Radiographs showed a scaphoid waist fracture Herbert type B1 (Fig. 17.1). The CT scan showed no angulation or displacement of the fracture fragments (Fig. 17.2). The advantages and disadvantages of conservative and operative treatment were discussed with the patient. The patient wanted to return to work as soon as possible and chose surgical treatment. When discussing the surgical plan with your residents, the question is raised: What is the optimal position of a screw in the scaphoid and how do you obtain it?

Herbert classified scaphoid fractures into acute stable (A), acute unstable (B), delayed union (C), and established nonunion (D). Stable acute fractures included fractures of the tubercle (A1) and incomplete unicortical "crack" fractures (A2). A type B1 is an acute unstable distal oblique fracture, a type B2 is a complete fracture of the waist, a type B3 is a proximal pole fracture, and a type B4 is a transscaphoid perilunate fracture dislocation of the carpus.

IMPORTANCE OF THE PROBLEM

Advantages of surgery for nondisplaced scaphoid fractures are quicker return to work and grip strength with similar long-term outcome compared with immobilization in a cast.[1,2] However, there is a higher risk of complications associated with surgical treatment, especially when there is suboptimal screw positioning.[1,2] Therefore, optimal screw placement is quintessential when scaphoid fractures are treated surgically. This can be challenging because of the shape of the scaphoid and its position in the wrist between the radius and other carpal bones.[3–5]

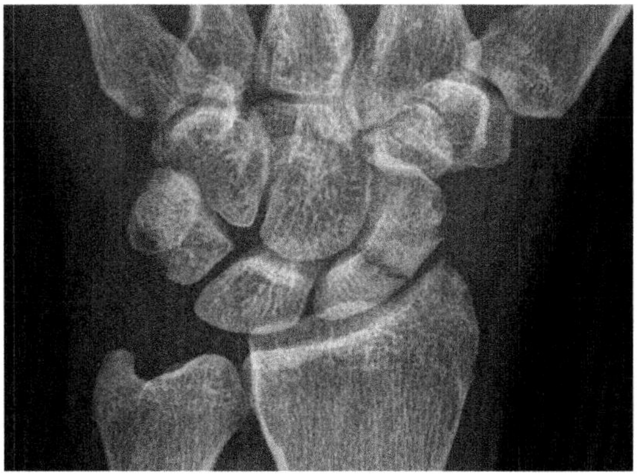

FIG. 17.1 Posteroanterior radiograph of the scaphoid with a horizontal oblique fracture at the waist.

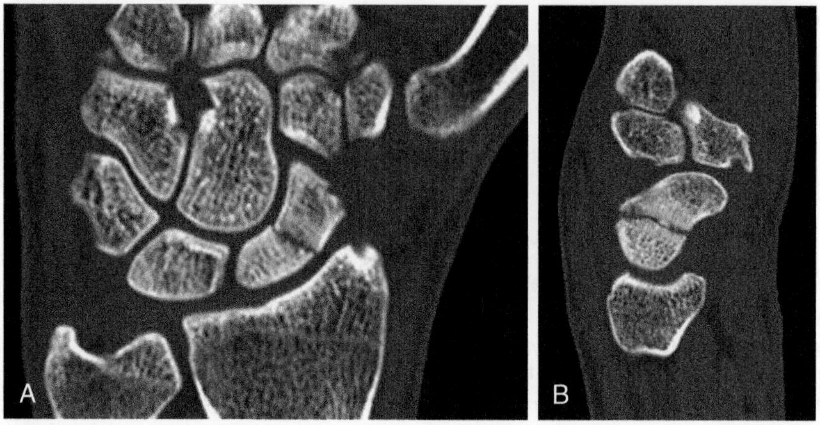

FIG. 17.2 **(A)** Coronal and **(B)** sagittal CT scan reconstructions of the same scaphoid show no significant displacement at the fracture site.

MAIN QUESTION

When treating a scaphoid fracture operatively, what is the optimal screw position and how can this be reliably achieved?

Current Opinion

Currently, fixation of a scaphoid fracture is performed using a cannulated headless screw, with a differential pitch. However, there is no consensus whether the screw should be placed central in the scaphoid or perpendicular to the fracture plane and which approach should be used to achieve this.

> The pitch of a screw thread is the distance from the crest of one thread to the next (Fig. 17.3). In differential pitch screws, the pitch of the trailing thread is smaller than the pitch of the leading thread. Because of this difference, the leading and trailing thread move a different distance with one rotation of 360 degrees and provide compression at the fracture site. The screws are headless so that they can be countersunk beneath the articular surface.

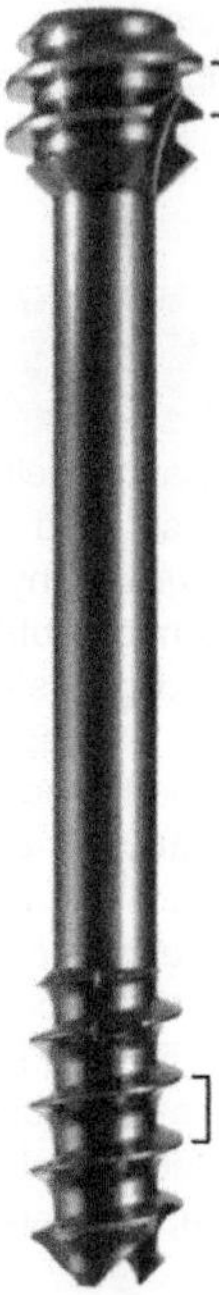

FIG. 17.3 Differential pitch screw with a shorter pitch at the trailing thread compared with the leading thread.

Finding the Evidence

- Cochrane database, with search term "scaphoid"
- Pubmed using keywords "scaphoid" and "fixation OR screw OR approach OR biomechanics"
- Pubmed clinical trial, metaanalysis, or review filter using keyword "scaphoid"
- Review of references of eligible studies
- Articles that were not in English, French, or German were excluded

Quality of the Evidence

Screw position

Level III:

Retrospective case-control studies: 3

Level V (basic science):

Computer models: 2

Human cadaveric biomechanical studies: 5

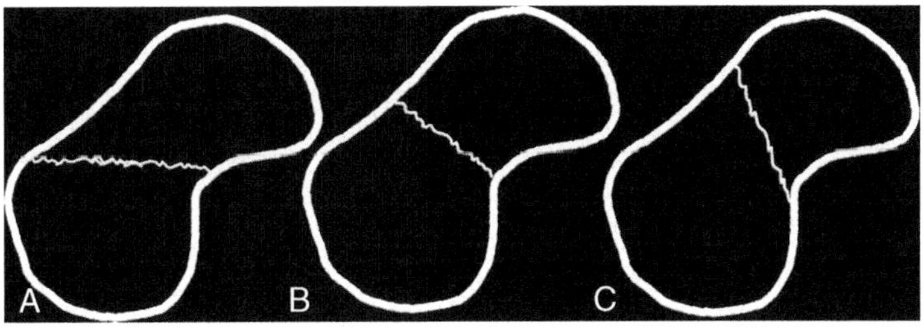

FIG 17.4 Classification of fractures at the level of the waist based on fracture plane orientation into horizontal **(A)** oblique, **(B)** transverse, and vertical **(C)** oblique fractures.

Approach

Level II:
- Metaanalysis of case studies: 1
- Randomized clinical trial with methodological limitations: 1

Level IV:
- Case series: 3

Level V:
- Expert opinion: 1
- Radiologic study: 1
- Human cadaveric studies: 9

FINDINGS

Screw Position

In a retrospective review of 34 patients treated for scaphoid nonunion, Trumble et al.[6] found that time to union was significantly shorter when the screw was placed in the central third of the proximal pole of the scaphoid ($P<.05$) and that the probability of a persistent nonunion was greater when the screw was placed more peripherally ($P<.01$). In a subsequent study, the same investigators looked at union in acute scaphoid fracture fixation. Because of the small numbers of eccentric screws in this subset of patients, these findings were not confirmed.[7]

Two biomechanical studies further explored positioning of a screw along the central long axis of the scaphoid. McCallister et al.[8] demonstrated superior biomechanical properties of single screw internal fixation when the screw was positioned in the central third of the proximal pole compared with eccentric placement at the proximal pole. Meermans et al.[9] demonstrated that central positioning at both the proximal and distal pole offered a biomechanical advantage compared with central positioning in only the proximal pole.

More recently, a retrospective review of 24 patients with an acute B1 or B2 scaphoid fracture that was treated surgically, demonstrated that time to union and persistent nonunion was correlated to the angle of the screw with the fracture plane.[10] The authors concluded that a screw placed perpendicular to the fracture plane could be superior to a screw placed along the long axis of the scaphoid.

Screw placement perpendicular to the fracture plane was also investigated in some in vitro studies. In a finite element analysis, Luria et al.[11] found that there was less motion at the fracture plane with screws placed perpendicular to this plane, especially in horizontal oblique type fracture (Herbert type B1). In a biomechanical study of a vertical oblique scaphoid fracture model, the same authors found no difference regarding stiffness and load to failure when comparing screws placed along the long axis of the scaphoid and screws placed perpendicular to the fracture plane.[12] Another biomechanical study looked at a horizontal oblique fracture model and also found no difference in load to failure comparing perpendicular with central screws.[13]

> Scaphoid waist fractures are classified according to the orientation of the fracture plane into horizontal oblique (HO), transverse (T), and vertical oblique (VO) fractures (Fig. 17.4). Regardless of the type of waist fracture, central screw positioning is possible using a modified volar or dorsal approach. Screw positioning perpendicular to the fracture plane from a volar approach is only possible for T and VO fractures. If the surgeon prefers screw placement perpendicular to the fracture plane in an HO type of fracture, the use of a dorsal approach will be necessary.

With regard to the maximum screw length, the design of the screw plays a major role. Screws with a leading thread diameter >3.0 mm, a trailing thread diameter >3.9 mm, increments of 2 or 2.5 mm, or placed through a dorsal approach were found to be significantly shorter.[14] Biomechanically, a longer screw provides significantly greater stability than a short screw, but screw prominence at the articular surface can lead to chondral damage.[15] The screw length should be as long as possible, but leave at least 2 mm of coverage at both ends of the scaphoid.

Approach

Seven studies[16–22] reporting on nonunion, functional outcome, grip strength, range of motion, postoperative complications, and pain were included in a recent metaanalysis, comparing the dorsal and volar percutaneous approaches in scaphoid fractures.[23] Pooling of data was only feasible for nonunion and postoperative complication rates, and no significant difference was found for these two outcomes. Analysis of overall functional outcome, postoperative pain, and grip strength revealed similar results for both approaches. Finally, no significant difference was found in the range of motion, except for ulnar deviation, which was significantly greater with the volar approach.

Two cadaveric studies examined the possibility to achieve central screw placement, comparing both approaches. Chan et al.[24] found no difference in the proximal or waist region between the two approaches, but the dorsal approach allowed for a more central position at the distal pole. Soubeyrand et al.[25] concluded that B2 type fractures can be adequately addressed by both approaches, but recommend the dorsal approach for B1 type fractures, because this approach permits screw alignment most perpendicular to the fracture plane. A modified volar, transtrapezial approach was proposed to allow for a more central screw placement throughout the scaphoid.[5] Three studies confirmed that this modified volar approach could reliably achieve central screw placement in the proximal and distal poles.[9,26,27]

The complication rates, up to 30%, are similar for both approaches, but the structures at risk are different (Table 17.1).[28,29] The structures at risk using the dorsal approach were investigated in two cadaveric studies, and they concluded that the extensor pollicis longus, extensor carpi radialis, extensor digitorum communis to index, extensor indicis proprius, and posterior interosseous nerve were particularly vulnerable.[30,31] This was confirmed by a case series combining arthroscopy and dorsal percutaneous fixation, where an iatrogenic rupture of the extensor pollicis longus tendon occurred in one of seven patients.[32] Similarly, two cadaveric studies described the anatomic structures at risk with the volar percutaneous technique: the flexor carpi radialis, superficial palmar branch of the radial artery, and the palmar cutaneous branch of the median nerve.[33,34] The authors of the four cadaveric studies examining the dorsal and volar approach all recommended dissection under direct

TABLE 17.1
Structures at Risk With Different Percutaneous Approaches

	Volar	Dorsal
Tendons	FCR	EPL
		ECRB
		EDC to index
		EIP
Nerves	Palmar cutaneous branch of the median nerve	Posterior interosseous nerve
Vessels	Superficial branch of the radial artery	

ECRB, extensor carpi radialis brevis; *EDC*, extensor digitorum communis; *EIP*, extensor indicis proprius; *EPL*, extensor pollicis longus; *FCR*, flexor carpi radialis.

supervision rather than a completely percutaneous technique.

Additionally, there have been concerns about scaphotrapezial (ST) joint degeneration after volar screw placement,[35–38] but this complication has also been reported in patients treated with a cast.[36,37] In a more recent case series using the transtrapezial technique, the authors did not find symptomatic ST degeneration at medium-term follow-up.[39] Some have suggested that ST joint degeneration is a minor complication, compared with the articular defect from the entry site of the screw in the radiocarpal joint created by the dorsal approach.[40]

RECOMMENDATION

When operating on patients with a scaphoid fracture, evidence suggests the following:

- When positioning a screw along the long axis of the scaphoid the screw should be in the center of the proximal and distal pole (=central axis) (overall quality: moderate).
- Biomechanically, there is no difference between screws placed along the central axis of the scaphoid or perpendicular to the fracture plane (overall quality: moderate).
- Both approaches can achieve central screw placement at the proximal pole, but a standard volar approach results in more eccentric screw placement at the distal pole (overall quality: high).
- The volar and dorsal approaches have similar outcomes regarding nonunion rate, function, grip strength, range of motion, postoperative complications, and pain (overall quality: moderate).

CONCLUSION

When treating a scaphoid fracture surgically, the screw should be positioned either along the central axis of the scaphoid or perpendicular to the fracture plane. Surgeons should carefully plan the operation and use either a (modified) volar or dorsal approach that allows them to achieve this goal.

PANEL 2
Author's Preferred Technique

In the aforementioned patient, the placement of a long headless bone screw through a transtrapezial volar approach was performed. Based on the current evidence, we aim to position the screw in the central one-third of the distal and proximal poles. This is also perpendicular to the fracture plane in transverse waist fractures (Fig. 17.5). Because central screw placement is hindered by the trapezium, manipulation and/or partial resection of the trapezium, or using a transtrapezial approach, is indicated.[3–5] We favor the latter because it allows a percutaneous approach without the risk of fracture displacement through manipulation and with minimal damage to the blood supply and soft tissues around the scaphoid. Careful fluoroscopic control in all planes (posteroanterior, lateral, and 45 degrees oblique pronated and supinated views) is essential to confirm the position of the guide wire and the final position and correct length of the screw. When the optimal screw position is obtained, early mobilization and return to function is allowed, with an expected union rate of over 95%.

Note 1: Most scaphoid waist fractures are transverse or horizontal oblique (Table 17.2).[41–46] A more recent study demonstrated that the average fracture plane at the waist is horizontal oblique rather than transverse.[47] This implies that a screw placed through the tuberosity would result in both an eccentric position at the distal pole and a more acute angle to the fracture plane compared with a dorsal or modified volar approach.[48]

Note 2: Using a dorsal approach is an alternative method to obtain central screw placement in scaphoid waist fracture treatment, but has some disadvantages. Full wrist flexion is necessary to obtain central placement of the guide wire, which hinders adequate fluoroscopic control of the position of the wire and may cause displacement of the fracture fragments into flexion. However, for proximal pole fractures, the dorsal approach is the preferred technique.

PANEL 3
Pearls and Pitfalls

PEARLS

- Before starting the procedure, carefully plan the position of the patient, the surgeon, and the fluoroscopy tube. Make sure the image on the monitor is oriented exactly as the limb of the patient in front of the surgeon. This will facilitate the procedure and placement of the implants.
- Position a guide wire on the skin along the central axis of the scaphoid in both planes and mark the position on the skin to provide a visual mark for guide wire insertion (Fig. 17.6).
- When using a transtrapezial approach, insert the guide wire in the trapezium first. If necessary, small adjustments in the direction of the guide wire can be made, by bringing the wrist into slight radial or ulnar deviation, before the guide wire is further advanced into the scaphoid.
- To minimize damage to the trapezium, use instruments (drill, length measurement device, and screwdriver) that have a long, narrow sleeve.
- When the screw is inserted, carefully check for screw protrusion on oblique fluoroscopy images and move the wrist through the full range of motion. Most often a grinding sensation can be felt, when the screw protrudes at the radiocarpal or ST joint (Fig. 17.7).
- As central screw placement provides a biomechanically solid fixation, it can also be used for a selected group of scaphoid delayed unions and nonunions, when no marked cyst formation (<5 mm), sclerosis, or deformity is present on radiographs or CT scans.
- Percutaneous, Transtrapezial Fixation without Bone Graft Leads to Consolidation in Selected Cases of Delayed Union of the Scaphoid Waist.[49]

PITFALLS

Removal of a screw positioned along the central axis of the scaphoid is also hindered by the trapezium and can therefore be complicated. Reinsertion of a guide wire and overdrilling of the trapezium will facilitate screw removal. If necessary, an angiocath needle can be slit over the guide wire, when it is advanced through the distal cortex of the scaphoid, to exert a retrograde force on the screw and facilitate removal. If this does not work, advancement of the screw through the proximal cortex and removal through a dorsal approach is the final salvage.

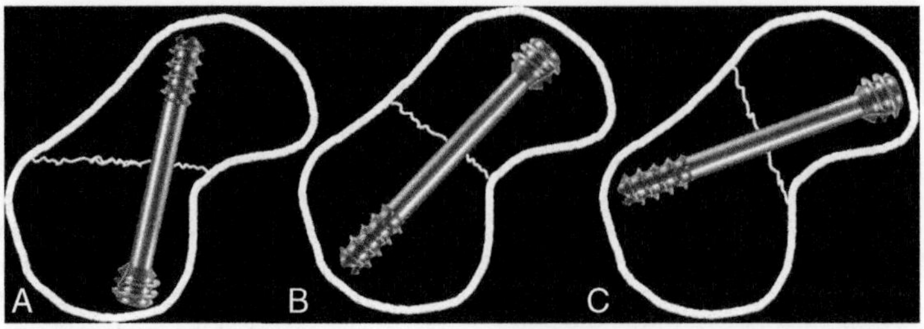

FIG. 17.5 Perpendicular screw placement according to different fracture plane orientation in a horizontal **(A)** oblique, **(B)** transverse, and vertical **(C)** oblique fracture types. The distal entry point is at the level of the scaphotrapezial joint in the horizontal oblique and transverse fracture type and at the tuberosity in the vertical oblique fracture type.

TABLE 17.2
Classification of Acute Scaphoid Waist Fractures Based on Fracture Plane Orientation

Author	Horizontal Oblique (%)	Transverse	Vertical Oblique
Böhler et al.[41]	47	50	3
Brøndum et al.[42]	43	53	4
Compson[43]	54.5	45.5	0
Garala et al.[44]	53.8	44.7	1.5
Russe[45]	35	60	5
Schunk et al.[46]	36	61	3

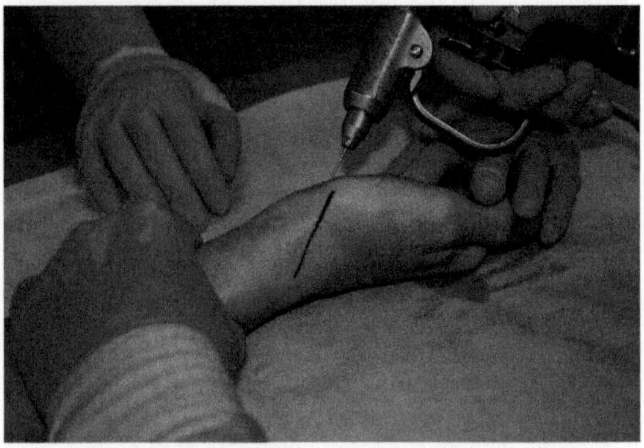

FIG. 17.6 Marking on the skin of the long axis of the scaphoid to aid guide wire placement.

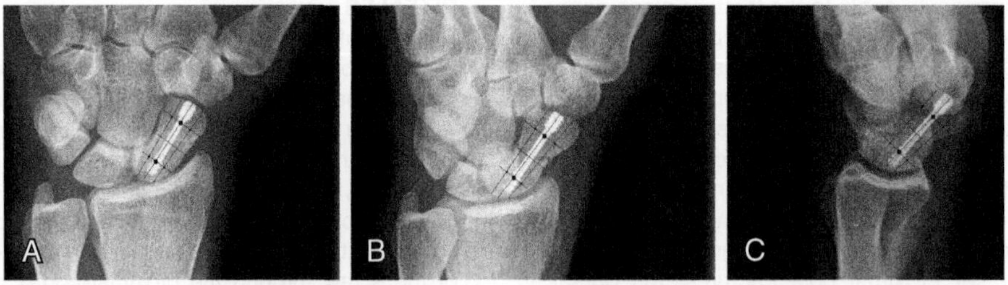

FIG. 17.7 Postoperative **(A)** posteroanterior, **(B)** oblique, and **(C)** lateral radiographs confirm central placement of the screw into the scaphoid.

REFERENCES

1. Buijze GA, Doornberg JN, Ham JS, Ring D, Bhandari M, Poolman RW. Surgical compared with conservative treatment for acute nondisplaced or minimally displaced scaphoid fractures: a systematic review and meta-analysis of randomized controlled trials. *J Bone Joint Surg Am*. 2010;92(6):1534–1544.
2. Ibrahim T, Qureshi A, Sutton AJ, Dias JJ. Surgical versus nonsurgical treatment of acute minimally displaced and undisplaced scaphoid waist fractures: pairwise and network meta-analyses of randomized controlled trials. *J Hand Surg Am*. 2011;36(11):1759–1768.
3. Leventhal EL, Wolfe SW, Walsh EF, Crisco JJ. A computational approach to the "optimal" screw axis location and orientation in the scaphoid bone. *J Hand Surg Am*. 2009;34(4):677–684.
4. Levitz S, Ring D. Retrograde (volar) scaphoid screw insertion-a quantitative computed tomographic analysis. *J Hand Surg Am*. 2005;30(3):543–548.
5. Meermans G, Verstreken F. A comparison of 2 methods for scaphoid central screw placement from a volar approach. *J Hand Surg Am*. 2011;36(10):1669–1674.
6. Trumble TE, Clarke T, Kreder HJ. Non-union of the scaphoid. Treatment with cannulated screws compared with treatment with Herbert screws. *J Bone Joint Surg Am*. 1996;78(12):1829–1837.
7. Trumble TE, Gilbert M, Murray LW, Smith J, Rafijah G, McCallister WV. Displaced scaphoid fractures treated with open reduction and internal fixation with a cannulated screw. *J Bone Joint Surg Am*. 2000;82(5):633–641.
8. McCallister WV, Knight J, Kaliappan R, Trumble TE. Central placement of the screw in simulated fractures of the scaphoid waist: a biomechanical study. *J Bone Joint Surg Am*. 2003;85-A(1):72–77.
9. Meermans G, Van Glabbeek F, Braem MJ, van Riet RP, Hubens G, Verstreken F. Comparison of two percutaneous volar approaches for screw fixation of scaphoid waist fractures: radiographic and biomechanical study of an osteotomy-simulated model. *J Bone Joint Surg Am*. 2014;96(16):1369–1376.
10. Mahmoud M, Hegazy M, Khaled SA, Abdelatif NM, Osman W, Elfar JC. Radiographic parameters to predict union after volar percutaneous fixation of Herbert type B1 and B2 scaphoid fractures. *J Hand Surg Am*. 2016;41(2):203–207.
11. Luria S, Hoch S, Liebergall M, Mosheiff R, Peleg E. Optimal fixation of acute scaphoid fractures: finite element analysis. *J Hand Surg Am*. 2010;35(8):1246–1250.
12. Luria S, Lenart L, Lenart B, Peleg E, Kastelec M. Optimal fixation of oblique scaphoid fractures: a cadaver model. *J Hand Surg Am*. 2012;37(7):1400–1404.
13. Faucher GK, Golden 3rd ML, Sweeney KR, Hutton WC, Jarrett CD. Comparison of screw trajectory on stability of oblique scaphoid fractures: a mechanical study. *J Hand Surg Am*. 2014;39(3):430–435.
14. Meermans G, Verstreken F. Influence of screw design, sex, and approach in scaphoid fracture fixation. *Clin Orthop Relat Res*. 2012;470(6):1673–1681.
15. Dodds SD, Panjabi MM, Slade 3rd JF. Screw fixation of scaphoid fractures: a biomechanical assessment of screw length and screw augmentation. *J Hand Surg Am*. 2006;31(3):405–413.
16. Drac P, Cizmar I, Manak P, et al. Comparison of the results and complications of palmar and dorsal miniinvasive approaches in the surgery of scaphoid fractures. A prospective randomized study. *Biomed Pap Med Fac Univ Palacky Olomouc Czech Repub*. 2014;158(2):277–281.
17. Drác P, Manák P, Cizmár I, Hrbek J, Zapletalová JA. Palmar percutaneous volar versus a dorsal limited approach for the treatment of non- and minimally-displaced scaphoid waist fractures: an assessment of functional outcomes and complications. *Acta Chir Orthop Traumatol Cech*. 2010; 77(2):143–148.
18. Gürbüz Y, Kayalar M, Bal E, Toros T, Küçük L, Sügün TS. Comparison of dorsal and volar percutaneous screw fixation methods in acute Type B scaphoid fractures. *Acta Orthop Traumatol Turc*. 2012;46(5):339–345.
19. Jeon IH, Micic ID, Oh CW, Park BC, Kim PT. Percutaneous screw fixation for scaphoid fracture: a comparison between the dorsal and the volar approaches. *J Hand Surg Am*. 2009;34(2):228–236.
20. Parajuli NP, Shrestha D, Dhoju D, Shrestha R, Sharma V. Scaphoid fracture: functional outcome following fixation with Herbert Screw. *Kathmandu Univ Med J*. 2011;9(36): 267–273.
21. Polsky MB, Kozin SH, Porter ST, Thoder JJ. Scaphoid fractures: dorsal versus volar approach. *Orthopedics*. 2002;25(8): 817–819.
22. Slade JF, Lozano-Calderón S, Merrell G, Ring D. Arthroscopic-assisted percutaneous reduction and screw fixation of displaced scaphoid fractures. *J Hand Surg Eur Vol*. 2008;33(3):350–354.
23. Kang KB, Kim HJ, Park JH, Shin YS. Comparison dorsal volar percutaneous approaches acute scaphoid fractures: a meta-analysis. *PLoS One*. 2016;11(9):e0162779.
24. Chan KW, McAdams TR. Central screw placement in percutaneous screw scaphoid fixation: a cadaveric comparison of proximal and distal techniques. *J Hand Surg Am*. 2004;29(1):74–79.
25. Soubeyrand M, Biau D, Mansour C, Mahjoub S, Molina V, Gagey O. Comparison of percutaneous dorsal versus volar fixation of scaphoid waist fractures using a computer model in cadavers. *J Hand Surg Am*. 2009;34(10): 1838–1844.
26. Kurahashi T, Shinohara T, Hirata H. Modified dorsal percutaneous screw fixation through a transtrapezial approach for scaphoid fractures. *J Hand Surg Eur Vol*. 2015;40(8):868–869.
27. Vaynrub M, Carey JN, Stevanovic MV, Ghiassi A. Volar percutaneous screw fixation of the scaphoid: a cadaveric study. *J Hand Surg Am*. 2014;39(5):867–871.
28. Dias JJ, Wildin CJ, Bhowal B, Thompson JR. Should acute scaphoid fractures be fixed? A randomized controlled trial. *J Bone Joint Surg Am*. 2005;87(10):2160–2168.

29. Bushnell BD, McWilliams AD, Messer TM. Complications in dorsal percutaneous cannulated screw fixation of nondisplaced scaphoid waist fractures. *J Hand Surg Am.* 2007;32(6):827–833.
30. Adamany DC, Mikola EA, Fraser BJ. Percutaneous fixation of the scaphoid through a dorsal approach: an anatomic study. *J Hand Surg Am.* 2008;33(3):327–331.
31. Weinberg AM, Pichler W, Grechenig S, Tesch NP, Heidari N, Grechenig W. The percutaneous antegrade scaphoid fracture fixation–a safe method? *Injury.* 2009;40(6):642–644.
32. Slade 3rd JF, Taksali S, Safanda J. Combined fractures of the scaphoid and distal radius: a revised treatment rationale using percutaneous and arthroscopic techniques. *Hand Clin.* 2005;21(3):427–441.
33. Evans S, Brantley J, Brady C, Salas C, Mercer D. Structures at risk during volar percutaneous fixation of scaphoid fractures: a cadaver study. *Iowa Orthop J.* 2015;35:119–123.
34. Kamineni S, Lavy CB. Percutaneous fixation of scaphoid fractures. An anatomical study. *J Hand Surg Br.* 1999;24(1):85–88.
35. Kehoe NJ, Hackney RG, Barton NJ. Incidence of osteoarthritis in the scapho-trapezial joint after Herbert screw fixation of the scaphoid. *J Hand Surg Br.* 2003;28(5):496–499.
36. Nicholl JE, Buckland-Wright JC. Degenerative changes at the scaphotrapezial joint following Herbert screw insertion: a radiographic study comparing patients with scaphoid fracture and primary hand arthritis. *J Hand Surg Br.* 2000;25(5):422–426.
37. Saedén B, Törnkvist H, Ponzer S, Höglund M. Fracture of the carpal scaphoid. A prospective, randomised 12-year follow-up comparing operative and conservative treatment. *J Bone Joint Surg Br.* 2001;83(2):230–234.
38. Vinnars B, Pietreanu M, Bodestedt A, Fa Ekenstam, Gerdin B. Nonoperative compared with operative treatment of acute scaphoid fractures. A randomized clinical trial. *J Bone Joint Surg Am.* 2008;90(6):1176–1185.
39. Geurts G, van Riet R, Meermans G, Verstreken F. Incidence of scaphotrapezial arthritis following volar percutaneous fixation of nondisplaced scaphoid waist fractures using a transtrapezial approach. *J Hand Surg Am.* 2011;36(11):1753–1758.
40. Slutsky DJ, Trevare J. Use of arthroscopy for the treatment of scaphoid fractures. *Hand Clin.* 2014;30(1):91–103.
41. Böhler L, Trojan E, Jahna H. The results of treatment of 734 fresh, simple fractures of the scaphoid. *J Hand Surg Br.* 2003;28(4):319–331.
42. Brøndum V, Larsen CF, Skov O. Fracture of the carpal scaphoid: frequency and distribution in a well-defined population. *Eur J Radiol.* 1992;15(2):118–122.
43. Compson JP. The anatomy of acute scaphoid fractures: a three-dimensional analysis of patterns. *J Bone Joint Surg Br.* 1998;80(2):218–224.
44. Garala K, Taub NA, Dias JJ. The epidemiology of fractures of the scaphoid: impact of age, gender, deprivation and seasonality. *Bone Joint J.* 2016;98-B(5):654–659.
45. Russe O. Fracture of the carpal navicular. Diagnosis, non-operative treatment, and operative treatment. *J Bone Joint Surg Am.* 1960;42-A:759–768.
46. Schunk K, Weber W, Strunk H, Regentrop H, Thelen R, Schild H. Traumatology and diagnosis of scaphoid fracture. *Radiologe.* 1989;29(2):61–67.
47. Luria S, Schwarcz Y, Wollstein R, Emelife P, Zinger G, Peleg E. 3-dimensional analysis of scaphoid fracture angle morphology. *J Hand Surg Am.* 2015;40(3):508–514.
48. Meermans G, Verstreken F. Letter regarding "Optimal fixation of oblique scaphoid fractures: a cadaver model". *J Hand Surg Am.* 2012;37(9):1957–1958.
49. Vanhees M, van Riet RRP, van Haver A, Kebrle R, Meermans G, Verstreken F. *J Wrist Surg.* 2017;6(3):183–187.

CHAPTER 18

Arthroscopy-Assisted Screw Fixation

JAN RAGNAR HAUGSTVEDT, MD, PHD • PETER JØRGSHOLM, MD, PHD •
HEBE DÉSIRÉE KVERNMO, MD, PHD, MHA

KEY POINTS

- Arthroscopy may be of value to evaluate a displaced scaphoid waist fracture, a comminuted waist fracture, a proximal pole fracture, or if a perilunate fracture dislocation is suspected.
- Arthroscopy may help diagnose concomitant soft tissue injuries with scaphoid fractures.
- Arthroscopy may help in the reduction and fixation of a scaphoid fracture.
- Arthroscopy-assisted screw fixation may give a faster rehabilitation with less damage to blood supply and innervation of bone and ligaments.

PANEL 1
Case Scenario 1

CASE 1

A 30-year-old, right-handed man with several previous injuries to his right hand, all of which he had recovered from, comes to the emergency room (ER) after hitting a punch ball on a stand, when he suddenly experienced pain in his wrist. He did not see a doctor until 4 weeks following the injury; at that time radiographs were taken, they were read as negative (Fig. 18.1A–B). Because of persistent pain, he was referred for new radiographs 6 weeks after the injury; these revealed a scaphoid fracture and he was referred to a hand surgeon. A CT-scan confirmed the diagnosis, there was a cyst in the scaphoid, and a possible malalignment was described (Fig. 18.2A–B). The patient told he did not smoke, however, was using "dipping tobacco" or "chewing tobacco." His wrist was hurting and he was unable to work.

Should this patient have a cast, should he be a candidate for open surgery with bone grafting, or is arthroscopy-assisted treatment an option?

CASE 2

A soccer player, a goalkeeper, seeks his family doctor the day after he was hit by a ball on his hand. His wrist was swollen; however, the doctor figured it was a bruised wrist and no further examination was performed. He came to the ER 6 weeks later, complained of pain, had reduced range of motion (ROM), and radiographs were performed. This was read as a healed distal radius fracture and the patient was instructed to perform exercises to strengthen the hand and increase the ROM in the wrist. Eight weeks later he went back to his family doctor because of persistent pain; at this time a proximal pole scaphoid fracture was diagnosed (Fig. 18.3). Because of doctor's delay, the patient was referred to and first seen by a hand surgeon 4 months following the original trauma. The patient experienced pain, had reduced ROM, and had a clearly visible proximal scaphoid fracture with a wide fracture line.

Should this patient be treated with open surgery with a vascularized bone graft, or could arthroscopy help in evaluation and treatment of the fracture?

CASE 3

A 32-year-old man, a former drug addict, seeks the ER immediately after a fall when landing on his left nondominant hand while snowboarding. Radiographs showed a scaphoid fracture, the displacement was considered as minimal, and the patient was put in a cast. A 2-week follow-up later revealed a cast that did not fit, the radiographs showed a gap over the fracture line and a displacement, and the SL interval seemed to be increased (Fig. 18.4). The patient had been without drugs for almost 1 year; however, he was still smoking 15–20 cigarettes a day.

Should this patient, as a former drug addict and still a smoker, have his cast changed and have conservative treatment, or should surgery be considered?

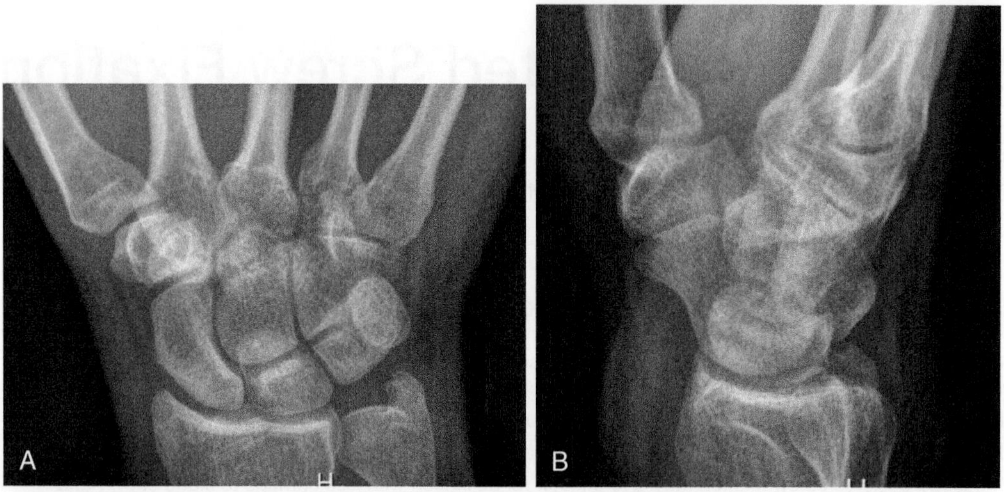

FIG. 18.1 Four weeks following the injury, the patient saw his doctor and these radiographs in **(A)** posterior-anterior and **(B)** lateral views were taken; the films were read as "negative."

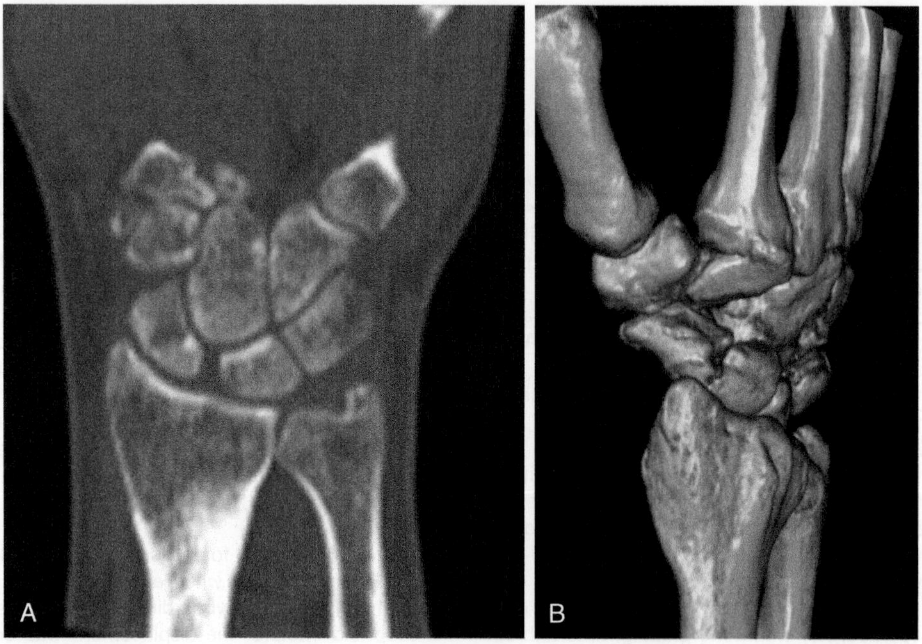

FIG. 18.2 Because of persistent pain, a CT scan was performed 2 weeks later. These films **(A** and **B)** revealed a scaphoid fracture.

IMPORTANCE OF THE PROBLEM

The indications for percutaneous screw fixation are the same as for open surgery: a proximal pole fracture, a waist fracture with more than 1 mm displacement or translation, angulated fractures, fractures with an oblique or vertical fracture line, and fractures with comminution.[1] Operative treatment is also recommended for combined injuries. In our experience, it could be difficult to understand the complete extent and nature of a lesion using different imaging modalities (radiographs, CT scans, and MRI studies) alone. Although radiographic examinations will

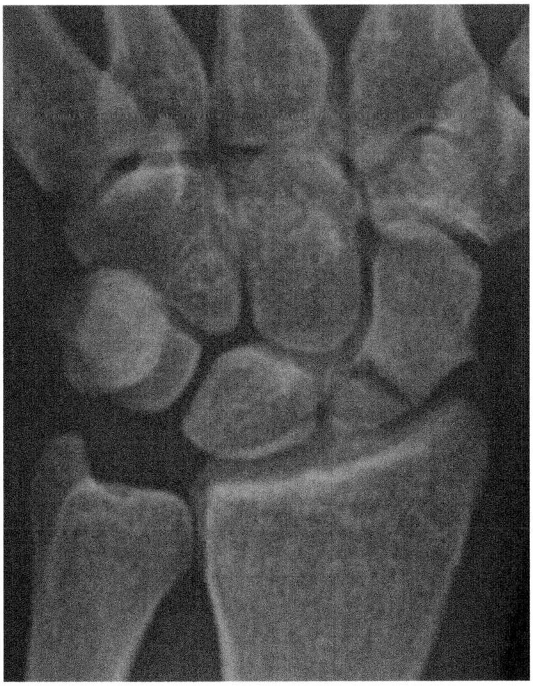

FIG. 18.3 This patient had a wrist trauma and saw his family doctor the following day. The doctor diagnosed a "bruised wrist" without any radiographs. Six weeks following the trauma, he came to the emergency room still complaining of wrist pain. At that time, radiographs were taken; these were interpreted as no scaphoid fracture, and the patient was sent home to exercise. His pain persisted and, 8 weeks later, he came back. New radiographs were performed that revealed the proximal pole fracture shown in this picture.

show an "image of the reality," the use of arthroscopy will reveal the entity of the bones and ligaments of the wrist and carpus and, thereby, "the reality." When a combined injury is suspected, when there is any displacement, comminution, or signs of instability, it may be advantageous to perform wrist arthroscopy.

This procedure aids us understanding the fracture itself and will help us diagnosing concomitant injuries. It will assist the surgeon to perform anatomic reduction and fixation of the scaphoid fracture with an arthroscopic-assisted bone grafting, if needed, as well as assist in the treatment of the concomitant injuries. This technique, where an arthroscopy-assisted screw fixation is used, should also be considered in an athlete, or where the patient for any reason is unable to wear a cast for up to 12 weeks, although there is no displacement, given the patient is informed about the risks involved in surgery.

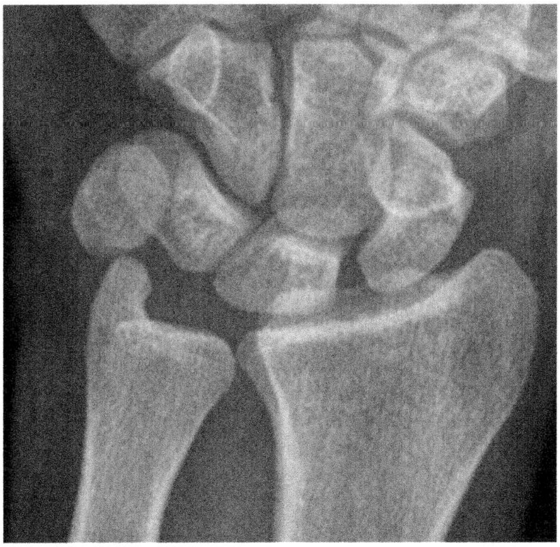

FIG. 18.4 The patient had radiographs the day after having sustained a fall on his outstretched hand while snowboarding. A scaphoid fracture was diagnosed and conservative treatment (cast) was initiated. Two weeks later, he came back to check his cast. The cast was "loose" and did not fit well; new radiographs showed a widening over the SL interval, as shown in this picture.

MAIN QUESTIONS

- Is there any role for arthroscopy in evaluation of a scaphoid fracture?
- Will minimal invasive surgery, or arthroscopy-assisted fixation of a scaphoid fracture, give a faster rehabilitation and better outcome?
- Are there any downsides from arthroscopy-assisted screw fixations?
- Is there any evidence showing improved outcome with arthroscopy-assisted screw fixation?

Current Opinion

- Most scaphoid fractures are treated conservatively with a cast based on the radiographic examinations (radiographs, CT scans, or MRIs).
- Many surgeons find no place for arthroscopy; the learning curve is steep, it takes extra time in many colleagues' opinion, and the results are not in favor of this "new" technique.
- If a comminuted fracture is found, or a displaced fracture is revealed, most surgeons will perform an open reduction and osteosynthesis.
- The authors feel that arthroscopy adds knowledge to the extent of the injury, the stability and displacement can be evaluated, bone grafting can be performed if

needed, and the treatment can be extended to include the instabilities and ligament injuries not visible in classic imaging modalities, thus enabling us for a precise treatment with a faster recovery.

Finding the Evidence

The search was performed with the help of our librarian. We performed the following searches:

- **Cochrane database.** Using "Scaphoid fracture" we had three hits in Cochrane; however, only one was a systematic overview. This overview looked at different imaging techniques and was thus not suitable for our study. The other two studies were a protocol and an overview that later was withdrawn. It showed up, however, 15 "Other reviews," that turned out to be "Systematic overviews" made by others than The Cochrane Collaboration.
- **Pubmed.** We tried the following search: (Scaphoid bone[mesh] OR scaphoid fracture*[tiab] OR scaphoid bone fracture*[tiab] OR scaphoid[tiab]) AND (operative treatment OR screw fixation* OR arthroscopy*). This gave 630 hits. When the search was reduced to "Systematic overviews," we had 16 hits.
- We then performed the following search: (Scaphoid fracture[tiab] OR scaphoid[tiab]) AND screw fixation) and had 590 hits. If the search was focused on "Systematic reviews," we had 9 hits.

Articles that were not in English, German, or French were excluded. We found some of the same articles in the different searches. We also checked the papers and found that a limited number dealt with the problem we wanted to focus on. The papers of interest, a total number of 16, were further studied.

Quality of the Evidence

The 16 papers we have considered should be classified as follows:

Level IA (systematic review of randomized controlled trials): 4
Level IIA (systematic review cohort studies): 8
Level IIIA (systematic review of case-controlled studies): 2
Level V (expert opinion): 2

FINDINGS

There was one study[2] (Level II) where patients with acute nondisplaced or minimally displaced scaphoid waist fractures were prospectively randomized to conservative or surgical treatment. Patients (24) in the conservative treatment group had a below-elbow thumb spica cast, whereas patients (14) in the group treated surgically had a percutaneous antegrade (through the proximal scaphoid pole) screw fixation. At 26 weeks, the patients treated in a cast had significantly better ROM with almost normal values; however, there were no significant differences concerning grip or pinch strengths. After 6 years, radiographic signs of arthritis in the radioscaphoid joint were more common in the surgically treated group (3 of 14 as opposed to 2 of the 21 available for follow-up in the conservative group); thus, in a nondisplaced waist fracture, conservative treatment is recommended.

In other papers reporting on minimally and/or nondisplaced waist fractures, the conclusions were that surgical treatment was favored in terms of fracture union, less nonunion rates, faster time to union, return to work, quicker recovery of function and grip strength, and better range of movement; however, the patients treated surgically had more complications; thus the long-term risks and short-term benefits of surgery should be weighed in clinical decision-making in these type of fractures.[3–9] In a displaced fracture of the scaphoid, nonunion is more likely if treated in a plaster cast; operative treatment may provide higher union rates.[10–11] Surgery might be considered more expensive than cast immobilization; however, in a young manual worker, these early expenses should be balanced with the shorter recovery time that will reduce workers' compensation costs.[12–13] For high-level athletes, screw fixation[1] or surgery[12] is suggested. Surgery is recommended for scaphoid fractures where the fracture line is more than 1 mm wide, where a translation is more than 1 mm, and where there is a multifragmented or comminuted fracture in the middle part, if there is a long, oblique fracture, a proximal fracture, or a fracture in combination with a perilunate dislocation.[14]

ANSWER TO THE MAIN QUESTIONS

Is there any role for arthroscopy in evaluation of a scaphoid fracture?

In a study to investigate diagnostic performance of radiographs and CT scans in patients with acute scaphoid waist fractures, the authors defined arthroscopy as the reference standard for displacement and instability and showed that CT was superior to radiographs by these means[15] (Level III). We will recommend arthroscopy for evaluation in selected cases.

Will minimal invasive surgery, or arthroscopy assisted fixation of a scaphoid fracture, give a faster rehabilitation and better outcome?

It has been referred (above) to studies showing surgical treatment might be favored in terms of faster time to union, less nonunion rates, return to work, quicker recovery of function and grip strength, and better range of movement. The blood supply to the scaphoid is through dorsal and palmar branches of the radial artery.[16–17] For better rehabilitation of patients with wrist injuries, one should pay respect to the importance of wrist joint proprioception; thus, if possible, the innervation of the wrist ligaments should be kept intact.[18] It is our belief that we could preserve blood supply and proprioception better if surgery is performed minimal invasive.

It has recently been suggested that there might be injuries more extensive than originally thought of; there is a higher incidence of intrinsic and extrinsic ligament injuries in scaphoid fractures, even perilunate dislocations.[19–20] There is no evidence; however, we believe that diagnosing and treating the scaphoid fracture and the concomitant injuries at the same time, using an arthroscopy-assisted technique, will leave the patients with less scar tissue and the possibility for a faster rehabilitation and a potential better outcome.

Are there any downsides from arthroscopy assisted screw fixations?

Within the last decades, percutaneous screw fixation of scaphoid fractures has become popular and was recommended as a treatment option in an athlete with a nondisplaced or minimally displaced fracture where early return to sport was a priority.[21] There are two possibilities for screw insertion: a volar or a dorsal approach. For retrograde insertion of the screw, excision of the volar tubercle of the trapezium was recommended.[21] The dorsal approach is recommended for proximal pole fractures, whereas the volar approach could be used for distal pole fractures.[1] The dorsal approach[2] will create a hole in the surface of the proximal pole of the scaphoid, whereas the volar approach[22] will affect the scaphotrapezial joint.[23] The same approaches are used for arthroscopy-assisted screw fixation. Although there are good control of reposition and stability of the osteosynthesis, arthroscopy is shown to be difficult and there is a significant learning curve with the technique. A survey based on 10,107 wrist arthroscopies showed that there was a failure of performing the procedure as planned for in 1.16% of the cases.[24] Other complications listed were nerve lesions, cartilage lesions, and complex regional pain syndrome, the complications being less when the procedure is performed by a surgeon with more than 5 years of experience and performing more than 25 wrist arthroscopies per year.

Is there any evidence showing the difference in outcome?

There is to date no study comparing arthroscopy-assisted screw fixation to minimally invasive/percutaneous approaches. In patients with posttraumatic radial wrist tenderness, it was shown that MRI revealed more fractures than radiographs and CT; however, it is not possible to conclude whether diagnosis or treatment of these injuries demonstrated on MRI only would improve the clinical outcome.[25] Arthroscopy may reveal more ligament injuries[19]; however, we do not know if there is any difference in outcome if these injuries are treated or not. In one study[2] (Level II), patients with acute nondisplaced or minimally displaced scaphoid waist fractures were prospectively randomized to conservative treatment or surgical treatment (wrist arthroscopy and percutaneous antegrade screw fixation). The authors conclude that operative treatment might give a better short-term result; however, a longer follow-up is needed to evaluate the risk of arthritis developing over time. In the study, more commonly radiographic signs of arthritis in the radioscaphoid joint were found in the group treated surgically. In another prospective randomized study comparing nonoperative with operative treatment of scaphoid fractures, a volar approach with a retrograde insertion of the screws was performed.[23] In this study a significant increase in the prevalence of osteoarthritis in the scaphotrapezial joint was found in the group that had been treated surgically. In neither of these studies, the documented signs of arthritis were shown to affect the subjective outcomes.

There are no prospective studies comparing arthroscopic evaluation of a scaphoid fracture diagnosing concomitant injuries to evaluate the outcome of surgical (arthroscopic assisted, minimal or percutaneous, or open) treatment to conservative treatment. This could be a potential study for the future; however, the question might arise whether it is ethical or not to diagnose an injury and not treat it. If a scaphoid fracture is treated using an arthroscopic-assisted screw fixation and then put in a cast, a potential ligament injury is treated with immobilization. An early mobilization may prevent the healing of the ligaments; however, if this will result in a difference in outcome has not been shown. It might, in our opinion, be difficult to perform such a study.

RECOMMENDATION

In patients with a displaced (≥1 mm) scaphoid waist fracture, in a comminuted or multifragmented waist fracture, in a late diagnosed scaphoid fracture with or without signs of cysts, in a combined injury, for instance a perilunate fracture dislocation, and in proximal pole fractures:

- Arthroscopic examination may be helpful to evaluate the nature, comminution, and stability of the fracture (overall quality: very low).
- Arthroscopic-assisted screw fixation of the fracture to give stability may allow for earlier mobilization (overall quality: very low).
- Arthroscopic-assisted evaluation of the wrist and midcarpal joints, with special focus on scapholunate ligament injuries, may give a more precise diagnosis and may be of value to treat any concomitant injuries at the same time as the fracture is treated (overall quality: very low).

CONCLUSION

Evidence regarding arthroscopy-assisted screw fixation for scaphoid fractures is still lacking. Indications for arthroscopic evaluation found in the literature include a scaphoid waist fracture with displacement and angulation, a comminuted fracture, and a proximal pole fracture, where a combination of injuries (scaphoid fracture and ligament injury) is suspected. The major advantage seems to be that concomitant injury can be detected early and treated appropriately. Disadvantages include extended time of surgery, a steep learning curve, and complications from arthroscopy.

EWAS classification of SL instability:
Stage I: No passage of hook in SL space but synovitis
Stage II: Passage in the SL space without widening
Stage III A: Volar partial widening at dynamic instability test from MC joint
Stage III B: Dorsal partial widening at dynamic instability test from MC joint
Stage III C: Complete widening of the space at dynamic test
Stage IV: Gap with passage of the arthroscope from midcarpal to radiocarpal joint
Stage V: Idem with radiographic abnormalities

PANEL 2
Case Scenario 2

CASE 1

Two months after injury, surgery was performed. Performing arthroscopy, we found continuity of the scaphoid with no dislocation, with a SL-instability grade II (per EWAS).[26] A synovectomy was performed over the SL interval and a retrograde screw was used to stabilize the fracture. (The technique for retrograde screw fixation is shown in Fig 18.5A–C.) The wrist was immobilized in a cast (SL injury). The patient quit using tobacco, the fracture healed, and the patient is back to work after healing of the fracture (Fig. 18.6A–C).

CASE 2

Because of doctor's delay, the surgery was performed 4 months after trauma. Arthroscopy was performed, the scaphoid was in continuity, and there is no widening of the fracture line and no ligament (or triangular fibrocartilage complex (TFCC)) injuries. This proximal pole fracture was addressed by a dorsal, antegrade screw fixation, and no bone was grafted (Fig. 18.7A–J). The fracture healed (Fig. 18.8) and at follow-up after 6 months quick-DASH was 0, and he had recovered 90% range of normal motion (contralateral side).

CASE 3

Because of the widening of the SL interval, and suspicion of soft tissue injuries, surgery was performed 3 weeks after the injury. We found a 1-mm step over the fracture line, an SL-instability grade III B (per EWAS), an LT-instability grade II, and a TFCC detachment from the capsule (Fig. 18.9). We performed a retrograde screw fixation, a TFCC reattachment, a synovectomy in the SL and LT intervals, and a transfixation of the SL and LT intervals (Fig. 18.10). He had cast for 10 weeks before the K-wires were removed and exercises were started. The fracture healed, and 4 months after surgery (Fig. 18.11A and B) he had minimal pain with good recovery of strength and range of motion.

PANEL 2
Author's Preferred Technique

- In patients with a displaced scaphoid waist fracture (≥1 mm), in a comminuted waist fracture, in a proximal pole fracture, or if a perilunate fracture dislocation is suspected, we perform wrist arthroscopy to evaluate the fracture and the soft tissue injuries.
- In a proximal pole fracture, we will recommend a dorsal approach with an antegrade screw fixation.
- In a waist fracture, a dorsal approach for antegrade fixation or a volar approach for a retrograde fixation is possible. The dorsal approach is made easier by the use of a traction tower that allows for wrist flexion.
- In a fracture of the distal part of the scaphoid, we recommend a retrograde screw fixation through a volar approach.
- In cases of comminution and instability, we will perform arthroscopically assisted bone grafting, in combination with screw fixation, or will add K-wires if necessary.
- If there is a combined lesion with a dorsal intercalated segment instability (DISI) deformity, we will reduce the DISI before stabilizing the scaphoid fracture.[3]
- If there is a concomitant soft tissue lesion, we will address this lesion at the same time. This will make immobilization in a cast postoperatively necessary.

PANEL 3
Pearls and Pitfalls

PEARLS

- If the fracture is angulated, we will use K-wires as joysticks to reduce the dislocation.
- If the fracture is comminuted, we will stabilize the fracture using more than one K-wire before entering the screw without compression.
- If a wide fracture line with cysts is found, we can use the arthroscopy-assisted technique, debride, and insert bone without any (potential) damages of ligaments, blood supply, or nerves.
- To avoid withdrawal of the guide wire when removing the drill, the K-wire could be drilled through the scaphoid (for instance over the ST joint for antegrade screw fixation).

PITFALLS

- The guide pin for the screw should be carefully inserted and the position checked in different views for correct alignment and position through the scaphoid.[3]
- When using a cannulated screw, the screw used should allow for a guide wire of at least 1 mm. A thinner guide wire is difficult to drill through the bone, as you might lose control of the direction while drilling.

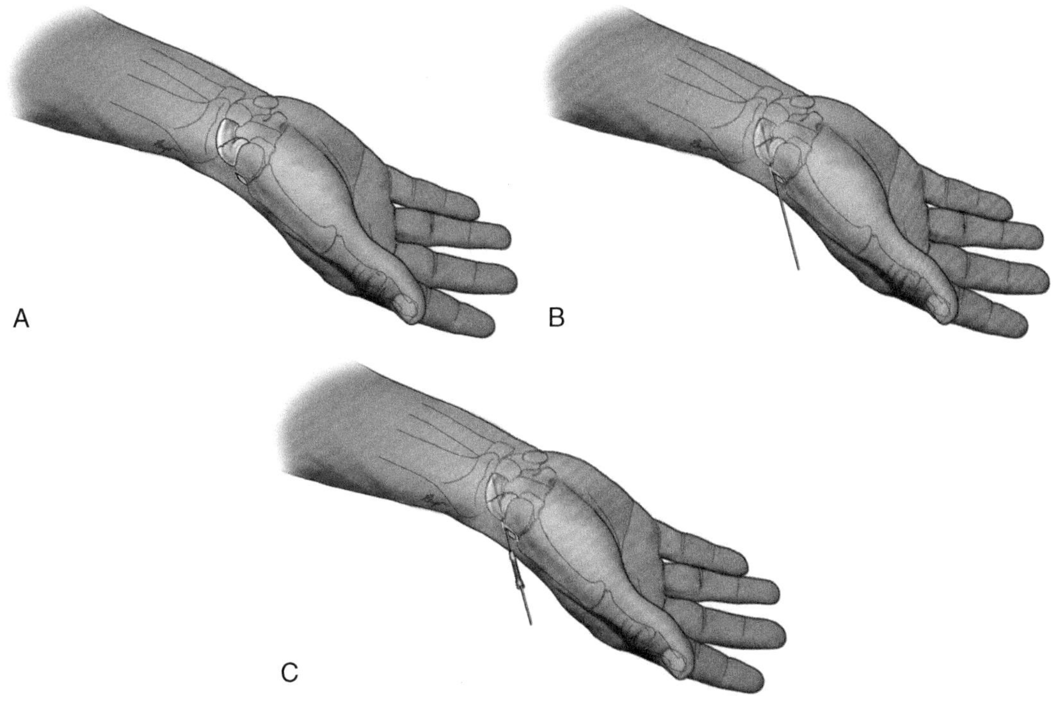

FIG. 18.5 Closed reduction of the scaphoid fracture is performed with the wrist in extension, supination and ulnar deviation. This is achieved by putting the forearm on a folded drape while pulling the thumb. We perform **(A)** a small incision where **(B)** the drill guide, K-wire, is inserted. When the position is good, we insert **(C)** the headless compression screw. (Courtesy of Haugstvedt JR, MD, PhD, Moss, Norway.)

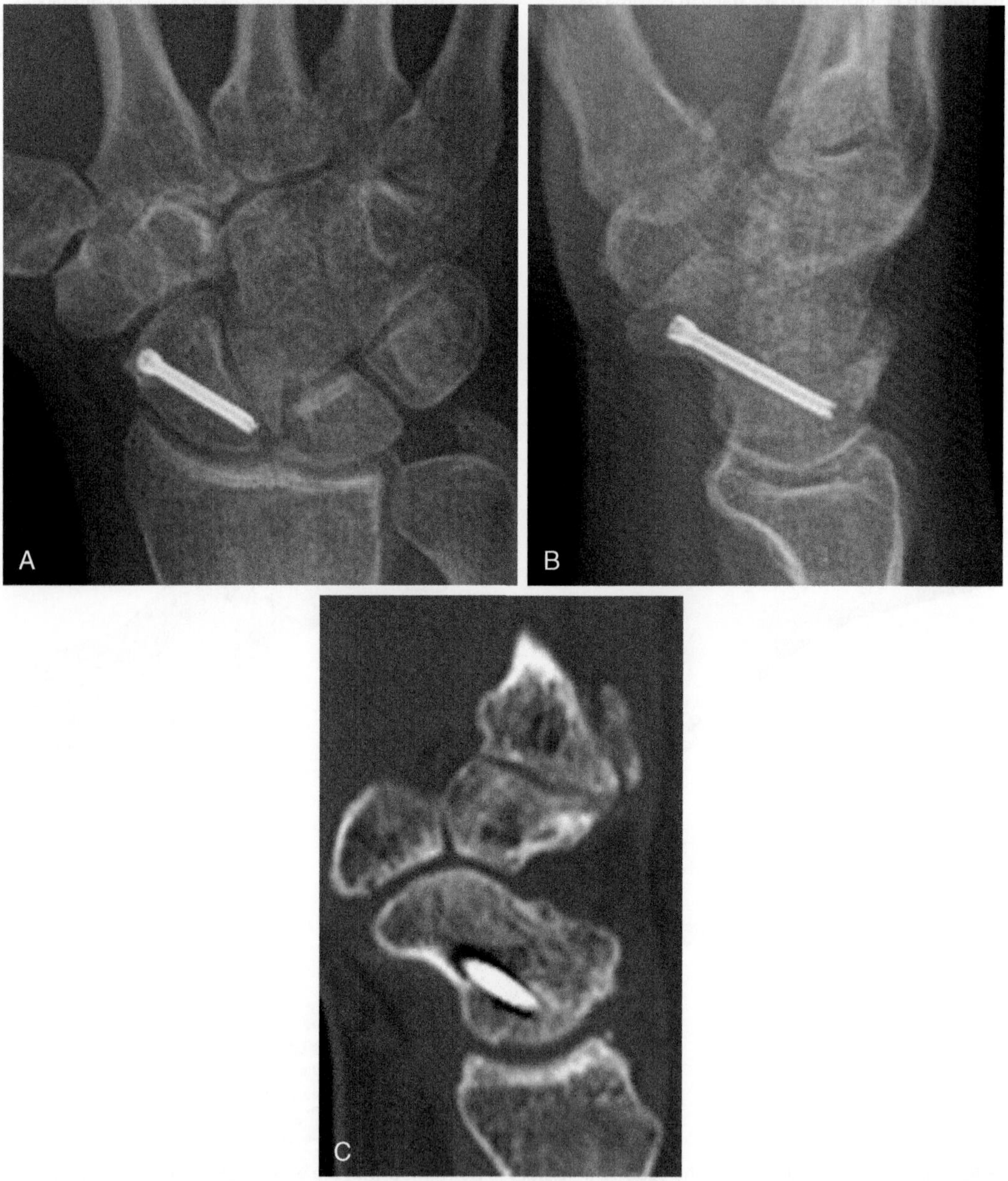

FIG 18.6 Healed scaphoid fracture after arthroscopy-assisted evaluation and retrograde screw fixation of the fracture; **(A)** posterior-anterior view, **(B)** lateral view, and **(C)** CT scan.

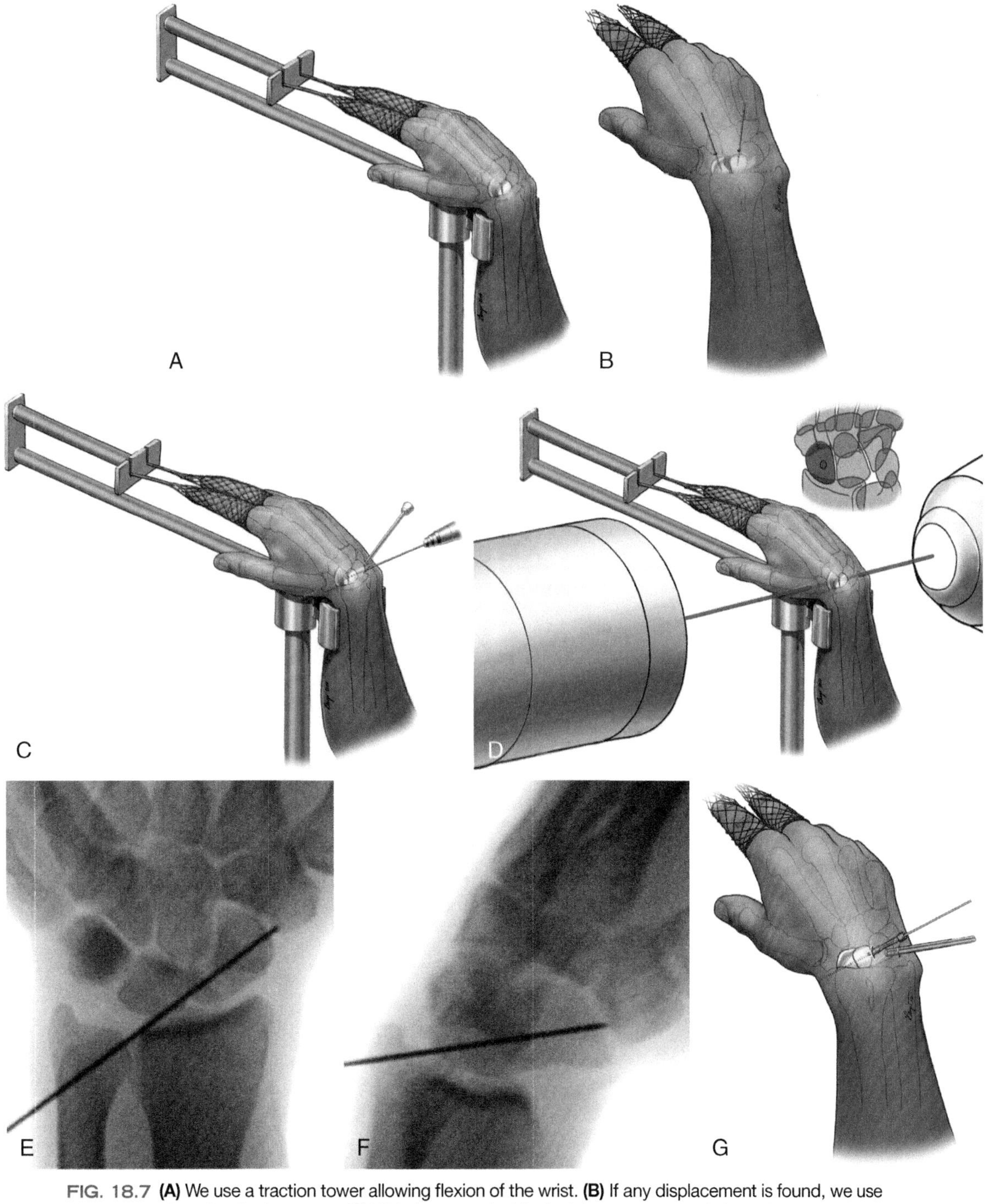

FIG. 18.7 **(A)** We use a traction tower allowing flexion of the wrist. **(B)** If any displacement is found, we use K-wires to reduce the displacement. **(C)** With the scope inside the joint, we can check the point where the K-wire (guide for the headless compression screw) should be inserted. For this, we keep the scope in the radiocarpal joint; however, to check the reposition of the fracture, we keep the scope in the midcarpal joint. **(D)** To insert the K-wire, we need imaging. With the wrist in a flexed and pronated position, we use a posterior-anterior view to identify the long axis of the scaphoid. In this view, the scaphoid could be viewed as a cylinder and the central axis of the scaphoid is the center of the circle. We aim for this center when inserting the K-wire; the entrance point in the proximal scaphoid is controlled with the scope in the radiocarpal joint. Having inserted the K-wire, the position is verified by imaging of the **(E)** posterior-anterior view and **(F)** lateral view. We check the reposition from the radiocarpal joint as well as from the midcarpal joint. **(G)** When the position is good, we perform the fixation using a headless compression screw.

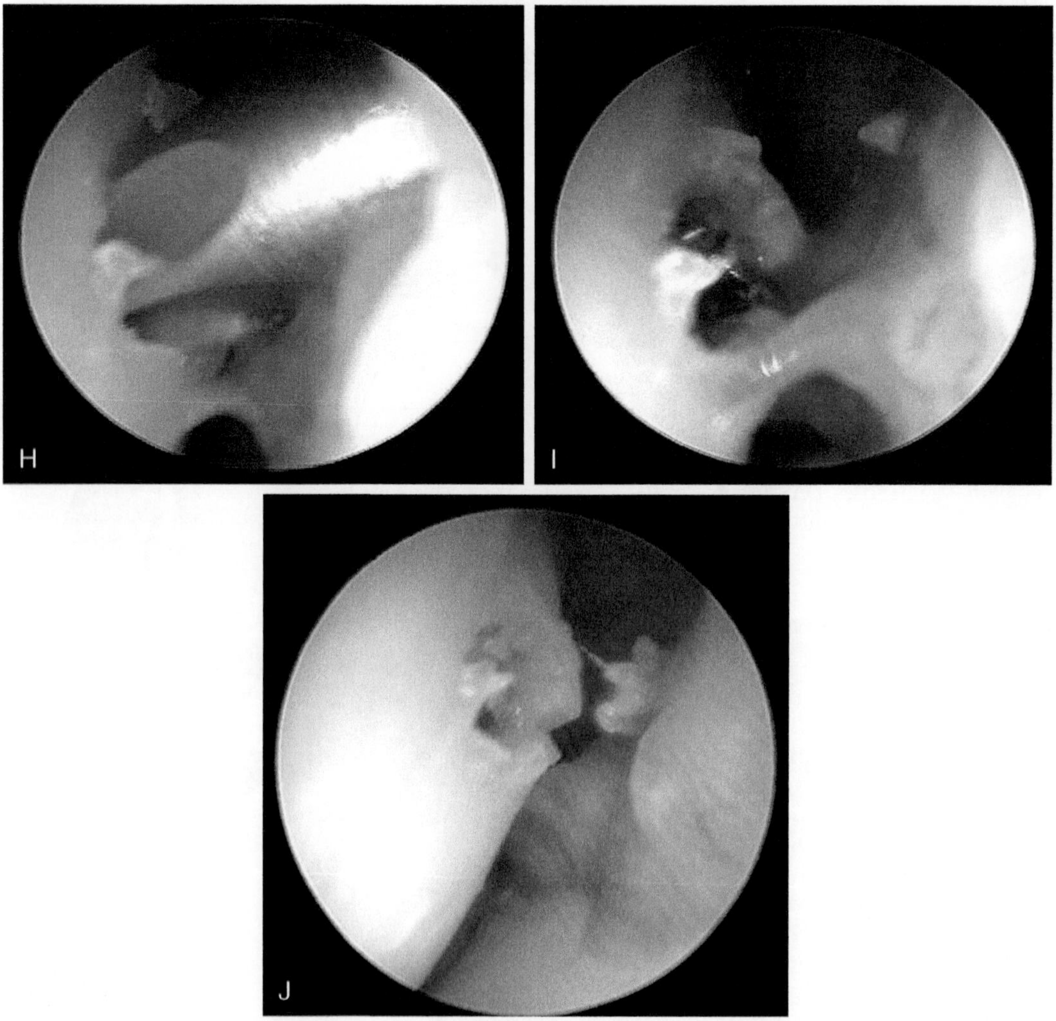

FIG. 18.7, cont'd **(H)** When the screw is inserted, we control the insertion through the scope. **(I)** We check the length of the screw and if there is any conflict with the cartilage, **(J)** the screw can be advanced further to be buried beneath the cartilage. ((A–D and G) Courtesy of Haugstvedt JR, MD, PhD, Moss, Norway.)

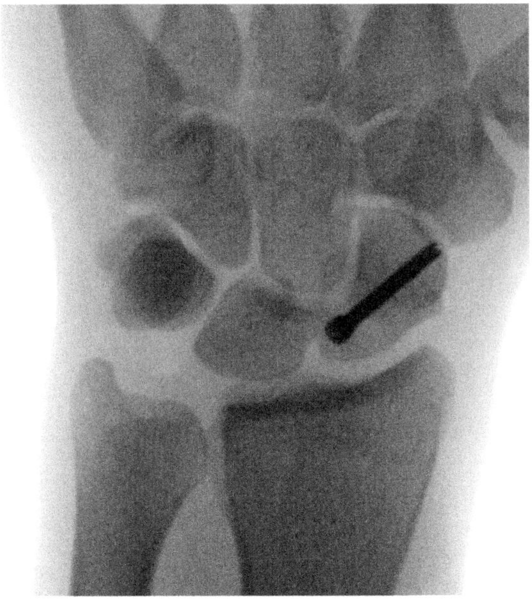

FIG. 18.8 The fracture healed.

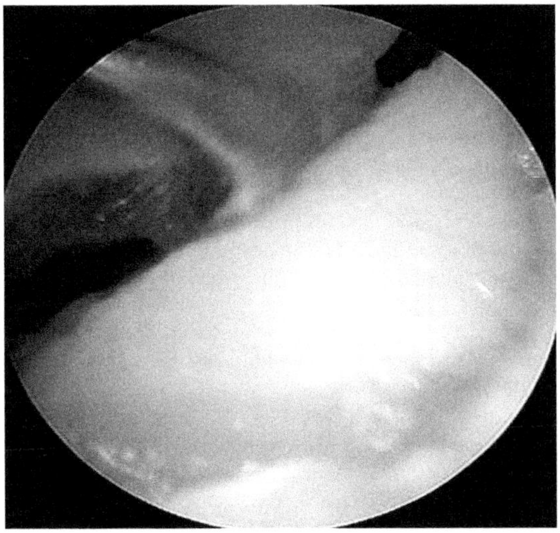

FIG. 18.9 From the midcarpal joint, the fracture was found unstable.

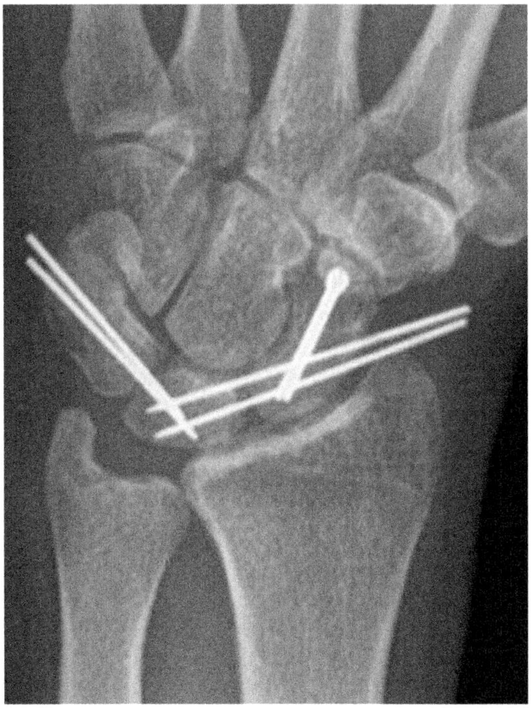

FIG. 18.10 Retrograde fixation of the scaphoid fracture with simultaneous pinning of the SL and LT intervals.

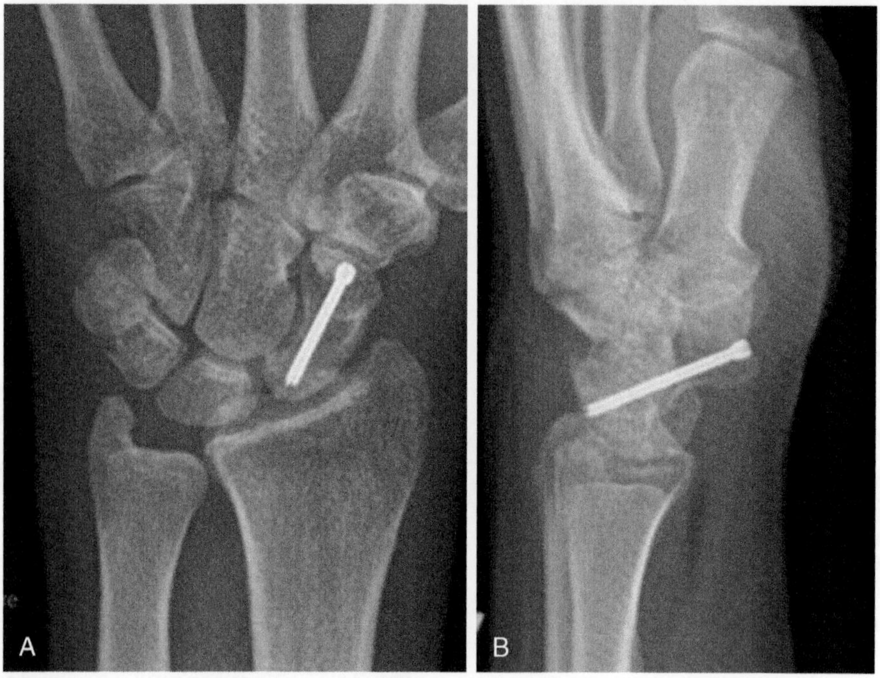

FIG. 18.11 Final result of treatment after removal of the K-wires; **(A)** posterior-anterior view and **(B)** lateral view.

REFERENCES

1. Slutsky DJ, Trevare J. Use of arthroscopy for the treatment of scaphoid fractures. *Hand Clin*. 2014;30:91–103.
2. Clementson M, Jørgsholm P, Besjako J, Thomsen N, Björkman A. Conservative treatment versus arthroscopic-assisted screw fixation of scaphoid waist fractures—a randomized trial with minimum 4-year follow-up. *J Hand Surg*. 2015;40:1341–1348.
3. Ibrahim T, Qureshi A, Sutton AJ, Dias JJ. Surgical versus nonsurgical treatment of acute minimally displaced and undisplaced scaphoid waist fractures: pairwise and network meta-analyses of randomized controlled trials. *J Hand Surg*. 2011;36:1759–1768.
4. Symes TH, Stothard J. A systematic review of the treatment of acute fractures of the scaphoid. *J Hand Surg*. 2011;36:802–810.
5. Buijze GA, Doornberg JN, Ham JS, Ring D, Bhandari M, Poolman RW. Surgical compared with conservative treatment for acute nondisplaced or minimally displaced scaphoid fractures. *J Bone Joint Surg Am*. 2010;92:1534–1544.
6. Alnaeem H, Aldekhayel S, Kanevsky J, Neel OF. A systematic review and meta-analysis examining the differences between nonsurgical management and percutaneous fixation of minimally and nondisplaced scaphoid fractures. *J Hand Surg*. 2016;41:1135–1144.
7. Shen L, Tang J, Luo C, Xie X, An Z, Zhang C. Comparison of operative and non-operative treatment of acute undisplaced or minimally-displaced scaphoid fractures: a meta-analysis of randomized controlled trials. *PLoS One*. 2015;10(5):e0125247. http://dx.doi.org/10.371/journal.pone.0125247.
8. Majeed H. Non-operative treatment versus percutaneous fixation for minimally displaced scaphoid waist fractures in high demand young manual workers. *J Orthop Traumatol*. 2014;15:239–244.
9. Grewal R, King GJ. An evidence-based approach to the management of acute scaphoid fractures. *J Hand Surg*. 2009;34:732–734.
10. Alshryda S, Shah A, Odak S, et al. Acute fractures of the scaphoid bone: systematic review and meta-analysis. *Surgeon*. 2012;10(4):218–229.
11. Singh HP, Taub N, Dias JJ. Management of displaced fractures of the waist of the scaphoid: meta-analyses of comparative studies. *Injury*. 2012;43:933–939.
12. Modi CS, Nancoo T, Powers D, Ho K, Boer R, Turner SM. Operative versus nonoperative treatment of acute undisplaced and minimally displaced scaphoid waist fracture-a systematic review. *Injury*. 2009;40:268–273.
13. Ram AN, Chung KC. Evidence-based management of acute nondisplaced scaphoid waist fractures. *J Hand Surg*. 2009;34:735–738.

14. Schädel-Höpfner M, Bickert B, Dumont C, et al. Die Frische Skaphoidfraktur. Management unter Berücksichtigung der neuen S3-Leitlinie. *Orthopade.* 2016;45:945–950.
15. Buijze GA, Jørgsholm P, Thomsen NO, Björkman A, Besjakov J, Ring D. Diagnostic performance of radiographs and computed tomography for displacement and instability of acute scaphoid waist fractures. *J Bone Joint Surg Am.* 2012;94:1967–1974.
16. Gelberman RH, Menon J. The vascularity of the scaphoid bone. *J Hand Surg.* 1980;5:508–513.
17. Oehmke MJ, Podranski T, Klaus R, et al. The blood supply of the scaphoid bone. *J Hand Surg.* 2009;34:351–357.
18. Hagert E. Proprioception of the wrist joint: a review of current concepts and possible implications on the rehabilitation of the wrist. *J Hand Ther.* 2010;23:2–16.
19. Jørgsholm P, Thomsen NO, Björkman A, Besjakov J, Abrahamsson SO. The incidence of intrinsic and extrinsic ligament injuries in scaphoid waist fractures. *J Hand Surg.* 2010;35:368–374.
20. Herzberg G. Perilunate injuries, not dislocated (PLIND). *J Wrist Surg.* 2013;2:337–345.
21. Geissler WB. Carpal fractures in athletes. *Clin Sports Med.* 2001;20:167–188.
22. Wong WYC, Ho PC. Minimal invasive management of scaphoid fractures: from fresh to nonunion. *Hand Clin.* 2011;27:291–307.
23. Vinnars B, Pietreanu M, Bodestedt A, Ekenstam F,Gerdin B. Nonoperative compared with operative treatment of acute scaphoid fractures. A randomized clinical trial. *J Bone Joint Surg Am.* 2008;90:1176–1185.
24. Leclercq C, Mathoulin C. Members of EWAS. Complications of wrist arthroscopy: a multicenter study based on 10,107 arthroscopies. *J Wrist Surg.* 2016;5:320–326.
25. Jørgsholm P, Thomsen NOB, Besjakov J, Abrahamsson SO, Björkman A. The benefit of Magnetic Resonance imaging for patients with posttraumatic radial wrist tenderness. *J Hand Surg.* 2013;38:29–33.
26. Messina JC, Van Overstraeten L, Luchetti R, Fairplay T, Mathoulin CL. The EWAS classification of scapholunate tears: an anatomical arthroscopic study. *J Wrist Surg.* 2013;2:105–109.

CHAPTER 19

Displaced Scaphoid Fracture Treatment

NICK JOHNSON MBCHB, FRCS • HARVINDER SINGH MBBS, FRCS, PHD • JOSEPH DIAS MBBS, FRCS, MD

KEY POINTS

- Displacement is seen in about 15% of scaphoid waist fractures.
- There is a four times higher risk of nonunion with a displaced fracture than with a nondisplaced fracture if treated in a plaster cast.
- Some evidence suggests that surgical fixation reduces nonunion rate.
- Long-term outcomes following operative and nonoperative treatment of displaced scaphoid fractures has not been established.

PANEL 1
Case Scenario

A 17-year-old male presented to the emergency department with radial-sided wrist pain after falling onto his outstretched left hand while playing football. Radiographs revealed a displaced scaphoid waist fracture. The patient would like a fast return to sporting activity but is unsure about undergoing surgery. He is concerned about potential complications and long-term outcomes. How best can you advise him? (Fig. 19.1A and B)

IMPORTANCE OF THE PROBLEM

A displaced fracture of the scaphoid is one in which the fragments have moved from their anatomic position or there is movement between them when stressed by physiologic loads.[1] Displacement is seen in about 15% of fractures of the waist of the scaphoid, although reported rates vary.[2] This is dependent on the radiologic investigation and the criteria used to identify displacement.

The four ways in which fractures can displace are translation, gap, angulation, and rotation. A scaphoid fracture is considered displaced if radiographs show an offset (step off) or gap of 1 mm or more.[1] However, difficulty with seeing a scaphoid fracture on radiographs is well recognized, reflecting the inclination of this bone. Computed tomography in the longitudinal axis of the scaphoid is a more reliable method for determining scaphoid displacement and has been discussed in Chapter 10.

Between 85% and 90% of fractures of the waist of the scaphoid will unite in a below-elbow plaster cast, but those with displacement have a higher incidence of nonunion.[3,4] Displacement of fractures of the waist of the scaphoid can result in malunion in flexion, but sometimes the distal fragment may heal in some pronation or ulnar translation.[5]

There is a four times higher risk of nonunion with a displaced fracture than with a nondisplaced fracture if treated in a plaster cast.[2] A large prospective study showed a nonunion rate of 14% in 74 displaced fractures of the waist of the scaphoid treated in a below-elbow plaster cast with the thumb left free.[4] In two small studies, nonunion was seen in 5 of 10 fractures of the waist of the scaphoid with a 1-mm gap or step treated with a cast.[1] Eddeland et al. observed nonunion in 23 (92%) of 25 scaphoid fractures with displacement > 1 mm, compared with 17 (19%) of 93 fractures with <1 mm displacement.[6] However, none of the patients with a nonunion in this study had been immobilized for the first 4 weeks, so this high incidence may reflect inadequate initial treatment. We do not know whether operative intervention reduces the risk of malunion or nonunion and subsequent osteoarthritis after a displaced scaphoid fracture.

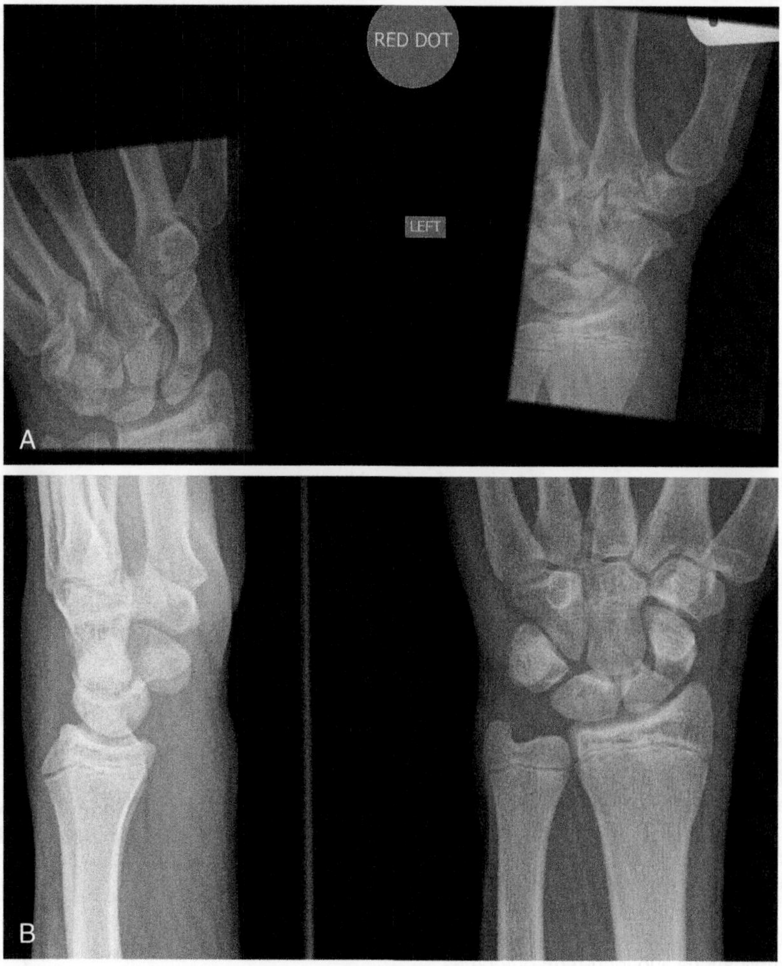

FIG. 19.1 (A and B) Acute displaced scaphoid waist fracture in a 17-year-old man.

QUESTION 1

In patients with displaced scaphoid fractures, does operative management compared with nonoperative management reduce nonunion rate or improve functional outcome?

Current Opinion

Many surgeons recommend reduction and internal fixation for displaced scaphoid fractures with the aim of preventing malunion, nonunion, and the development of osteoarthritis along with allowing earlier mobilization and return to work and normal activities (Fig. 19.2(A and B)).

Search Strategy

Embase

(((exp "SCAPHOID FRACTURE"/OR exp "SCAPHOID BONE FRACTURE"/OR ((exp "SCAPHOID BONE"/ OR (scaphoid).ti,ab OR (navicular AND (carpus OR hand OR wrist)).ti,ab) AND (FRACTURE/OR (fracture).ti,ab))) AND ("FRACTURE TREATMENT"/OR "ORTHOPEDIC SURGERY"/OR (surgery).ti,ab OR "FRACTURE FIXATION"/OR ("open reduction internal fixation" OR orif).ti,ab)) AND ("FRACTURE NONUNION"/OR "FRACTURE UNION DELAY"/OR (displace* OR maluni* OR non-union OR unstable OR (delayed ADJ4 union)).ti,ab)) AND ("CONSERVATIVE TREATMENT"/OR "CAST, PLASTER"/OR "EXTERNAL FIXATOR"/OR SPLINT/OR (non-surgical).ti,ab OR (non-operative).ti,ab OR (immobili*).ti,ab OR IMMOBILIZATION/OR (conservative).ti,ab)

Medline

(((("SCAPHOID BONE"/OR (scaphoid).ti,ab OR (navicular AND(carpus OR hand OR wrist)).ti,ab)

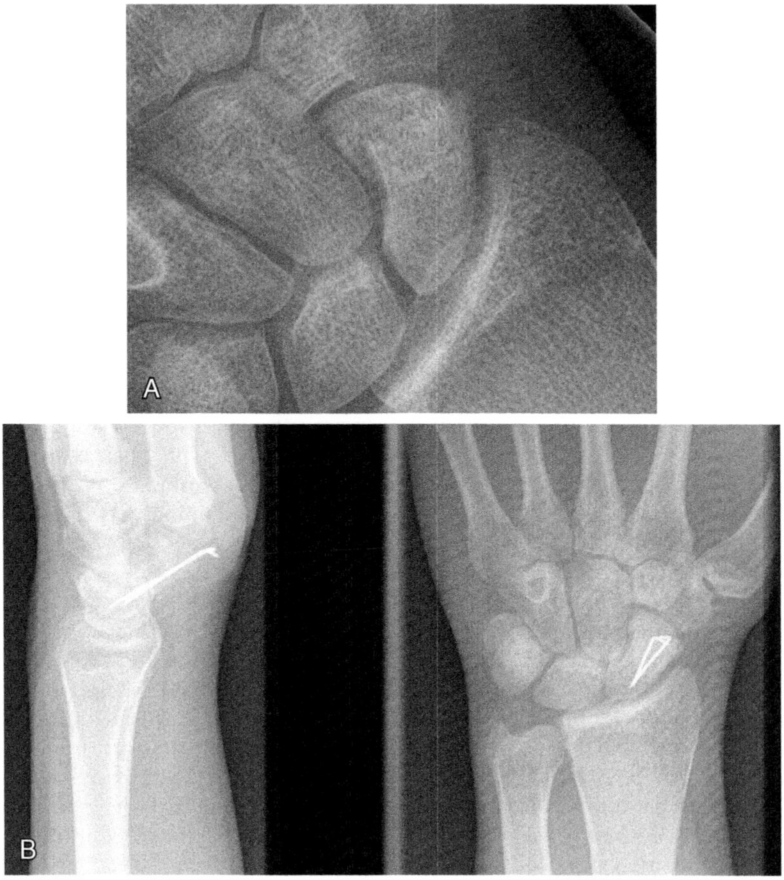

FIG. 19.2 (A and B) Displaced scaphoid fracture in a 26-year-old man treated with open reduction and internal fixation with two Kirschner wires.

AND ((fracture).ti,ab OR exp"FRACTURES, BONE"/)) AND ((("SCAPHOID BONE"/OR(scaphoid).ti,ab OR (navicular AND (carpus OR hand ORwrist)).ti,ab) AND ((fracture).ti,ab OR exp "FRACTURES, BONE"/))AND (displace* OR maluni* OR non-union OR unstable OR (delayed ADJ4 union)).ti,ab)) AND ("SURGICAL PROCEDURES, OPERATIVE"/OR "FRACTURE FIXATION"/OR "ORTHOPEDIC PROCEDURES"/OR (fracture xation).ti,ab OR (orif OR "open reduction internal xation").ti,ab OR (stabili*).ti,ab)) AND ((conservative).ti,ab OR "EXTERNAL FIXATORS"/OR "CASTS, SURGICAL"/OR (non-operative).ti,ab OR (non-surgical).ti,ab OR (splint*).ti,ab OR SPLINTS/OR (immobili*).ti,ab OR IMMOBILIZATION/)

Quality of the Evidence

Level III: 1
Level IV: 13

Findings

Singh et al. performed a systematic review comparing surgical treatment with plaster treatment of displaced fractures of the waist of the scaphoid.[2] Seven published case series were identified for surgical fixation of displaced scaphoid waist fractures with headless screws.[7–12] The studies were all case series and two studies were based on the same data reported separately. Metaanalysis was therefore not possible.

Analysis of the pooled results of the six studies reporting separate data revealed 157 patients with displaced scaphoid waist fractures fixed surgically (range 14–67). Follow-up ranged from 1 to 4 years. Only two (2%) fractures did not unite. In the nonoperative group, eight articles were included in a metaanalysis because they reported results after plaster cast treatment for both displaced and nondisplaced fractures.[1,3,4,6,13–16] One study was subsequently excluded because patients had inadequate initial treatment with no cast immobilization for the first 4 weeks after injury. In the remaining seven studies, 207 displaced scaphoid waist fractures (range 7–74) were seen with 37 (18%) fractures failing to unite. Follow-up ranged from 0.5 to 7 years. There was a 4.4 times higher risk of fracture nonunion for displaced fractures (RR 4.40, 95% CI = 2.23–8.67; $I^2 = 54\%$) compared with nondisplaced fractures. An I^2 value of 54% suggests heterogeneity between studies. Some of the included studies were carried out over 30 years ago; the definition of displacement was not standardized and treatment involved different types of casts for different durations.

A two-way contingency table analysis was used to compare nonunion rates of those treated surgically with nonoperatively. This showed an odds ratio of 16.9 of nonunion with plaster cast treatment compared with fixation ($P < .001$).

QUESTION 2

In patients with displaced scaphoid fractures, does surgical treatment using a volar approach compared with a dorsal approach reduce nonunion rate/complications or improve functional outcome?

Current Opinion

The current consensus is that fractures of the proximal third are approached from the dorsum of the wrist and fractures of the distal two-thirds are approached from the volar approach. However, there is great variation in surgical approaches determined mainly by surgical preference.

Search Strategy

As above, using keywords:

SURGICAL APPROACH ROUTE, SURGICAL APPROACH, VOLAR APPROACH, DORSAL APPROACH

Quality of the Evidence

Level IV: 4

Findings

There are no randomized controlled trials investigating the outcome following surgical treatment of displaced acute scaphoid fractures using a volar approach compared with a dorsal approach. All studies identified were small case series.

Slade et al. retrospectively reviewed 20 patients with displaced scaphoid fractures who were treated with arthroscopic-assisted percutaneous screw fixation.[12] Seven patients had volar percutaneous screw insertion and 13 underwent dorsal percutaneous screw insertion. They reported that there were no complications and all fractures were healed at 18-month (range 6–48 months) follow-up.

Bain et al. describe a novel approach of dorsal plating for displaced scaphoid fractures.[17] They suggest that a dorsal plate uses the tension side of the bone to create compression and is biomechanically superior to a screw or volar plating. Resistance to torsion and collapse makes it useful for displaced and comminuted fractures. In a series of 10 displaced fractures and nonunions, they report that one patient had delayed union. All other fractures united.

QUESTION 3

In patients with displaced scaphoid fractures, does surgical treatment with open reduction compared with percutaneous or arthroscopic-assisted reduction reduce the rate of nonunion and complications or improve functional outcome?

Current Opinion

In practice, we use distraction to align the fragments and assist this using the wire introduced into the distal fragment. Radial deviation of the wrist will use the scaphoid facet of the distal radius to help reduce a step at the fracture line. It is very uncommon to need direct manipulation of the displaced fracture to reduce a step. A gap of >1 mm is dealt with using precompression before advancing the screw threads across the fracture. At present we do not usually pay particular attention to angulation or rotation, and this does need more definition.

Search Strategy

As above, using keywords:

OPEN REDUCTION, ARTHROSCOPIC REDUCTION, PERCUTANEOUS REDUCTION, FRACTURE FIXATION, INTERNAL, ARTHROSCOPY

Quality of the Evidence

Level IV: 3

Findings

There are no randomized controlled trials investigating the outcome following surgical treatment of displaced acute scaphoid fractures using open reduction compared with a percutaneous approach or arthroscopic-assisted reduction. All studies identified were small case series.

In a retrospective review, Trumble et al. treated 35 patients with an acute displaced fracture of the scaphoid waist with open reduction through a volar approach and

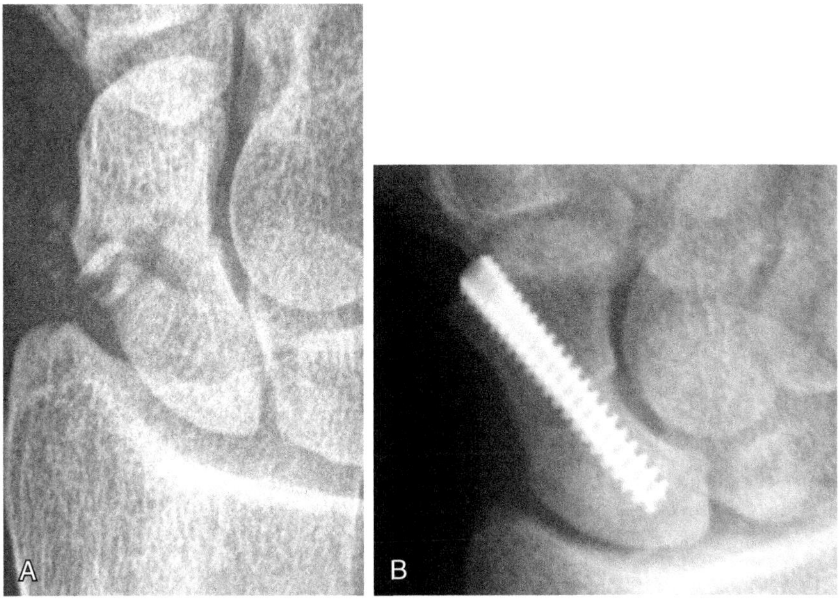

FIG. 19.3 **(A** and **B)** Displaced, comminuted scaphoid waist fracture in a 33-year-old male patient, which was treated with open reduction and screw fixation and united uneventfully.

internal fixation using a cannulated screw.[8] All fractures united. Screw placement and reduction was accurate. Functional results in terms of grip strength and range of movement were satisfactory. Rettig et al. described open reduction of 14 displaced scaphoid waist fractures.[7] A volar approach was used in 12 patients and a dorsal approach in 2 patients. Bone grafting was performed in 10 cases due to comminution. Fixation was achieved with compression screws in eight patients and Kirschner wires (K-wires) in six patients. Only one fracture failed to unite and no evidence of carpal instability was seen. Functional range of motion and grip strength was achieved in all patients.

Using an arthroscopic-assisted reduction, Slade et al. treated 20 consecutive displaced scaphoid fractures with percutaneous screw fixation.[12] There were no implant problems and all fractures united. Patients had good functional outcome. They suggested an arthroscopic-assisted reduction, and percutaneous screw fixation avoids the need for an open exposure in displaced scaphoid fractures and may preserve blood supply and reduce wrist ligament injury.

QUESTION 4

In patients with displaced scaphoid fractures, does surgical fixation using a screw compared with wires reduce nonunion rate/complications or improve functional outcome?

Current Opinion

Internal fixation using a single headless screw is currently the most frequently used method of stabilization for displaced scaphoid fractures after reduction (Fig. 19.3A and B).

Search Strategy

As above, using keywords:

BONE SCREW, SCREW, BONE PLATE, BONE WIRE, KIRSCHNER WIRE, K-WIRE

Quality of the Evidence

Level IV: 6

Findings

There are no randomized controlled trials investigating the outcome following surgical treatment of displaced acute scaphoid fractures using screws compared with wires. All studies identified were small case series reporting on one method of fixation (n = 3–35) or biomechanical studies.

In a retrospective study of 35 patients, Trumble et al. compared two different types of screws used for fixation of displaced scaphoid fractures following open reduction. Of those, 16 patients were treated with a Herbert-Whipple screw and 19 with a 3.5-mm AO/ASIF screw.[8] There was no difference in functional or radiologic outcome between the groups. They concluded that cannulated screws were a safe and effective treatment for displaced scaphoid fractures.

Dodds et al. assessed the biomechanical stability of unstable scaphoid fractures fixed with short screws, long screws, and long screws with K-wire augmentation.[18] They created 3-mm volarly based osteotomies in cadaveric scaphoids to produce a displaced fracture model. After physiologically applied loading, it was demonstrated that the long screw provided significantly less interfragmentary motion than the short screw. Addition of a K-wire seemed to improve stability, but this was not statistically significant. They recommended that optimum fixation was using a long screw sited deep into subchondral bone down the central axis of the scaphoid.

QUESTION 5

In patients with displaced scaphoid fractures, does internal fixation affect the rate of malunion and osteoarthritis?

Current Opinion

Many surgeons advocate reduction and internal fixation for displaced scaphoid fractures to prevent malunion or the development of osteoarthritis, although long-term outcome is poorly understood (Fig. 19.4(A-C)).

Search Strategy

As above, using keywords:

MALUNION, POSITION, ALIGNMENT, DISPLACEMENT, MALALIGNMENT, OSTEOARTHRITIS, ARTHRITIS

Quality of the Evidence

Level IV: 2

Findings

There are no randomized controlled trials investigating the effect of internal fixation of displaced acute scaphoid fractures on malunion and the development of osteoarthritis.

Whether operative intervention reduces the risk of osteoarthritis after a displaced scaphoid fracture is unknown. At mean follow-up of 93 months, no statistical difference was seen in the rate of radioscaphoid osteoarthritis in 71 patients with an acute minimally or nondisplaced fracture of the scaphoid who had been randomized to cast treatment or surgical fixation.[19]

Raudasoja et al. retrospectively evaluated 63 patients with displaced scaphoid fractures at a mean of 54 months after nonoperative treatment.[20] One-third of patients developed osteoarthritis. This was associated with age of the patient and humpback deformity but did not correlate with pain or grip strength. Of those, five (8%) patients demonstrated dorsal intercalated segment instability. Malalignment was not associated with adverse functional outcome.

RECOMMENDATION

In patients with a displaced scaphoid fracture:

- There is a higher risk of fracture nonunion for displaced scaphoid fractures compared with nondisplaced fractures treated nonoperatively (overall quality: low to moderate).
- There is weak evidence that surgical fixation reduces nonunion rate (overall quality: low).
- There is minimal evidence to suggest which surgical approach has the best outcome for displaced scaphoid fractures (overall quality: very low).
- There is little evidence to suggest whether an open, percutaneous, or arthroscopic-assisted approach produces the best outcome (overall quality: low)
- Screw fixation produces satisfactory results (overall quality: low).

CONCLUSION

Further research is required to investigate the effect of internal fixation of displaced acute scaphoid fractures on malunion and the development of osteoarthritis. Long-term outcome has not been established. Radiologic outcome does not appear to correlate with functional outcome. Displaced scaphoid fractures have a four times higher risk of nonunion compared with nondisplaced fractures treated nonoperatively. There is some evidence that nonunion rate is reduced by surgical fixation. This should be explained to the patient when discussing treatment options and prognosis.

There is minimal evidence to suggest which surgical approach has the best outcome or whether an open, percutaneous, or arthroscopic-assisted approach improves outcome. Further high-quality research is needed. Small case series have reported promising results regarding union rate, complication

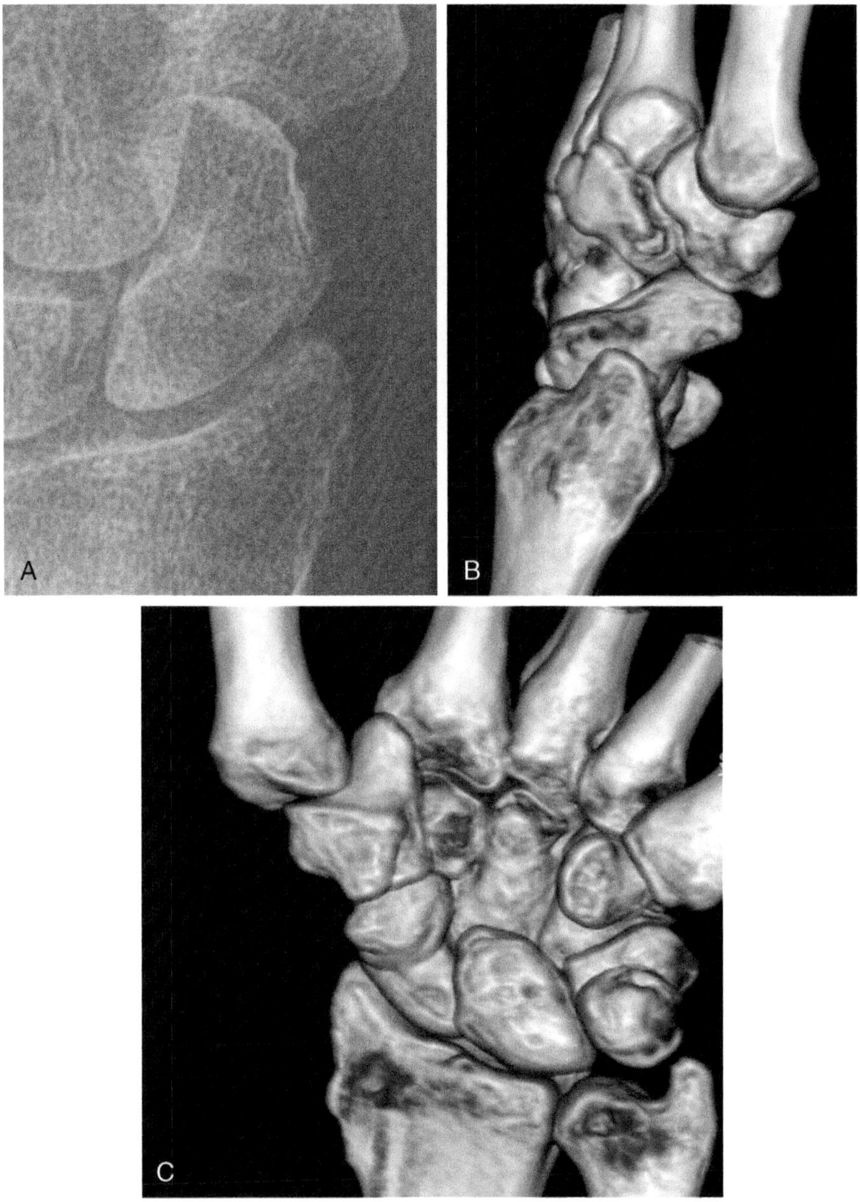

FIG. 19.4 **(A–C)** A 58-year-old woman presented with a displaced scaphoid fracture, which was treated nonoperatively. Subsequent CT scans showed that the fracture had healed with a mild humpback deformity.

rate, and functional outcome for open reduction and internal fixation and arthroscopic-assisted percutaneous fixation. There is little evidence to suggest which fixation device produces the best outcome. Biomechanically, a long screw in the central axis of the scaphoid produces a stable fixation in displaced scaphoid fractures. Further research is required to investigate the effect of internal fixation of displaced acute scaphoid fractures on malunion and the development of osteoarthritis. Long-term outcome has not been established. Radiologic outcome does not appear to correlate with functional outcome.

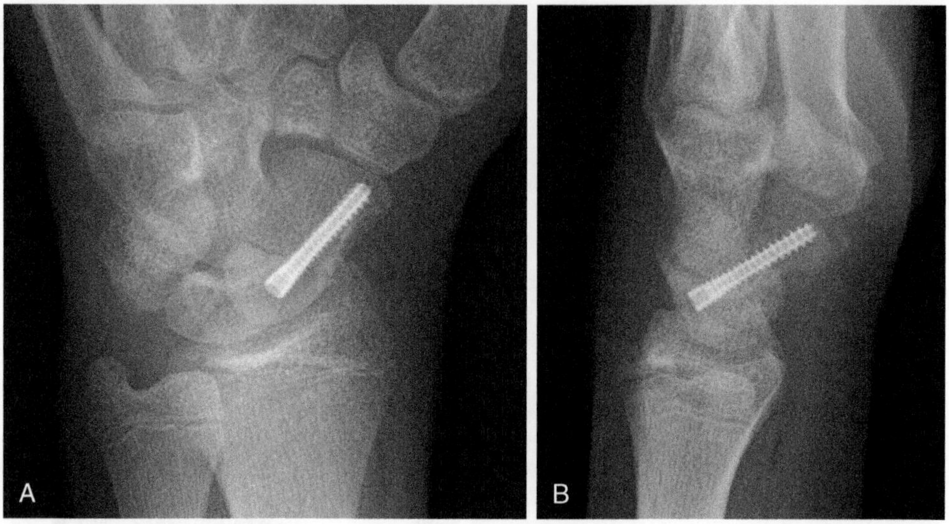

FIG. 19.5 **(A and B)** Healed displaced scaphoid waist fracture in a 17-year-old male, which was treated by internal fixation with a single screw.

PANEL 2
Author's Preferred Technique (Related to Case Scenario)

In this case of a displaced scaphoid waist fracture in a young, healthy patient, the fracture was treated with internal fixation. After discussion with the patient regarding risks and benefits of the treatment options, this method was chosen because of the potential lower nonunion rate and the patient's wishes to return to sport as soon as possible. Radial deviation of the wrist was applied to use the scaphoid facet of the distal radius to help reduce a step in the fracture and a percutaneous approach chosen. Precompression was applied to reduce the fracture gap and a single screw advanced over a guide wire placed in the central axis of the scaphoid (Fig. 19.5A and B).

PANEL 3
Pearls and Pitfalls

PEARLS

- Most fractures with a step can have their position improved by distraction or by using the adjacent articular surfaces of the radius and capitate to assist reduction.
- An intra-articular lever introduced from the 3/4 portal (either an arthroscopic cannula or an elevator) can assist reduction without the need to open the joint.
- During reduction of very unstable fractures, separate wires in the proximal and distal poles can be placed percutaneously. Once the step is reduced, angular reduction is accomplished by pushing the wires in the appropriate direction, at which point a third K-wire is drilled percutaneously across the fracture as close as possible to the axis of the scaphoid.
- At least four threads of the screw should engage each fracture fragment. Rotation of the fragments during tightening of the screw may be countered using a derotation wire or using a tap.

PITFALLS

- Failure to pass a central guide wire will lead to eccentric screw placement and risks exaggerating the step or angle as the screw is tightened.
- Anterior placement of a screw can worsen humpback deformity as the screw is advanced.
- Selection of a screw that is too long may lead to protrusion into the joint or distraction of the fracture, rather than compression, when it is advanced and the far end pushes against subchondral bone.

REFERENCES

1. Cooney WP, Dobyns JH, Linscheid RL. Fractures of the scaphoid: a rational approach to management. *Clin Orthop*. 1980;(149):90–97.
2. Singh HP, Taub N, Dias JJ. Management of displaced fractures of the waist of the scaphoid: meta-analyses of comparative studies. *Injury*. 2012;43(6):933–939.
3. Bhat M, McCarthy M, Davis TRC, Oni JA, Dawson S. MRI and plain radiography in the assessment of displaced fractures of the waist of the carpal scaphoid. *J Bone Joint Surg Ser B*. 2004;86(5):705–713.
4. Clay NR, Dias JJ, Costigan PS, Gregg PJ, Barton NJ. Need the thumb be immobilised in scaphoid fractures? A randomised prospective trial. *J Bone Joint Surg Br*. 1991;73(5):828–832.
5. Fernandez DL, Martin CJ, Gonzalez del Pino J. Scaphoid malunion. the significance of rotational malalignment. *J Hand Surg Br*. 1998;23(6):771–775.
6. Eddeland A, Eiken O, Hellgren E, Ohlsson N. Fractures of the scaphoid. *Scand J Plast Reconstr Surg*. 1975;9(3):234–239.
7. Rettig ME, Kozin SH, Cooney WP. Open reduction and internal fixation of acute displaced scaphoid waist fractures. *J Hand Surg*. 2001;26(2):271–276.
8. Trumble TE, Gilbert M, Murray LW, Smith J, Rafijah G, McCallister WV. Displaced scaphoid fractures treated with open reduction and internal fixation with a cannulated screw. *J Bone Joint Surg Ser A*. 2000;82(5):633–641.
9. Shih J, Lee H, Hou Y, Tan C. Results of arthroscopic reduction and percutaneous fixation for acute displaced scaphoid fractures. *Arthroscopy*. 2005;21(5):620–626.
10. Chen AC, Chao E, Hung S, Lee MS, Ueng SW. Percutaneous screw fixation for unstable scaphoid fractures. *J Trauma*. 2005;59(1):184–187.
11. Martinache X, Mathoulin C. Osteosynthese percutanee des fractures du scaphoide carpien avec assistance arthroscopique Percutaneous fixation of scaphoid fractures with arthroscopic assistance. *Chir Main*. 2006:25.
12. Slade JF, Lozano-Calderon S, Merrell G, Ring D. Arthroscopic-assisted percutaneous reduction and screw fixation of displaced scaphoid fractures. *J Hand Surg Eur Vol*. 2008;33(3):350–354.
13. Bohler L, Trojan E, Jahna H. The results of treatment of 734 fresh, simple fractures of the scaphoid. *J Hand Surg Br*. 2003;28(4):319–331.
14. Leslie IJ, Dickson RA. The fractured carpal scaphoid. natural history and factors influencing outcome. *J Bone Joint Surg Br*. 1981;63-B(2):225–230.
15. Alho A, Kankaanpaa U. Management of fractured scaphoid bone. A prospective study of 100 fractures. *Acta Orthop Scand*. 1975;46(5):737–743.
16. Thorleifsson R, Karlsson J, Sigurjonsson K. Fractures of the scaphoid bone A follow-up study. *Arch Orthop Trauma Surg*. 1984;103(2):96–99.
17. Bain GI, Turow A, Phadnis J. Dorsal plating of unstable scaphoid fractures and nonunions. *Tech Hand Upper Extrem Surg*. 2015;19(3):95–100.
18. Dodds SD, Panjabi MM, Slade JF. Screw fixation of scaphoid fractures: a biomechanical assessment of screw length and screw augmentation. *J Hand Surg*. 2006;31(3):405–413.
19. Dias JJ, Dhukaram V, Abhinav A, Bhowal B, Wildin CJ. Clinical and radiological outcome of cast immobilisation versus surgical treatment of acute scaphoid fractures at a mean follow-up of 93 months. *J Bone Joint Surg Br*. 2008;90(7):899–905.
20. Raudasoja L, Rawlins M, Kallio P, Vasenius J. Conservative treatment of scaphoid fractures: a follow up study. *Ann Chir Gynaecol*. 1999;88(4):289–293.

CHAPTER 20

Transscaphoid Perilunate Injuries

JONG-PIL KIM, MD, PHD

KEY POINTS

- The key to successful treatment for transscaphoid perilunate injuries is early surgical intervention to restore normal carpal alignment besides fracture healing.
- Controversy still exists on optimum treatment for transscaphoid injuries.

PANEL 1
Case Scenario

A 35-year-old man injured his right wrist in a motor vehicle collision. At initial presentation, he complained of severe wrist pain and swelling with median nerve paresthesia. Wrist radiographs showed a dorsal perilunate fracture-dislocation with a scaphoid waist fracture. Fractures at the radial styloid and triquetrum were also noted on the plane radiographs (Fig. 20.1). A closed reduction method for dorsal perilunate reduction was attempted.[1] However, postreduction computed tomography scan showed that the lunate was still located out of the lunate fossa with a proximal fragment of the scaphoid (Fig. 20.2).

What is the preferred treatment option for this patient (open reduction and internal fixation with dorsal, palmar, or combined approaches/closed reduction or arthroscopic-assisted reduction and percutaneous pinning) and should the carpal tunnel be released?

IMPORTANCE OF THE PROBLEM

Transscaphoid perilunate injuries refers to perilunate dislocations with a concomitant scaphoid fracture. Basically, perilunate injuries are highly unstable carpal dissociations, characterized by a complete loss of contact between the lunate and surrounding carpal bones. Perilunate injuries are also referred to as lesser arc injuries when ligaments around the lunate are involved only, whereas dislocations associated with fractures (perilunate fracture-dislocations) are referred to as greater arc injuries (Fig. 20.3).[3] Greater arc injuries most commonly involve fractures through the scaphoid (transscaphoid perilunate fracture-dislocation), accounting for approximately 95% of perilunate fracture-dislocations, and this corresponds to 5% of wrist fractures.[4] Greater arc injuries may involve any bone in sequence, such as the radial styloid, capitate, hamate, triquetrum, or lunate.

Perilunate injuries are caused by high-energy impact, such as falls from a height, motor vehicle accidents, or play injury from contact sports. The mechanism of these injuries includes forceful hyperextension, ulnar deviation, and intercarpal supination of the wrist along with axial load. The force is applied to the scaphoid (causing a transscaphoid fracture) or to the scapholunate ligament (causing a scapholunate dissociation). The force then progresses through the scaphocapitate and capitolunate joint or capitate, finally reaching the lunotriquetral ligament or triquetrum. Based on these pathomechanics, Mayfield et al.[5] described a spectrum of injuries characterized by four distinct stages (see Box 20.1).

Transscaphoid injuries are usually associated with disruption of the lunotriquetral ligament or triquetrum and/or ulnar styloid fracture. However, specific variation of this injury such as scaphocapitate syndrome, which includes both scaphoid and capitate fractures, can be noted. In a stage type IV transscaphoid injury, the lunate with the proximal fragment of the scaphoid is pushed into the carpal canal through the *space of Poirier*, which is the weakest area over the capitolunate articulation between the radioscaphocapitate and long radiolunate ligaments, whereas the distal fragment of the scaphoid attached to the distal carpal low is remained in the radial articular fossa (Fig. 20.4).

The opposite pattern referred to palmar perilunate fracture-dislocation can be seen with hyperflexion

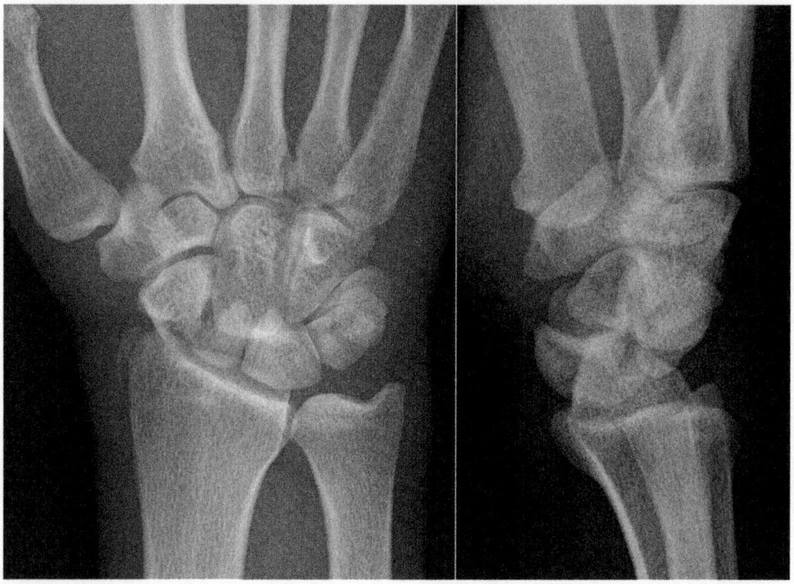

FIG. 20.1 **Posteroanterior and Lateral Radiographs for the Case, Showing a Transscaphoid Perilunate Fracture-Dislocation.** The injury also involved fractures at the radial styloid and triquetrum.

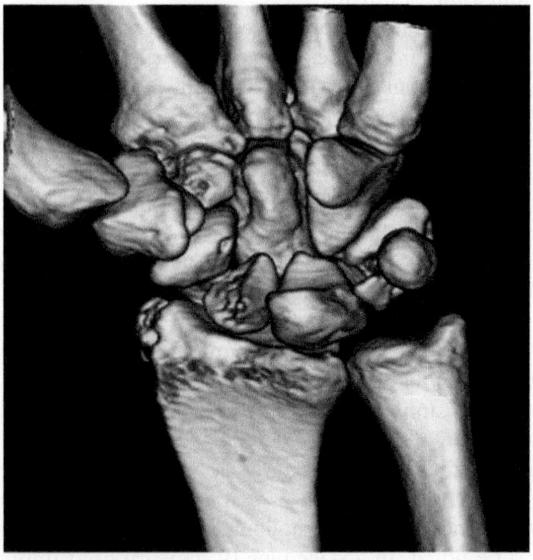

FIG. 20.2 **Three-Dimensional CT Image After Attempting a Closed Reduction.** Note that the lunate was still located out of the lunate fossa with a proximal fragment of the scaphoid.

injuries of the wrist. This represents only 10% of perilunate injuries.[6]

Patients with perilunate injury typically present with pain, swelling, and decreased range of motion. Neurologically, patients may present with acute median neuropathy (carpal tunnel syndrome). The incidence of carpal tunnel syndrome has been reported to be approximately 25%, ranging from 16% to 46%.[7] Posteroanterior (PA) view of standard wrist radiographs may show scaphoid fractures and disruption of the Gilula lines, which are formed by the proximal and distal articular surfaces of the proximal row and the proximal cortical margins of the capitate and hamate.[8] The lunate can appear triangular, which may be displaced depending on the extent of energy imparted.[9] A symmetric widening of the intercarpal joint spaces and fractures of the triquetrum, capitate, ulnar styloid, or distal radius may be seen on PA radiographs. A radiograph in gravity traction or with a small weight may facilitate evaluation, as it may effectively unmask an intercarpal dissociation if it is suspected.[10] Lateral radiograph can commonly reveals loss of colinearity between the capitate, lunate, and radius.[11] The capitate may be displaced in a dorsal direction, whereas the lunate displaced palmarly. Three-dimensional reconstruction of CT images can provide excellent visual information about the orientation of fracture fragments and dislocation.[1] Nonetheless, studies have shown that, even with adequate radiographic images, the diagnosis of perilunate injuries can be missed in up to 25% of cases, resulting in delayed treatment and disabling wrist arthritis.[4] Given the high-energy nature of these injuries, their detection

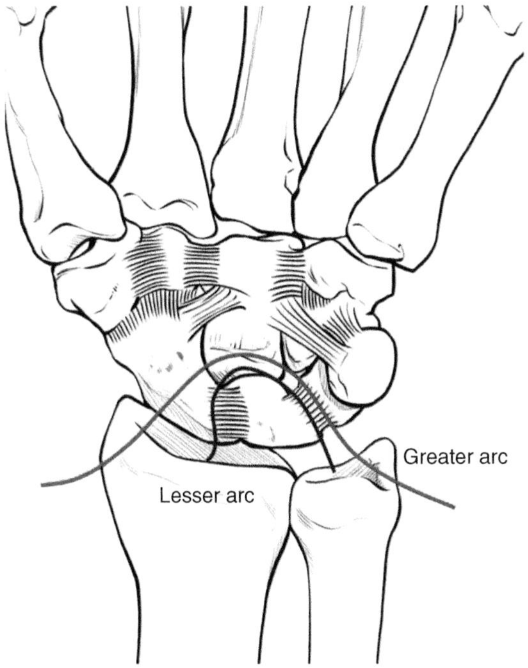

FIG. 20.3 **Patterns of Greater Arc and Lesser Arc Injuries.** Greater arc injuries involve a fracture of any bone in the sequence of the radial styloid, scaphoid, capitate, hamate, or triquetrum, whereas lesser arc injuries involve pure ligaments around the lunate.

BOX 20.1
Mechanism of Perilunate Injuries

Stage I: The scapholunate ligament and the radioscapholunate ligament are torn.

Stage II: The force is transmitted to the lunocapitate articulation where the capitate dislocates and the radioscaphocapitate ligament, dorsal intercarpal ligament, and radial collateral ligament are injured.

Stage III: Energy propagates into the lunotriquetral joint, resulting in the lunotriquetral ligament tear and a triquetral dislocation.

Stage IV: The lunate dislocates volarly and no longer remains within the lunate fossa as a result of ulnotriquetral and dorsal radiocarpal ligament tears.

Adaped from Mayfield JK, Johnson RP, Kilcoyne RK. Carpal dislocations: pathomechanics and progressive perilunar instability. *J Hand Surg Am*. 1980;5:226–241, with permission.

requires a high index of suspicion and a thorough upper-extremity examination.

The key to a successful treatment of perilunate injuries is early surgical intervention to restore normal alignment of carpal bones and stability because late treatment of unreduced perilunate injuries can lead to difficult wrist problems.[12] Treatments of transscaphoid perilunate injuries include closed reduction and cast immobilization or percutaneous or external fixation, open reduction and internal fixation, and arthroscopic-assisted reduction and percutaneous fixation. Among them, open reduction and internal fixation of the fractures and ligament repair or reconstruction through either dorsal or palmar approach or both has been generally accepted.[2,9,13,12–15] Recent arthroscopic techniques as a minimal invasive treatment have emerged with results similar to or better than those of open approach, as well as having less posttraumatic arthrosis.[15–17] However, the feasibility of arthroscopic technique in presence of median nerve dysfunction and whether intercarpal ligaments can achieve reliable healing that is sufficient enough to maintain carpal stability without a direct repair are uncertain and debatable.

MAIN QUESTIONS

1. How long would a delayed injury be repairable?
2. Do surgical methods affect the union rates in transscaphoid perilunate fracture dislocation? Closed reduction and percutaneous fixation, open reduction with internal fixation, or arthroscopic treatment appropriate?
3. What is the preferred operative exposure for open reduction and internal fixation: dorsal, palmar, or combined?
4. What is the ideal treatment for transscaphoid perilunate injuries in terms of functional outcomes and posttraumatic arthritis?
5. Should the carpal tunnel be released in transscaphoid perilunate injuries with acute carpal tunnel syndrome?

Question 1: How long would delayed injury be repairable?

Current opinion

Reestablishment of carpal alignment with repair of scaphoid fracture is possible a few weeks after injury.

Finding the evidence

- The following electronic databases were searched: Cochrane Database, Pubmed MEDLINE, Ovid MEDLINE, EMBASE, and SCOPUS. The medical subject headings and key words included "perilunate injury" OR "carpal dislocation" OR "trans-scaphoid" AND "treatment" or "management."
- Bibliography of eligible articles

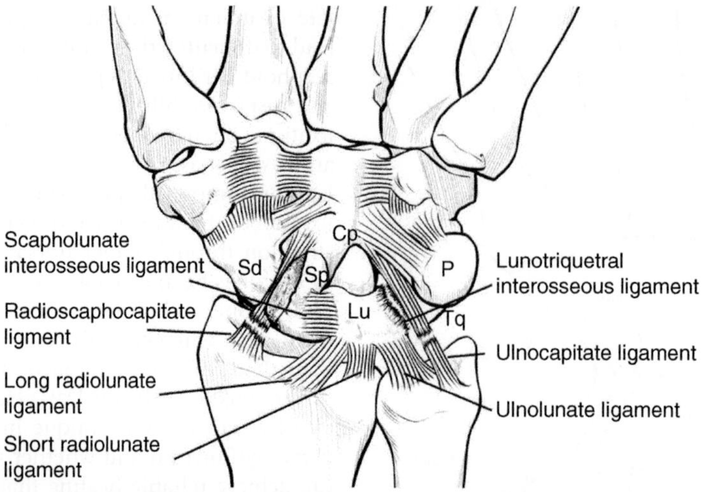

FIG. 20.4 **Volar Perspective of the Transscaphoid Perilunate Injury.** In a stage type IV transscaphoid injury, the lunate with the proximal fragment of the scaphoid is pushed palmar until it dislocates through the *space of Poirier*, which is the weakest area over the capitolunate articulation between the radioscaphocapitate and long radiolunate ligaments, while the carpal row attached with the distal fragment of the scaphoid is remained in the radial articular fossa. *Cp*, capitate; *Lu*, lunate; *Sp*, proximal fragment of the scaphoid; *Sd*, distal fragment of the scaphoid; *P*, pisiform; *Tq*, triquetrum.

- Articles that were not in English, French, or German and relevant with case reports, review, and surgical techniques were excluded

Quality of the evidence

Level III:
Retrospective comparative studies: 1[18]
Level IV:
Case series: 7[4,19–21]
Level V: Expert opinion[13,22–25]

Findings

Siegert et al.[26] reported on 16 chronic perilunate dislocations and fracture-dislocations with definite treatment being delayed up to 35 weeks after injury. They reported that all patients were completely treated by open reduction and internal fixation with satisfactory outcomes. They also found that late open reduction could be accomplished at up to 35 weeks postinjury. However, Inoue and Shionoya[21] performed open reduction and internal fixation through combined palmar and dorsal approach for six patients with perilunate injuries that were untreated for a minimum of 6 weeks (range, 6–52 weeks). Results with a mean follow-up of 6.8 years revealed that three patients who were treated at more than 2 months after injury had poor functional outcomes with midcarpal arthritis. However, favorable outcomes of proximal row carpectomy were found in 16 patients treated at more than 2 months after injury. Weir[19] reported poor functional and radiologic outcomes for five cases with perilunate dislocation and fracture-dislocation treated with open reduction at 2 weeks or more after the injury. In the study of Herzberg et al.,[4] 21 cases treated with either closed reduction with or without percutaneous pinning or open reduction and internal fixation at 7 days or later after injury showed significantly worse clinical scores than 51 cases treated within 1 week.

In a retrospective case-control study conducted by Komurcu et al.,[18] the outcomes of early treatment (within 3 days) and delayed treatment (after 3 days or more) in 12 patients with transscaphoid perilunate injuries were compared. They found that early treatment resulted in better functional and radiologic outcomes.

Question 2: Do surgical methods such as closed reduction and percutaneous fixation versus open reduction with internal fixation or arthroscopic treatment affect the union rates in transscaphoid perilunate fracture-dislocation?

Current opinion

Closed reduction with either immobilization or pin fixation has inferior union rates than open or arthroscopic-assisted reduction technique because this technique cannot restore normal anatomy, which is critical to optimum healing of ligaments and fractured bone.[13,27,28]

Finding the evidence

As above including subheadings of treatment methods such as percutaneous, screw, repair, arthroscopy, and dorsal or volar approach.

Quality of the evidence

Level III:
 Retrospective comparative studies: 2[29,30]
Level IV:
 Case series: 18[16–18,29,31–44]

Findings

A total of 20 studies (308 wrists, range 4–28 wrists) were identified and included in the review.[18,29,31–39] Fourteen articles reported surgical outcomes of open reduction and internal fixation with either dorsal, palmar, or combined approaches.[16,18,29–36,40–43] Three articles reported closed reduction and percutaneous fixation[37,38,44] and three articles reported arthroscopic-assisted reduction and percutaneous fixation.[17,29,39] There was only one comparative study between the open technique using dorsal approach and arthroscopic treatment.[29]

A total of 226 cases were treated with open reduction and internal fixation using either dorsal, palmar, or a combined approach. Their mean age was 31 years (range, 14–67 years). For fixation of the scaphoid fracture, a headless screw was used in eight articles, K-wires were used in one article, and either aheadless screw or K-wires were used in four articles. For closed reduction and percutaneous fixation group, a total of 52 cases with mean patient age of 33 years (range, 18–49 years) were reported. A headless screw was placed for the fixation of scaphoid fracture in two articles, whereas K-wires were used in one article. For the arthroscopic treatment group, a total of 30 cases were reported with a mean age of 33 years (range, 19–39 years). For fixation of the scaphoid fracture, either a headless screw or K-wires were used.

Regarding the success rate in treatment for scaphoid fracture, 212 of 226 cases had union, yielding a union rate of 94% (range, 85%–100%) in the open reduction group. For the closed reduction group, 48 of 52 cases had union, yielding a union rate of 92% (range, 71%–96%). In the arthroscopic group, only 3 of 30 cases reported nonunion, yielding a union rate of 90% (range, 87%–100%). In only one comparative study by Oh et al.,[29] scaphoid union was noted in 11 of 11 wrists (100%) treated with arthroscopic assisted technique and 8 of 9 patients (89%) treated with open approach.

Question 3: What is the preferred operative exposure for open reduction and internal fixation of transscaphoid perilunate injuries: Dorsal, palmar, or combined?

Current opinion

Dorsal only, palmar only, or a combined approach can be used.

Finding the evidence

As above including subheadings of treatment methods such as percutaneous, screw, repair, and dorsal or volar approach.

Quality of the evidence

Level III:
 Retrospective comparative studies: 1[29]
Level IV:
 Case series: 10[18,29,31–36]

Findings

A total of 156 cases with a mean patient age of 31 years (range, 14–67 years) were found in eight articles. Surgical outcomes of open reduction and internal fixation with either dorsal, palmar, or combined approaches for transscaphoid perilunate injury were reported.[18,29,31–36] Surgical approaches were dorsal only in two articles,[29,35] dorsal and combined in five articles,[18,31,33,34,36] and palmar only and combined in one article.[32] Direct comparative studies between different operative approaches for perilunate injuries have not been reported. All three open exposures (dorsal, volar, and combined) appeared to result in satisfactory functional outcomes. However, four of six articles, which used combined approach, reported a total of 41 (34%) patients with posttraumatic arthritis in either midcarpal or radiocarpal joint.

Inoue and Kuwahata[45] have reported satisfactory results of a palmar approach with several advantages, including direct repair of palmar capsular ligament and accurate reduction of fracture alignment. A long-term outcome study by Knoll et al.[35] for 25 transscaphoid perilunate fracture-dislocations treated by dorsal approach with direct repair of the lunotriquetral ligament has shown 91% recovery for wrist range of motion and scaphoid union in all cases. The combined dorsal and volar approach offers the advantages of both approaches. It is the preferred choice of the senior author, as it allows access to all injured structures. However, it should be noted that improvement in exposure increases the possibility of postoperative fibrosis and stiffness.

Question 4: What is the ideal treatment for transscaphoid perilunate injuries in terms of functional outcomes and posttraumatic arthritis?

Current opinion

Transscaphoid perilunate injuries can be treated by closed reduction and immobilization, closed reduction and percutaneous or external fixation, open reduction and fixation with K-wires or screws, and arthroscopic-assisted reduction and percutaneous fixation.[9,15] However, given the advantage of full visualization of the injury with particular attention to the median nerve and secure stabilization of scaphoid fracture and dislocated lunate, open procedure has been preferred.[7,9,42,46,47]

Finding the evidence

As above including subheadings of treatment methods such as arthritis, percutaneous, screw, repair, arthroscopy, and dorsal or volar approach.

Quality of the Evidence

Level III:
  Retrospective comparative studies: 1[29]
Level IV:
  Case series: 10[18,29,31–39]

Findings

A total of 11 studies with 261 wrists (range, 4–28) were identified for inclusion in the review. [18,29,31–39] Among them, 10 studies were level IV (241 wrist, range 4–28) and one study was Level III with retrospective case series (20 wrists). Seven articles reported surgical outcomes of open reduction and internal fixation with either dorsal, palmar, or combined approach.[18,29,31–36] Two articles reported closed reduction and percutaneous fixation.[37,38] Two articles reported arthroscopic-assisted reduction and percutaneous fixation.[29,39]

A total of 201 cases treated with open reduction and internal fixation using either dorsal, palmar, or combined approach were reported. Their mean age was 30 years (range, 14–67 years), and the percentage of males was 87% (range, 54–100%). For fixation of the scaphoid fracture, a headless screw was used in six studies, K-wires in one study, and either a headless screw or K-wires in one study. In seven of eight studies, the lunotriquetral joint was stabilized using K-wires with or without lunotriquetral ligament repair. For the closed reduction and percutaneous fixation group, a total of 45 cases were reported with a mean age of 31 years (range, 19–49 years) and 68% males (range, 54–81%). For arthroscopic treatment group, a total of 15 cases were reported with a mean age of 31 years (range, 20–39 years), and all patients were male. For fixation of the scaphoid fracture, either K-wires or a headless screw was used. The lunotriquetral joint was stabilized with percutaneous K-wires.

Functional outcomes of open reduction were reported with a mean follow-up of 36 months (range, 6–134 months). The wrist range of motion at final follow-up was recorded in six of eight articles. The average flexion-extension arc was 112 degrees (range, 105–170 degrees). The Modified Mayo Wrist Score (MMWS) was reported in seven of eight articles with an average score of 74 (range, 25–95). For the closed reduction, functional outcomes were reported at a mean follow-up of 41 months (range, 13–67 months). The average flexion-extension arc at final follow-up was 143 degrees (range, 141–144 degrees). The average MMWS was 81.5 (range, 65–93). For arthroscopic treatment, functional outcomes were reported at a mean follow-up of 34 months (range, 12–72 months). The average flexion-extension arc at final follow-up was 125 degrees (range, 87–144 degrees) and the average MMWS was 81 (range, 70–87).

Posttraumatic arthrosis was reported in five of eight studies. A total of 47 cases progressed to midcarpal and/or radiocarpal arthritis (23%) in the open reduction group. In the closed reduction group, 4 of 45 cases (9%) reported posttraumatic arthritis, including two midcarpal, one radiocarpal, and one scaphotrapezial arthritis. The arthroscopic treatment group reported 4 midcarpal arthritis among the 15 wrists (27%).

Although there is not enough evidence to determine the best method for these injuries, the data published on closed and arthroscopic-assisted reduction and percutaneous fixation suggest that they are not inferior to the open technique.

Question 5: Should the carpal tunnel be released in transscaphoid perilunate injuries with acute carpal tunnel syndrome?

Current opinion

Acute median nerve compression can lead to long-term nerve deficits, hand stiffness, and, potentially, a complex regional pain syndrome. If preoperative history and examination are consistent with acute carpal tunnel syndrome associated with transscaphoid perilunate fracture-dislocation, open reduction using an extended palmar approach is preferred.

Finding the evidence

As above including subheadings of treatment methods such as carpal tunnel syndrome, percutaneous, screw, repair, arthroscopy, and dorsal or volar approach.

Quality of the evidence

Level IV:

Case series: 9[17,31,32,34–37,40,41]

Findings

Acute carpal tunnel syndrome was reported in nine studies.[18,29,31–39] All studies were Level IV, and a total of 64 of 233 wrists (28%) showed acute median nerve dysfunction clinically. Carpal tunnel release through a palmar or combined approach was performed for 46 wrists in six studies, which resulted in complete relief of symptoms. For 18 wrists in the other three studies, carpal tunnel release was not performed besides definite procedures such as closed reduction and percutaneous fixation method, arthroscopic-assisted management, and open reduction through a dorsal approach. However, complete resolution of acute neuropathic symptoms was obtained for all patients.

Evidence suggests that if restoration of carpal anatomy can be achieved through either open or percutaneous approach and maintained by rigid fixation, palmar approach for carpal tunnel release is unnecessary.

RECOMMENDATION

In patients with transscaphoid perilunate injury, evidence suggests the following:

- Open reduction can be performed electively within 2 months. However, it is recommended to repair perilunate injuries as soon as possible, preferably within a week after the injury (overall quality: low to moderate).
- If the scaphoid is securely fixed, closed reduction can provide union rate equal to open reduction and arthroscopic-assisted reduction (overall quality: low to moderate).
- Surgical approach can be based on the surgeon's preference and individualized to the patient (overall quality: low).
- Outcomes of percutaneous reduction with either closed or arthroscopic assisted technique are comparable with those of open reduction technique. The surgical approach should be based on the surgeon's preference and can be individualized for the patient (overall quality: low to moderate).

In patients with acute carpal tunnel syndrome associated with transscaphoid perilunate fracture dislocation, evidence suggests the following:

- Carpal tunnel release is not required if restoration of carpal anatomy can be achieved through either open or percutaneous technique (overall quality: low).

CONCLUSION

Repair of transscaphoid perilunate injuries should be performed within a week of the injury, although open reduction can be performed electively within 2 months. Functional and radiologic outcomes of percutaneous fixation through closed or arthroscopic-assisted reduction and open reduction and internal fixation are comparable. Therefore, surgical approach can be based on the surgeon's preference and can be individualized for the patient. Carpal tunnel release is not required if restoration of carpal anatomy can be achieved through open or percutaneous technique.

PANEL 2
Author's Preferred Technique

For this patient with transscaphoid perilunate fracture-dislocation, where the gross reduction is not amenable to the initial closed reduction, repeating this maneuver is not recommended as to prevent further cartilage or soft tissue damage. We prefer an arthroscopic technique to allow for visualization of the radiocarpal and midcarpal joints and precise anatomic reduction of intercarpal articulations. It also facilitates the healing of fractures and torn ligaments through minimizing capsular and adjacent soft tissue injuries. This is crucial to prevent arthritis in author's opinion. We prefer to wrap the forearm with a compressive elastic bandage to minimize fluid extravasation.

After clot and debris are removed through 3–4 and 4–5 portals, we commonly find the torn palmar capsular ligaments interposed between the lunate and scaphoid and the capitate, which can prevent gross reduction by a closed manipulation (Fig. 20.5). In these cases, the volarly dislocated lunate with the proximal scaphoid can be effectively reduced by pulling them dorsally using a probe (Fig. 20.6). If the carpal alignment is precisely reduced and fixed, we do not need to open the carpal tunnel for patients with acute carpal tunnel syndrome.

Entering the midcarpal space is feasible if the proximal carpal row is adequately reduced (Fig. 20.7). We focus on thorough removal of osteochondral fragments from the capitate or scaphoid and debridement of frayed edges of torn palmar capsular ligaments to facilitate precise reduction of the carpus and prevent posttraumatic arthritis.

We use two K-wires driven into the distal fragment and a probe, respectively, to reduce the scaphoid fragments by manipulating them while viewing the articular surface through the midcarpal portal. K-wires in the

Continued

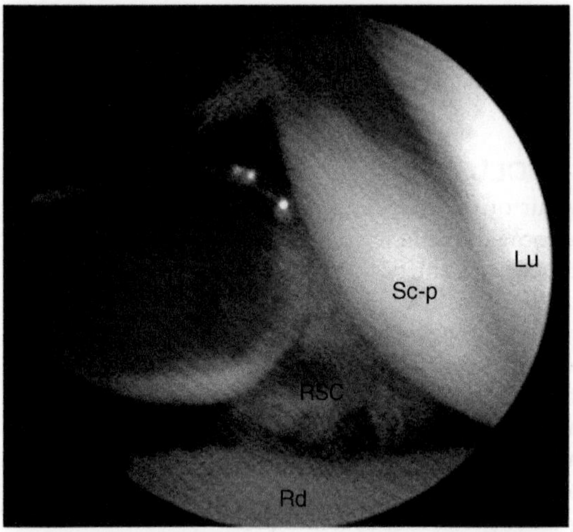

FIG. 20.5 Arthroscopic Finding of Unreduced Transscaphoid Perilunate Injury. Palmar capsular ligaments are torn and interposed between the lunate and proximal fragment of the scaphoid and the capitate, which prevented a gross reduction by a closed manipulation. *Lu*, lunate; *Sc-p*, proximal fragment of the scaphoid; *Sc-d*, distal fragment of the scaphoid; *Rd*, radius; *RSC*, radioscaphocapitate ligament; *SLIL*, scapholunate interosseous ligament.

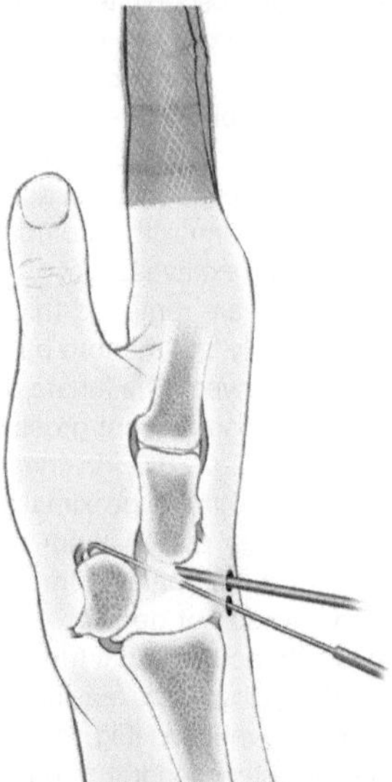

FIG. 20.6 Arthroscopic Reduction of the Dislocated Lunate. The palmarly dislocated lunate with proximal scaphoid can be effectively reduced by pulling them dorsally using a special sharp-hooked probe.

PANEL 2
Author's Preferred Technique—cont'd

distal pole are introduced to the lunate after a congruous articular surface is obtained. We prefer a cannulated headless screw to definitely fix the scaphoid. We use two percutaneous K-wires of 1.2 mm to fix the lunotriquetral joint or triquetrum fracture (Fig. 20.8). Sometimes we use a supplemental capitotriquetral K-wire fixation for highly unstable midcarpal joint because scaphocapitate K-wire fixation is tricky when a headless screw is introduced into the scaphoid (Fig. 20.9). We prefer to remove K-wires at 10–12 weeks followed by intensive physiotherapy (Figs. 20.10 and 20.11).

PANEL 3
Pearls and Pitfalls

PEARLS

- In transscaphoid perilunate injuries, scaphoid fracture is commonly comminuted and interposed by palmar capsular ligament, making it difficult to obtain anatomic reduction. Thorough debridement of interposed ligament and removal of small fracture fragments should be performed prior to reduction of scaphoid fracture and intercarpal joints.
- If the fracture is proximal in the scaphoid, it is highly unstable. We prefer to introduce an additional K-wire on the dorsum of the proximal fragment to use as a joystick with two K-wires driven into the distal fragment. After obtaining precise articular reduction, distal K-wires are advanced into the proximal fragment through the fracture site. One of two distal pins can be used as antirotation pin while a headless screw is placed in the scaphoid (Fig. 20.12A).
- We reduce the lunotriquetral joint using provisional K-wires introduced into the triquetrum and a probe, viewing through the 4–5 portal, which provide a better repositioning of torn intercarpal ligaments in our experience (Fig. 20.12B).

PITFALLS

- Although it is important to place the screw as close as possible to the central axis of the scaphoid, surgeons should attempt to place the screw slightly dorsal because transscaphoid perilunate injuries are commonly comminuted. Otherwise, it may compress the fracture back into volarly flexed angulation (i.e., humpback deformity).
- We prefer buried K-wire fixation of the lunotriquetral and triquetrocapitate intervals because restoration of intercarpal integrity has been shown to be a key determinant of outcome.[2]

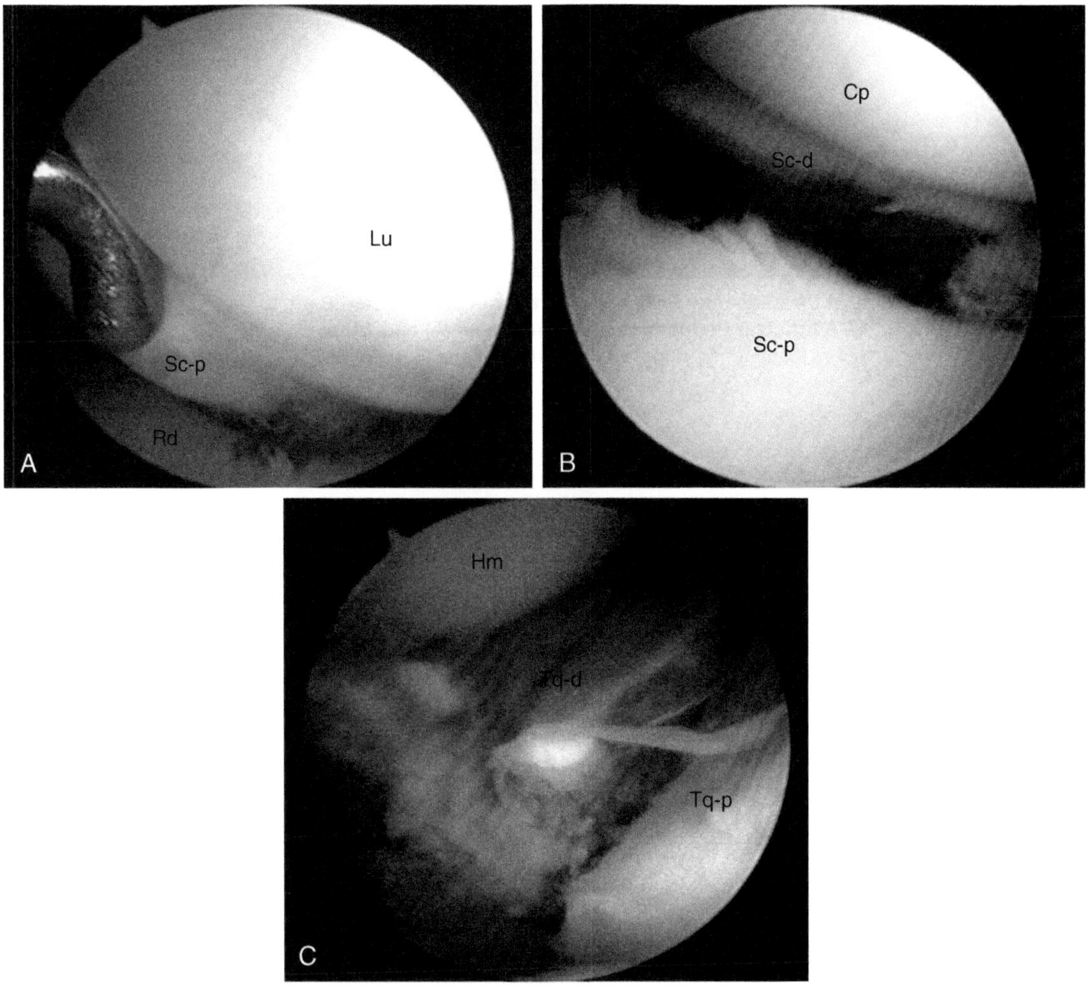

FIG. 20.7 **Findings After Reduction of the Lunate and Proximal Scaphoid by Viewing Through the Radiocarpal Joint (A) and Midcarpal Joint (B and C).** *Lu*, lunate; *Sc-p*, proximal fragment of the scaphoid; *Rd*, radius; *Cp*, capitate; *Hm*, hamate; *Tq-p*, proximal fragment of the triquetrum; *Tq-d*, distal fragment of the triquetrum.

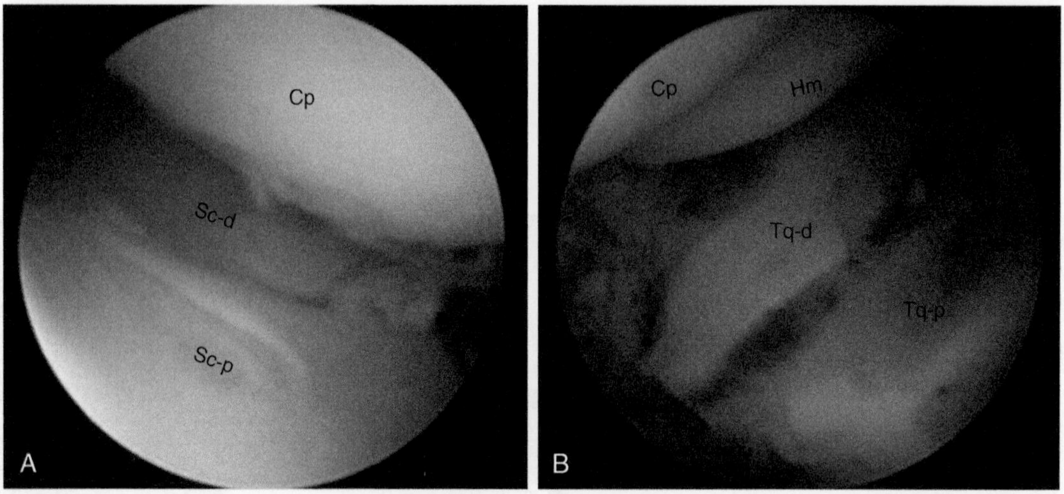

FIG. 20.8 **Findings at the Midcarpal Portal After Arthroscopic-Assisted Reduction and Percutaneous Fixation. Accurate Articular Reductions of the Scaphoid (A) and Triquetrum (B) Can be Obtained.** *Cp*, capitate; *Hm*, hamate; *Tq-p*, proximal fragment of the triquetrum; *Tq-d*, distal fragment of the triquetrum.

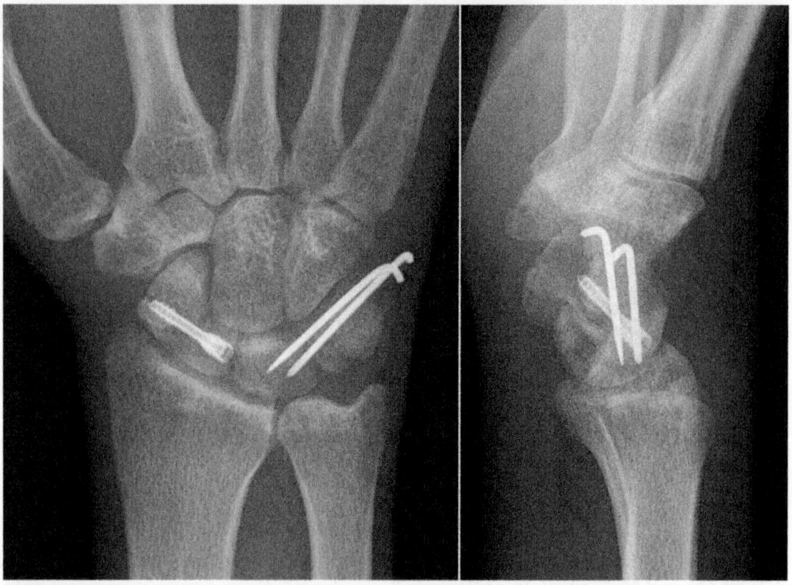

FIG. 20.9 **Postoperative Radiographs Showing Well-Established Carpal Alignment With Anatomic Reduction of the Scaphoid Fracture.**

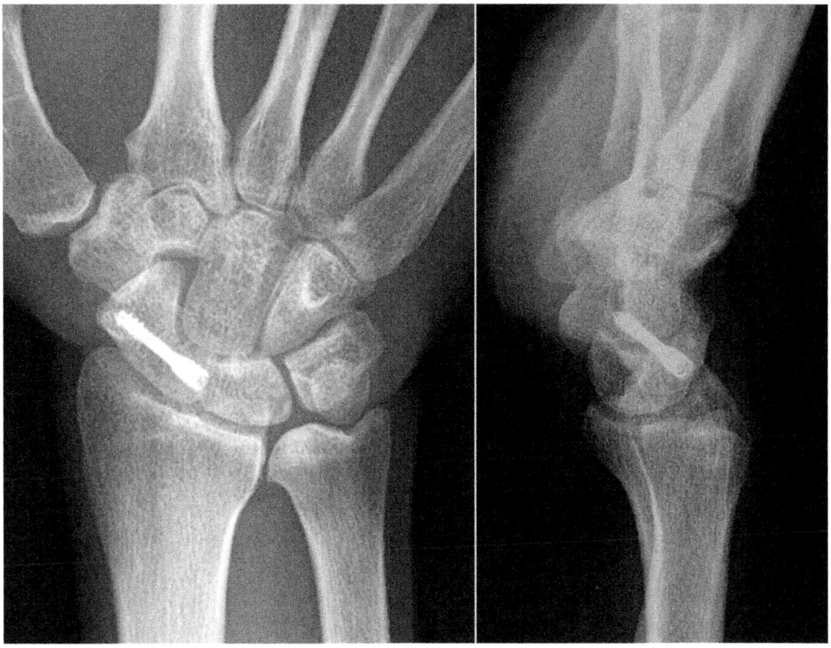

FIG. 20.10 **Twenty-Four-Month Follow-Up Radiographs Showing Union of Fractures Without Evidence of Arthritis.**

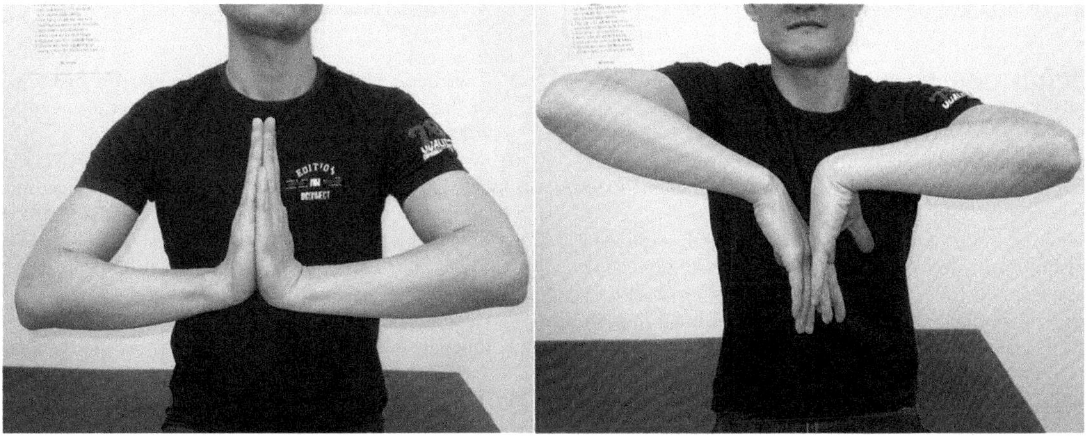

FIG. 20.11 **The Patient had a Similar Wrist Extension Arc, but Mild Limitation of Flexion Compared to the Contralateral Side Without Pain.**

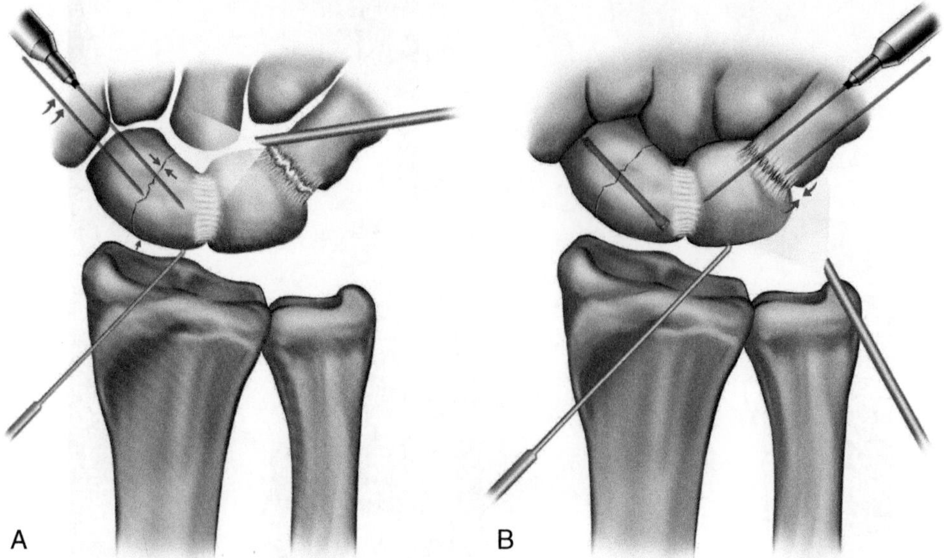

FIG. 20.12 **Arthroscopic Techniques.** We prefer to introduce two K-wires on the distal fragment and a probe at the radiocarpal portal. A additional K-wire on the dorsum of the proximal fragment is used as a joystick. After precise articular reduction, distal K-wires are advanced from the fracture site into the proximal fragment followed by a headless screw while viewing through the midcarpal ulnar portal (Fig. 20.12A). The lunotriquetral joint can be reduced by using provisional K-wires introduced into the triquetrum and a probe while viewing through the 4–5 portal, which can provide better reposition of torn intercarpal ligaments during percutaneous pinning (Fig. 20.12B).

REFERENCES

1. Scalcione LR, Gimber LH, Ho AM, Johnston SS, Sheppard JE, Taljanovic MS. Spectrum of carpal dislocations and fracture-dislocations: imaging and management. *AJR Am J Roentgenol*. 2014;203:541–550.
2. Vitale MA, Seetharaman M, Ruchelsman DE. Perilunate dislocations. *J Hand Surg Am*. 2015;40:358–362;quiz 362.
3. Mayfield JK, Johnson RP, Kilcoyne RK. Carpal dislocations: pathomechanics and progressive perilunar instability. *J Hand Surg Am*. 1980;5:226–241.
4. Herzberg G, Comtet JJ, Linscheid RL, Amadio PC, Cooney WP, Stalder J. Perilunate dislocations and fracture-dislocations: a multicenter study. *J Hand Surg Am*. 1993;18:768–779.
5. Mayfield JK, Johnson RP, Kilcoyne RK. Carpal dislocations: pathomechanics and progressive perilunar instability. *J Hand Surg Am*. 1980;5:226–241.
6. Deleted in review
7. Trumble T, Verheyden J. Treatment of isolated perilunate and lunate dislocations with combined dorsal and volar approach and intraosseous cerclage wire. *J Hand Surg Am*. 2004;29:412–417.
8. Gilula LA, Destouet JM, Weeks PM, Young LV, Wray RC. Roentgenographic diagnosis of the painful wrist. *Clin Orthop Relat Res*. 1984:52–64.
9. Sawardeker PJ, Kindt KE, Baratz ME. Fracture-dislocations of the carpus: perilunate injury. *Orthop Clin North Am*. 2013;44:93–106.
10. Kwon BC, Choi SJ, Song SY, Baek SH, Baek GH. Modified carpal stretch test as a screening test for detection of scapholunate interosseous ligament injuries associated with distal radial fractures. *J Bone Joint Surg Am*. 2011;93:855–862.
11. Green DP, O'Brien ET. Classification and management of carpal dislocations. *Clin Orthop Relat Res*. 1980:55–72.
12. Herzberg G, Forissier D. Acute dorsal trans-scaphoid perilunate fracture-dislocations: medium-term results. *J Hand Surg Br*. 2002;27:498–502.
13. Budoff JE. Treatment of acute lunate and perilunate dislocations. *J Hand Surg Am*. 2008;33:1424–1432.
14. Cooney WP, Bussey R, Dobyns JH, Linscheid RL. Difficult wrist fractures. Perilunate fracture-dislocations of the wrist. *Clin Orthop Relat Res*. 1987:136–147.
15. Park MJ, Ahn JH. Arthroscopically assisted reduction and percutaneous fixation of dorsal perilunate dislocations and fracture-dislocations. *Arthroscopy*. 2005;21:1153.
16. Herzberg G, Burnier M, Marc A, Merlini L, Izem Y. The role of arthroscopy for treatment of perilunate injuries. *J Wrist Surg*. 2015;4:101–109.
17. Kim JP, Lee JS, Park MJ. Arthroscopic reduction and percutaneous fixation of perilunate dislocations and fracture-dislocations. *Arthroscopy*. 2012;28:196–203.e192.

18. Komurcu M, Kurklu M, Ozturan KE, Mahirogullari M, Basbozkurt M. Early and delayed treatment of dorsal transscaphoid perilunate fracture-dislocations. *J Orthop Trauma*. 2008;22:535–540.
19. Weir IG. The late reduction of carpal dislocations. *J Hand Surg Br*. 1992;17:137–139.
20. Kim JP, Lee JS, Park MJ. Arthroscopic treatment of perilunate dislocations and fracture dislocations. *J Wrist Surg*. 2015;4:81–87.
21. Inoue G, Shionoya K. Late treatment of unreduced perilunate dislocations. *J Hand Surg Br*. 1999;24:221–225.
22. Sauder DJ, Athwal GS, Faber KJ, Roth JH. Perilunate injuries. *Hand Clin*. 2007;26:145–154.
23. Herzberg G. Perilunate and axial carpal dislocations and fracture-dislocations. *J Hand Surg Am*. 2008;33:1659–1668.
24. Pappas 3rd ND, Lee DH. Perilunate injuries. *Am J Orthop (Belle Mead NJ)*. 2015;44:E300–E302.
25. Muppavarapu RC, Capo JT. Perilunate dislocations and fracture dislocations. *Hand Clin*. 2015;31:399–408.
26. Siegert JJ, Frassica FJ, Amadio PC. Treatment of chronic perilunate dislocations. *J Hand Surg Am*. 1988;13:206–212.
27. Weil WM, Slade 3rd JF, Trumble TE. Open and arthroscopic treatment of perilunate injuries. *Clin Orthop Relat Res*. 2006;445:120–132.
28. Adkison JW, Chapman MW. Treatment of acute lunate and perilunate dislocations. *Clin Orthop Relat Res*. 1982:199–207.
29. Oh WT, Choi YR, Kang HJ, Koh IH, Lim KH. Comparative outcome analysis of arthroscopic-assisted versus open reduction and fixation of trans-scaphoid perilunate fracture dislocations. *Arthroscopy*. 2017;33:92–100.
30. Souer JS, Rutgers M, Andermahr J, Jupiter JB, Ring D. Perilunate fracture-dislocations of the wrist: comparison of temporary screw versus K-wire fixation. *J Hand Surg Am*. 2007;32:318–325.
31. Herzberg G, Forissier D. Acute dorsal trans-scaphoid perilunate fracture-dislocations: medium-term results. *J Hand Surg Br*. 2002;27:498–502.
32. Inoue G, Imaeda T. Management of trans-scaphoid perilunate dislocations. Herbert screw fixation, ligamentous repair and early wrist mobilization. *Arch Orthop Trauma Surg*. 1997;116:338–340.
33. Israel D, Delclaux S, Andre A, et al. Peri-lunate dislocation and fracture-dislocation of the wrist: retrospective evaluation of 65 cases. *Orthop Traumatol Surg Res*. 2016;102:351–355.
34. Kara A, Celik H, Seker A, Kilinc E, Camur S, Uzun M. Surgical treatment of dorsal perilunate fracture-dislocations and prognostic factors. *Int J Surg*. 2015;24:57–63.
35. Knoll VD, Allan C, Trumble TE. Trans-scaphoid perilunate fracture dislocations: results of screw fixation of the scaphoid and lunotriquetral repair with a dorsal approach. *J Hand Surg Am*. 2005;30:1145–1152.
36. Moneim MS, Hofammann 3rd KE, Omer GE. Transscaphoid perilunate fracture-dislocation. Result of open reduction and pin fixation. *Clin Orthop Relat Res*. 1984:227–235.
37. Wong TC, Ip FK. Minimally invasive management of trans-scaphoid perilunate fracture-dislocations. *Hand Surg*. 2008;13:159–165.
38. Chou YC, Hsu YH, Cheng CY, Wu CC. Percutaneous screw and axial Kirschner wire fixation for acute transscaphoid perilunate fracture dislocation. *J Hand Surg Am*. 2012;37:715–720.
39. Jeon IH, Kim HJ, Min WK, Cho HS, Kim PT. Arthroscopically assisted percutaneous fixation for trans-scaphoid perilunate fracture dislocation. *J Hand Surg Eur Vol*. 2010;35:664–668.
40. Capo JT, Corti SJ, Shamian B, et al. Treatment of dorsal perilunate dislocations and fracture-dislocations using a standardized protocol. *Hand (N Y)*. 2012;7:380–387.
41. Krief E, Appy-Fedida B, Rotari V, David E, Mertl P, Maes-Clavier C. Results of perilunate dislocations and perilunate fracture dislocations with a minimum 15-year follow-up. *J Hand Surg Am*. 2015;40:2191–2197.
42. Forli A, Courvoisier A, Wimsey S, Corcella D, Moutet F. Perilunate dislocations and transscaphoid perilunate fracture-dislocations: a retrospective study with minimum ten-year follow-up. *J Hand Surg Am*. 2010;35:62–68.
43. Massoud AH, Naam NH. Functional outcome of open reduction of chronic perilunate injuries. *J Hand Surg Am*. 2012;37:1852–1860.
44. Savvidou OD, Beltsios M, Sakellariou VI, Papagelopoulos PJ. Perilunate dislocations treated with external fixation and percutaneous pinning. *J Wrist Surg*. 2015;4:76–80.
45. Inoue G, Kuwahata Y. Management of acute perilunate dislocations without fracture of the scaphoid. *J Hand Surg Br*. 1997;22:647–652.
46. Viegas SF, Bean JW, Schram RA. Transscaphoid fracture/dislocations treated with open reduction and Herbert screw internal fixation. *J Hand Surg Am*. 1987;12:992–999.
47. Melone CP Jr, Murphy MS, Raskin KB. Perilunate injuries. Repair by dual dorsal and volar approaches. *Hand Clin*. 2000;16:439–448.

CHAPTER 21

Pediatric Scaphoid Fractures

JOSEPH S. KHOURI, MD • ALEXANDER Y. SHIN, MD

KEY POINTS

1. Despite being the most common carpal injury in the pediatric patient population, scaphoid fractures have remained relatively rare, and because radiographs are difficult to interpret in the immature carpus, there is a high rate of misdiagnosis of these injuries.
2. Previously thought to be epidemiologically unique, recent epidemiologic data have shown that scaphoid fracture pattern presentation in children has come to resemble that of the adult population.
3. Children and adolescents, who display union at midterm follow-up, will achieve excellent outcomes, with no difference in outcomes between cast immobilization and surgical fixation.
4. Cast immobilization or nonremovable splinting is the standard of care for nondisplaced or minimally displaced scaphoid fractures and should be instituted for 2 weeks with follow-up radiographic examination. The duration of cast immobilization depends on the fracture location and acuity; the more proximal the fracture and the later the presentation, the longer the requisite period of immobilization
5. Failure of casting to produce union is an indication for surgical treatment and the presence of osteonecrosis as well as late/chronic fracture presentation are independent predictors of a worse upper limb function.

PANEL 1
Case Scenario

A 12-year-old man visited the emergency department several days after a fall onto his outstretched hand with complaints of left wrist pain. He is a competitive swimmer, with plans to compete in the next 4–6 weeks. Parents are stressing the importance of the upcoming swimming competition and see no need for prolonged immobilization if the child's symptoms are decreased by then. Radiographs initially show no osseous pathology (Fig. 21.1). What clinical treatment strategy will you decide on and how will you follow this patient's course with this modality?

IMPORTANCE OF THE PROBLEM

A scaphoid fracture in a patient who has an open physeal growth plate of the distal radius and ulna is considered a pediatric scaphoid fracture.[1] Despite being the most common carpal injury in the pediatric patient population, scaphoid fractures have remained relatively rare, accounting only for 0.45% of all pediatric upper extremity fractures and 0.34% of all fractures in children.[1–4] Because these injuries are relatively rare and radiographs are difficult to interpret in the immature carpus, there is a high rate of misdiagnosis of these injuries.[1] The patterns of injury of scaphoid fractures differ in children.[5,6] Secondary to the changes that occur at the ossification center of the scaphoid during maturation,[1,4,7–9] the endochondral ossification center forms distally and grows eccentrically during the early stages of growth. During this period, the scaphoid is more susceptible to soft tissue and avulsion fractures, explaining why the most common pattern of scaphoid fracture in children has been the distal pole fracture.[1,10,11] As ossification progresses proximally, the fracture patterns becomes similar to adult scaphoid fractures. Recently, epidemiologic data have shown that scaphoid fracture pattern presentation in children has come to resemble that of the adult population.[3,10] Overall, these patients tend to do fairly well.[11–14] Outcome depends on achieving union, as it has been shown that children and adolescents who display union at midterm follow-up will achieve excellent outcomes, with no difference in outcomes between cast immobilization and surgical fixation.[13]

MAIN QUESTION

What is the preferred treatment for pediatric scaphoid fractures?

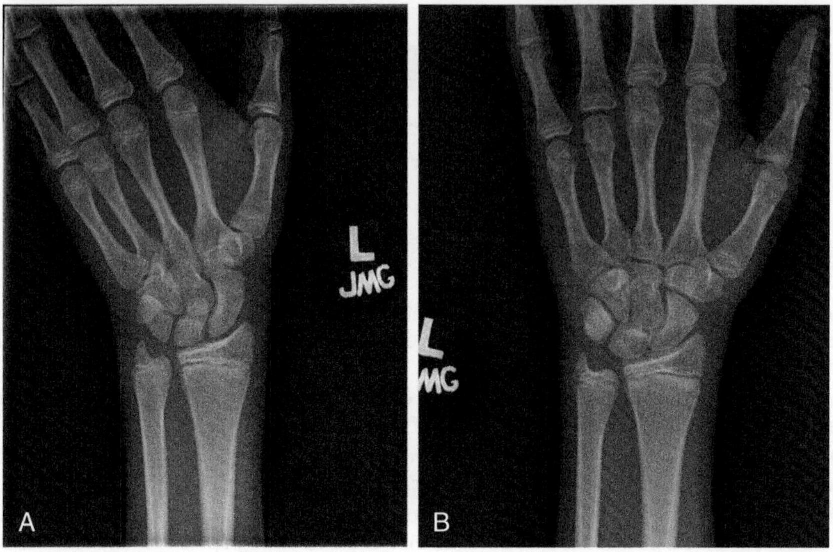

FIG. 1 Scaphoid **(A)** and posteroanterior **(B)** views of left wrist at presentation showing no fracture.

Pediatric Scaphoid Fractures	
Patient	Any patient with a scaphoid fracture who has an open physeal growth plate of the distal radius and ulna
Intervention	Surgical treatment of the scaphoid
Control	Immobilization and long-term follow-up
Outcome	Union rate, functional outcomes

Current Opinion

The primary treatment strategy for acute, nondisplaced fractures of the scaphoid in this pediatric population has been cast immobilization.[1,3,4,11,15–17] In contrast, the recommended treatment for patients presenting with acute displaced fracture or a chronic nonunion is open reduction and internal fixation.[13,14] Recently published data suggest a change in previous opinions on scaphoid fracture patterns in the pediatric population; specifically,[3,10,13,14,18] pediatric scaphoid fracture patterns more closely resemble adult patterns with the majority affecting the scaphoid waist.[13,14] Historically, most pediatric scaphoid fractures were thought to involve the distal pole and required neither surgical treatment nor long-term follow-up and were recognized to heal secondary to the superior blood flow in the distal pole region.[1,13,15,17,19]

Finding the Evidence

- Cochrane search: Pediatric Scaphoid Fracture
- Pubmed (Medline): ("Pediatric Scaphoid Bone" [Mesh] OR pediatric scaphoid fracture*[tiab] OR pediatric scaphoid bone Fracture*[tiab] OR pediatric carpal bone OR pediatric carpal bone fracture OR scaphoid[tiab]) AND ("classification" [Subheading] OR fracture*)
- Bibliography of eligible articles
- Articles that were not in English were excluded

Quality of the Evidence

Level II: This evidence is sparse in the literature with only two cohort studies encountered.[20,21]

Level III: Two Level III retrospective comparative studies are found in the literature.[13,14]

Level IV: Most of the evidence in the literature comes in the form of Level IV case series.[3,4,6,7,15,17,18,22–43]

Level V: There were two Level V expert opinion articles found.[11,45]

FINDINGS

There have been many studies delineating the anatomic distribution of pediatric scaphoid fractures (Table 21.1), healing times with immobilization of pediatric scaphoid fractures (Table 21.2) and locations of nonunions in pediatric scaphoid fractures (Table 21.3).

In contrast to Level IV studies, where 30 were identified, there is a paucity of higher level studies, with only two Level III evidence studies.

Level II

Evenski et al. reviewed 104 pediatric wrists with high clinical suspicion but no radiographic evidence of scaphoid fracture on initial examination

TABLE 21.1
Anatomic Distribution of Pediatric Scaphoid Fractures

Author(s)	No. of Fractures	Age Range (Year)	Distribution (%)	Year	Evidence Level
Mussbichler[23]	100	8–15	52 avulsion distal (52), 33 distal (33), 15 waist (15)	1961	IV
Grundy[24]	8	10–15	2 tuberosity (25), 53 distal (38), 3 waist (37)	1969	IV
Vanhvanen and Westerlund[17]	108	6–14	52 avulsion distal (38), 53 distal (49), 13 waist (12)	1980	IV
Greene et al.[15]	9	6–14	1 tuberosity (11), 5 distal (56), 3 waist (33)	1984	IV
Christodoulou and Colton[4]	64	8–14	21 tuberosity (33), 17 distal (27), 24 waist (37), 2 proximal (3)	1986	IV
Wulff and Schmidt[25]	33	7–16	4 avulsion distal (12), 17 distal (53), 12 waist (36)	1998	IV
Johnson et al.[21]	16	6–15	6 distal pole, 4 waist, 3 lower pole, 3 transverse through length of scaphoid	2000	II
Fabre et al.[6]	23	6–17	5 avulsion distal (22), 17 middle and distal (74), 1 proximal (4)	2001	IV
D'Arienzo[11]	39	8–15	5 tuberosity (13), 31 distal (79), 3 waist (8)	2002	V
Gholson et al.[14]	351	7–18	81 distal pole (23), 22 proximal pole (6), 248 waist (71)	2011	III
Ahmed et al.[3]	56	9–13	45 distal pole (80), 1 proximal pole (2), 10 waist (18)	2014	IV

and noted that 31 (30%) of them had radiographically evident scaphoid fracture at follow-up. They concluded that volar scaphoid tenderness, pain with radial deviation, and pain with active wrist range of motion were physical examination findings that suggested scaphoid fracture when present at initial evaluation. They recommend that all clinically suspected pediatric scaphoid fractures be immobilized with repeat radiographs and physical examination at 2 weeks.[20]

Johnson et al. used MRI results obtained within 10 days of injury to dictate management of pediatric scaphoid fractures in a prospective cohort study of 57 scaphoid fractures that presented in skeletally immature patients. They diagnosed 16 (28%) scaphoid fractures by MRI. When they reviewed radiographs of those patients with positive MRI, they noted that 75% if the original radiographic reports indicated that a fracture was not seen. They conclude that radiographs are a poor discriminator of scaphoid injuries in pediatric patients and recommend a two-stage work-up: when the history and examination suggest scaphoid fracture, the patient should have radiographs with four views of the scaphoid; if no fracture is observed and clinical suspicion persists, the patient should be referred for MRI as early as possible; if no MRI is available, the patient would be casted and seen after 2 weeks for

TABLE 21.2
Healing Times With Immobilization of Pediatric Scaphoid Fractures

Author(s)	Location	Healing Time (Week)	Year
Mussbichler[23]	Distal avulsion	3–6	1961
	Distal	4–7	
	Waist	4–7	
Vahvanen and Westerlund[17]	Distal avulsion	3	1980
	Distal	4–8	
	Waist	4–16	
	Proximal avulsion	3	
Gamble and Simmons[26]	Tuberosity	3–4	1982
	Distal	5	
	Waist	7–8	
D'Arienzo[11]	Tuberosity	3–4	2002
	Distal	5	
	Waist	7–8	
Toh et al.[18]	NA	4–6	2003
Gholson[14]	Distal pole	5–7	2011
	Proximal pole	8–23	
	Waist	7–10	

TABLE 21.3
Location of Pediatric Scaphoid Nonunions

Author(s)	No. of Nonunions	Location	Study Level	Year
Mussbichler[23]	2	NA	IV	1961
Southcott and Rosman[27]	8	Waist	IV	1977
Vahvanen and Westerlund[17]	1	Waist	IV	1980
Maxted and Owen[28]	2	Waist	IV	1982
Onuba and Ireland[29]	2	Waist	IV	1983
McCoy et al.[30]	1	Waist	IV	1987
Pick and Segal[31]	1	Waist	IV	1983
Greene et al.[15]	2	1 waist, 1 distal pole	IV	1984
Christodoulou and Colton[4]	1	Waist	IV	1986
Larson et al.[35]	1	Waist	IV	1987
Wilson-MacDonald[7]	1	NA	IV	1987
De Boeck et al.[33]	1	Waist	IV	1991
Horii et al.[34]	46	44 waist, 1 proximal, 1 distal pole	IV	1994
Littlefield et al.[36]	2	Waist	IV	1995
Mintzer and Waters[36]	13	Waist	IV	1999
Fabre et al.[6]	2	NA	IV	2001
Garcia-Mata[37]	4	Waist	IV	2002
Waters and Stewart[38]	3	Proximal Pole	IV	2002
Henderson and Letts[39]	20	Waist	IV	2003
Toh et al.[18]	46	44 waist, 1 distal pole, 1 proximal pole	IV	2003
Duteille and Dautel[40]	11	9 waist, 2 distal pole	IV	2004
Chloros et al.[41]	12	Waist	IV	2007
Kapoor[42]	1	Distal pole	IV	2013
Reigstad et al.[43]	12	10 middle third, 1 proximal third	IV	2013
Ben-Amotz[44]	1	NA	IV	2015

follow-up examination and possibly radiograph. If repeat radiographs are normal and clinical examination indicates scaphoid fracture, then MRI should be performed.[21] Cost analysis, loss of wages (although mostly not applicable to pediatric population), and change in ultimate outcome were not evaluated.

Level III

Gholson et al. identified 351 pediatric scaphoid fractures over a 15-year period and had follow-up data on 312 fractures. They found 71% of fractures occurring at the scaphoid waist, 23% at the distal pole, and 6% at the proximal pole. 90% union rate was noted with casting alone in cases of acute nondisplaced fractures. Chronic fractures treated with casting alone, displaced fractures, and proximal fractures were associated with lower union rates and required immobilization for up to 3 months. Chronic fractures, displaced fractures, proximal fractures, and patients with osteonecrosis were characteristics associated with longer time to union. Surgery produced 96.5% union rate.[14]

Bae et al. reviewed the functional outcomes in 63 children and adolescents after treatment of scaphoid fractures using Disability of the Arm, Shoulder, and Hand (DASH) inventory, DASH work and sports modules, and the Modified Mayo Wrist Score (MMWS) at a median follow-up of 6.3 years (2.6–17.7 years). They report that 95% of children and adolescents with scaphoid fractures achieve excellent or good functional outcomes. They note that osteonecrosis or chronic nonunion are more likely to have a worse outcome. In their study, surgical intervention did not predict poorer outcomes and this supported their use of open reduction with internal fixation—with or without bone grafting—as the preferred treatment modality for acute displaced fractures as well as chronic malunions.[13]

Level IV

Gajdobranski et al. concluded that conservative therapy of acute scaphoid fractures is an acceptable treatment for pediatric patients that yielded excellent functional results. 31 (91%) children with acute scaphoid fractures were immobilized for an average of 51 days. Functional results determined by the MMWS were excellent.[22]

NONUNION

Pediatric scaphoid nonunion has been shown to develop, even in properly managed scaphoid fractures.[4,30,31,33,36,40] The overwhelming number of pediatric nonunions will occur at the scaphoid waist (Table 21.3). There have not been many cases of avascular necrosis or total scaphoid avascular necrosis in this patient population.[35,38,39,41] It is important to rule out a bipartite scaphoid when encountering a possible pediatric scaphoid nonunion—which will present bilaterally and with no relation to trauma and will have similar bone fragment densities, but the bone will exhibit nodular rounded edges.[44] Treatment modalities to achieve union have included casting alone,[31] casting with electromagnetic field treatment,[47] Matti-Russe procedure,[26] iliac crest bone graft,[34,46] open reduction with bone grafting alone,[48] bone grafting with Kirschner wire,[27,49] open reduction with internal screw fixation and bone graft,[34] and vascularized bone graft.[35,46] In nearly all studies, the diagnosis of "healing" was made through radiographic examination alone, and the role or necessity of CT imaging was not elaborated on.

ROLE OF VASCULARIZED BONE GRAFT

Vascularized bone graft from the distal radius,[46] pronator quadratus–based muscle pedicle bone graft,[36] and medial femoral condyle[35] have been used to treat scaphoid nonunions in children after development of avascular necrosis and nonunion. Nonvascularized and vascularized bone grafts used for scaphoid nonunion reconstruction have been prospectively compared in the adult population.[50] With exception of radius vascularized grafts showing superior radial deviation compared with contralateral side, no statistical difference in wrist movements, grip strength, or bone union was seen.[50] Although new data exist regarding the long-term outcomes of vascularized bone graft reconstruction in the pediatric population, the few case reports that exist in the literature report that all fractures went onto achieve successful graft incorporation.

COST ANALYSIS OF ADVANCED IMAGING

The cost-effectiveness of obtaining early MRI imaging versus traditional immobilization and radiographic follow-up has been investigated in Europe and Australia for adult scaphoid fractures.[51–56] Each of these studies concluded that MRI was a cost-effective adjunct to the treatment of suspected scaphoid fractures in the adult populations. A cost analysis of traditional splint and follow-up protocol versus MRI for radiographically occult adult scaphoid fractures found that the cost to exclude a fracture was lower in the MRI group versus traditional immobilization and radiographic follow-up group, although the average overall cost of treatment of patients with MRI was higher.[56] Several studies take into account the cost to society associated with unnecessary immobilization and the benefit associated with early fracture exclusion.[51,53–55] Although the literature does not currently contain a cost analysis of the use of early MRI versus 2-week immobilization and radiographic follow-up in the pediatric scaphoid fracture population, it is presumable that "productivity lost" and "workdays missed" are not a significant healthcare cost concerns in this population and that cast immobilization is much more cost-effective treatment modality. MRI should be judiciously utilized and is indicated if there is unusual or atypical pain, especially on the ulnar side of the wrist.

RECOMMENDATION

In pediatric patients that present with clinical suspicion of scaphoid fracture, evidence suggests the following:

- Cast immobilization or nonremovable splinting should be instituted for 2 weeks with a follow-up radiographic examination. However, there is no consistent evidence to show that 7–10 days of immobilization is superior to repeat clinical examination (with selective repeated radiography only) as a modality of treatment in cases in which there is a clinical suspicion. Splinting/casting is a means to ensure or emphasize that the patient and family return for repeat examination and radiographs (overall quality: low).

In pediatric patients with an acute nondisplaced scaphoid fracture, evidence suggests the following:

- Cast immobilization provides excellent chance of union (overall quality: moderate).

In pediatric patients with an acute displaced or chronic scaphoid fracture, evidence suggests the following:

- Excellent functional outcomes for surgically treated patients (overall quality: low).

In pediatric patients with nonunion and avascular necrosis of the scaphoid, evidence suggests the following:

- The use of open reduction with internal fixation and nonvascularized bone grafting provides for excellent rates of union (overall quality: moderate).
- Vascularized bone graft is a viable option for pediatric scaphoid nonunions with avascular necrosis (overall quality: low).

CONCLUSION

Cast immobilization remains the gold standard of care for most nondisplaced or minimally displaced scaphoid fractures (<1 mm) in pediatric populations, resulting in a union rate of >90%.[1,14,16,17] The duration of cast immobilization depends on the fracture location and acuity; the more proximal the fracture and the later the presentation, the longer the requisite period of immobilization.[1,14,18,20]

- Avulsion and incomplete fractures are treated for 4–6 weeks in a short-arm thumb spica cast; a long-arm cast may be used in a younger child to prevent falling off or excessive activity.
- 6–8 weeks of immobilization is recommended for waist and transverse fractures.
- Rare cases such as proximal third fractures or instances with bony resorption are treated with a longer period of immobilization (8–12 total weeks) that starts with 6 weeks of long thumb spica and then with another 6 weeks of short thumb spica.[1,17]

Failure of cast immobilization to produce union is a clear indication for surgical treatment.[1,18,20–22] The presence of osteonecrosis as well as late/chronic fracture presentation are independent predictors of a worse upper limb function.[13] Operative reduction and internal fixation—with or without bone grafting and with correction of the humpback deformity—is the preferred treatment in pediatric patients with displaced acute injuries or established nonunions.[13] Vascularized bone grafts have been proven to be feasible in cases of avascular necrosis of the scaphoid.[35,36,46].

PANEL 2
Case Scenario

You decided to treat the patient with 2 weeks of cast immobilization. At 2-week follow-up, scaphoid fracture is clearly visualized (Fig. 21.2). After long discussion regarding treatment options and competitive swimming schedule, the patient was then placed in short-arm thumb spica cast for 4–6 weeks.

PANEL 3
Case Scenario

After 6 weeks of short-arm thumb spica cast immobilization, the scaphoid fracture is healed, which can be confirmed by CT scan (Fig. 21.3).

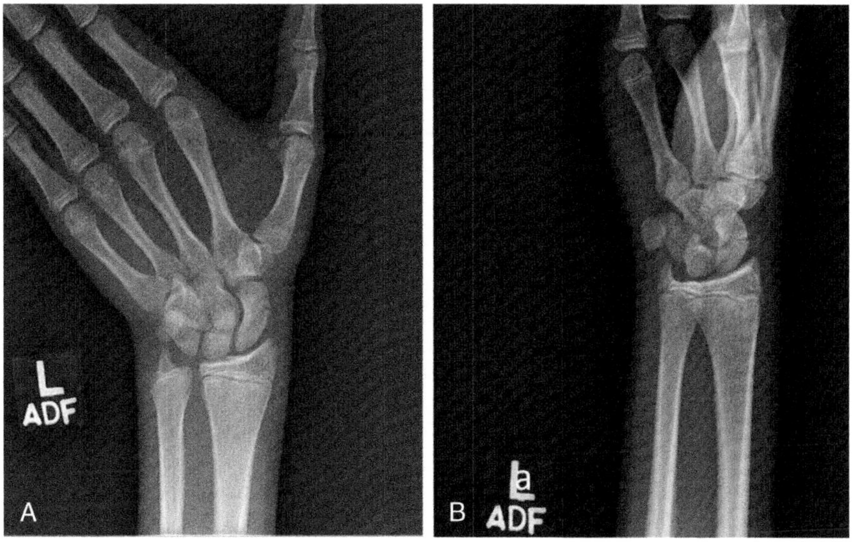

FIG. 2 Scaphoid **(A)** and lateral **(B)** views of left wrist after 2 weeks of splint immobilization clearly show scaphoid waist fracture.

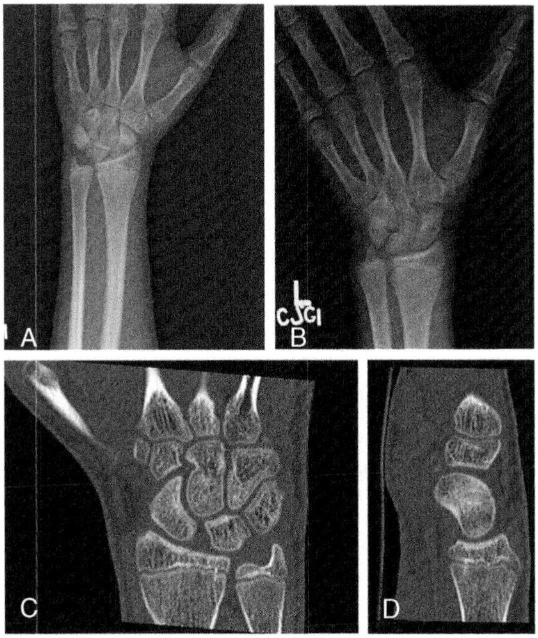

FIG. 3 AP **(A)** and scaphoid **(B)** radiographic views indicating fracture union at 6 weeks. Coronal **(C)** and sagittal **(D)** CT scans confirm osseous healing of the scaphoid.

REFERENCES

1. Elhassan BT, Shin AY. Scaphoid fracture in children. *Hand Clin*. 2006;22:31–41.
2. Beatty E, Light TR, Belsole RJ, Ogden JA. Wrist and hand skeletal injuries in children. *Hand Clin*. 1990;6:723–738.
3. Ahmed I, Ashton F, Tay WK, Porter D. The pediatric fracture of the scaphoid in patients aged 13 years and under: an epidemiological study. *J Pediatr Orthop*. 2014;34:150–154.
4. Christodoulou AG, Colton CL. Scaphoid fractures in children. *J Pediatr Orthop*. 1986;6:37–39.
5. Leslie IJ, Dickson RA. The fractured carpal scaphoid. Natural history and factors influencing outcome. *J Bone Joint Surg Br*. 1981;63-B:225–230.
6. Fabre O, De Boeck H, Haentjens P. Fractures and nonunions of the carpal scaphoid in children. *Acta Orthop belg*. 2001;67:121–125.
7. Wilson-MacDonald J. Delayed union of the distal scaphoid in a child. *J Hand Surg*. 1987;12:520–522.
8. Cockshott WP. Distal avulsion fractures of the scaphoid. *Br J Radiol*. 1980;53:1037–1040.
9. Williams AA, Lochner HV. Pediatric hand and wrist injuries. *Curr Rev Musculoskelet Med*. 2013;6:18–25.
10. Stanciu C, Dumont A. Changing patterns of scaphoid fractures in adolescents. *Can J Surg J Can Chir*. 1994;37:214–216.
11. D'Arienzo M. Scaphoid fractures in children. *J Hand Surg Edinb Scotl*. 2002;27:424–426.
12. Anz AW, Bushnell BD, Bynum DK, Chloros GD, Wiesler ER. Pediatric scaphoid fractures. *J Am Acad Orthop Surg*. 2009;17:77–87.

13. Bae DS, Gholson JJ, Zurakowski D, Waters PM. Functional outcomes after treatment of scaphoid fractures in children and adolescents. *J Pediatr Orthop*. 2016;36:13–18.
14. Gholson JJ, Bae DS, Zurakowski D, Waters PM. Scaphoid fractures in children and adolescents: contemporary injury patterns and factors influencing time to union. *J Bone Joint Surg Am*. 2011;93:1210–1219.
15. Greene MH, Hadied AM, LaMont RL. Scaphoid fractures in children. *J Hand Surg*. 1984;9:536–541.
16. Stewart MJ. Fractures of the carpal navicular (scaphoid); a report of 436 cases. *J Bone Joint Surg Am*. 1954;36-A:998–1006.
17. Vahvanen V, Westerlund M. Fracture of the carpal scaphoid in children. A clinical and roentgenological study of 108 cases. *Acta Orthop Scand*. 1980;51:909–913.
18. Toh S, et al. Scaphoid fractures in children: problems and treatment. *J Pediatr Orthop*. 2003;23:216–221.
19. Hove LM. Epidemiology of scaphoid fractures in Bergen. *Nor Scand J Plast Reconstr Surg Hand Surg*. 1999;33:423–426.
20. Evenski AJ, Adamczyk MJ, Steiner RP, Morscher MA, Riley PM. Clinically suspected scaphoid fractures in children. *J Pediatr Orthop*. 2009;29:352–355.
21. Johnson KJ, Haigh SF, Symonds KE. MRI in the management of scaphoid fractures in skeletally immature patients. *Pediatr Radiol*. 2000;30:685–688.
22. Gajdobranski D, et al. Scaphoid fractures in children. *Srp Arh Celok Lek*. 2014;142:444–449.
23. Grundy M. Fractures of the carpal scaphoid in children. A series of eight cases. *Br J Surg*. 1969;56:523–524.
24. Mussbichler H. Injuries of the carpal scaphoid in children. *Acta Radiol*. 1961;56:361–368.
25. McCoy GF, Graham HK, Piggot J. Non-union of fracture of the carpal scaphoid in a child. *Ulster Med J*. 1987;56:66–68.
26. Southcott R, Rosman MA. Non-union of carpal scaphoid fractures in children. *J Bone Joint Surg Br*. 1977;59:20–23.
27. Maxted MJ, Owen R. Two cases of non-union of carpal scaphoid fractures in children. *Injury*. 1982;13:441–443.
28. Pick RY, Segal D. Carpal scaphoid fracture and non-union in an eight-year-old child. Report of a case. *J Bone Joint Surg Am*. 1983;65:1188–1189.
29. Horii E, Nakamura R, Watanabe K, Tsunoda K. Scaphoid fracture as a 'puncher's fracture'. *J Orthop Trauma*. 1994;8:107–110.
30. Larson B, Light TR, Ogden JA. Fracture and ischemic necrosis of the immature scaphoid. *J Hand Surg*. 1987;12:122–127.
31. De Boeck H, Van Wellen P, Haentjens P. Nonunion of a carpal scaphoid fracture in a child. *J Orthop Trauma*. 1991;5:370–372.
32. Garcia-Elias M, Bishop AT, Dobyns JH, Cooney WP, Linscheid RL. Transcarpal carpometacarpal dislocations, excluding the thumb. *J Hand Surg*. 1990;15:531–540.
33. Henderson B, Letts M. Operative management of pediatric scaphoid fracture nonunion. *J Pediatr Orthop*. 2003;23:402–406.
34. Chloros GD, et al. Pediatric scaphoid nonunion. *J Hand Surg*. 2007;32:172–176.
35. Ben-Amotz O, Ho C, Sammer DM. Reconstruction of scaphoid non-union and total scaphoid avascular necrosis in a pediatric patient: a case report. *Hand N Y N*. 2015;10:477–481.
36. Kapoor S, Pawar I, Kapoor S. Posttraumatic osteonecrosis and nonunion of distal pole of scaphoid. *Indian J Orthop*. 2013;47:425–428.
37. Wulff RN, Schmidt TL. Carpal fractures in children. *J Pediatr Orthop*. 1998;18:462–465.
38. Duteille F, Dautel G. Non-union fractures of the scaphoid and carpal bones in children: surgical treatment. *J Pediatr Orthop B*. 2004;13:34–38.
39. Moritomo H, Tada K, Yoshida T, Masatomi T. The relationship between the site of nonunion of the scaphoid and scaphoid nonunion advanced collapse (SNAC). *J Bone Joint Surg Br*. 1999;81:871–876.
40. Louis DS, Calhoun TP, Garn SM, Carroll RE, Burdi AR. Congenital bipartite scaphoid-fact or fiction? *J Bone Joint Surg Am*. 1976;58:1108–1112.
41. Littlefield WG, Friedman RL, Urbaniak JR. Bilateral nonunion of the carpal scaphoid in a child. A case report. *J Bone Joint Surg Am*. 1995;77:124–126.
42. Espinosa GA, et al. Osteonecrosis of the distal pole of the carpal navicular following fracture. *Mil Med*. 1986;151:663–665.
43. Sherman SB, Greenspan A, Norman A. Osteonecrosis of the distal pole of the carpal scaphoid following fracture–a rare complication. *Skeletal Radiol*. 1983;9:189–191.
44. García-Mata S. Carpal scaphoid fracture nonunion in children. *J Pediatr Orthop*. 2002;22:448–451.
45. Gamble JG, Simmons SC. Bilateral scaphoid fractures in a child. *Clin Orthop*. 1982:125–128.
46. Waters PM, Stewart SL. Surgical treatment of nonunion and avascular necrosis of the proximal part of the scaphoid in adolescents. *J Bone Joint Surg Am*. 2002;84-A:915–920.
47. Godley DR. Nonunited carpal scaphoid fracture in a child: treatment with pulsed electromagnetic field stimulation. *Orthopedics*. 1997;20:718–719.
48. Caputo AE, Watson HK, Nissen C. Scaphoid nonunion in a child: a case report. *J Hand Surg*. 1995;20:243–245.
49. Reigstad O, Thorkildsen R, Grimsgaard C, Reigstad A, Rokkum M. Excellent results after bone grafting and K-wire fixation for scaphoid nonunion surgery in skeletally immature patients: a midterm follow-up study of 11 adolescents after 6.9 years. *J Orthop Trauma*. 2013;27:285–289.
50. Braga-Silva J, Peruchi FM, Moschen GM, Gehlen D, Padoin AV. A comparison of the use of distal radius vascularised bone graft and non-vascularised iliac crest bone graft in the treatment of non-union of scaphoid fractures. *J Hand Surg Eur Vol*. 2008;33:636–640.
51. Bergh TH, et al. Costs analysis and comparison of usefulness of acute MRI and 2 weeks of cast immobilization for clinically suspected scaphoid fractures. *Acta Orthop*. 2015;86:303–309.

52. Karl JW, Swart E, Strauch RJ. Diagnosis of occult scaphoid fractures: a cost-effectiveness analysis. *J Bone Joint Surg Am*. 2015;97:1860–1868.
53. Kelson T, Davidson R, Baker T. Early MRI versus conventional management in the detection of occult scaphoid fractures: what does it really cost? A rural pilot study. *J Med Radiat Sci*. 2016;63:9–16.
54. Patel NK, Davies N, Mirza Z, Watson M. Cost and clinical effectiveness of MRI in occult scaphoid fractures: a randomised controlled trial. *Emerg Med J EMJ*. 2013;30:202–207.
55. Brooks S, et al. Cost effectiveness of adding magnetic resonance imaging to the usual management of suspected scaphoid fractures. *Br J Sports Med*. 2005;39:75–79.
56. Gooding A, Coates M, Rothwell A, Accident Compensation Corporation. Cost analysis of traditional follow-up protocol versus MRI for radiographically occult scaphoid fractures: a pilot study for the Accident Compensation Corporation. *N Z Med J*. 2004;117:U1049.

FURTHER READING

1. Mintzer CM, Waters PM. Surgical treatment of pediatric scaphoid fracture nonunions. *J Pediatr Orthop*. 1999;19:236–239.
2. Masquijo JJ, Willis BR. Scaphoid nonunions in children and adolescents: surgical treatment with bone grafting and internal fixation. *J Pediatr Orthop*. 2010;30:119–124.

CHAPTER 22

Predicting Union of Scaphoid Fractures

JASON A. STRELZOW, BSc, MD, FRCSC • RUBY GREWAL, MSc, MD, FRCSC

KEY POINTS

- Prompt diagnosis and initiation of treatment is of paramount importance to ensure optimal opportunity for union. CT scan investigation provides an accurate tool to assess radiographic predictors of scaphoid union.
- Modern CT-based studies suggest low rates of nonunion following treatment for nondisplaced (0%–12%) scaphoid waist and distal pole fractures.
- A careful understanding of how patient factors and fracture characteristics influence union will help us better predict outcomes of scaphoid fractures.
- Delays in treatment, displaced fractures (translation > 1 mm, fracture gap > 3 mm, or presence of a humpback deformity), and proximal pole fractures are established predictors of delayed time to union and/or nonunion. Patient factors such as smoking and diabetes also affect union.

PANEL 1
Case Scenario

A 23-year-old male smoker falls off his motorbike at moderate speed while attempting to avoid traffic. He is seen in the emergency department at a local hospital and diagnosed clinically and radiographically with a nondisplaced midwaist scaphoid fracture.

After a discussion with the patient, he states that his friend had a similar injury and was only immobilized in a cast for 4 weeks. The patient would like to know the chances he will heal and how long it may take him to unite. How will you counsel the patient and determine if he has healed?

IMPORTANCE OF THE PROBLEM

Fracture union is at the heart of orthopedic management. This biologic and mechanical process requires a complex repair cascade resulting in a healed fracture allowing for the transmission of mechanical load across a bone.[1,2] Adequate cellular vascularity, mechanical stability, appropriate progenitor cells, and bone-on-bone contact must be present for the process of fracture union to occur.[3] A lack or disruption in any one of these factors may lead to nonunion or delayed union.

Fracture healing can occur through either of two processes, primary or secondary healing, which occur depending on the fracture pattern, fracture location, and treatment strategies. Primary bone healing involves the process of short gap formation and cutting cone mechanisms, thereby producing little, if any, callus.[1,4] A fracture gap of <0.01 mm with minimal strain is optimal for primary bone healing while a gap > 1 mm is substantially more likely not to heal through direct bone healing methods. By contrast, secondary healing occurs through various stages of callus formation and maturation to produce a united fracture.[3]

Nonunion or delayed union typically occurs through a disruption in the normal healing processes by either mechanical or biologic causes.[3] A biologically inappropriate environment may lead to an absence or suppression of the normal milieu of required enzymes and nutrients. Micromotion at a fracture site, including shear, can lead to nonunion through the deposition of fibrous tissue rather than bony union.[5] As there is a "link" between the distal and proximal row of the carpus, the scaphoid has a particularly tenuous mechanical environment when fractured. The distal pole has a tendency to flex with the distal row, whereas the proximal fragments are typically under extension load through the lunate.[6–8] This interplay of forces generates a central bending/shear force present within the waist of the scaphoid itself and may play a role in the development of nonunion if left uncontrolled.

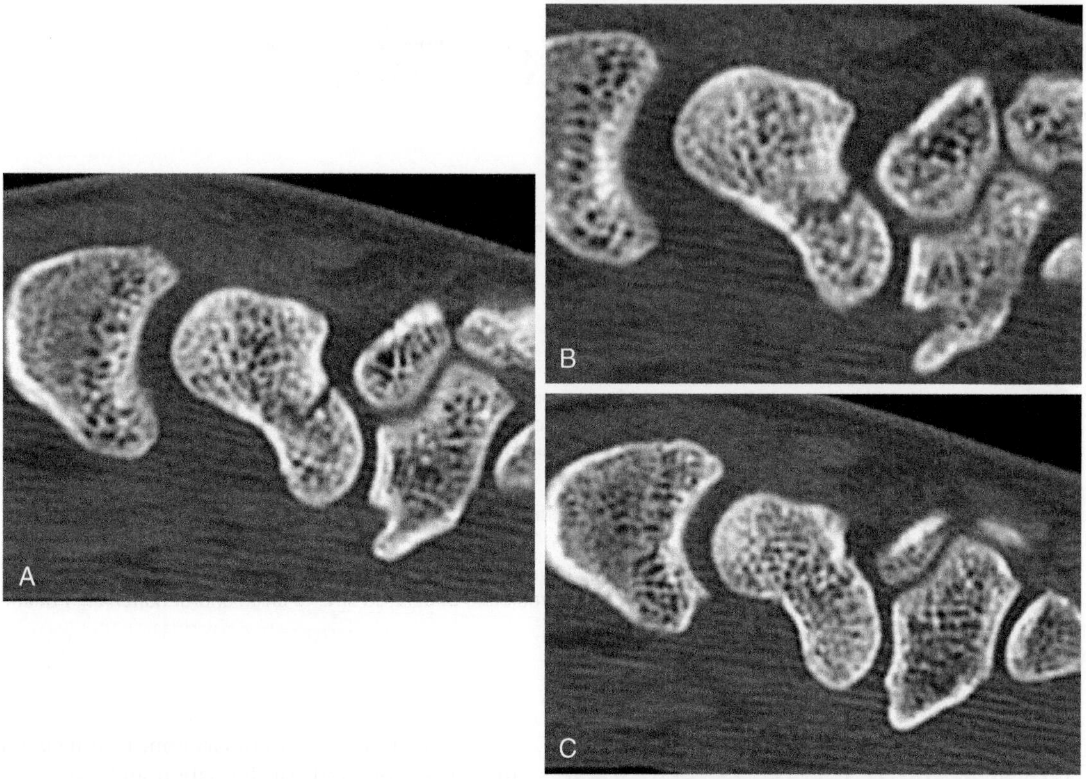

FIG. 22.1 CT scan images illustrating partial union of a scaphoid fracture as seen on sequential cuts across the bone. (A) A sagittal CT scan of the scaphoid demonstrates a partial union of the scaphoid with volar cortical healing and a dorsal fracture line still visible. (B) An additional sagittal cut demonstrating a clearly visible fracture at this location. (C) A subsequent sagittal CT scan view demonstrating healing across the fracture along both the dorsal and volar cortices.

Considering the complexity of the process, it is not, therefore, surprising that multiple definitions exist to define and assess union. The definition of union may be clinical, mechanical, or radiographic.[4] Clinically and mechanically, a pain- and displacement-free fracture site placed under physiologic loading (distraction and torsional forces) suggests union. Radiographically, union has been defined as bridging fracture callus visualized at three cortices on at least two orthogonal radiographs.[9]

These definitions are not immune to controversy, particularly when applied to certain anatomic locations such as the scaphoid. Dias (2001) produced the most ubiquitous and generic definition for union of the scaphoid: "the restoration of bony architecture across the fracture site."[10] Singh and colleagues[11] suggested a radiographic assessment of union of the scaphoid based on CT evaluation of percentage of union at the fracture, thereby enabling the diagnosis of partial union. This concept helps to explain the phenomenon of apparent fracture union discovered intraoperatively when plain films suggested nonunion[12] (Fig. 22.1).

The anatomy and location of the scaphoid challenges our evaluation of scaphoid fractures and healing. Multiple radiographic techniques and imaging modalities have been developed to optimize our ability to diagnose and assess fractures of the scaphoid. Currently, scaphoid-specific radiographic views are the first study of choice. The radiographs are a semipronated oblique view or 45 degrees anteroposterior pronated view.[13,14] Lateral radiographs can also be useful. Additional modalities of investigation include helical CT scan and MRI in which each have high inter- and intraobserver reliability.[14–19] Serial radiographs, the most commonly utilized modality for monitoring healing progression in most published research trials, demonstrate poor interobserver reliability at 12 weeks postinjury.[20–23] CT scan evaluation of the percentage of scaphoid healing at the fracture site as reviewed by Singh et al.[11] and Grewal et al.[25] demonstrate high interrater reliability.[11,24,25] These methods should be utilized in the clinical and research setting to standardize the assessment of union and guide treatment. Although concern regarding total effective radiation load is a current and appropriate concern, modern CT extremity protocols have documented a low effective radiation dose to the patient (0.03 mSv) or less than half the equivalent background radiation exposure for 1 week.[26]

Predicting scaphoid union remains an elusive topic and frustrates the clinician's ability to inform and guide patient care. The variability in imaging modalities used in prior studies on scaphoid union has limited the generalizability and reliability of many of these results.[27] Predicting scaphoid union requires an understanding of the bony anatomy and the implications of patient characteristics, injury pattern, and treatment modalities.

MAIN QUESTION

How do we predict a patient's likelihood of and time to scaphoid union after fracture?

Current Opinion

Nondisplaced acute scaphoid waist or distal pole fractures in otherwise healthy young patients treated appropriately are considered at low risk for developing nonunion. Displaced fractures, chronic fractures, fractures with signs of avascular necrosis, and patients who smoke or have extensive comorbidities are at increased risk of developing a nonunion.

Proximal pole fractures are considered at high risk for nonunion, delayed union, and poor outcome. These injuries are, therefore, typically treated with ORIF. Conversely, pediatric scaphoid fractures are considered at low risk for nonunion and almost universally treated with immobilization. Nondisplaced fractures are currently treated according to patient preference and surgeon comfort, as outcomes are comparable.

Finding the Evidence

- Cochrane database search: Scaphoid Union
- Pubmed: ("Scaphoid Union" [Mesh] OR "Scaphoid Non-union" OR "Scaphoid Healing")
- Bibliography of eligible articles
- Foreign language articles not written in English were excluded from review

Quality of the Evidence

Level I:

Metaanalysis/systematic reviews: 2

Level II:

Randomized trials with methodological limitations: 1

Level III:

Retrospective cohort studies: 3

Level IV:

Consecutive case series: 15

FINDINGS

Predicting scaphoid union requires an understanding of the injury pattern, fracture location and characteristics, bone quality, vascularity, and patient comorbidities. These factors have complex interactions that contribute to a specific patient's nonunion risk. A thorough understanding of these factors allows the surgeon to formulate a generalized risk of delayed or nonunion. This perceived nonunion risk may help in the development of a treatment plan.

Fracture Location: Proximal/Waist/Distal

Only one large systematic review exists addressing the question of predicting union rates after scaphoid fracture.[28] A total of 67 proximal pole fractures treated nonoperatively met eligibility for this metaanalysis. The authors found proximal pole fractures had a relative risk of nonunion of 7.5 compared with waist and distal pole scaphoid fractures (95% confidence interval [CI], 4.9–11.5). Based on this small sample set, Eastley et al. (2013) suggest that nearly 34% of acute proximal pole fractures managed nonoperatively will not unite (n = 67). The results of this metaanalysis must be considered based on the strength of the included studies, which have a number of limitations including historical and outdated treatment protocols (articles as early as 1934 are included), the use of plain radiographs to assess union in nine of the included studies, and the inconsistent outcomes reported by various authors. Four studies have supported the conclusion that proximal pole fractures are at increased risk (nonunion rates of 15% [n = 7], 14% [n = 28], 50% [n = 22], 41% [n = 30])[29–32]; however, a recent CT-based study showed that nonunion rates in proximal pole fractures was not as high as previously reported (nonunion rate 10%, n = 53)[31] In a separate retrospective series of 219 scaphoid fractures treated in cast alone, Grewal et al. found an overall union rate of 95% but longer time to union based on location (16 ± 16 weeks proximal pole, 9 ± 8 weeks waist, 8 ± 4 weeks for distal pole fractures).[33] This study did not report a statistically higher nonunion rate; however a trend was noted. Schuind et al.[32] found an increased nonunion rate depending on fracture location. Their review of 138 nonunions undergoing surgical treatment found no nonunions of the distal tubercle and significantly more in the proximal pole. Interestingly, the duration of treatment in acute nondisplaced fractures may not be as long as historical evidence would suggest. Geoghegan et al. have shown treatment success and radiographic union of nondisplaced waist fractures at the 4-week mark after immobilization.[34] Forty-four percent of their patient cohort were removed from cast at the 4-week mark after CT scan evaluation documented successful union (Figs. 22.2 and 22.3).

Fracture Characteristics

Clementson et al.[35] evaluated union rates between two cohorts of scaphoid waist fractures (n = 39) using CT assessment. After assessing nonoperative and arthroscopically assisted fixation groups, they found high rates of union at 6 weeks for both groups (90% vs. 82%). Prolonged time to union (10–14 weeks) in the conservatively treated cohort correlated with fracture comminution, particularly when a radial cortical fragment was identified, a finding supported by other authors.[33,35] Comminution with fragmentation was a common finding in their population, seen in 34% of fractures. This study was underpowered to detect a relationship between displacement and fracture union; however, a trend was seen toward longer time to union with displacement >1 mm. Grewal et al. demonstrated a small but positive correlation between time to union and translation ($r = 0.24$, $P < .001$) with a significant increase in the attributable risk of nonunion with translation >1 mm.[33] Eight studies have suggested an increase in time to union with displaced fractures.[15,29–31,34,36–38] These studies are limited by small sample sizes (n = 28–248) and lack statistical power for definitive conclusions. Two retrospective case series quantified displacement (translation >1.5 mm) and the risk of nonunion (odds ratio of 3.4, 95% CI: 1–11.3).[33,36] A fracture gap of greater than 3 mm evaluated at 4 weeks postinjury carried an odds ratio of nonunion of 9.9 (95% CI: 1.7–56.3).[36] The presence of a humpback deformity also resulted in lower union rates in a retrospective series of 219 nonoperatively treated scaphoid fractures (odds ratio of 6.9, 95% CI: 1.9–25.7)[33] (Table 22.1).

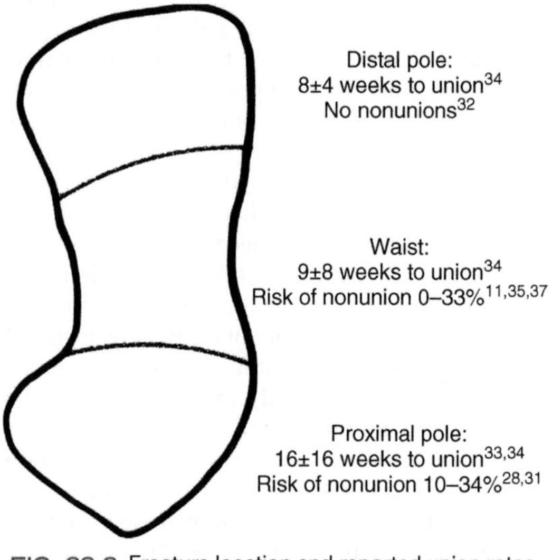

FIG. 22.2 Fracture location and reported union rates.

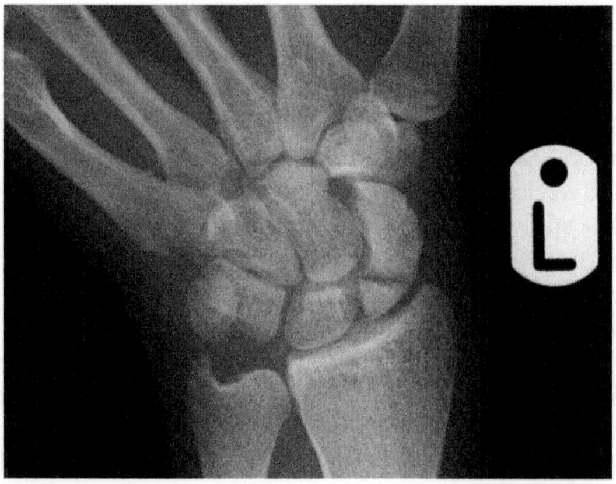

FIG. 22.3 Typical appearance of a scaphoid fracture of the proximal pole. This demonstrates minimal translation; however, CT scan evaluation is required for a more reliable critic of fracture displacement.

Only two case series have evaluated the importance of fracture line sclerosis finding no increased rates of nonunion.[33,36] Conflicting evidence exists regarding the impact of cystic changes and fracture resorption on union rates. Two small case series (n = 53 and n = 219) documented no significant effect of fracture edge resorption on the rate of union, whereas a third study (n = 31) reported resorption of greater than 50% of the fracture cross section purported an increased nonunion risk.[33,36,37] Grewal et al. recently documented an increased time to union when cystic resorption was identified on CT scans but not an increased risk of nonunion.[39]

Treatment Timing

A timely and accurate diagnosis is critical to facilitate the early initiation of treatment. A high index of suspicion and the use of additional cross-sectional imaging can be useful to ensure diagnostic clarity.[11,19,24,25] Unfortunately, diagnosis and early management remains problematic[40,41] (Fig. 22.4). The importance of early initiation of treatment has been demonstrated in seven studies. Langhoff and Andersen provided early case series evidence that a delay in treatment (>4 weeks) significantly increased nonunion rates.[38] Early diagnosis and treatment in their study leads to a nonunion rate of 3% compared with nearly 40%

TABLE 22.1
Impact of Fracture Location and Characteristics on Time to Union and Rate of Nonunion

Study	Number of Patients	Diagnostic Investigation	Method of Treatment	Union	Nonunion	Delayed Union	Time to Union	Comments
FRACTURE LOCATION								
Eastley et al. (Metanalysis)[28]	162 proximal pole	Radiologic and clinical	Nonoperative and operative	131	25	6 (>4 mo to union)	No specified	
Eddeland et al.[29]	7 proximal	Radiologic and clinical	Nonoperative and operative	6	1	Not reported	19 weeks	
	14 waist			12	2		14 weeks	
	2 distal			2	0		12 weeks	
Grewal et al.[31]	52 proximal	CT scan	Nonoperative and operative	47	5	Not reported	14 ± 8 weeks surgical 14 ± 12 weeks cast alone	
FRACTURE DISPLACEMENT								
Clementson et al.[35]	52 nondisplaced	CT scan	Mixed operative and nonoperative	52	0	1	82% at 6 weeks 97% at 14 weeks	1 nonunion at 1 year despite surgical intervention. Fracture comminution and displacement significant risk for delayed union.
	13 displaced (>1.5 mm)			9	1	4	80% at 6 weeks 94% at 10 weeks	
Grewal et al.[33]	160 nondisplaced	CT scan	Nonoperative	145	15	Not reported	10 ± 10 weeks (no humpback) 9 ± 8 weeks (no translation)	Presence of comminution had effect on time to union adding 29 days to the average time to union (48 days) if present. Factors were found to be additive to union rate and time to union.
	59 displaced (humpback or translation > 1.5 mm)			50	9		12 ± 8 weeks (presence of humpback) 15 ± 13 weeks (presence of translation)	
Amirfeyz et al.[36]	13 nondisplaced	CT scan	Nonoperative	13	0	Not reported	Not reported (median immobilization) 11 (4–13) weeks	CT scan evaluation of displacement was evaluated at 4 weeks postinjury.
	18 displaced (>2 mm)			8	10			

continued

TABLE 22.1
Impact of Fracture Location and Characteristics on Time to Union and Rate of Nonunion—cont'd

Study	Number of Patients	Diagnostic Investigation	Method of Treatment	Union	Nonunion	Delayed Union	Time to Union	Comments
Bhat et al.[15]	40 nondisplaced	MRI and radiographs	Nonoperative	40	0			Demonstrated poor reproducibility and specificity in detection of displacement between observers using plain radiographs for diagnosis.
	9 displaced (>1 mm)			6	3			
Desai et al.[23]	134 nondisplaced	X-ray only	Nonoperative	120	14	Not reported	Not reported	Additional found no effect of comminution or location of the fracture site (proximal, waist, distal) on time to union.
	17 displaced (>1 mm)			15	2			
Geoghegan et al.[33]	59 nondisplaced	26 X-rays and 3 CT scans	Nonoperative	53	6	Not reported	22/26 united on CT at 4 weeks	
	16 displaced (≥1 mm)			11	5		11/16 united on CT at 4 weeks	

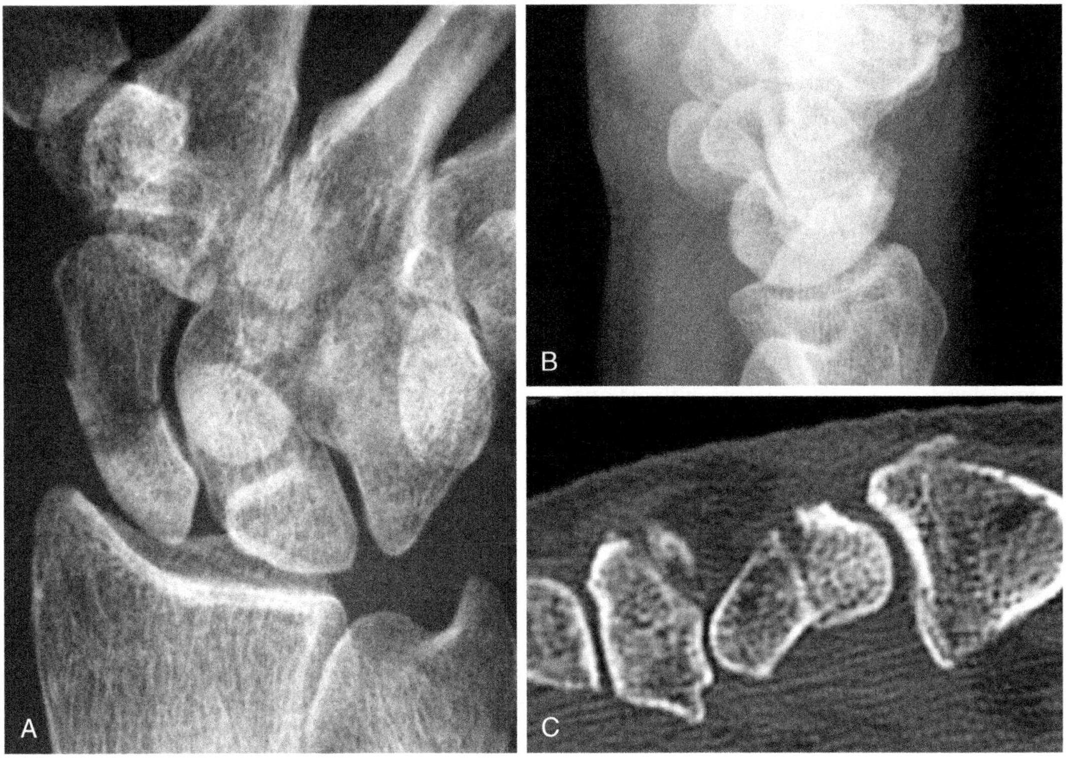

FIG. 22.4 Apparent minimally displaced scaphoid fracture visualized on AP **(A)** and lateral **(B)** plain X-rays. CT scan documents significant fracture displacement with flexion at the fracture site **(C)**.

in the late treatment cohort. Four additional studies have examined timing of treatment and the effect on union.[30–32,37] Grewal et al. reported their experience (n = 28) with fractures identified and treated between 6 weeks and 6 months with a nonunion rate of 17.9% and a prolonged time to union between approximately 11–14 weeks of immobilization depending on the location of injury.[37] A retrospective review of 351 adolescent and pediatric scaphoid injuries documented a 29.7 times higher rate of developing nonunion when chronic injuries (mean time to treatment, 26.8 ± 34.3 weeks) were treated with casting compared with acute injuries.[30,37] A multicenter retrospective case study (n = 138) examining prognostic factors for healing in scaphoid nonunion surgery identified time from injury and time to definitive treatment as the only factors affecting success (odds ratio of 0.31, 95% CI: 0.2–0.8 for successful union with increased time to treatment).[32] A recently published review (n = 138) supports this finding documenting a significant correlation between the time from fracture until immobilization and time until union.[39]

Patient Factors

Multiple patient factors have been implicated in the general inhibition of fracture healing, including patient comorbidities (diabetes mellitus, hypothyroidism, and malnutrition), nonsteroidal antiinflammatory drugs, corticosteroids, smoking, and potentially some classes of antibiotics.[37,42] Smoking may have a profound effect on the success rates of scaphoid healing; however, data are conflicting. A recent metaanalysis and retrospective case series reported an odds ratio of 10.1 (95% CI: not reported) and relative risk of 3.4 for persistent nonunion in smokers despite operative management for established nonunion.[43,44] A retrospective study demonstrated a delayed time to union in diabetics with an additional 25 days that were required for union ($P = .04$).[39] A history of osteonecrosis has been suggested to increase the risk of nonunion; however, recent available literature suggests this may not be a risk factor.[45] This is supported by Dawson et al.[46] who documented no increased risk of nonunion in patients with proximal pole hypovascularity diagnosed on gadolinium enhanced MRI.

RECOMMENDATIONS

- Modern CT-based studies suggest low rates of nonunion following treatment for nondisplaced (0%–12%) and displaced (0%–33%) scaphoid fractures (overall quality: moderate).
- Displaced fractures (translation >1 mm, fracture gap > 3 mm, or presence of a humpback deformity) are at an increased risk of nonunion or delayed time to union (overall quality: moderate).
- Nondisplaced fractures have a high rate of union when treated (95%–100% regardless of operative or nonoperative treatment strategy) (overall quality: moderate).
- Proximal pole fractures (proximal one-fifth of bone) are at significantly increased risk of developing a nonunion or requiring prolonged time to union (overall quality: low evidence).
- Delay to definitive treatment may increase the risk of nonunion or prolong the time to union (overall quality: low).
- Fracture comminution may delay time to union (overall quality: low).
- Fracture line sclerosis, cystic change, and hypovascularity of the proximal pole seen on contrast-enhanced MRI may not effect union rates or time to union. The literature shows that the presence of cystic changes observed on CT scan has conflicting evidence regarding the importance (overall quality: low).
- Patient factors such as smoking and diabetes have a negative effect on fracture union (overall quality: low).
- Nondisplaced waist fractures in patients without significant risk factors for nonunion should be assessed clinically, and if indicated by an equivocal examination or ongoing pain, they should be assessed with cross-sectional imaging (CT or MRI) between 4 and 6 weeks. Union must be confirmed before discontinuing immobilization and the authors feel that union is most accurately detected with CT scan. In our experience, collaboration with radiologists has ensured that, for purposes of detecting union, only a focused CT scan of the scaphoid is performed (rather than a standard wrist CT scan), allowing this to be an efficient, cost-effective modality at our center (overall quality: low).

CONCLUSION

Multiple factors appear to play a role in the potential for union of scaphoid fractures. Factors may be categorized as patient, injury, or treatment related. Although there is ample research on the topic of scaphoid fracture epidemiology, diagnosis, and management, our understanding and evidence for predicting which fractures will successfully unite remains relatively elementary. Current literature would suggest a dynamic interplay between elements that play a role in predicting scaphoid fracture union. Fracture union rate and likelihood of union is most probably affected in an additive way with the compounding of each additional risk factor for union.[30,33] Rates of union for acute nondisplaced distal and waist fractures approach 100% with operative or nonoperative strategies.[27,47] In contrast, chronic displaced fractures of the waist and proximal pole may have rates of union as low as 2% with cast treatment alone.[30] Patients should be assessed for suspected risk factors and be counseled accordingly. Overall, the literature, although extensive, is of low quality and has not focused on reliable, established methods for assessing and predicting union utilizing standardized research protocols. Definitive conclusions remain elusive and further investigation is required.

PANEL 2
Author's Preferred Technique

In the case of our nondisplaced waist fracture in a young patient, there is a high likelihood of union based on the location and position of the fracture. Additional cross-sectional imaging with scaphoid-specific CT scan images is recommended to accurately assess fracture characteristics (i.e., comminution, displacement) and thereby more reliably predict union risk. Current evidence would suggest that CT scan confirmed nondisplaced scaphoid fractures have high rates of union **within 4–10 weeks**. Displaced, comminuted, or proximal pole fractures have increased time to union and rates of nonunion. The patient should be counseled regarding smoking cessation because this has a detrimental impact on bony union. Open reduction and internal fixation should be discussed with the patient because it is a viable option that may or may not shorten time to union.[48–50]

PANEL 3
Pearl's and Pitfalls

PEARLS

- Patients with scaphoid fractures should be evaluated with CT scan to assess for translation and gapping at the fracture site to diagnose and guide treatment and predict possibility of union.
- Early reevaluation with CT scan at 4–6 weeks can be a useful tool to calculate the amount of union to guide the need for additional immobilization. Recent

PANEL 3
Pearl's and Pitfalls—cont'd

studies suggest that union time may be as short as 4–6 weeks for scaphoid waist fractures that have been proven to be nondisplaced by CT scan.

PITFALLS

- Discontinuing immobilization without a radiographic and clinical assessment of union may lead to inadequate immobilization, consequently leading to the development of persistent nonunion or the late development of a SNAC wrist. In the setting of nonunion risk factors or an equivocal clinical examination, cross-sectional imaging (CT/MRI) may be required for adequate assessment of the fracture site.
- Failure to consider fracture morphology and location in the context of the risk of delayed or nonunion increases the risk of inadequate treatment.
- Chronic scaphoid fractures with displacement or gapping >1 mm treated with immobilization alone may develop ongoing nonunion without additional treatment.

REFERENCES

1. Marsell R, Einhorn TA. The biology of fracture healing. *Injury*. 2011;42(6):551–555. http://dx.doi.org/10.1016/j.injury.2011.03.031.
2. Einhorn TA. The cell and molecular biology of fracture healing. *Clin Orthop Relat Res*. 1998;(355 suppl):S7–S21.
3. Brinker MR, OConnor DP. The biological basis for nonunions. *JBJS Rev*. 2016;4(6):e3. http://dx.doi.org/10.2106/JBJS.RVW.15.00078.
4. Oryan A, Monazzah S, Bigham-Sadegh A. Bone injury and fracture healing biology. *Biomed Environ Sci*. 2015;28(1):57–71. http://dx.doi.org/10.3967/bes2015.006.
5. Augat P, Burger J, Schorlemmer S, Henke T, Peraus M, Claes L. Shear movement at the fracture site delays healing in a diaphyseal fracture model. *J Orthop Res*. 2003;21(6):1011–1017. http://dx.doi.org/10.1016/S0736-0266(03)00098-6.
6. Garcia-Elias M. Kinetic analysis of carpal stability during grip. *Hand Clin*. 1997;13(1):151–158.
7. Kobayashi M, Garcia-Elias M, Nagy L, et al. Axial loading induces rotation of the proximal carpal row bones around unique screw-displacement axes. *J Biomech*. 1997;30(11–12):1165–1167.
8. Smith DK, Cooney III WP, An KN, Linscheid RL, Chao EYS. The effects of simulated unstable scaphoid fractures on carpal motion. *J Hand Surg Am*. 1989;14(2):283–291. http://dx.doi.org/10.1016/0363-5023(89)90022-1.
9. Whelan DB, Bhandari M, McKee MD, et al. Interobserver and intraobserver variation in the assessment of the healing of tibial fractures after intramedullary fixation. *J Bone Joint Surg Br*. 2002;84(1):15–18.
10. Dias JJ. Definition of union after acute fracture and surgery for the fracture nonunion of the scaphoid. *J Hand Surg*. 2001;26(4):321–325. http://dx.doi.org/10.1054/jhsb.2001.0596.
11. Singh H, Singh HP, Forward D, et al. Partial union of acute scaphoid fractures. *J Hand Surg*. 2005;30(5):440–445. http://dx.doi.org/10.1016/j.jhsb.2005.05.007.
12. Barton NJ. Apparent and partial non-union of the scaphoid. *J Hand Surg Br*. 1996;21(4):496–500.
13. Cooney WP, Dobyns JH, Linscheid RL. Fractures of the scaphoid: a rational approach to management. *Clin Orthop Relat Res*. 1980;149:90–97.
14. Ring D, Lozano-Calderón S. Imaging for suspected scaphoid fracture. *J Hand Surg Am*. 2008;33(6):954–957. http://dx.doi.org/10.1016/j.jhsa.2008.04.016.
15. Bhat M, McCarthy M, Davis TRC, Oni JA, Oni JA, Dawson S. MRI and plain radiography in the assessment of displaced fractures of the waist of the carpal scaphoid. *J Bone Joint Surg Br*. 2004;86(5):705–713. http://dx.doi.org/10.1302/0301-620X.86B5.14374.
16. Lozano-Calderón S, Blazar P, Zurakowski D, Lee S-G, Ring D. Diagnosis of scaphoid fracture displacement with radiography and computed tomography. *J Bone Joint Surg Am*. 2006;88(12):2695–2703. http://dx.doi.org/10.2106/JBJS.E.01211.
17. Temple CLF, Ross DC, Bennett JD, Garvin GJ, King GJW, Faber KJ. Comparison of sagittal computed tomography and plain film radiography in a scaphoid fracture model. *J Hand Surg Am*. 2005;30(3):534–542. http://dx.doi.org/10.1016/j.jhsa.2005.01.001.
18. Imaeda T, Nakamura R, Miura T, Makino N. Magnetic resonance imaging in scaphoid fractures. *J Hand Surg Br*. 1992;17(1):20–27.
19. Bain GI. Clinical utilization of computed tomography of the scaphoid. *Hand Surg*. 1999;4(1):3–9. http://dx.doi.org/10.1142/S0218810499000198.
20. Dias JJ, Taylor M, Thompson J, Brenkel IJ, Gregg PJ. Radiographic signs of union of scaphoid fractures. An analysis of inter-observer agreement and reproducibility. *J Bone Joint Surg Br*. 1988;70(2):299–301.
21. Hackney LA, Dodds SD. Assessment of scaphoid fracture healing. *Curr Rev Musculoskelet Med*. 2011;4(1):16–22. http://dx.doi.org/10.1007/s12178-011-9072-0.
22. Buijze GA, Buijze GA, Wijffels MME, et al. Interobserver reliability of computed tomography to diagnose scaphoid waist fracture union. *J Hand Surg Am*. 2012;37(2):250–254. http://dx.doi.org/10.1016/j.jhsa.2011.10.051.
23. Desai VV, Davis TR, Barton NJ. The prognostic value and reproducibility of the radiological features of the fractured scaphoid. *J Hand Surg Br*. 1999;24(5):586–590. http://dx.doi.org/10.1054/jhsb.1999.0197.
24. Bain GI, Bennett JD, Richards RS, Slethaug GP, Roth JH. Longitudinal computed tomography of the scaphoid: a new technique. *Skeletal Radiol*. 1995;24(4):271–273. http://dx.doi.org/10.1007/BF00198413.

25. Grewal R, Frakash U, Osman S, McMurtry RY. A quantitative definition of scaphoid union: determining the inter-rater reliability of two techniques. *J Orthop Surg Res*. 2013;8(1):28. http://dx.doi.org/10.1186/1749-799X-8-28.
26. Biswas D, Bible JE, Bohan M, Simpson AK, Whang PG, Grauer JN. Radiation exposure from musculoskeletal computerized tomographic scans. *J Bone Joint Surg Am*. 2009;91(8):1882–1889. http://dx.doi.org/10.2106/JBJS.H.01199.
27. Buijze GA, Doornberg JN, Ham JS, Ring D, Bhandari M, Poolman RW. Surgical compared with conservative treatment for acute nondisplaced or minimally displaced scaphoid fractures: a systematic review and meta-analysis of randomized controlled trials. *J Bone Joint Surg Am*. 2010;92(6). http://dx.doi.org/10.2106/JBJS.I.01214.
28. Eastley N, Singh H, Dias JJ, Dias JJ, Taub N. Union rates after proximal scaphoid fractures; meta-analyses and review of available evidence. *J Hand Surg Eur Vol*. 2013;38(8):888–897. http://dx.doi.org/10.1177/1753193412451424.
29. Eddeland A, Eiken O, Hellgren E, Ohlsson NM. Fractures of the scaphoid. *Scand J Plast Reconstr Surg*. 1975;9(3):234–239.
30. Gholson JJ, Bae DS, Zurakowski D, Waters PM. Scaphoid fractures in children and adolescents: contemporary injury patterns and factors influencing time to union. *J Bone Joint Surg Am*. 2011;93(13). http://dx.doi.org/10.2106/JBJS.J.01729.
31. Grewal R, Lutz K, MacDermid JC, Suh N. Proximal pole scaphoid fractures: a computed tomographic assessment of outcomes. *J Hand Surg Am*. 2016;41(1):54–58. http://dx.doi.org/10.1016/j.jhsa.2015.10.013.
32. Schuind F, Haentjens P, Van Innis F. Prognostic factors in the treatment of carpal scaphoid nonunions. *J Hand Surg Am*. 1999;24(4):761–776. http://dx.doi.org/10.1053/jhsu.1999.0761.
33. Grewal R, Suh N, MacDermid JC. Use of computed tomography to predict union and time to union in acute scaphoid fractures treated nonoperatively. *J Hand Surg Am*. 2013;38(5):872–877. http://dx.doi.org/10.1016/j.jhsa.2013.01.032.
34. Geoghegan JM, Woodruff MJ, Bhatia R, et al. Undisplaced scaphoid waist fractures: is 4 weeks' immobilisation in a below-elbow cast sufficient if a week 4 CT scan suggests fracture union? *J Hand Surg Eur Vol*. 2009;34(5):631–637. http://dx.doi.org/10.1177/1753193409105189.
35. Clementson M, Jorgsholm P, Besjakov J, Bjorkman A, Thomsen N. Union of scaphoid waist fractures assessed by CT scan. *J Wrist Surg*. 2015;4(1):049–055. http://dx.doi.org/10.1055/s-0034-1398472.
36. Amirfeyz R, Bebbington A, Downing ND, Oni JA, Davis TRC. Displaced scaphoid waist fractures: the use of a week 4 CT scan to predict the likelihood of union with nonoperative treatment. *J Hand Surg Eur Vol*. 2011;36(6):498–502. http://dx.doi.org/10.1177/1753193411403092.
37. Grewal R, Suh N, Suh N, MacDermid JC, MacDermid J. The missed scaphoid fracture–outcomes of delayed cast treatment. *J Wrist Surg*. 2015;4(4):278–283. http://dx.doi.org/10.1055/s-0035-1564983.
38. Langhoff O, Andersen JL. Consequences of late immobilization of scaphoid fractures. *J Hand Surg Br*. 1988;13(1):77–79.
39. Grewal R, Suh N, MacDermid JC. Is casting for non-displaced simple scaphoid waist fracture Effective? A CT based assessment of union. *Open Orthop J*. 2016;10(1):431–438. http://dx.doi.org/10.2174/1874325001610010431.
40. Lindström G, Nystrom P. Natural history of scaphoid non-union, with special reference to "asymptomatic" cases. *J Hand Surg*. 1992;17(6):697–700. http://dx.doi.org/10.1016/0266-7681(92)90204-F.
41. Wong K, Schroeder von HP. Delays and poor management of scaphoid fractures: factors contributing to non-union. *J Hand Surg Am*. 2011;36(9):1471–1474. http://dx.doi.org/10.1016/j.jhsa.2011.06.016.
42. Gaston MS, Simpson A. Inhibition of fracture healing. *Bone Joint J*. 2007. http://dx.doi.org/10.1302/0301-620X.89B12.
43. Ditsios K, Konstantinidis I, Agas K, Christodoulou A. Comparative meta-analysis on the various vascularized bone flaps used for the treatment of scaphoid non-union. *J Orthop Res*. March 2016. http://dx.doi.org/10.1002/jor.23242.
44. Dinah AF, Vickers RH. Smoking increases failure rate of operation for established non-union of the scaphoid bone. *Int Orthop*. 2006;31(4):503–505. http://dx.doi.org/10.1007/s00264-006-0231-7.
45. Tait MA, Bracey JW, Gaston RG. Acute scaphoid fractures: a critical analysis review. *JBJS Rev*. 2016;4(9):e3. http://dx.doi.org/10.2106/JBJS.RVW.15.00073.
46. Dawson JS, Dawson JS, Martel AL, Davis TRC, Davis TR. Scaphoid blood flow and acute fracture healing. *J Bone Joint Surg*. 2001;83(6):809–814. http://dx.doi.org/10.1302/0301-620X.83B6.11897.
47. Gregory JJ, Mohil RS, Ng AB, Warner JG, Hodgson SP. Comparison of Herbert and Acutrak screws in the treatment of scaphoid non-union and delayed union. *Acta Orthop Belg*. 2008;74(6):761–765.
48. Modi CS, Nancoo T, Powers D, Ho K, Boer R. Operative versus nonoperative treatment of acute undisplaced and minimally displaced scaphoid waist fractures—a systematic review. *Injury*. 2009;40.
49. McQueen MM, Gelbke MK, Wakefield A, Will EM, Gaebler C. Percutaneous screw fixation versus conservative treatment for fractures of the waist of the scaphoid: a prospective randomised study. *J Bone Joint Surg Br*. 2008;90(1):66–71. http://dx.doi.org/10.1302/0301-620X.90B1.19767.
50. Suh N, Benson EC, Faber KJ, MacDermid J, Grewal R. Treatment of acute scaphoid fractures: a systematic review and meta-analysis. *Hand*. 2010;5(4):345–353. http://dx.doi.org/10.1007/s11552-010-9276-6.

CHAPTER 23

Value of Pulsed Electromagnetic Stimulation in Acute Scaphoid Fractures

PASCAL F.W. HANNEMANN, MD, PHD • MARTIJN POEZE, MD, PHD • PETER R.G. BRINK, MD, PHD

KEY POINTS

- A significant number of orthopedic trauma surgeons incorporate bone growth stimulation into their treatment regimes for long-bone fractures.
- The use of pulsed electromagnetic stimulation for treatment of nondisplaced scaphoid waist fractures does not lead to accelerated bone healing.
- From a socioeconomic perspective, pulsed electromagnetic stimulation in acute scaphoid fractures cannot be considered as cost-effective.
- There is insufficient evidence to justify routine use of bone growth stimulation in the treatment of acute scaphoid fractures to reduce the number of nonunions.

PANEL 1
Case Scenario

A 37-year-old healthcare worker visited the emergency department with complaints of left wrist pain after a hyperextension trauma of the wrist incurred during a soccer match. Radiographs show a left-sided scaphoid fracture. The CT scan shows a minimally displaced scaphoid waist fracture without comminution (Fig. 23.1). Because the fracture is a nondisplaced (or minimally displaced) waist fracture, 6 weeks of cast immobilization is proposed. The patient suggests the application of pulsed electromagnetic field bone growth stimulation because he wants to shorten his period of sick leave and improve functional outcome on short-term. Do you agree that this might be a good idea?

IMPORTANCE OF THE PROBLEM

The primary goals of scaphoid fracture treatment, regardless of treatment mode, are to achieve consolidation and maximize functional outcome, while minimizing socioeconomic consequences. Scaphoid fractures can be treated either conservatively, with immobilization in a cast, or operatively. Given the high risk of nonunion, functional treatment of radiographically proven scaphoid fractures is not recommended.

Surgical treatment of nondisplaced fractures of the scaphoid waist has been shown to lead to earlier return of function and to sport and full work compared with nonoperative treatment.[1,2] However, a statistically significant difference in union rates between surgery and conservative treatment of acute minimally displaced and nondisplaced scaphoid waist fractures has not been reported in the literature to date.[3] In addition, surgery of scaphoid waist fractures is associated with a significantly higher risk of complications.[3,4] A recent meta-analysis on surgical versus conservative treatment of minimally displaced and nondisplaced scaphoid waist fractures revealed a significantly increased risk of complications of surgical treatment, with a pooled odds ratio of 7.69 (95% confidence interval [CI]: 2.16–27.4, $P=.02$, $I^2=0\%$).[3] Therefore, controversy still surrounds the best treatment for minimally displaced and nondisplaced scaphoid waist fractures because failed treatment and complicated healing of scaphoid fractures may have severe personal, economic, and social consequences in the mainly young, working population affected.[5] As

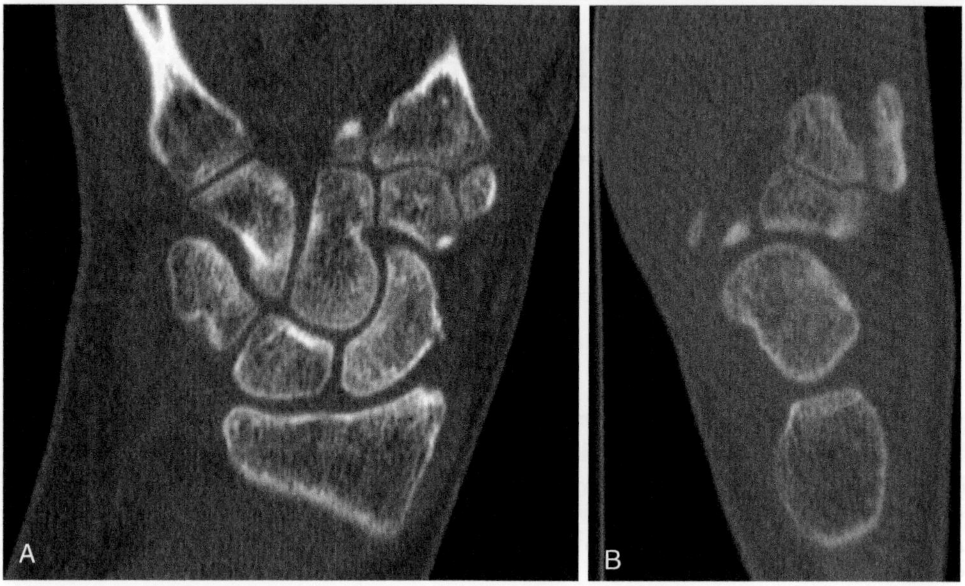

FIG. 23.1 Coronal **(A)** and sagittal **(B)** multiplanar reconstruction CT scan views of a minimally displaced scaphoid waist fracture.

a consequence, other adjunct treatment options have been under consideration.

Adjunct interventions, such as electrophysical bone growth stimulation, are frequently used to facilitate and accelerate fracture repair and healing of long-bone fractures.[6,7] A 2008 survey of 450 Canadian trauma surgeons revealed that 45% of surgeons incorporated bone growth stimulators into their treatment regimes for long-bone fractures.[8] One of the most used electrophysical techniques for acceleration of fracture repair is pulsed electromagnetic field (PEMF) stimulation. PEMF has been used widely to accelerate fracture repair and has been shown to reduce osteoclast resorption, to induce osteoid formation, to enhance bone mineralization, and to stimulate angiogenesis.[9,10] Although the potential efficacy of PEMF bone growth stimulation is supported by numerous clinical and basic research studies, Level I or II evidence to support the addition of PEMF to the conservative treatment of acute scaphoid fractures to accelerate bone healing is very limited.

MAIN QUESTION

What is the added value of pulsed electromagnetic field stimulation in the treatment of acute scaphoid fractures when considering the effect on fracture healing, functional outcome, and cost-effectiveness?

Current Opinion

Although PEMF bone growth stimulation has been used extensively to accelerate fracture repair, the efficacy of this technique in acute scaphoid fractures has never been thoroughly investigated. Therefore, no recommendations regarding the use of this technique for treatment of acute scaphoid fractures can be made.

Finding the Evidence

- Cochrane search: "scaphoid" AND "Pulsed electromagnetic" OR "pulsed electromagnetic field" OR "PEMF"
- Pubmed (Medline): "Scaphoid Bone" [Mesh] OR "Scaphoid" [tiab] OR "Scaphoid Fracture" [tiab] AND "Pulsed electromagnetic" [tiab] OR "Pulsed electromagnetic field" [tiab] OR "PEMF" [tiab]
- Only articles written in English, French, or German were included

Quality of the Evidence

Level I:

Randomized controlled trials: 3[11–13]

Level IV:

Case series: 2[14,15]

FINDINGS

Two of the randomized, double-blind, placebo-controlled trials reported on time to radiologic union,

	PEMF			Placebo				Mean Difference
Study or Subgroup	**Mean**	**SD**	**Total**	**Mean**	**SD**	**Total**	**Weight**	**IV, Random, 95% CI**
Hannemann 2012	10.375	10.781	24	7.552	6.184	29	35.7%	2.82 [−2.04, 7.69]
Hannemann 2014	10.429	12.5	51	7.74	4.289	51	64.3%	2.69 [−0.94, 6.32]
Total (95% CI)			**75**			**80**	**100.0%**	**2.74 [−0.17, 5.64]**

Heterogeneity: $Tau^2 = 0.00$; $Chi^2 = 0.00$, df = 1 (P=.97); $I^2 = 0\%$
Test for overall effect: Z = 1.84 (P=.07)

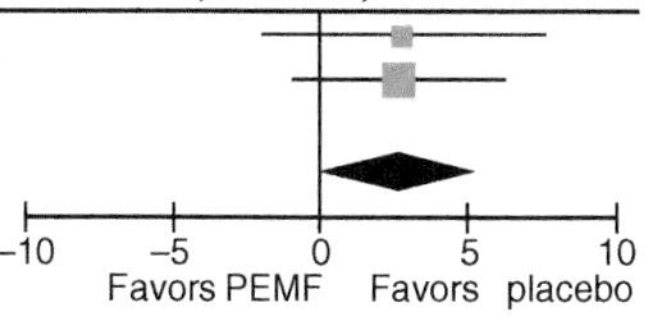

FIG. 23.2 Time until clinical union based on the absence of anatomic snuffbox tenderness for pulsed electromagnetic field (PEMF) treatment versus placebo treatment.

	PEMF			Placebo				Mean Difference
Study or Subgroup	**Mean**	**SD**	**Total**	**Mean**	**SD**	**Total**	**Weight**	**IV, Random, 95% CI**
Hannemann 2012	10.292	13.309	24	5.448	3.856	29	34.3%	4.84 [−0.66, 10.35]
Hannemann 2014	7.235	3.622	51	7.235	3.573	51	65.7%	0.00 [−1.40, 1.40]
Total (95% CI)			**75**			**80**	**100.0%**	**1.66 [−2.85, 6.17]**

Heterogeneity: $Tau^2 = 7.53$; $Chi^2 = 2.79$, df = 1 (P=.09); $I^2 = 64\%$
Test for overall effect: Z = 0.72 (P=.47)

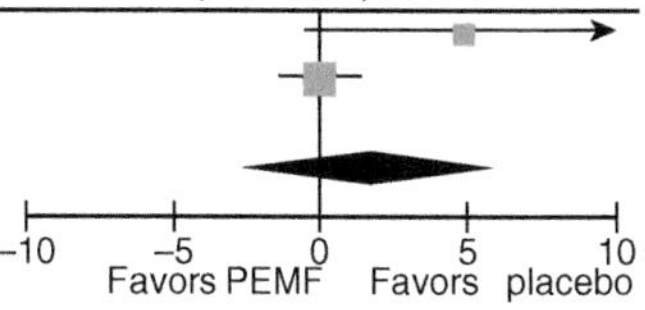

FIG. 23.3 Time until clinical union based on the absence of pain with longitudinal compression of the scaphoid for pulsed electromagnetic field (PEMF) treatment versus placebo treatment.

comparing PEMF with placebo as an adjunct to conservative treatment for acute scaphoid fractures.[12,13] Data could not be successfully pooled because outcome parameters were determined differently. One study used scaphoid radiographs to conform the presence of union[13] and the other study used multiplanar reconstruction CT scans.[12] Both studies, however, revealed no significant difference in time to radiologic union between the two groups (PEMF or placebo) as a result from log-rank analysis ($\chi^2 = 0.03$, $P = .32$[13] and $\chi^2 = 0.001$, $P = .975$,[12] respectively).

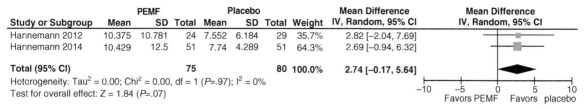

For time to clinical union, two of the randomized trials used the absence of anatomic snuffbox tenderness and the absence of pain with longitudinal compression of the scaphoid bone as clinical criteria for assessment of fracture consolidation.[12,13] Data for both tests could be successfully pooled for both studies. Concerning anatomic snuffbox tenderness, analysis based on homogenous groups revealed no significant difference in treatment effect for PEMF or placebo (MD = 2.74, 95% CI = −0.17 to 5.64, $P = .07$, $I^2 = 0\%$) (Fig. 23.2).

Concerning pain on longitudinal compression of the scaphoid, again no significant difference in treatment effect was observed between PEMF and placebo when considering time until clinical union. However, groups were quite heterogeneous (MD = 1.66, 95% CI = −2.85 to 6.17, $P = .47$, $I^2 = 64\%$) (Fig. 23.3).

All three randomized trials reported on functional outcome, comparing PEMF with placebo.[11–13] Two studies assessed functional outcome in terms of loss of wrist movement.[12,13] In both studies, wrist movement returned to normal at 12 weeks for both the PEMF and the placebo groups (<25% loss of wrist movement, $P = .92$ and $P = .54$, respectively).

One study used the Patient-Rated Wrist/Hand Evaluation (PRWHE) questionnaire to assess the level of fracture-related functional deficit and pain level from the patient's perspective.[11] No significant differences were found between the active PEMF group and the control group at any of the chosen time points (6, 9, 12, 24, and 52 weeks after injury) for the 102 included patients.

> The Patient Rated Wrist/Hand Evaluation (PRWHE) is a 15-item questionnaire that allows patients to rate the level of wrist pain and disability in activities of daily living via a 10-point categorical scale from 0 (no complaint) to 10 (worst possible complaint).[16]

In one randomized trial, a prospective economic evaluation of PEMF bone growth stimulation for acute scaphoid fractures was carried out from a social perspective.[11] All costs of PEMF treatment, including medical costs and costs due to productivity loss, were measured during 1 year and compared with costs of conservative treatment (care as usual) for nondisplaced, acute scaphoid fractures. A significant difference in costs at the expense of the PEMF group could be attributed entirely to the use of the PEMF device (difference of €719, 95% CI = €652–€772). Indeed, no significant differences in the amount of lost workdays were observed between the two groups (9.8 days for the PEMF group vs. 12.9 days for the placebo group, $P = .651$).

	PEMF		Placebo			Risk Ratio
Study or Subgroup	Events	Total	Events	Total	Weight	M-H, Fixed, 95% CI
Hannemann 2012	1	24	1	29	31.2%	1.21 [0.08, 18.32]
Hannemann 2014	4	51	2	51	68.8%	2.00 [0.38, 10.44]
Total (95% CI)		**75**		**80**	**100.0%**	**1.75 [0.43, 7.14]**
Total events	5		3			

Heterogeneity: $Chi^2 = 0.10$, df = 1 (P=.76); $I^2 = 0\%$
Test for overall effect: Z = 0.78 (P=.43)

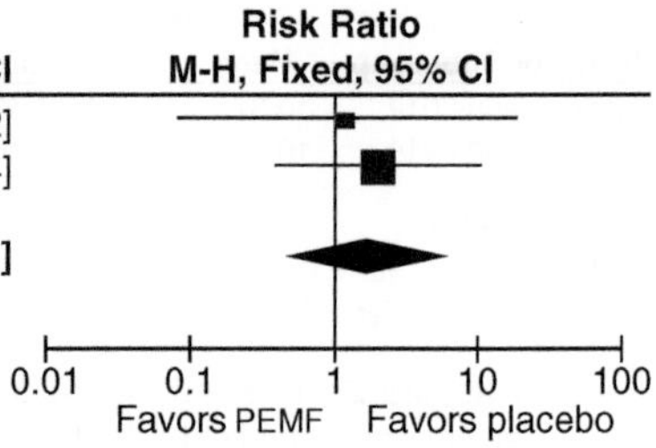

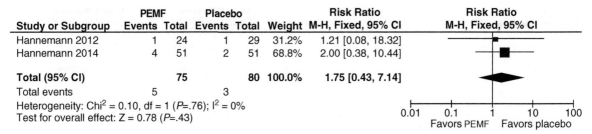

FIG. 23.4 Number of nonunions for pulsed electromagnetic field (PEMF) treatment versus placebo treatment.

Two randomized trials reported on the number of radiologically confirmed nonunions.[12,13] Data of both studies could be successfully pooled with homogeneous groups. There was no significant difference in the rate of nonunion for both groups across both studies (RR = 1.75, 95% CI = 0.43–7.14, P = .43, I^2 = 0%) (Fig. 23.4).

RECOMMENDATION

In patients with a nondisplaced fracture of the scaphoid, evidence suggests the following:

- Bone growth stimulation in acute scaphoid fractures by means of PEMF does not lead to accelerated healing of the fracture (overall quality: high).
- Bone growth stimulation in acute scaphoid fractures by means of PEMF does not lead to improved functional outcome at 1 year after injury (overall quality: high).
- Bone growth stimulation in acute scaphoid fractures by means of PEMF does not lead to a reduction in the number of nonunions (overall quality: high).
- Bone growth stimulation in acute scaphoid fractures by means of PEMF cannot be considered as a cost-effective treatment because it does not reduce the number of workdays lost with significantly higher treatment costs (overall quality: high).

CONCLUSION

Available Level I evidence has not demonstrated significant advantage from the use of PEMF treatment to justify routine application of PEMF bone growth stimulation in acute scaphoid fractures. We conclude that neither time to full union nor the number of nonunions in scaphoid fractures is significantly influenced by the use of PEMF. Because the length of unemployment in patients treated with PEMF is not significantly shorter than in patients treated conservatively in a below-elbow cast, PEMF treatment for acute scaphoid fractures is an inferior treatment compared with care as usual, when considering cost-effectiveness.

PANEL 2
Author's Preferred Technique (Related to Case Scenario)

In the represented case, conservative treatment in a below elbow cast is preferred over pulsed electromagnetic field bone growth stimulation. A CT scan is recommended prior to start of the treatment to rule out displacement, proximal pole localization, or comminution, because these factors are associated with an increased risk of nonunion after conservative treatment. In case of a nondisplaced scaphoid waist fracture, cast immobilization is recommended for 4–6 weeks. For evaluation of consolidation, again a CT-scan is recommended because radiographs are insufficiently reliable and accurate to diagnose union or nonunion after (conservative) treatment of scaphoid fractures.

DISCLOSURE

All named authors declare that they have no commercial or financial conflicts of interest to disclose, and none of the authors received any funding sources for this work.

REFERENCES

1. McQueen MM, Gelbke MK, Wakefield A, Will EM, Gaebler C. Percutaneous screw fixation versus conservative treatment for fractures of the waist of the scaphoid: a prospective randomised study. *J Bone Joint Surg Br Vol*. 2008;90(1):66–71.
2. Bond CD, Shin AY, McBride MT, Dao KD. Percutaneous screw fixation or cast immobilization for nondisplaced scaphoid fractures. *J Bone Joint Surg Am Vol*. 2001;83-A(4):483–488.
3. Ibrahim T, Qureshi A, Sutton AJ, Dias JJ. Surgical versus nonsurgical treatment of acute minimally displaced and undisplaced scaphoid waist fractures: pairwise and network meta-analyses of randomized controlled trials. *J Hand Surg*. 2011;36(11):1759–1768.e1751.

4. Buijze GA, Doornberg JN, Ham JS, Ring D, Bhandari M, Poolman RW. Surgical compared with conservative treatment for acute nondisplaced or minimally displaced scaphoid fractures: a systematic review and meta-analysis of randomized controlled trials. *J Bone Joint Surg Am Vol.* 2010;92(6):1534–1544.
5. van der Molen AB, Groothoff JW, Visser GJ, Robinson PH, Eisma WH. Time off work due to scaphoid fractures and other carpal injuries in The Netherlands in the period 1990 to 1993. *J Hand Surg Br.* 1999;24(2):193–198.
6. Mollon B, da Silva V, Busse JW, Einhorn TA, Bhandari M. Electrical stimulation for long-bone fracture-healing: a meta-analysis of randomized controlled trials. *J Bone Joint Surg Am Vol.* 2008;90(11):2322–2330.
7. Hannemann PF, Mommers EH, Schots JP, Brink PR, Poeze M. The effects of low-intensity pulsed ultrasound and pulsed electromagnetic fields bone growth stimulation in acute fractures: a systematic review and meta-analysis of randomized controlled trials. *Arch Orthop Trauma Surg.* 2014;134(8):1093–1106.
8. Busse JW, Morton E, Lacchetti C, Guyatt GH, Bhandari M. Current management of tibial shaft fractures: a survey of 450 Canadian orthopedic trauma surgeons. *Acta Orthop.* 2008;79(5):689–694.
9. Otter MW, McLeod KJ, Rubin CT. Effects of electromagnetic fields in experimental fracture repair. *Clin Orthop Relat Res.* 1998;(355):S90–S104.
10. Jansen JH, van der Jagt OP, Punt BJ, et al. Stimulation of osteogenic differentiation in human osteoprogenitor cells by pulsed electromagnetic fields: an in vitro study. *BMC Musculoskelet Disord.* 2010;11:188.
11. Hannemann PF, Essers BA, Schots JP, Dullaert K, Poeze M, Brink PR. Functional outcome and cost-effectiveness of pulsed electromagnetic fields in the treatment of acute scaphoid fractures: a cost-utility analysis. *BMC Musculoskelet Disord.* 2015;16:84.
12. Hannemann PF, van Wezenbeek MR, Kolkman KA, et al. CT scan-evaluated outcome of pulsed electromagnetic fields in the treatment of acute scaphoid fractures: a randomised, multicentre, double-blind, placebo-controlled trial. *Bone Joint J.* 2014;96-B(8):1070–1076.
13. Hannemann PF, Gottgens KW, van Wely BJ, et al. The clinical and radiological outcome of pulsed electromagnetic field treatment for acute scaphoid fractures: a randomised double-blind placebo-controlled multicentre trial. *J Bone Joint Surg Br Vol.* 2012;94(10):1403–1408.
14. Adams BD, Frykman GK, Taleisnik J. Treatment of scaphoid nonunion with casting and pulsed electromagnetic fields: a study continuation. *J Hand Surg.* 1992;17(5):910–914.
15. Frykman GK, Taleisnik J, Peters G, et al. Treatment of nonunited scaphoid fractures by pulsed electromagnetic field and cast. *J Hand Surg.* 1986;11(3):344–349.
16. MacDermid JC, Turgeon T, Richards RS, Beadle M, Roth JH. Patient rating of wrist pain and disability: a reliable and valid measurement tool. *J Orthop Trauma.* 1998;12(8):577–586.

CHAPTER 24

Diagnosing the Malunited Scaphoid

TIMOTHY A. COUGHLIN, BMBS, BMEDSCI, MRCS • FAIZ S. SHIVJI, BMBS, BMEDSCI, MRCS • MICHAEL R. GALE, MA, MBBCHIR, FRCS (TR&ORTH) • DAREN P. FORWARD, MA, FRCS, DM

KEY POINTS

- The malunited scaphoid waist fracture usually results in a humpback deformity.
- The humpback deformity consists of flexion of the distal fragment in the sagittal plane, ulnar deviation of the distal fragment in the frontal plane, and pronation of the distal fragment.
- The best imaging modality to determine scaphoid malunion is using CT scan with the slices taken in the true longitudinal axis of the scaphoid.
- The measurable parameters on a CT scan relevant to scaphoid malunion are the lateral intrascaphoid angle (LISA), anteroposterior intrascaphoid angle (APISA), height to length ratio (HLR), and the dorsal cortical angle (DCA).
- Abnormal scaphoid morphology has not yet been shown to correlate with outcome, but if the malunion results in dorsal intercalated segment instability (DISI), this is associated with poorer outcomes.

PANEL 1
Case Scenario

A 35-year-old male manual worker visited the elective hand clinic with complaints of radial-sided right wrist pain for the past 6 months. He describes the pain as mild to moderate, but it does not prevent him from working. He "sprained" his wrist 2 years ago, but never sought medical advice. Radiographs show a united scaphoid waist fracture with slight dorsal intercalated segment instability. A CT scan suggests the presence of a malunited fracture of the scaphoid with a "humpback" deformity shown by an increased lateral intrascaphoid angle of 40 degrees and height to length ratio of 0.8.

The decision was made to undertake corrective scaphoid osteotomy with Russe anterior corticocancellous bone grafting. The fracture went on to unite, although at 2 years there was evidence of moderate radiocarpal and scaphotrapezial arthritis. The patient was nonetheless happy with his result and has returned to work in his heavy manual job.

Was the decision to operate the key to his good clinical outcome? Could the development of arthritis have been mitigated by either an earlier presentation or a different surgical strategy (and does it matter)?

IMPORTANCE OF THE PROBLEM

Scaphoid fractures that unite usually go on to good outcomes, but in some patients there are persisting symptoms.[1,2] Most acute scaphoid fractures are nondisplaced and therefore go on to asymptomatic union.[3] It is fractures where there is early displacement that either goes on to nonunion or malunion. Up to 40% of scaphoid fractures are missed at initial presentation, so inevitably some of those with early displacement are missed.[4]

The typical deformity of a malunited scaphoid waist fracture includes flexion of the distal fragment in the sagittal plane, ulnar deviation of the distal fragment in the frontal plane, and pronation of the distal fragment. The resulting deformity is referred to as the humpback deformity.[5] As shown in Fig. 24.1A and B, the result of this deformity is an overall shortening of the scaphoid length and an increase in the height as seen in the sagittal plane with a resultant increase in the HLR.

Early diagnosis is sadly not a solution to the problem of malunion. Even in patients where the fracture is promptly diagnosed and surgery is performed, malunion is not uncommon. Filan[6] reported a malunion rate of only 2% in their series of 431 patients treated with Herbert screw fixation, whereas Jiranek[7] reported

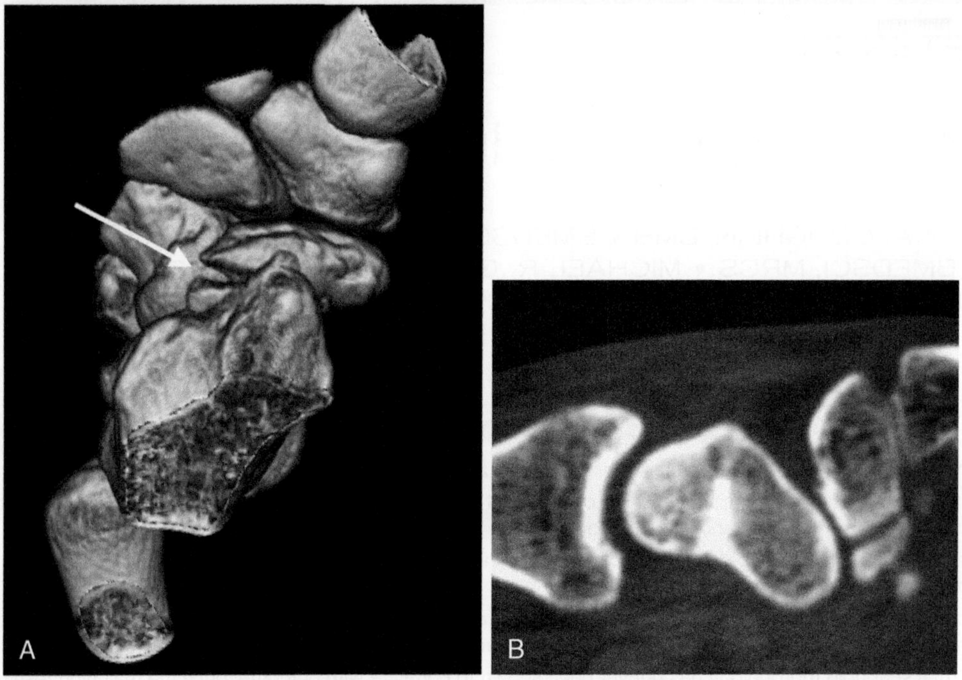

FIG. 24.1 **(A)** CT reconstruction of a fractured scaphoid showing the preunion position of displacement as shown by the white arrow, which leads to the humpback deformity. **(B)** CT scan of malunited scaphoid fracture exhibiting the foreshortening and flexion classical of the humpback deformity.

a malunion rate of 50% in 25 patients treated with Russe anterior corticocancellous bone grafting. It would be reasonable to assume that a patient surgically treated who has an equal degree of eventual malunion as a patient treated nonoperatively will have a worse outcome because of increased adhesions and scar tissue formation. There is no published incidence of scaphoid fracture malunion, but it is likely underdiagnosed.

The consequences of malunion are not easy to predict. Amadio et al. reported in their series of 45 patients that malunited scaphoid fractures elicit poorer clinical and radiographic outcomes.[8] Patients with greater than 45 degrees of LISA had a satisfactory clinical outcome only 27% (4 of 15 patients) of the time. Of these 15 patients, 54 developed posttraumatic arthritis. However, Forward et al. concluded that there was no significant relationship between outcome measures (grip strength, Patient Evaluation Measure, Disabilities of the Arm, Shoulder and Hand [DASH] scores) and degrees of malunion (HLR, the DCA, and the LISA) in 42 patients at 1 year.[9]

Malunion is known to cause carpal collapse with development of DISI.[5,10] Wrists with a scaphoid malunion perform less well on tests of range of movement and grip strength and develop radiocarpal and scaphotrapezial arthritis in a predictable pattern.[7,11]

Scaphoid malunion is an unfortunate consequence of some scaphoid fractures, whether diagnosed acutely and appropriately managed or occurring in patients with a delayed presentation. The key is therefore to demonstrate how best to diagnose the complication and to demonstrate the parameters that lead to poorer outcomes and should therefore lead to consideration of intervention.

MAIN QUESTION

What is the best imaging modality to diagnose a malunited scaphoid fracture and what parameters should be used to assess the need for surgical intervention?

Current Opinion

CT is the imaging modality of choice used to assess scaphoid malunion. The CT images should be taken in the long axis of the scaphoid. The parameters that can be measured are as follows:

1. LISA
2. APISA

3. HLR
4. DCA

There is insufficient evidence to demonstrate that any of these parameters are associated with poorer outcomes.

In addition, extrascaphoid measurements can be made on either CT or radiographs:

1. Radiolunate (RL) angle
2. Scapholunate (SL) angle

There is some evidence suggesting that an abnormal radiolunate angle correlates with poor outcome measures.

Finding the Evidence

Cochrane: Search strategy: "scaphoid" (studies identified: 1)
Pubmed (review): Search strategy: "scaph*" AND malun*" (studies identified: 25)
Pubmed: Search strategy: "scaph*" AND malun*" (studies identified: 112)
Embase: Search strategy" "scaph* AND malun*" (studies identified: 100)
Articles that were not in English were excluded.

Quality of the Evidence

Level I:
Randomized trials: 2
Level II:
Cohort studies: 5
Level IV:
Case series: 10
Level V:
Expert opinion: 7

FINDINGS

Choice of Imaging Modality

Sanders established that CT scanning the wrist in the true longitudinal axis of the scaphoid allows a full assessment of its anatomy, deformity, and fracture pattern.[12] Although this was a case series of just three patients, this method is now widely recognized as the imaging technique of choice. Most studies of accuracy and reliability of the various imaging techniques focus on diagnosing displacement in the acute fracture, but this information can probably be extended to the assessment of malunion.

Compared with plain radiography, CT yields higher sensitivity and specificity, along with better intra- and interobserver reliability (moderate to good vs. poor to moderate-poor) when assessing displacement of scaphoid fractures.[13]

Bone scintigraphy has been shown to be extremely sensitive in diagnosing acute fracture (in some studies 100%), but of little use in assessing scaphoid morphology.[14]

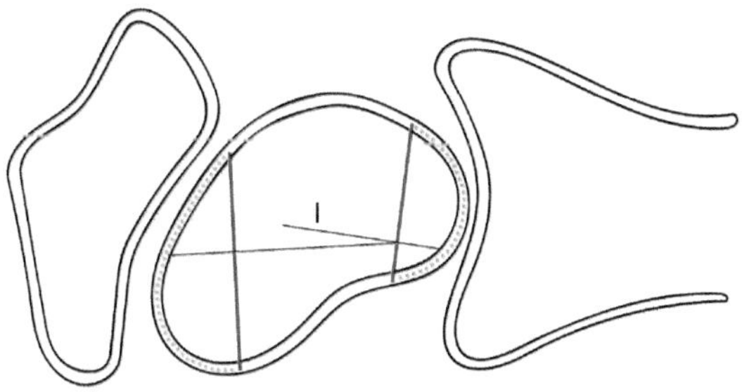

FIG. 24.2 The lateral intrascaphoid angle (I) is the angle between two perpendicular lines drawn from the proximal and distal articular joint surfaces, respectively.

Comparing CT with MRI, de Zwart et al. showed that MRI is more sensitive in diagnosing acute fractures, especially trabecular fractures where no cortical break exists.[14] In the context of malunion, MRI can also be used to determine scaphoid morphology with reasonable reliability, but it ultimately loses out to CT because of difficulties in identifying joint surface margins with less clear delineation of the cortex and lower fidelity images.

Bain et al. have described the optimal patient positioning to allow such an image to be produced, with minimum patient discomfort.[15] Patients are positioned prone in the scanner, with the wrist placed above their head, and lying in a pronated, radially deviated, and neutrally flexed position. The scanning plane is directed along the thumb metacarpal, which corresponds to the scaphoid longitudinal axis.

Measurable Parameters

Various measurements have been described to determine the degree of malunion. The majority of these are based on CT, although they can be applied to MRI images.

Lateral Intrascaphoid Angle

The LISA is determined on CT from the central longitudinal slice on a sagittal view. Lines are drawn perpendicular to the proximal and distal articular surfaces as shown in Fig. 24.2.

Amadio et al. reviewed 46 scaphoid fractures at a mean of 44.7 months postunion (range 6–108 months).[8] Patients with a LISA of more than 45 degrees (n = 15) had a satisfactory outcome 27% (four patients) of the time, and 54% (nine patients) developed posttraumatic arthritis. This study therefore suggested that a malunion causing a LISA of more than 35 degrees is unacceptable.

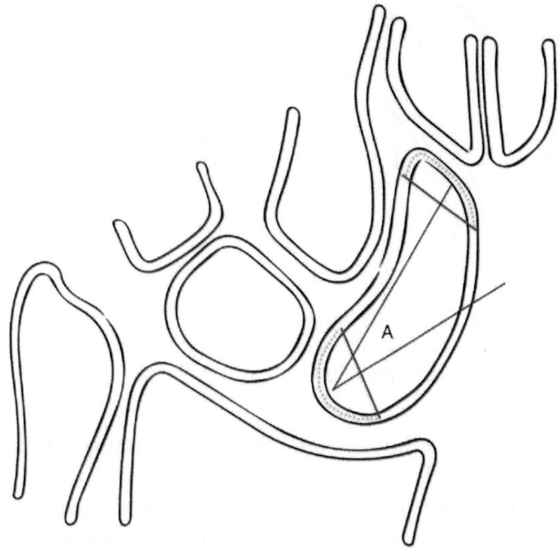

FIG. 24.3 The anteroposterior intrascaphoid angle (A) is the angle between two perpendicular lines drawn from the proximal and distal articular joint surfaces, respectively, in the same way as for the lateral intrascaphoid angle but from coronal CT cuts.

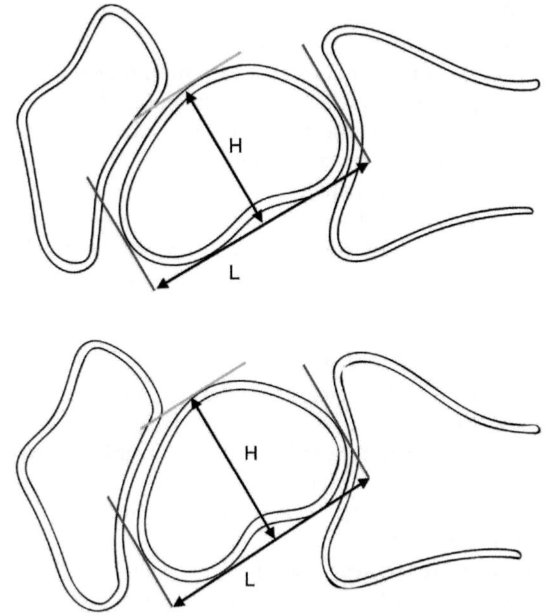

FIG. 24.4 **(A)** The height to length ratio (HLR) is measured using a baseline along the volar scaphoid with the length (L) being represented by two lines at right angles from the most proximal and distal points and the height (H) measures at right angles to the most dorsal point. **(B)** In the humpback deformity the height is increased and the length is decreased. Malunion is considered to have occurred if the HLR is >0.6.

Anteroposterior Intrascaphoid Angle

The APISA is measured by the intersection of the two perpendicular lines drawn from the distal and proximal scaphoid articular surfaces on a coronal view as shown in Fig. 24.3.[16] Most studies concentrate on the other measurements that are taken on the single sagittal view.

It has been difficult to establish an accurate normal value for the APISA, but 40 degrees (range 32–46 degrees) has been suggested. Amadio found that, in his group of patients, half of those with a poor outcome had a normal APISA.[8]

Height to Length Ratio

Using the central slice of the sagittal longitudinal reconstruction, the HLR is measured by measuring a line drawn along the palmar aspect of the scaphoid with two perpendicular lines intersecting it at the most proximal and distal extent of the scaphoid cortex to give a value for length (L) as shown in Fig. 24.4A. The maximum height of the scaphoid is measured with a third perpendicular line drawn to the maximum extent of the dorsal cortex to give height (H). The ratio is calculated by dividing the height by the length.

ten Berg et al. have produced normal ranges for the HLR in the sagittal and coronal planes. CT scans from 74 uninjured wrists were used to calculate the mean HLR in sagittal and coronal planes.[17] This was compared with the mean HLRs for 26 fibrous nonunions. The mean HLR for uninjured wrists in the sagittal plane was 0.61 with a 95% normal range from 0.54 to 0.69 and in the coronal plane 0.42 with a range from 0.36 to 0.48. The HLRs for nonunions were significantly larger than the uninjured wrists. This paper suggested that by calculating the HLR in both planes, the detection rate for malunion could be increased. However, in this paper the difference was not significant. With these data and previous literature, the normal HLR, when measured from the most central longitudinal slice in the sagittal plane of the CT, can be described as equal to or less than 0.6.[9,18]

When malunion and a humpback deformity has occurred, the HLR is increased as the length decreases and height increases as shown in Fig. 24.4B. Recent research suggests that an HLR of >0.73 can be associated with the development of DISI.[19]

The HLR has been shown to be more reproducible than the LISA and DCA.[13,20] Intraobserver reliability is reported as moderate with interobserver reliability moderate to excellent.[9,13,15] Level IV evidence from Lee et al. showed excellent interobserver reliability

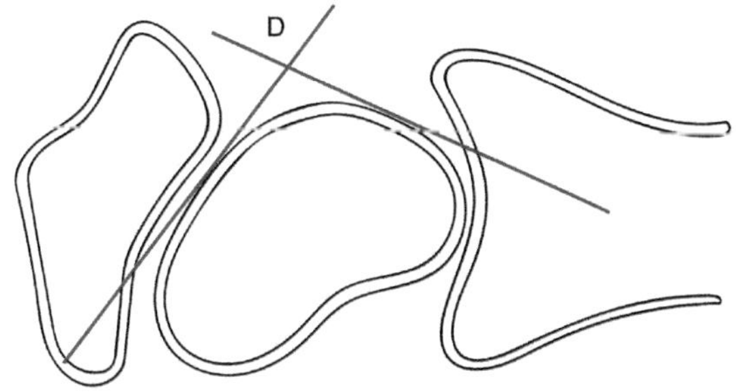

FIG. 24.5 The dorsal cortical angle (D) is the angle between two lines drawn along the proximal and distal cortices of the dorsal aspect of the scaphoid.

(ICC = 0.826) with 2 observers assessing 25 malunited scaphoids.[18]

The HLR has not been found to correlate with clinical outcomes. Lee et al. found no correlation between HLR and pain, Mayo scores, DASH scores, or the Patient Evaluation Measure in patients with a mean follow-up of 81 months.[18] Similar results were found by Forward and Afshar.[9,16]

Dorsal Cortical Angle

The DCA is measured by two intersecting lines drawn along the dorsal cortices of the proximal and distal scaphoid as shown in Fig. 24.5. Bain et al. described the normal DCA in a small series as 139 ± 25 degrees.[20] A retrospective study comparing 17 normal scaphoids versus fractured contralateral scaphoids again showed the normal DCA to be 139.1 ± 1 degree.[16] Unfortunately, there is little high-quality additional evidence to prove what the normal DCA range should be.

The DCA was also shown to have excellent intraobserver reliability and moderate interobserver reliability by Bain.[20] However, in a more recent study involving 15 normal patients with CT scans in three different planes (radial, ulna, and intermediate), the intraobserver and interobserver reliability was poor.[13] Poor reproducibility was also found by Bhat in a series of 50 patients.[3] Similarly, reproducibility of the DCA measured via CT by Forward et al. in a study of 42 scaphoid waist fractures was so poor that the authors felt it was impossible to define the "normal" ranges for the DCA using their data.[9]

In a series of 65 scaphoid fractures treated with internal fixation, Megerle et al. found a mean DCA of 106.9 degrees (range 50–145 degrees).[21] At a mean of 45-month follow-up, the DCA was found not to significantly correlate with range of movement, grip strength, pain, or progression to carpal collapse. Afshar et al. also found no correlation between the DCA and clinical outcomes.[16]

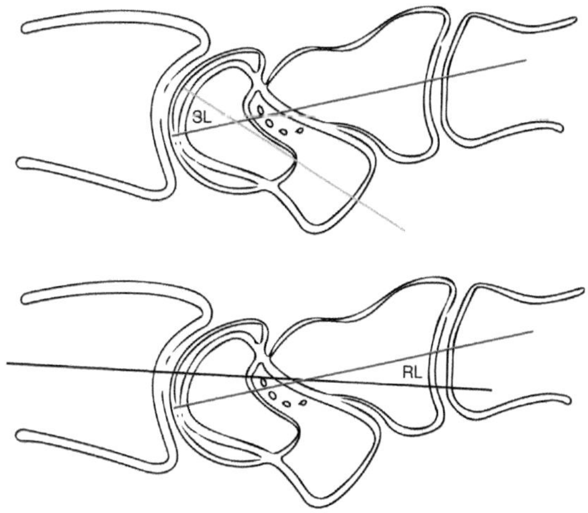

FIG. 24.6 The scapholunate angle (SL) is measured on a true lateral radiograph by the angle formed from intersecting lines along the axis of the lunate and the scaphoid. The radiolunate angle (RL) is taken from the same view as the intersection of the long axis of the radius and lunate.

Carpal Alignment

In contrast to intrascaphoid measurements, the gross carpal alignment measured on lateral radiographs has been shown to correlate significantly with the aforementioned wrist outcome measures. The two parameters that can be measured are the SL and RL angles as shown in Fig. 24.6. The upper limit of normal for the RL angle is 10 degrees of dorsal angulation and for the SL angle is 60 degrees.

A radiolunate angle of more than 10 degrees, indicating a DISI, led to a significantly lower grip strength, worse DASH and Mayo scores, and higher pain scores.[21–23] The authors concluded that a DISI deformity, as evidenced by a high RL angle, suggests carpal instability and poor outcomes. von Steiger and Sennwald found higher rates of symptomatic arthritis in patients with DISI deformity than in those without DISI deformity 25 years after scaphoid fixation.[24] Indeed, there is some evidence that reducing DISI deformity by scaphoid corrective osteotomy can improve wrist pain and function.[5]

RECOMMENDATIONS

- The best imaging modality to diagnose a malunited scaphoid is CT. To make a complete assessment of the six parameters, the slices need to be taken or reformatted to the long axis of the scaphoid sagittally, a coronal view and a sagittal view in the long axis of the forearm (overall quality: moderate).

- The intrascaphoid parameters that can be measured are the LISA, APISA, HLR, and DCA (overall quality: moderate).
- In essence, the intrascaphoid parameters measure the presence of a humpback deformity, but even the presence of the deformity, putting aside the problems with quantifying it, cannot be proven to result in poorer outcomes (overall quality: moderate).
- What may be relevant to outcome is the degree of DISI deformity produced (or allowed) by the scaphoid malunion (overall quality: low).

CONCLUSION

Evidence for each measurement of malunion as an independent indication for corrective surgery has not yet been demonstrated. From the evidence presented in this chapter, it is possible to suggest that with a combination of a LISA of >35 degrees, an HLA of >0.73, and an RL angle of >10 degrees, corrective surgery is easier to justify with the aim of improving function if not preventing arthritis.

REFERENCES

1. Hambidge JE, Desai VV, Schranz PJ, Compson JP, Davis TRC, Barton NJ. Acute fractures of the scaphoid. Treatment by cast immobilisation with the wrist in flexion or extension? *J Bone Joint Surg Eur*. 1999;81:91–92.
2. Lindstrom G, Nystrom A. Incidence of post-traumatic arthrosis after primary healing of scaphoid fractures: a clinical and radiological study. *J Hand Surg Eur*. 1990;15:11–13.
3. Bhat M, McCarthy M, Davis TRC, Oni JA, Dawson S. MRI and plain radiography in the assessment of displaced fractures of the waist of the carpal scaphoid. *J Bone Joint Surg Eur*. 2004;86:705–713.
4. Waizenegger M, Barton NJ, David TR, Waistie ML. Clinical signs in scaphoid fractures. *J Hand Surg Br*. 1994;19:743–746.
5. Nakamura P, Imaeda T, Miura T. Scaphoid malunion. *J Bone Joint Surg Eur*. 1991;73:134–137.
6. Filan SL, Herbert TJ. Herbert screw fixation of scaphoid fractures. *J Bone Joint Surg Br*. 1996;78(4):519–529.
7. Jiranek WA, Ruby LK, Millender LB, Bankoff MS, Newberg A. Long-term results after Russe bone-grafting: the effect of malunion of the scaphoid. *J Bone Joint Surg Am*. 1992;74:1217–1228.
8. Amadio PC, Berquist TH, Smith DK, Ilstrup DM, Cooney 3rd WP, Linscheid RL. Scaphoid malunion. *J Hand Surg Am*. 1989;14(4):679–687.
9. Forward DP, Singh HP, Dawson S, Davis TRC. The clinical outcome of scaphoid malunion at 1 year. *J Hand Surg Eur Vol*. 2009;34E(1):40–46.
10. Linscheid RL, Dobyns JH, Beabout JW, Bryan RS. Traumatic instability of the wrist. Diagnosis, classification, and pathomechanics. *J Bone Joint Surg Am*. 1972;54(8):1612–1632.
11. Burgess RC. The effect of a simulated scaphoid malunion on wrist motion. *J Hand Surg Am*. 1987;12(5):774–776.
12. Sanders WE. Evaluation of the humpback scaphoid by computed tomography in the longitudinal axial plane of the scaphoid. *J Hand Surg*. 1988;13(2):182–187.
13. Ring D, Patterson JD, Levitz S, Wang C, Jupiter JB. Both scanning plane and observer affect measurements of scaphoid deformity. *J Hand Surg Am*. 2005;30:696–701.
14. de Zwart AD, Beeres FJP, Rhemrev SJ, et al. Comparison of MRI, CT and bone scintigraphy for suspected scaphoid fractures. *Eur J Trauma Emerg Surg*. 2016;42:725.
15. Bain GI, Bennett JD, Richards RS, Slethaug GP, Roth JH. Longitudinal computed tomography of the scaphoid: a new technique. *Skeletal Radiol*. 1995;24(4):271–273.
16. Afshar A, Mohammadi A, Zohrabi K, Navaeifar N, Sami SH, Taleb H. Correlation of reconstructed scaphoid morphology with clinical outcomes. *Arch Bone Joint Surg*. 2015;3(4):244–249.
17. ten Berg PW, Dobbe JG, Strackee SD, Streekstra GJ. Quantifying scaphoid malalignment based upon height-to-length ratios obtained by 3-dimensional computed tomography. *J Hand Surg Am*. 2015;40(1):67–73.
18. Lee CH, Lee KH, Lee BG, Kim DY, Choi WS. Clinical outcome of scaphoid malunion as a result of scaphoid fracture nonunion surgical treatment: a 5-year minimum follow-up study. *Orthop Traumatol Surg Res*. 2015;101(3):359–363.
19. Kim JH, Lee KH, Lee BG, Lee CH, Kim SJ, Choi WS. Dorsal intercalated segmental instability associated with malunion of a reconstructed scaphoid. *J Hand Surg Eur Vol*. 2017;42(3):240–245.
20. Bain GI, Bennett JD, MacDermid JC, Slethaug GP, Richards RS, Roth JH. Measurement of the scaphoid humpback deformity using longitudinal computed tomography: intra- and interobserver variability using various measurement techniques. *J Hand Surg Am*. 1998;23(1):76–81.
21. Megerle K, Harenberg PS, Germann G, Hellmich S. Scaphoid morphology and clinical outcomes in scaphoid reconstructions. *Injury*. 2012;43(3):306–310.
22. Alho A, Kankaanpää U. Management of fractured scaphoid bone. A prospective study of 100 fractures. *Acta Orthop Scand*. 1975;46(5):737–743.
23. Roh YH, Noh JH, Lee BK, et al. Reliability and validity of carpal alignment measurements in evaluating deformities of scaphoid fractures. *Arch Orthop Trauma Surg*. 2014;134(6):887–893.
24. Steiger von R, Sennwald G. Late results of operated scaphoid pseudoarthroses. *Handchir Mikrochir Plast Chir*. 1990;22:152–155.

CHAPTER 25

Three-Dimensional Planning of Scaphoid Malunion and Nonunion Correction

PAUL W.L. TEN BERG, MD • SIMON D. STRACKEE, MD, PHD

KEY POINTS

- The importance of restoring scaphoid alignment in nonunion surgery and the advisability of an osteotomy in malunion treatment are currently areas of debate.
- Evidence suggests that three-dimensional (3D) surgical planning may improve the precision of fragment realignment in a subset of scaphoid nonunions.
- Based on our literature search, there are no reports on the 3D surgical planning in the treatment of scaphoid malunions.
- Planning software enables assessing fragment malalignment, both pre- and postoperatively, which may improve investigating the relationship between reconstructed scaphoid morphology and clinical outcome in future studies.

PANEL 1
Case Scenario

A right-handed 15-year-old boy was referred to the plastic surgery department because of a left-sided scaphoid waist nonunion with a *dorsal intercalated segment instability* deformity, as shown on radiographs (Fig. 25.1). An additional computed tomography (CT) scan showed an evident *humpback deformity* and cystic changes in the nonunion area (Fig. 25.2). Might three-dimensional (3D) CT-based planning help guiding the reconstruction with a structural bone graft?

IMPORTANCE OF THE PROBLEM

In scaphoid waist nonunions, fragment displacement, often manifested as *a humpback deformity*, is common. Osseous union with the proximal and distal scaphoid pole in a displaced configuration results in a so-called malunion.[1] It remains a surgical challenge to restore the anatomy of a scaphoid nonunion or malunion by realigning the fragments, because of the small and complex anatomy of the scaphoid.[2] Moreover, fragment displacement is a 3D problem.[3–5] Besides a flexion deformity in the sagittal plane, there may also be a rotational deformity in the axial plane, which may be difficult to assess on standard radiography or fluoroscopy.

There is much controversy about the clinical consequences of a scaphoid malunion.[6] Some clinical series suggested that a scaphoid malunion will lead to pain, loss of motion, and an increased risk of carpal osteoarthritis in the long-term.[7–10] Contrary, other clinical studies observed no relationship of malunion with range of motion and grip strength, nor with patient satisfaction.[6,11] It is likely that this controversy can be explained by the less reliable use of standard two-dimensional imaging tools to evaluate the level of scaphoid malalignment.[12–14] The importance of restoring scaphoid alignment in scaphoid nonunion surgery and the advisability of osteotomy in malunion treatment remain, therefore, areas of debate.[14] Nevertheless, it seems that in the treatment of scaphoid nonunions, many surgeons agree that a restoration as close as possible to the original anatomy would benefit patient outcome and should be pursued in additional to fracture healing.[4]

In the past decades, radiologic software developments have enabled planning scaphoid reconstructions,

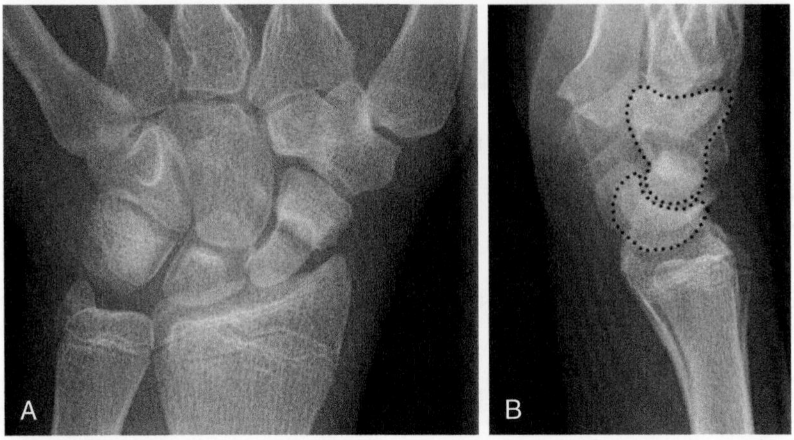

FIG. 25.1 Preoperative radiographs of a left-sided wrist following a scaphoid waist nonunion, with an approximate duration of 4 years. **(A)** Anteroposterior and **(B)** lateral views. In the lateral view, a pathologic extended posture of the lunate (*dotted line*) relative to the capitate (*dotted line*) is notable.

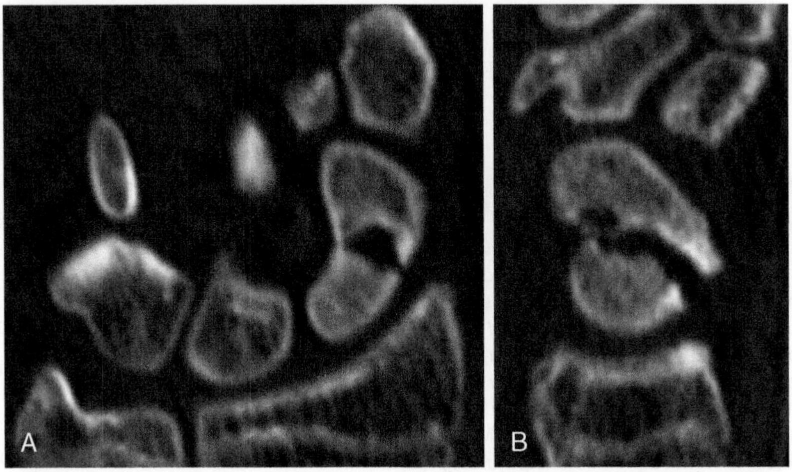

FIG. 25.2 Preoperative CT scan showing cystic changes around the nonunion area in the waist area. **(A)** Coronal and **(B)** sagittal CT slice. The sagittal slice clearly shows a *humpback* deformity.

which become increasingly accessible for clinical use. This may help guiding anatomic fragment reduction and improving the anatomic restoration. The operative plan, however, only works effectively if it can be transferred to the actual surgical procedure. *Rapid prototyping* may offer a solution, by creating patient-specific physical parts, including reduction guides, based on 3D CT-based patient computer data. In this chapter, a review of medical literature is conducted on the existing evidence of the surgical benefits of 3D planning techniques in scaphoid reconstructions.

The humpback deformity is a typical deformity associated with scaphoid waist nonunions in which the distal scaphoid fragment lies in a flexed position relative to the proximal fragment. This deformity is the result of a disturbed carpal equilibrium caused by the breakage of the bony link between the first and second carpal rows. The proximal fragment now acts as an extension of the lunate, which may follow its natural tendency to extend, whereas the distal scaphoid fragment rotates into flexion. The pathologic extended posture of the lunate is also known as *dorsal intercalated segment instability* deformity.

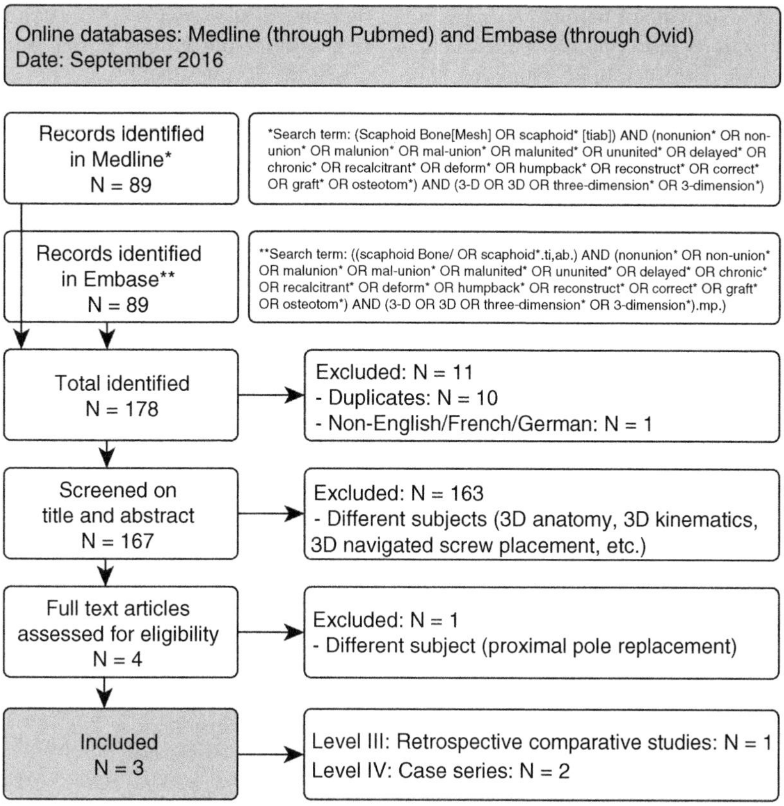

FIG. 25.3 Flow chart of the online search strategy in Medline and Embase databases.

> *Rapid prototyping* comprises several techniques used to rapidly manufacture scale models of physical parts or prototypes based on virtual 3D computer information, which have become available in the late 1980s. Medical research using rapid prototyping was initially focused on craniofacial and dental surgery to improve planning strategies. Currently, the manufacturing of models is usually done with 3D printers and is used in many surgical specialties, including orthopedic and hand/wrist surgery.

MAIN QUESTION

What is the additional value of 3D planning on the precision of fragment reduction in scaphoid malunion and nonunion corrections?

Current Opinion

There is currently no consensus about the optimal strategy for corrective surgery in scaphoid nonunion treatment.[15] Three-dimensional surgical planning strategies may result in a more precise fragment reduction than conventional reduction techniques. It is unclear whether the potential incremental surgical benefits are worth the costs.

Finding the Evidence

An online literature search was conducted in the Cochrane database of systematic reviews and both the Medline and Embase databases through Pubmed and Ovid search engines, respectively.

- In the Cochrane database, the following search term was used: "scaphoid."
- In Medline and Embase databases, we used Medical Subject Headings (MeSH) (=scaphoid bone) or Subject Heading (=scaphoid bone), respectively, using free search terms in title and abstract with (=scaphoid*), and using free search terms in all fields with truncation. The search strategy in Medline and Embase is described in Fig. 25.3.
- After removing duplicates in EndNote X7 (Thomas Reuter, London, United Kingdom), all titles and abstracts were retrieved for eligibility assessment. If eligibility criteria were met, articles were obtained and reviewed.

- *Inclusion criteria* were (1) clinical reports focusing on scaphoid reconstructions including the realignment of the proximal and distal scaphoid segments; (2) reports including techniques using 3D planning software and/or custom manufactured patient-specific operative tools; and (3) availability of postoperative data regarding the precision of the fragment reduction or carpal realignment.
- *Exclusion criteria* were (1) reports focusing on conventional planning strategies including standard preoperative radiography and CT, or intraoperative fluoroscopy; (2) languages other than English, French, and German.
- After final selection, all articles were reviewed with special attention to the applied planning strategy, reduction outcome, and the quality of the study.

Quality of the Evidence

Level III:

Retrospective comparative studies: 1 (2016[16])

Level IV:

Case series: 2 (2005,[17] 2016[18])

FINDINGS

No relevant articles were found in the Cochrane database. In the Medline and Embase databases, three articles[16–18] met the inclusion criteria (Fig. 25.3). In the three articles, the described preoperative plan included the usage of a virtual mirrored 3D model of the contralateral intact scaphoid as anatomic template to find the optimal post-reduction position of the scaphoid nonunion fragments. All articles included scaphoid nonunions with a fracture in the middle third or at the junction between the middle and proximal third. The articles, however, used different reduction techniques and outcome measures and are therefore discussed separately.

In a retrospective comparative studies, Schweizer et al.[16] experimented on fragment repositioning using patient-specific intraoperative 3D printed reduction guides based on virtual planning. To this end, a newly developed reduction technique was applied in nine scaphoid nonunion patients (case group) and compared with the outcome of 13 scaphoid nonunion patients treated with a conventional freehand reduction technique (control group). The new reduction technique was based on two consecutive guides. A prereduction guide, which snugly fitted the scaphoid surfaces, was used to find the insertion points of two parallel K-wires into both fragments. A postreduction guide was then used to manipulate the K-wires to define the reduced fragment position, as virtually planned. The study outcome was based on 3D CT analysis of residual fragment displacement based on the difference in position of the distal part between the operated and contralateral scaphoid, relative to the position of the proximal part, in 3D space. This is comparable with the technique as described in Fig. 25.4. In the case group, fragment reduction was significantly more precise in terms of the residual angulation/rotation ($P = .001$). This study,[16] however, showed considerable methodological limitations, regarding the selection of the cases and controls. Cases and controls were recruited in different periods and were not comparable indicating a potential selection bias. More controls showed osteonecrosis of the proximal pole and carpal osteoarthritis at baseline. In addition, most controls were treated with vascularized and structural grafts, whereas most cases were treated with compressed cancellous bone grafts. These limitations hamper reliably comparing outcome between groups, lowering the quality of evidence.

In a single patient case, after a preliminary cadaveric study, Haefeli et al.[18] experimented on a titanium printed guide to define the reduced fragment positions as virtually planned. This single patient-specific guide consisted of a proximal and distal pad, which also snuggly fitted the scaphoid surfaces and were connected by a small bridge crossing the nonunion gap. The study outcome included 3D CT analysis of residual fragment displacement based on a distance map between the reduced fragment models and the superimposed contralateral intact scaphoid model. Maximum surface-to-surface differences were less than 1.5 mm, which were interpreted as an indication for a good repositioning. Based on the preliminary cadaveric study,[18] the authors noted that finding the correct position was especially difficult in models with a small proximal pole.

In a clinical series of seven scaphoid nonunion patients, Murase et al.[17] used full-sized stereolithography models to visually interpret the optimal reduced fragment configuration during surgery. These patient-specific models included models of the scaphoid nonunion with the fragments in displaced configuration, models with the fragments in reduced configuration as virtually planned, and models of the contralateral intact scaphoid. Outcome measures included the level of carpal realignment on pre- and postoperative radiographs. The scapholunate angle (SLA) normalized from 70 to 50 degrees, the radiolunate angle (RLA) from −6 to 5 degrees, and the capitolunate angle (CLA) from −4 to 4 degrees. The mean SLA, RLA, and CLA of the contralateral wrist were 50, 5 and 9 degrees. In addition, in three patients, models of the estimated bone defect

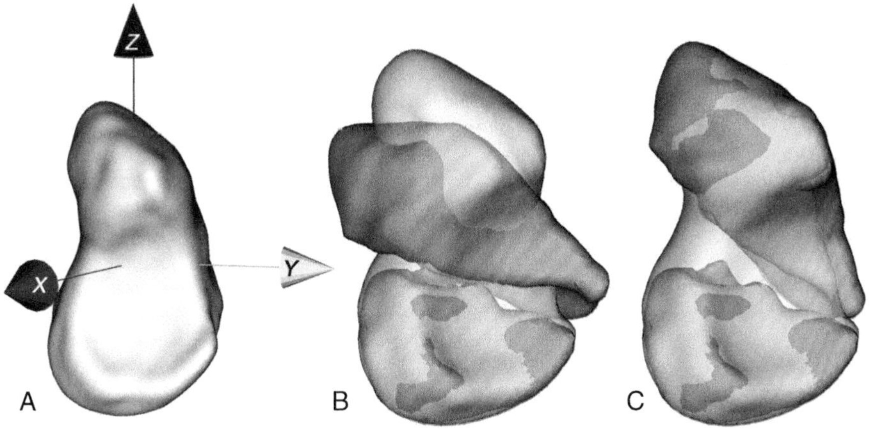

FIG. 25.4 Radioulnar views of the virtual planning of the scaphoid nonunion reconstruction using 3D CT models, based on the preoperative scan as shown in Fig. 25.2. **(A)** A model of the contralateral intact scaphoid (white model) serves as virtual reduction template; based on its inertial properties a local coordinate system is set resulting in three axes corresponding to (1) radioulnar axis (*X*), (2) the palmodorsal axis (*Y*), and the proximodistal axis (*Z*). **(B)** After superimposing the proximal nonunion fragment (orange model) and the intact proximal pole, the level of displacement of the distal fragment (orange model) can be quantified based on the difference with the position of the intact distal pole in 3D space: the flexion deformity of the distal fragment is 27 degrees, with a proximal translation of 3.8 mm. **(C)** After superimposing the distal nonunion fragment and the intact distal pole, both fragments are reduced in optimal position.

were created to guide shaping the graft. The actual bone graft was larger than the estimated bone defect due to resection of the sclerotic bone of the nonunion sites to visible bleeding. The intrinsic scaphoid morphology was not assessed postoperatively.

RECOMMENDATION

- Three-dimensional surgical planning may improve the precision of fragment reduction in a subset of scaphoid nonunions—most likely in waist nonunions with relatively large, intact proximal and distal surfaces, allowing a proper fit with the reduction guide (overall quality: very low).
- There are no reports on the 3D surgical planning in the treatment of scaphoid malunions (overall quality: evidence nonexistent).

CONCLUSION

It is currently not clear if patient-specific reduction techniques based on 3D planning lead to superior results in terms of fragment reduction and/or carpal realignment compared with conventional techniques. As resources are always limited, the potential advantages of these advanced techniques must be critically compared with standard practice in future clinical controlled studies.

PANEL 2
Authors' Preferred Technique

In this case showing evident dorsal intercalated segment instability (DISI) deformity on the preoperative images (Fig. 25.1), reconstructive surgery was predominantly directed at restoring the normal lunate stance. Three-dimensional (3D) CT-based planning software enabled quantifying the humpback deformity and virtually reducing the fragments in 3D space by matching the proximal and distal fragments with the contralateral intact scaphoid, serving as anatomic template (Fig. 25.4). This helps guiding the reconstruction with a structural bone graft. A surgical technique as previously described by Tomaino was used.[19] This technique included transfixing the lunate to the radius in neutral position, opening the nonunion site by extending the wrist, and inserting the graft, resulting in correction of the DISI stance and scaphoid humpback deformity (Figs. 25.5 and 25.6). Postoperative evaluation with 3D CT-based planning software showed overlengthening of the scaphoid, which is the result of using a nonanatomically sized graft—also

Continued

PANEL 2
Authors' Preferred Technique—cont'd

known as scaphoid overstuffing (Fig. 25.7).[20–22] To adequately restore the lunate alignment sometimes requires scaphoid overlengthening, thus deviating from the preoperative plan. Long-term follow-up assessment is required to investigate the relation between the reconstructed scaphoid morphology and (further) carpal osteoarthritic development.

In retrospect, we also manufactured 3D printed models of the contralateral intact scaphoid and of the nonunion with the fragments in malaligned position and with the fragments in realigned position as virtually planned (Fig. 25.8). Besides the potency to guide and improve fragment reduction, 3D printed models can also be utilized to educate surgical residents and to improve communication with patients. As the newest 3D printers produce durable models within hours in a hospital setting, the use of such models becomes an interesting area for future clinical research.

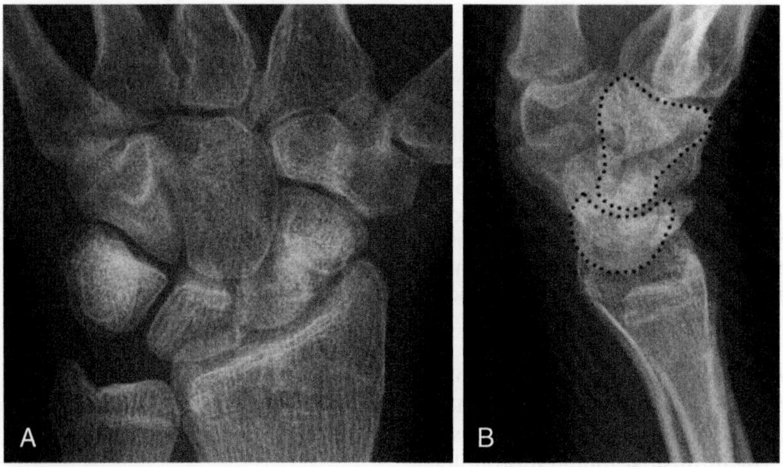

FIG. 25.5 Postoperative radiographs of the same case as in Figs. 25.1, 25.2, and 25.4, 8 months after the reconstructive surgery showing fracture consolidation. **(A)** Anteroposterior and **(B)** lateral views. Although the lateral image was taken with the wrist in slightly dorsiflexed position, carpal realignment was confirmed. based on the configuration of the lunate (dotted line) and capitate (dotted line).

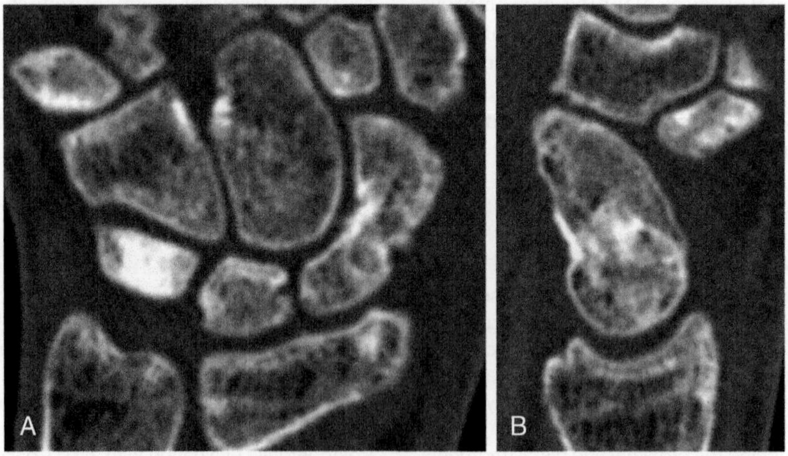

FIG. 25.6 Postoperative CT scan 9 months after the reconstructive surgery showing fracture consolidation by trabecular bridging and absence of the fracture gap. **(A)** Coronal and **(B)** sagittal CT slice. The sagittal slice clearly shows a correction of the *humpback* deformity.

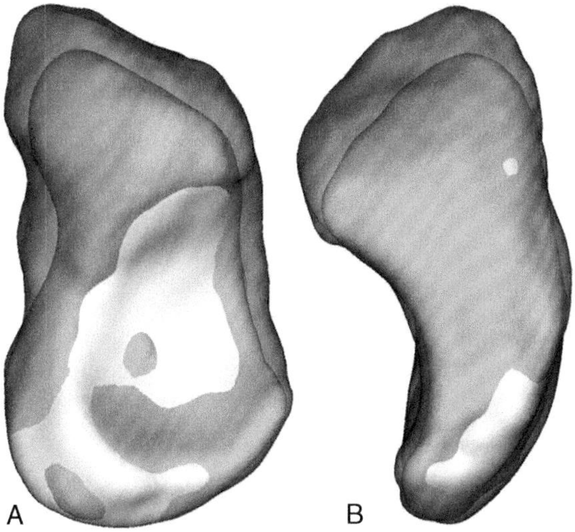

FIG. 25.7 Postoperative evaluation of the scaphoid nonunion correction using 3D CT models, based on the postoperative scan as shown in Fig. 25.5. **(A)** Radioulnar view and **(B)** dorsopalmar view. The length of the restored scaphoid (orange model) is 2.2 mm longer than the length of the contralateral scaphoid (white model), indicating a slight overcorrection.

PANEL 3
Pearls and Pitfalls

PEARLS

- In the treatment of scaphoid waist nonunions, restoring the intrinsic scaphoid anatomy may be enhanced by preoperative 3D planning strategies.
- Planning software enables assessing scaphoid deformity both pre- and postoperatively. This may benefit future investigations on the relationship between the level of scaphoid malunion and clinical outcome, which is currently to a large degree speculative.
- The continuing development efforts for easy-to-use planning software and the increasing availability of 3D printers in hospital setting will enhance utilizing these advanced techniques, also in less specialized clinics.

PITFALLS

- Restoration of the intrinsic scaphoid anatomy does not ensure adequate correction of the DISI stance of the lunate, nor restoration of the normal carpal kinematics.
- The exact amount of sclerotic margin at the nonunion sites to be removed is often determined intraoperatively. This hampers planning the optimal size of a structural bone graft preoperatively.
- Proximal scaphoid nonunions are likely less suitable for 3D printed reduction guides because it is difficult to obtain a unique fit of the guide with the smooth surface of the small proximal pole.

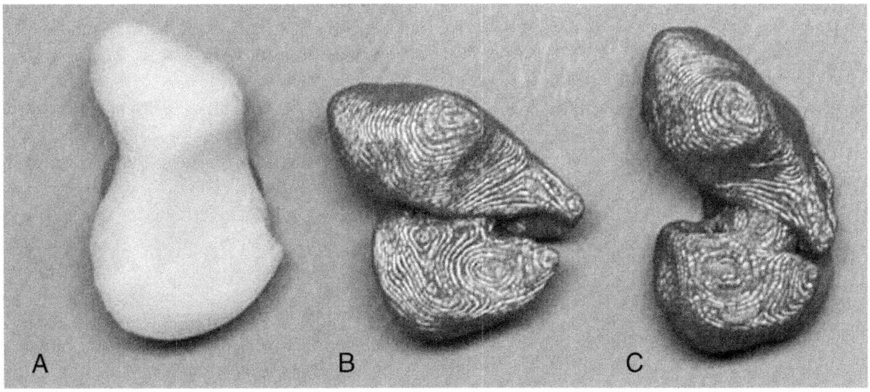

FIG. 25.8 Three-dimensional printed models based on the preoperative bilateral CT scan, including the model of **(A)** the contralateral intact scaphoid and of the nonunion with **(B)** the fragments in malaligned position and **(C)** with the fragments in realigned position as virtually planned, as also shown in Fig. 25.4.

CONFLICT OF INTEREST

Each author certifies that he or she has no commercial associations (e.g., consultancies, stock ownership, equity interest, patent/licensing arrangements) that might pose a conflict of interest in connection with the submitted article.

REFERENCES

1. Buijze GA, Ochtman L, Ring D. Management of scaphoid nonunion. *J Hand Surg Am*. 2012;37(5):1095–1100.
2. van de Giessen M, Foumani M, Streekstra GJ, et al. Statistical descriptions of scaphoid and lunate bone shapes. *J Biomech*. 2010;43(8):1463–1469.
3. Moritomo H, Viegas SF, Elder KW, et al. Scaphoid nonunions: a 3-dimensional analysis of patterns of deformity. *J Hand Surg Am*. 2000;25(3):520–528.
4. Schweizer A, Furnstahl P, Nagy L. Three-dimensional computed tomographic analysis of 11 scaphoid waist nonunions. *J Hand Surg Am*. 2012;37(6):1151–1158.
5. Ten Berg PW, Dobbe JG, Horbach SE, Gerards RM, Strackee SD, Streekstra GJ. Analysis of deformity in scaphoid non-unions using two- and three-dimensional imaging. *J Hand Surg Eur Vol*. 2016;41(7):719–726.
6. Forward DP, Singh HP, Dawson S, Davis TR. The clinical outcome of scaphoid fracture malunion at 1 year. *J Hand Surg Eur Vol*. 2009;34(1):40–46.
7. Amadio PC, Berquist TH, Smith DK, Ilstrup DM, Cooney 3rd WP, Linscheid RL. Scaphoid malunion. *J Hand Surg Am*. 1989;14(4):679–687.
8. Lynch NM, Linscheid RL. Corrective osteotomy for scaphoid malunion: technique and long-term follow-up evaluation. *J Hand Surg Am*. 1997;22(1):35–43.
9. Nakamura P, Imaeda T, Miura T. Scaphoid malunion. *J Bone Joint Surg Br*. 1991;73(1):134–137.
10. Lindstrom G, Nystrom A. Incidence of post-traumatic arthrosis after primary healing of scaphoid fractures: a clinical and radiological study. *J Hand Surg Br*. 1990; 15(1):11–13.
11. Jiranek WA, Ruby LK, Millender LB, Bankoff MS, Newberg AH. Long-term results after Russe bone-grafting: the effect of malunion of the scaphoid. *J Bone Joint Surg Am*. 1992;74(8):1217–1228.
12. Bain GI, Bennett JD, MacDermid JC, Slethaug GP, Richards RS, Roth JH. Measurement of the scaphoid humpback deformity using longitudinal computed tomography: intra- and interobserver variability using various measurement techniques. *J Hand Surg Am*. 1998;23(1):76–81.
13. Bhat M, McCarthy M, Davis TR, Oni JA, Dawson S. MRI and plain radiography in the assessment of displaced fractures of the waist of the carpal scaphoid. *J Bone Joint Surg Br*. 2004;86(5):705–713.
14. Ring D, Patterson JD, Levitz S, Wang C, Jupiter JB. Both scanning plane and observer affect measurements of scaphoid deformity. *J Hand Surg Am*. 2005;30(4): 696–701.
15. Pinder RM, Brkljac M, Rix L, Muir L, Brewster M. Treatment of scaphoid nonunion: a systematic review of the existing evidence. *J Hand Surg Am*. 2015;40(9):1797–1805.
16. Schweizer A, Mauler F, Vlachopoulos L, Nagy L, Furnstahl P. Computer-assisted 3-dimensional reconstructions of scaphoid fractures and nonunions with and without the use of patient-specific guides: early clinical outcomes and postoperative assessments of reconstruction accuracy. *J Hand Surg Am*. 2016;41(1):59–69.
17. Murase T, Moritomo H, Goto A, Sugamoto K, Yoshikawa H. Does three-dimensional computer simulation improve results of scaphoid nonunion surgery? *Clin Orthop Relat Res*. 2005;(434):143–150.
18. Haefeli M, Schaefer DJ, Schumacher R, Muller-Gerbl M, Honigmann P. Titanium template for scaphoid reconstruction. *J Hand Surg Eur Vol*. 2015;40(5):526–533.
19. Tomaino MM, King J, Pizillo M. Correction of lunate malalignment when bone grafting scaphoid nonunion with humpback deformity: rationale and results of a technique revisited. *J Hand Surg Am*. 2000;25(2):322–329.
20. Bindra R, Bednar M, Light T. Volar wedge grafting for scaphoid nonunion with collapse. *J Hand Surg Am*. 2008; 33(6):974–979.
21. Capito AE, Higgins JP. Scaphoid overstuffing: the effects of the dimensions of scaphoid reconstruction on scapholunate alignment. *J Hand Surg Am*. 2013;38(12): 2419–2425.
22. Eggli S, Fernandez DL, Beck T. Unstable scaphoid fracture nonunion: a medium-term study of anterior wedge grafting procedures. *J Hand Surg Br*. 2002;27(1):36–41.

CHAPTER 26

Corrective Osteotomy for Scaphoid Malunion

MICHAEL B. GOTTSCHALK, MD • SANJEEV KAKAR, MD, MRCS

KEY POINTS

- Scaphoid malunion can be assessed using the height (H) to length (L) ratio, dorsal cortical angle (DCA), and lateral intrascaphoid angle (LISA).
- Scaphoid malunion that results in associated carpal instability may produce pain, early arthritis, and wrist dysfunction.
- Although prior case series report favorable results with scaphoid osteotomy, recent studies demonstrate similar outcomes with nonoperative treatment.

PANEL 1
Case Scenario

A 28-year-old man was referred with continued wrist pain after undergoing open reduction internal fixation of a scaphoid waist fracture elsewhere. Preoperative radiographs demonstrated a displaced scaphoid waist fracture (Fig. 26.1). Postoperative radiographs demonstrated a healed fracture with significant flexion deformity and associated volar intercalated instability without lunotriquetral symptomatology (Fig. 26.2). A CT of the wrist confirmed a scaphoid malunion as demonstrated by altered height to length ratio, dorsal cortical angle, and lateral intrascaphoid angles (Fig. 26.3). The patient inquires as to whether there is anything that can be done to reduce his pain and improve his range of motion. Could you improve his pain, range of motion, and function by performing a corrective osteotomy for this symptomatic deformity?

IMPORTANCE OF THE PROBLEM

The incidence of scaphoid malunions is rare and most likely underdiagnosed. It most commonly arises from incorrect reduction and fixation of an acute scaphoid fracture, transscaphoid perilunate, or chronic scaphoid nonunion.[1–6] There is a paucity of data about the natural history of scaphoid malunion with most information arising from small case series.

Patients may present with a prior history of a scaphoid fracture or surgical fixation of the scaphoid with continued pain, loss of motion, decreased grip strength, and disability of the hand/wrist. Plain radiographs and CT scans can help define altered scaphoid morphology as evidenced by changes in H/L ratio, DCA, and LISA.

The H/L ratio is calculated by using the midcut of a sagittal CT scan (based on the axis of the scaphoid) where a baseline is drawn on the volar aspect of the scaphoid (length) and a perpendicular line is then drawn to calculate the height. H/L ratios vary widely and normal values are thought to be less than 0.6 or 0.5 (Fig. 26.4A).[4,7] The DCA can also be measured on the midcut of a sagittal CT and is measured by the angle formed by the two dorsal cortical intersecting lines (Fig. 26.4B). DCA angles vary widely and there is no normal value although malunions have ranged from 15 to 150 degrees, demonstrating its significant variability.[7] LISA can also be measured on the midcut of the CT and is derived from the perpendicular lines drawn from the articular surface of the proximal and distal poles of the scaphoid (Fig. 26.4C). Acceptable LISAs have been thought to be less than 35 degrees.

The diagnosis may include signs and symptoms of carpal instability, loss of motion, and pain. Radiographs and CT scans should be used to quantify the nature of the malunion for which the H/L, DCA, and LISA can be useful. Studies have shown, however, that their intra- and interobserver reliability can be varied.[7]

Controversy remains about the sequelae of scaphoid malunions. Several authors have demonstrated minimal to no correlation between scaphoid malunion and subjective outcomes.[4,8,9] However, others have demonstrated that parameters, such as H/L, DCA, and LISA,

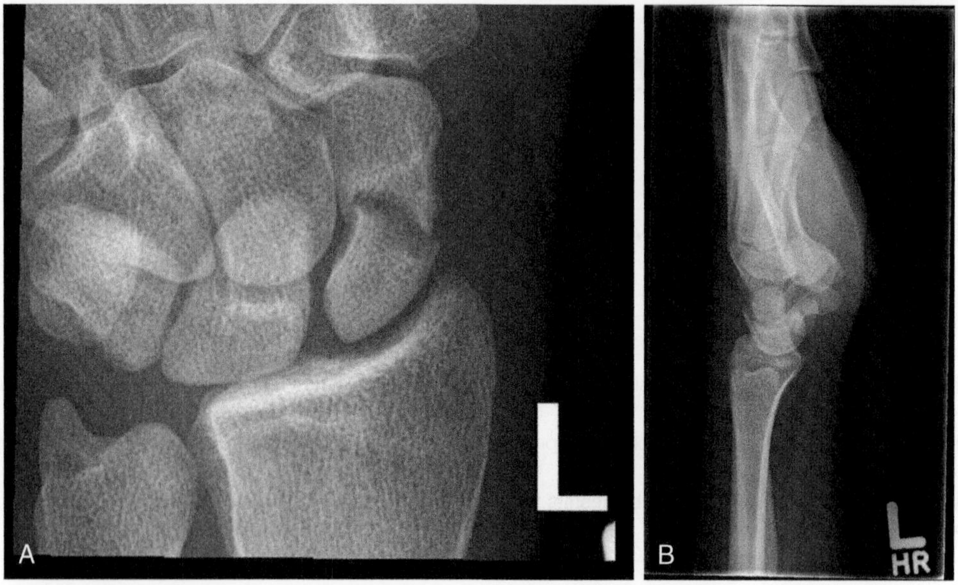

FIG. 26.1 (**A** and **B**) Posteroanterior and lateral preoperative radiographs demonstrating a displaced scaphoid waist fracture. (Courtesy of Sanjeev Kakar, Mayo Clinic, Rochester, MN.)

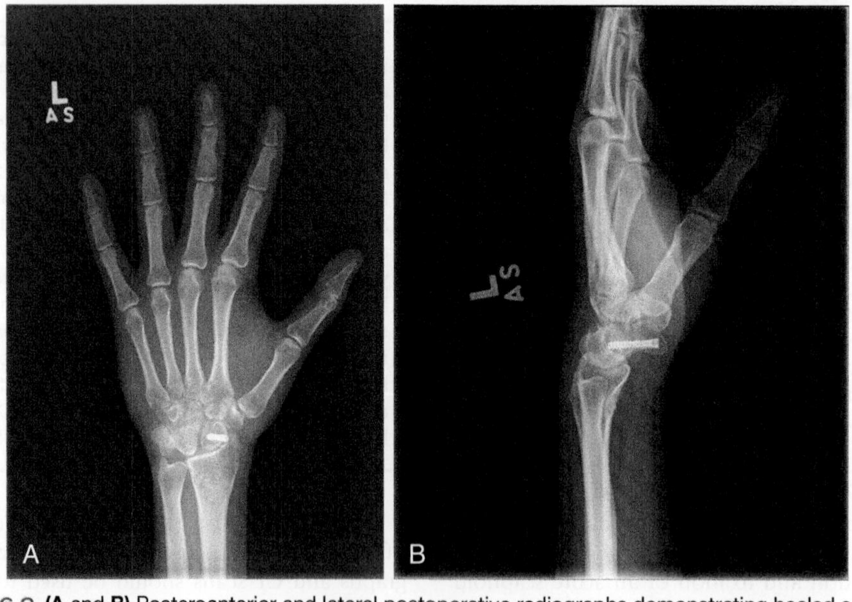

FIG. 26.2 (**A** and **B**) Posteroanterior and lateral postoperative radiographs demonstrating healed scaphoid waist fracture with flexion deformity. (Courtesy of Sanjeev Kakar, Mayo Clinic, Rochester, MN.)

are not predicative of outcome compared with associated carpal deformity as measured by the radiolunate and capitolunate angles.[6] Most recently Gillette and colleagues reported on the outcomes of 17 patients with an average follow-up of 21 years. Regardless of the treatment (corrective osteotomy, salvage procedures or observation), functional outcomes were similar between the patients.[10]

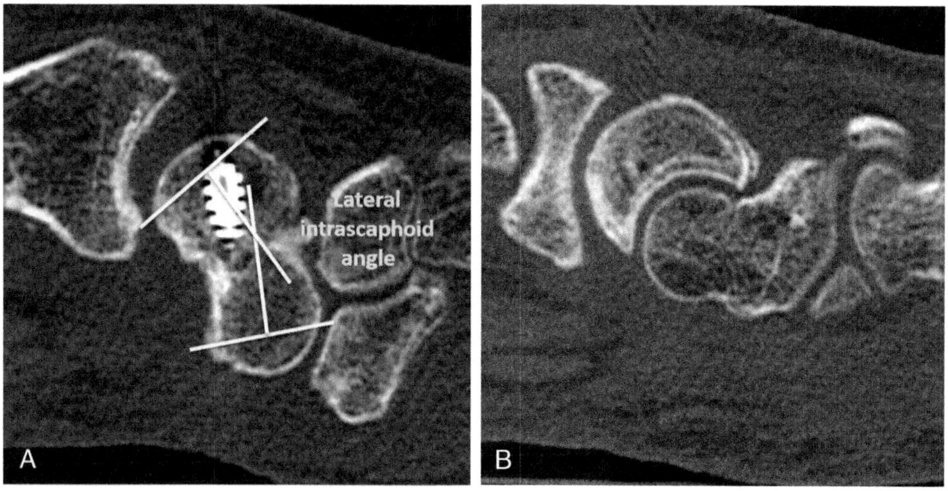

FIG. 26.3 **(A)** Sagittal cut of the postoperative CT scan demonstrating an increased lateral intrascaphoid angle. **(B)** Sagittal cut of the postoperative CT scan demonstrating volar intercalated instability deformity. (Courtesy of Sanjeev Kakar, Mayo Clinic, Rochester, MN.)

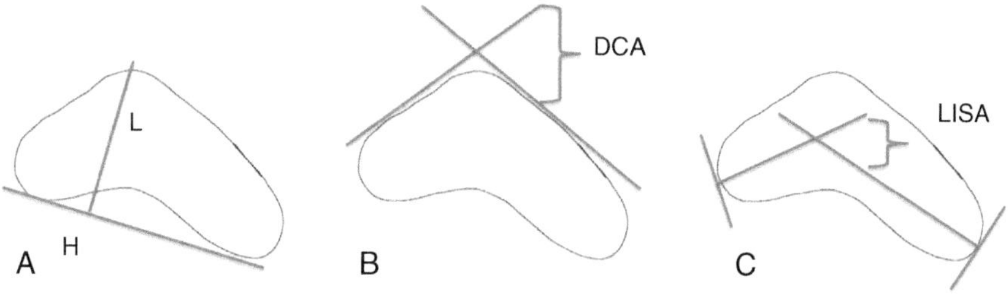

FIG. 26.4 **(A–C)** Midcut CT scan of a scaphoid with height to length (H/L) ratio, dorsal cortical angle (DCA), and lateral intrascaphoid angle (LISA) depictions. (Courtesy of Michael Gottschalk, Emory University School of Medicine, Dunwoody, GA.)

MAIN QUESTION

What is the relative effect of corrective osteotomy versus conservative treatment in patient functional outcome and disability in malunions of the scaphoid?

Current Opinion

Depending on the degree of scaphoid malunion, controversy exists regarding the appropriate management. In those that are asymptomatic, expectant management may be of order as opposed to those that have concomitant carpal instability, where a corrective osteotomy may be indicated. This can be defined as radiolunate angle > 10 degrees or capitolunate angles < 0 or > 15 degrees.

Finding the Evidence

- Pubmed: Search ("Scaphoid Malunion" [Mesh])
- Articles that were not in English were excluded

Quality of the Evidence

Level IV:
 Case series: 14
Level V:
 Technique/cadaveric: 2

FINDINGS

Several studies have reported on the outcomes of patients with scaphoid malunions.[1,4–6,8,9] Forward et al. reported on 42 nonoperatively treated fractures that then went on to union and correlated scaphoid morphologic parameters (H/L, DCA, and LISA) and patient-reported outcomes (range of motion, Patient Evaluation Measure and Disabilities of the Arm, Shoulder, and Hand [DASH] scores) after 1 year from the injury.[4] Scaphoid malunion was defined as H/L ratio of >0.60. The authors noted that there was no correlation between scaphoid malunion and patient-reported outcomes.[4] Amadio et al. studied 46 scaphoid fractures more then 6 months after union.[1] The authors defined a malunion as a LISA of >35 degrees. Twenty patients had normal anatomy (e.g., LISA <35) and 26 patients had a malunion as defined by a LISA of >35 degrees. Of the 20 normal scaphoids, 7 were treated with surgery and 13 were treated nonoperatively. Similarly, of the 26 patients with a malunion, 20 patients underwent operative intervention. Those with a LISAof <35 degrees were appeared to have an effect in clinical outcome, exhibiting 83% satisfactory outcomes and only posttraumatic arthritis in 22%. Those with LISA>45 degrees had satisfactory clinical outcome in only 27% and posttraumatic arthritis in 54%. The authors report that union alone is an insufficient criterion for success based on the fact that patients with a united scaphoid but abnormal LISA defined as >45 degrees (e.g., humpback deformity) had significant posttraumatic arthritis and less successful outcomes. Megerle et al. reviewed 65 patients at a mean of 45 months after scaphoid nonunion fixation. The authors measured and correlated H/L ratio, LISA, DCA, scapholunate (SL) angle, and radiolunate (RL) angle and compared these scaphoid parameters to wrist ROM, grip strength, Visual Analog Pain Scale, Mayo scores, and DASH scores. Patients with a RL angle of >10 degrees correlated with decreased wrist ROM and grip strength and increased pain levels.[6] Similar to other studies, however, there was no correlation between SL angle, LISA, DCA, and H/L ratio and Mayo and DASH scores. The authors concluded that osseous union alone was insufficient to provide satisfactory clinical results and that restoration of normal carpal angles is imperative for successful results.

In performing a scaphoid corrective osteotomy, it is important to understand its effects on carpal kinematics. In a cadaver model, Burgess demonstrated that there was a loss of radiocarpal extension that occurred at 15 degrees of volar angulation at the scaphoid waist (e.g., increasing LISA by 15 degrees), whereas loss of midcarpal extension occurred at 30 degrees of volar angulation.[2] The site of malunion will determine the nature of corrective osteotomy required. Most are the result of a humpback deformity where the scaphoid is shortened with apex dorsal angulation around the radioscaphocapitate ligament. Through a volar approach, Birchard et al. described a Russe-type opening wedge osteotomy with iliac crest bone grafting in two patients with scaphoid malunion.[11] Both patients had carpal instability symptoms with increased SL angles and lunocapitate angles (patient 1 with 75 and 48 degrees, respectively, and patient 2 with 74 and 15 degrees, respectively). Correction improved SL and lunocapitate angles to 60 and 17 degrees for patient 1 and 60 and 0 degrees for patient 2, respectively. Nakamura et al. reviewed 10 patients with associated scaphoid malunion and dorsal intercalated segment instability (DISI) deformity who underwent seven corrective osteotomies with anterior wedge bone grafting and internal fixation. The authors noted that the restriction of flexion-extension and grip strength correlated with the DISI deformity, specifically the radiolunate angle, which following correction of deformity resulted in improvement of those parameters.[12] Postoperatively, they demonstrated an improvement in average flexion-extension from 95 to 137 degrees and grip strength from 54% to 89%. The single patient who underwent styloidectomy alone did not demonstrate any improvement even after 7 years. The authors concluded that the residual symptoms after a scaphoid malunion are due to carpal instability and if corrected to within normal parameters, patients may have satisfactory results. Linscheid et al. described a similar technique with tricortical iliac crest bone graft, which provided a structural support for the osteotomy.[13] The approach was through a radial palmar incision at the snuffbox. The extensor pollicis brevis and longus were retracted dorsally and the abductor pollicis longus retracted volarly. The terminal branches of the cephalic vein and radial artery were identified and retracted. After performing a radial styloidectomy, a corrective scaphoid osteotomy and iliac crest wedge graft was inserted. As noted in Table 26.1, there was an improvement in range of motion and grip strength at 9 years of follow-up.[14] A similar case series by El Karef et al., which prospectively reviewed 13 patients who underwent correction of a malunited B2, demonstrated similar results as depicted in Tables 26.2 and 26.3.[15] Two other case series have demonstrated similar results with improvement of range of motion, pain, and grip strength.[12,16]

Most recently, Gillette, Amadio, and Kakar reported on the outcomes of 17 patients over a 30-year period.[10] Four patients underwent corrective osteotomy, five had a cheilectomy and/or radial styloidectomy, two had a scaphoid excision and intercarpal fusion, and six were treated nonoperatively. After an average follow-up of 21 years, the authors noted that the final mean Patient-Rated Wrist Evaluation and QuickDASH scores for corrective osteotomy, salvage procedures, and nonoperative treatment were 23 and 6, 18 and 10, and 33 and 22, respectively. Overall, the patients had similar long-term outcome scores regardless of the treatment type.

RECOMMENDATION

- Associated carpal malalignment/instability with scaphoid malunion correlates with wrist symptomatology (overall quality: low to moderate).

TABLE 26.1
Preoperative and Postoperative Clinical Results After Scaphoid Malunion Correction With Tricortical Iliac Crest Bone Graft

	PREOPERATIVE		POSTOPERATIVE	
Variable	**Mean**	**Range**	**Mean**	**Range**
Flexion (degrees)	47	20–85	60	20–76
Extension (degrees)	35	25–47	46	34–64
Radial deviation (degrees)	20	5–25	20	16–28
Ulnar deviation (degrees)	25	15–30	30	22–56
Total active motion (degrees)	127	95–165	156	95–214
Grip (kg)	26	14–35	37	24–48

Data from Lynch NM, Linscheid RL. Corrective osteotomy for scaphoid malunion: technique and long-term follow-up evaluation. *J Hand Surg*. 1997;22(1):35–43.

TABLE 26.2
Clinical Morphologic Results After B2 Malunion Correction

	PREOPERATIVE		LAST VISIT	
	Mean (Range)	**Percent of Uninvolved**	**Mean (Range)**	**Percent of Uninvolved**
Active movements				
Dorsiflexion (degrees)	41 (25–48)	47	57 (55–85)[a]	73[a]
Palmar flexion (degrees)	75 (65–80)	89	79 (60–85)	94[a]
Pronation (degrees)	80 (70–85)	91	87 (70–90)	96
Supination (degrees)	74 (40–80)	70	81 (65–90)[a]	89[a]
Ulnar deviation (degrees)	18 (20–25)	64	22 (18–25)	84
Radial deviation (degrees)	12 (10–15)	48	16 (14–22)	82
Grip strength (kg)	19 (13–30)	47	32 (26–36)[a]	79[a]

[a]Significant differences between the preoperative and last visit means.
Data from El-Karef EA. Corrective osteotomy for symptomatic scaphoid malunion. *Injury.* 2005;36(12):1440–1448.

TABLE 26.3
Radiographic Measurements After B2 Malunion Correction

	PREOPERATIVE		LAST VISIT	
	Mean	**Range**	**Mean**	**Range**
Scapholunate angle (degrees)	60	50–85	55	40–70
Radiolunate angle (degrees)	16	0–20	7	0–12[a]
Capitolunate angle (degrees)	20	0–30	9	0–15[a]
Lateral intrascaphoid angle (degrees)	59	53–65	34	29–39[a]
Dorsal cortical angle (degrees)	139	135–143	147	139–156
Height to length ratio	0.62	0.58–0.66	0.53	0.51–0.53

[a]Significant differences between the pre operative and last visit means.
Data from El-Karef EA. Corrective osteotomy for symptomatic scaphoid malunion. *Injury.* 2005;36(12):1440–1448.

- Scaphoid osteotomy should be reserved for patients with scaphoid malunion and associated symptomatic carpal malalignment (overall quality: low).
- Nonoperative and operative treatments provide similar results for scaphoid malunions (overall quality: low).

CONCLUSION

Nonoperative treatment for scaphoid malunions can be considered when the patients are asymptomatic, and the deformity is not associated with carpal malalignment. Scaphoid corrective osteotomy may provide improved functional outcomes when associated with carpal malalignment. In planning a corrective osteotomy, preoperative templating from the uninjured wrist can be helpful because, oftentimes, the degree and site of scaphoid malunion may be subtle..

PANEL 2
Authors' Preferred Technique

In the case presented, there is a symptomatic scaphoid malunion with a humpback deformity and carpal instability. Given the site of malunion within the scaphoid, a volar Russe approach allows correction of the deformity and placement of the bone graft. Dorsal osteotomies may be needed if the scaphoid is shortened with a loss of the lateral intrascaphoid angle. Preoperative CT templating from the contralateral scaphoid may assist in planning the osteotomy and placement of the graft. Our preference is to use cannulated screw fixation with structural bone grafts if feasible. On follow up, a CT is recommended to ensure final healing (Fig. 26.5).

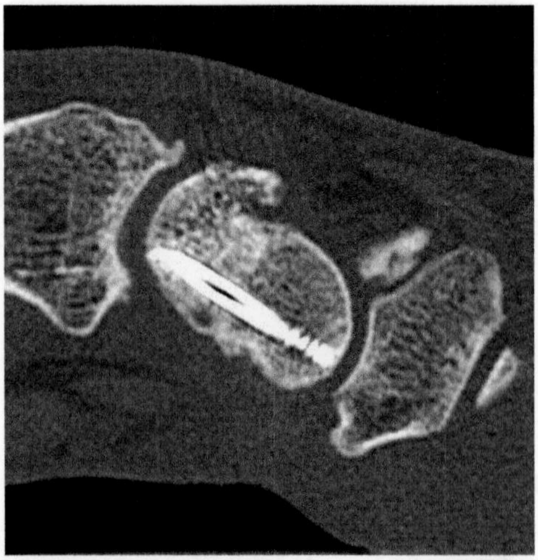

FIG. 26.5 Midcut CT scan demonstrating the healed osteotomy with cannulated screw.

PANEL 3
Pearls and Pitfalls

PEARLS

- A detailed history and physical examination should be performed to ascertain the degree of disability experienced by a scaphoid malunion.
- Without symptomatic carpal instability, a cheilectomy with a radial styloidectomy may be indicated if patients are symptomatic secondary to impingement with radial deviation.
- Patients should be counseled that the goal of surgery is to correct scaphoid malunion, which may or may not improve their symptoms.
- In planning a scaphoid osteotomy, we recommend obtaining a CT scan with 3D reconstructions of the injured side and contralateral side.

PITFALLS

- Correction of a malunited scaphoid with associated carpal malalignment may not fully correct the carpal kinematics if there is also associated ligamentous disruption (e.g., may have to address both the scaphoid malunion and the ligamentous disruption).

REFERENCES

1. Amadio PC, Berquist TH, Smith DK, Ilstrup DM, Cooney 3rd WP, Linscheid RL. Scaphoid malunion. *J Hand Surg.* 1989;14(4):679–687.
2. Burgess RC. The effect of a simulated scaphoid malunion on wrist motion. *J Hand Surg.* 1987;12(5 Pt 1):774–776.
3. Fernandez DL, Eggli S. Scaphoid nonunion and malunion. How to correct deformity. *Hand Clin.* 2001;17(4). 631–646, ix.
4. Forward DP, Singh HP, Dawson S, Davis TR. The clinical outcome of scaphoid fracture malunion at 1 year. *J Hand Surg Eur Vol.* 2009;34(1):40–46.
5. Lee CH, Lee KH, Lee BG, Kim DY, Choi WS. Clinical outcome of scaphoid malunion as a result of scaphoid fracture nonunion surgical treatment: a 5-year minimum follow-up study. *Orthop Traumatol Surg Res.* 2015;101(3):359–363.
6. Megerle K, Harenberg PS, Germann G, Hellmich S. Scaphoid morphology and clinical outcomes in scaphoid reconstructions. *Injury.* 2012;43(3):306–310.
7. Ring D, Patterson JD, Levitz S, Wang C, Jupiter JB. Both scanning plane and observer affect measurements of scaphoid deformity. *J Hand Surg.* 2005;30(4):696–701.
8. Afshar A, Mohammadi A, Zohrabi K, Navaeifar N, Sami SH, Taleb H. Correlation of reconstructed scaphoid morphology with clinical outcomes. *Arch Bone Jt Surg.* 2015;3(4): 244–249.
9. Jiranek WA, Ruby LK, Millender LB, Bankoff MS, Newberg AH. Long-term results after Russe bone-grafting: the effect of malunion of the scaphoid. *J Bone Joint Surg Am Vol.* 1992;74(8):1217–1228.

10. Gillette Blake P, Amadio PC, Kakar S. Long-term outcomes of scaphoid malunion. *Hand*. 2016;12(1):26–30.
11. Birchard D, Pichora D. Experimental corrective scaphoid osteotomy for scaphoid malunion with abnormal wrist mechanics. *J Hand Surg*. 1990;15(6):863–868.
12. Nakamura P, Imaeda T, Miura T. Scaphoid malunion. *J Bone Joint Surg Br Vol*. 1991;73(1):134–137.
13. Linscheid RL, Lynch NM. Scaphoid osteotomy for malunion. *Tech Hand Up Extrem Surg*. 1998;2(2):119–125.
14. Lynch NM, Linscheid RL. Corrective osteotomy for scaphoid malunion: technique and long-term follow-up evaluation. *J Hand Surg*. 1997;22(1):35–43.
15. El-Karef EA. Corrective osteotomy for symptomatic scaphoid malunion. *Injury*. 2005;36(12):1440–1448.
16. Fernandez DL, Martin CJ, Gonzalez del Pino J. Scaphoid malunion. The significance of rotational malalignment. *J Hand Surg*. 1998;23(6):771–775.

CHAPTER 27

Diagnosing Vascularity Issues of the Scaphoid

DR. KARL-JOSEF PROMMERSBERGER, MD • DR. RAINER SCHMITT, MD • DR. KARLHEINZ KALB, MD • DR. GEORGIOS CHRISTOPOULOS, MD

KEY POINTS

- For scaphoid nonunion the viability of the proximal fragment is a critical issue in the outcome of surgical treatment of nonunion.
- Preiser disease is an avascular necrosis (AVN) of the scaphoid, involving only a proximal part or the entire scaphoid.
- Gadolinium-enhanced MRI is used to investigate the vascularity and viability of bones and soft tissues.

PANEL 1
Case Scenario

A 23-year-old man presented with persistent radial-sided pain of the right wrist during sports and daily activities 1 year after a scooter accident. At the time, no medical care was sought. He is right hand dominant. Radiographs showed a midwaist scaphoid nonunion (Fig. 27.1). To decide on the most appropriate treatment option, you want to be informed about the vascularity and viability of the proximal pole. What is the most accurate diagnostic method for this issue?

IMPORTANCE OF THE PROBLEM

There are two issues where the vascularity of the scaphoid is of special interest, scaphoid nonunion, and AVN (Preiser disease). For scaphoid nonunion, especially after failed scaphoid reconstruction, the presence of AVN of the proximal fragment has been shown to be a critical issue in the outcome of surgical treatment of nonunion. In an illustrative case series of seven patients with persisting nonunion after operative treatment of scaphoid nonunion with bone grafting and internal fixation using a Herbert screw, one had a moderate ischemia, two had a severe ischemia, and four had a necrosis of the proximal fragment as rated intraoperatively after tourniquet release by the amount of punctate bleeding.[1] Patients with a Preiser disease in whom MRI signal changes of necrosis and/or ischemia involve the entire scaphoid have a propensity for scaphoid deterioration, while patients having MRI signal changes involving only part of the scaphoid show fewer tendencies toward scaphoid fragmentation.[2]

MAIN QUESTION

How are vascularity issues of the scaphoid best diagnosed?

Current Opinion

In both conditions, scaphoid nonunion and Preiser disease, assessment of scaphoid vascularity offers valuable information to the treating surgeon. An imaging modality that can depict preoperatively the vascularity and the viability of the proximal pole in scaphoid nonunion and the scaphoid in Preiser disease greatly facilitates the selection of the most appropriate treatment.

Finding the Evidence

- Cochrane search: Scaphoid Fracture
- Pubmed (Medline): ("Scaphoid Bone" [Mesh] OR scaphoid fracture*[tiab] OR scaphoid bone Fracture*[tiab] OR scaphoid[tiab]) AND ("vascularity" [Subheading] OR viability OR proximal pole)
- Bibliography of eligible articles
- Articles that were not in English or German language were excluded

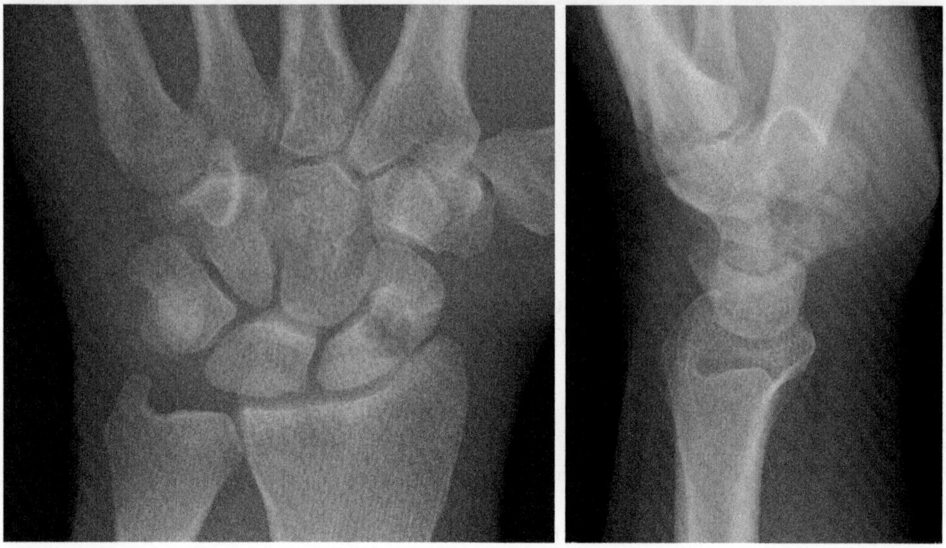

FIG. 27.1 Posteroanterior and lateral radiographs showed a midwaist scaphoid nonunion without degenerative changes.

Quality of the Evidence

Level IIb:

Cohort study/low-quality randomized controlled trial: 8

Level III:

Retrospective comparative studies: 2

Level IV:

Case series: 5

Level V:

Expert opinion: 6

FINDINGS

Assessment of Scaphoid Vascularity and Viability

There are several approaches to assess the vascularity and viability of the scaphoid, respectively, of the proximal fragment in a scaphoid nonunion: imaging, surgical inspection with visualization of bleeding points, and bone biopsy examination.

Imaging approaches to assess the scaphoid vascularity include conventional radiographs, computed tomography (CT), bone scintigraphy, unenhanced MRI, and gadolinium-enhanced MRI. Increased bone density on conventional radiographs and CT has been assumed as an imaging parameter of osteonecrosis. In scaphoid nonunion, increased bone density may be mimicked by dorsal rotation of the proximal fragment, leading to misinterpretation in projection radiography.[3] Furthermore, radiographs may depict a sclerotic proximal pole, but do not provide detailed information on its vascularity. Osseous sclerosis may be a transient phenomenon related to reduced bone remodeling from transient ischemia, indicating revascularization rather than ongoing AVN.[4,5] Radiologically sclerotic proximal pole can bleed,[4] whereas a normal one may be completely ischemic intraoperatively.[6]

Smith et al. showed that increased radiodensity of the proximal pole and absence of any converging trabeculae between the fracture fragments in a preoperative longitudinal CT of scaphoid nonunion correlate with histologic evidence of AVN of the proximal pole.[7] In addition, increased radiodensity of the proximal pole statistically correlated with postoperative union rates ($P<.05$), while the presence of bridging trabeculae trended toward correlation with postoperative union, but did not reach statistical significance ($P=.08$). In contrast, Bervian et al. did not found a correlation between CT evaluation and scaphoid proximal fragment necrosis. The vascular status of the proximal scaphoid was determined intraoperatively by the presence or absence of punctate bone bleeding and confirmed by pathologic examination of harvested samples.[8]

A "cold spot" in technetium 99m bone scan is also deemed as an indicator for an AVN. However, bone scintigraphy is suffering from both limited spatial resolution and specificity.

Many recent studies provide data to support the use of MRI for assessment of the vascularity of the scaphoid. In unenhanced MRI, bone viability is assumed in the presence of unaffected bone marrow signal.

Normal bone viability is displayed by high signal intensity in both T1- and T2-weighted sequences. Viable bone marrow is also assumed in the presence of a bone marrow edema, presenting with high signal intensity in fat-suppressed T2-weighted images. The underlying theory is that bone marrow edema can only develop if the blood supply of the bone is either unaffected or only minimally compromised with residual perfusion being preserved.[9] In contrast, it has been suggested that low signal intensity on T1- and T2-weighted sequences is highly predictive of AVN.[6,9] Unfortunately, low signal intensity in the bone marrow is recognized in necrosis, ischemia, and even viable bone.[1,10] Furthermore, T2-weighted images have the lowest accuracy in assessing AVN.[1,10] In addition, Fox et al. reported that the use of STIR images in addition to T1-weighted images were not beneficial in determining proximal pole viability.[11]

In 2000 Cerezal et al. showed that gadolinium-enhanced MRI is the best technique for detecting proximal pole AVN.[1] Thirty patients with a scaphoid nonunion were prospectively examined with unenhanced and gadolinium-enhanced MRI. Using the surgical findings as the gold standard, sensitivity, specificity, and accuracy of both MRI techniques were calculated. Although there was no correlation between the surgical findings and the findings in unenhanced MRI, the correlation between gadolinium-enhanced MRI and the surgical findings was good ($P<.0001$). Furthermore, global sensitivity, specificity, and accuracy of gadolinium-enhanced MRI were superior to those of unenhanced MRI.

Schmitt et al. compared the preoperative findings of unenhanced and gadolinium-enhanced MRI of 88 patients suffering from symptomatic scaphoid nonunion with the intraoperative punctate bleeding of the proximal fragment after tourniquet release. Intraoperatively, 17 necrotic proximal fragments were found. In 29 the blood supply was compromised, and in 42 it was deemed normal. In unenhanced MRI bone viability was judged necrotic in 1 patient, compromised in 20 patients, and unaffected in 67 patients. Gadolinium-enhanced MRI revealed 14 necrotic, 21 compromised, and 53 normal proximal fragments. Using surgical findings as standard of reference, in unenhanced MRI, the sensitivity was 6.3%, specificity 100%, positive prediction value 100%, negative prediction value 82.6%, and accuracy 82.9%. For gadolinium-enhanced MRI, sensitivity was 76.5%, specificity 98.6%, positive prediction value 92.9%, negative prediction value 94.6%, and accuracy 94.3%. Sensitivity for detecting avascular proximal fragments was significantly better ($P<.001$) in gadolinium-enhanced MRI in comparison to unenhanced MRI. Based on their imaging findings, they recommended application of intravenous gadolinium for diagnosing vascularity issues of the scaphoid[12] and described three viability patterns (Fig. 27.2): completely preserved viability of the proximal fragment, but bone marrow edema (pattern A); partial osteonecrosis of the proximal fragment (pattern B); and complete osteonecrosis of the proximal fragment (pattern C).

Larribe et al. evaluated the usefulness of dynamic gadolinium-enhanced MRI for assessing the viability of the proximal pole of the scaphoid in patients with acute scaphoid fracture. Using the histologic findings of a cylindrical specimen of the proximal pole obtained during surgery as the standard of reference, gadolinium-enhanced MRI achieved the best results for sensitivity, specificity, and positive and negative predictive values showing that dynamic gadolinium-enhanced imaging with time-intensity curve analysis does not provide additional predictive value over standard delayed enhanced imaging for acute scaphoid fracture.[13] In a similar study Donati et al. also found that dynamic gadolinium-enhanced MR imaging in the evaluation of scaphoid viability was inferior to that of a standard MRI protocol and concluded that dynamic acquisition may not be needed in patients with nonunion of scaphoid fractures.[14]

Dailiana et al. used unenhanced and gadolinium-enhanced MRI to assess union, graft viability, and proximal pole bone marrow status in 15 patients treated for a scaphoid nonunion with vascularized bone grafts from the distal radius.[15] Both plain and contrast-enhanced MRI obtained 3 months postoperative showed viability of the bone graft in all cases. Three months postoperative according to plain radiographs union was established on both sides of the graft in 12 patients and between the graft and the proximal pole in 3 patients. In contrast, plain MRI showed five nonunion, two between the graft and the proximal pole, two distally, and one on both sides of the graft, whereas gadolinium-enhanced MRI revealed one case of nonunion proximally. In four patients, who were considered to have osteonecrosis of the proximal pole intraoperatively, contrast-enhanced MRI showed 3 months after surgery reversal of necrotic changes in all four scaphoids. Dailiana et al. concluded that gadolinium-enhanced MRI is able to demonstrate early union after treatment of scaphoid nonunion with vascularized bone grafts, thus allowing earlier mobilization. In addition, MRI can be used to assess the viability of the proximal pole and the graft postoperatively. In a similar study Anderson et al. also found MRI useful to determine vascularized bone graft incorporation and revascularization of the proximal pole of the scaphoid in the setting of avascular scaphoid nonunion.[16]

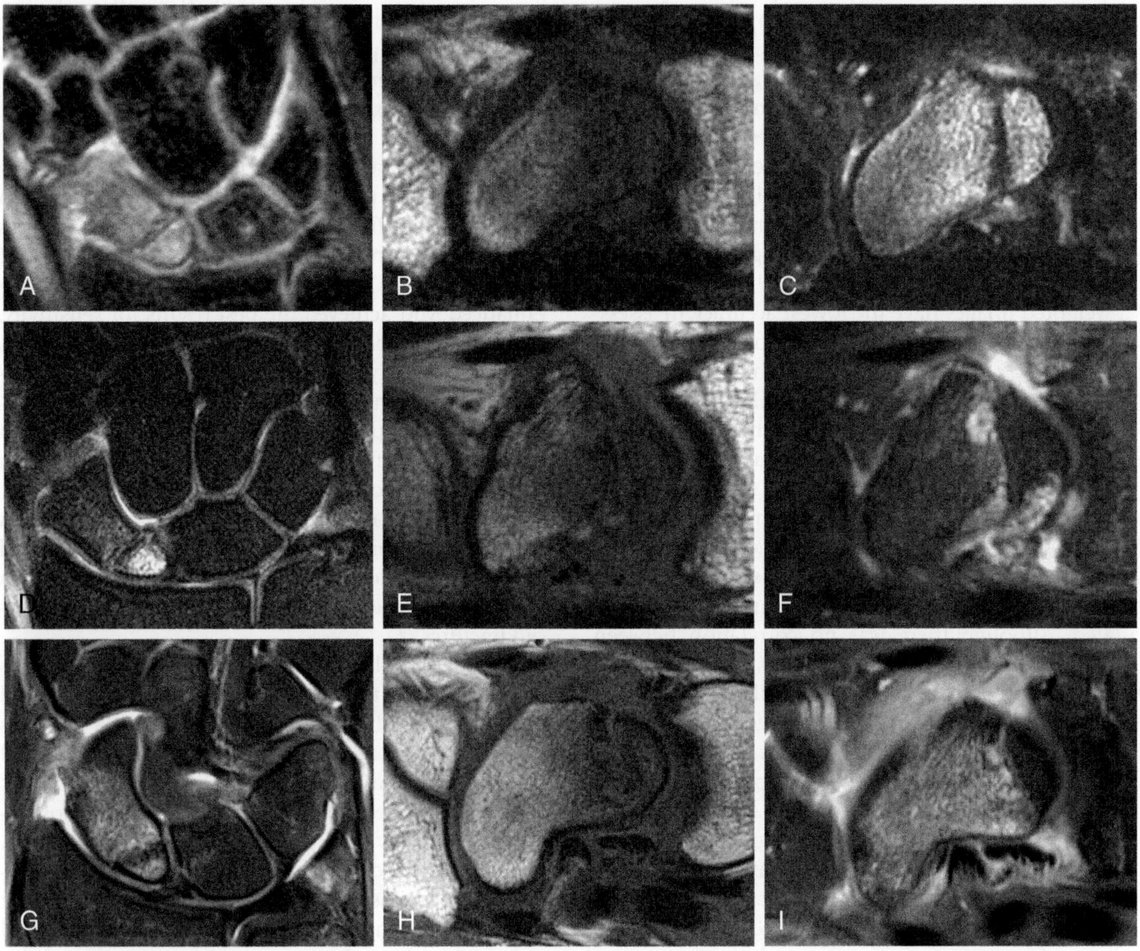

FIG. 27.2 MRI patterns of vascularity issues in three different patients with proximal scaphoid nonunion. Image arrangement is as follows: coronal fat-saturated proton density (PD)-weighted fast spin-echo (FSE) images in the left column **(A**, **D**, and **G)**, plain sagittal-oblique, T1-weighted FSE images in the middle column **(B**, **E**, and **H)**, and plain sagittal-oblique, contrast-enhanced T1-weighted FSE images with fat saturation in the right column **(C**, **F**, and **I)**. MRI pattern A (image row **A–C**): scaphoid nonunion with completely preserved vascularity of the proximal fragment. Bone marrow edema is evident in both fragments **(A)**, while decreased signal intensity of the proximal fragment and the adjacent segment of the distal fragment is decreased in the plain T1-weighted sequence **(B)**. Hypervascularity in both fragments is clearly visible after intravenous gadolinium **(C)**. MRI pattern B (image row **D–F**): scaphoid nonunion with partial osteonecrosis of the proximal fragment. Bone marrow edema is present in the proximal fragment and slightly the adjacent distal fragment **(D)**. The entire proximal fragment is of low signal height in the plain T1-weighted sequence **(E)** with hypervascularization limited to its palmar zone, but missing in the dorsal zone **(F)**. **(G–I)** MRI pattern C (image row **G–I**): scaphoid nonunion with total osteonecrosis of the proximal fragment. Bone marrow edema is present in both the proximal and distal fragments **(G)**. In the proximal fragment, signal height is decreased in the plain T1-weighted sequence **(H)** and remains completely low in the contrast-enhanced T1-weighted image **(I)**.

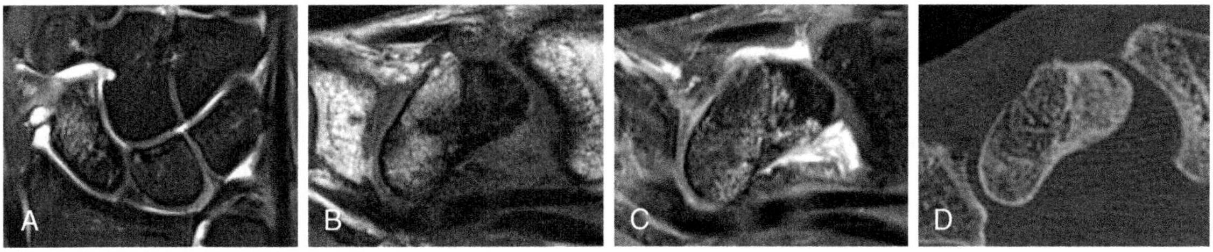

FIG. 27.3 MRI and CT findings in primary osteonecrosis of the scaphoid (Preiser disease). In the coronal fat-saturated PD-weighted image, there is moderate bone marrow edema in the middle and distal scaphoid segments, whereas the proximal pole appears of normal signal height **(A)**. In the plain T1-weighted sequence, the proximal scaphoid pole is of significant low signal height, indicating loss of fatty bone marrow cells, whereas bone-marrow signals are preserved to a wide extent in the middle and distal thirds **(B)**. In the contrast-enhanced, fat-saturated T1-weighted image, contrast enhancement after intravenous gadolinium is completely missing in the proximal scaphoid pole, and diffuse, but inhomogeneous, hypervascularization is evident in the middle and distal scaphoid zones **(C)**. A sagittal-oblique CT image (slice thickness 0.6 mm) visualizes an osteosclerotic proximal pole within a scaphoid of preserved shape and contour. Trabecular structure is slightly altered in the middle and distal parts, but without evidence of a previous scaphoid fracture **(D)**.

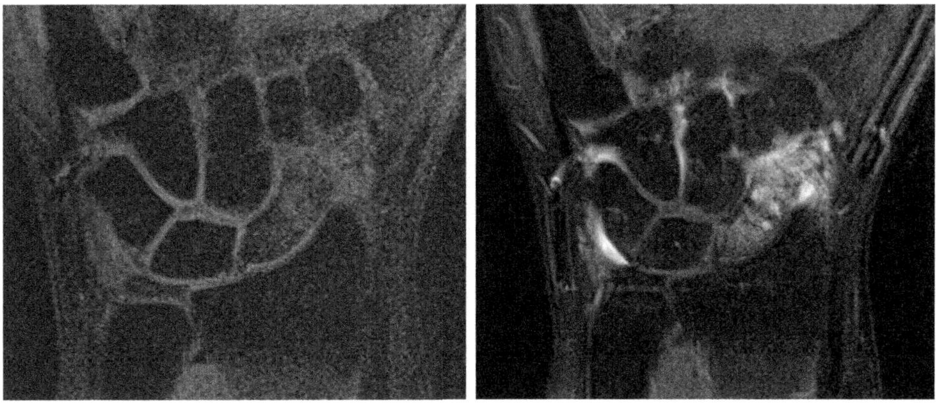

FIG. 27.4 Fat-saturated T1-weighted coronal images were achieved before (left) and after (right) administration of gadolinium, showing that the proximal pole was viable.

Preiser Disease

Idiopathic AVN of the scaphoid, first described by Preiser[17] in 1910, is a rare condition of ischemia and necrosis of the scaphoid that occurs in the absence of a previous scaphoid fracture or nonunion. Until yet, neither the etiology nor the pathology of this uncommon entity is entirely understood. Kalinov et al. described two different patterns of Preiser disease. In type 1 MRI signal changes of necrosis and/or ischemia involves 100% of the scaphoid, whereas in type 2 MRI changes involves only part of the scaphoid.[2] 63% of type 2 patients reported a history of wrist trauma before the onset of their wrist pain. However, no acute scaphoid fracture was diagnosed or identified in these patients. In contrast, only 9% type 1 patients reported a precipitating wrist injury. Regardless of the treatment used, type 1 scaphoids were fragmented and collapsed. In type 2 cases, scaphoid architecture was altered minimally after similar treatment methods.

Schmitt described the imaging in Preiser disease of the scaphoid and reported gadolinium-enhanced MRI findings in Preiser disease (Fig. 27.3) comparable with those he described for Kienböck disease at the lunate.[18,19] Ten patients with primary osteonecrosis of the scaphoid underwent plain radiography, CT imaging, and gadolinium-enhanced MRI. In all patients, osteosclerosis and bone marrow were most intense at the proximal scaphoid pole. A three-layered architecture was found with the zone of osteonecrosis located most proximally, followed by a zone of repair in the middle, and a zone of viable bone marrow in the distal part of the scaphoid. From the morphologic aspect, there were three stages. The initial stage is characterized by proximal sclerosis, but unchanged shape of the scaphoid. At the advanced stage, there are pathologic fractures and volume loss of the proximal pole. Finally, the entire scaphoid is necrotic.

The findings by Schmitt et al. that Preiser disease shows a pattern similar to the pattern of Kienböck disease is supported by the observation of Budoff[20] and Bhardwaj et al.,[21] describing concomitant Kienböck and Preiser disease.

RECOMMENDATION

In patients with a scaphoid nonunion, evidence suggests the following:

- Gadolinium-enhanced MRI achieved the best results for sensitivity, specificity, and positive and negative predictive values of proximal pole viability (overall quality: moderate).

CONCLUSION

Patients with scaphoid nonunion in whom the vascularity of the proximal fragment is suspicious to be compromised and patients with a suspected Preiser disease should be diagnosed in addition to conventional radiography and CT imaging by gadolinium-enhanced MRI. The vascularity of the proximal pole plays an important role regarding the prognosis in long-standing scaphoid nonunion and persisting nonunion following operative treatment of a scaphoid fracture, even more of a scaphoid nonunion. Patients with a Preiser disease with involvement of the entire scaphoid have a higher risk for fragmentation of the scaphoid as patients with involvement only part of the scaphoid.

PANEL 2
Author's Preferred Technique

The primary radiologic diagnostics for all scaphoid pathologies is a conventional radiography in three planes (dorsopalmar, lateral, and Stecher's views). If there is a scaphoid fracture or a scaphoid nonunion or if a scaphoid fracture cannot be ruled out, a CT scan is performed. With the patient in prone position on the CT table and the arm over the head ("superman's position"), a dedicated volume data set is acquired with the imaging plane sagittal-oblique in orientation and parallel to the longitudinal axis of the scaphoid (Fig. 27.3D). Slice thickness is 0.6 mm, field of view (FOV) is 60 mm. High-resolution images are calculated at 0.4 mm increments with applying a high-resolution kernel. In the postprocessing of the volumetric data set, coronal-oblique images are reconstructed using the multiplanar reconstruction mode and geometric parameters as applied during acquisition (FOV 60 mm, increment 0.4 mm, high-resolution kernel). If conventional radiographs and/or CT imaging are suspected of a Preiser disease or an osteonecrosis of the proximal fragment and in cases with a longstanding scaphoid nonunion, as well as in cases of a failed scaphoid reconstruction, an MRI scan is taken using a multichannel phased-array wrist coil. The following sequences are applied: fat-saturated PD-weighted FSE in both the coronal and sagittal planes, T1-weighted SE in the sagittal-oblique plane parallel to the longitudinal axis of the scaphoid unenhanced, as well as contrast enhanced and fat saturated after intravenous application of gadolinium. For all sequences a FOV of 80 mm and slice thickness of 2 mm without slice gap are recommended.

PANEL 3
Case Scenario (Continued)

In this case, a gadolinium-enhanced MRI was performed to assess the viability of the proximal pole. Fat-saturated T1-weighted coronal images were achieved before and after administration of gadolinium, showing that the proximal pole was viable (Fig. 27.4). Based on these findings, a nonvascularized graft reconstruction was opted.

REFERENCES

1. Cerezal L, Abascal A, Garcia-Valutille R, et al. Usefulness of gadolinium-enhanced MR Imaging in the evaluation of the vascularity of scaphoid nonunion. *AJR Am J Roentgenol*. 2000;174:141–149.
2. Kalainov DM, Cohen MS, Hendrix RW, et al. Preiser's disease: identification of two patterns. *J Hand Surg Am*. 2003;28:767–778.
3. Schmitt R, Heinze A, Fellner F, et al. Imaging and staging of avascular osteonecrosis at the wrist and hand. *Eur J Radiol*. 1997;25:92–103.
4. Green DP. The effect of avascular necrosis on Russe bone grafting for scaphoid nonunion. *J Hand Surg Am*. 1985;10:597–605.
5. Büchler U, Nagy L. The issue of vascularity in fractures and non-union of the scaphoid. *J Hand Surg Br*. 1995;20:726–735.
6. Perlik PC, Guilford WB. Magnet resonance imaging to assess vascularity of scaphoid nonunions. *J Hand Surg Am*. 1991;16:498–504.

7. Smith ML, Bain GI, Chabrel N, et al. Using computed tomography to assist with diagnosis of avascular necrosis complicated chronic scaphoid nonunion. *J Hand Surg Am.* 2009;34:1037–1043.
8. Bervian MR, Ribak S, Livani B. Scaphoid fracture nonunion: correlation of radiographic imaging, roximal fragment histologic viability evaluation, and estimation of viability at surgery: diagnosis of scaphoid pseudarthrosis. *Int Orthop.* 2015;39:67–72.
9. Trumble TE. Avascular necrosis after scaphoid fracture: correlation of magnetic resonance imaging and histology. *J Hand Surg Am.* 1990;15:557–564.
10. Desser TS, McCarthy S, Trumble T. Scaphoid fractures and Kienbock's disease of the lunate: MR imaging with histopathologic correlation. *Magn Reson Imaging.* 1990;8:357–361.
11. Fox MG, Gaskin CM, Chhabra AB, et al. Assessment of scaphoid viability with MRI: a reassessment of findings on unenhanced MR images. *AJR Am J Roentgenol.* 2010;195:W281–W286.
12. Schmitt R, Christopolous G, Wagner M, et al. Avascular necrosis (AVN) of the proximal fragment in scaphoid nonunion: is intravenous contrast agent necessary in MRI? *Eur J Radiol.* 2011;77:222–227.
13. Larribe M, Gay A, Freire V, et al. Usefulness of dynamic contrast-enhanced MRI in the evaluation of the viability of acute scaphoid fracture. *Skeletal Radiol.* 2014;43:1697–1703.
14. Donati OF, Zanetti M, Nagy L, et al. Is dynamic gadolinium enhancement needed in MR imaging for the preoperative assessment of scaphoidal viability in patients with scaphoid nonunion. *Radiology.* 2011;260:808–816.
15. Dailiana ZH, Zachos V, Varitimidis S, et al. Scaphoid nonunions treated with vascularized bone grafts: MRI assessment. *Eur J Radiol.* 2004;50:217–224.
16. Anderson SE, Steinach LS, Tschering-Vogel D, et al. MR imaging of avascular scaphoid nonunion before and after vascularized bone grafting. *Skeletal Radiol.* 2005;34:314–320.
17. Preiser G. Eine typische posttraumatische und zur Spontanfraktur führende Ostitis des Naviculare carpi. *Fortschr Geb Roentgenstr.* 1910;15:189–197.
18. Schmitt R, Fröhner S, van Schoonhoven J, et al. Idiopathic osteonecrosis of scaphoid (Preiser's disease) – MRI gives new insights into etiology and pathology. *Eur J Radiol.* 2011;77:228–234.
19. Schmitt R, Kalb K. Imaging in Kienböck's disease. *Handchir Mikrochir Plast Chir.* 2010;42:162–170.
20. Budolff JE. Concomitant Kienböck's and Preiser's disease: a case report. *J Hand Surg Am.* 2006;31:1149–1153.
21. Bharwaj P, Sharma C, Sabapathy SR. Concomitant avascular necrosis of the scaphoid and lunate. *Hand Surg.* 2012;17:239–241.

CHAPTER 28

Three-Dimensional Analysis of Nonunion Patterns

KUNIHIRO OKA, MD • HISAO MORITOMO, MD

KEY POINTS

- 3D analysis elucidates that natural history and carpal deformity of scaphoid nonunion is classified into two patterns based on the fracture location relative to the dorsal scaphoid apex.
- 3D computed tomography (CT) simplifies the identification of the dorsal scaphoid apex.

PANEL 1
Case Scenarios

Case 1: A 63-year-old man had a scaphoid fracture for 6 months. His wrist pain and restriction in wrist motion was severe and continuous. Radiographs revealed nonunion at the midthird, i.e., waist of the scaphoid and dorsal intercalated segment instability (DISI) deformity (Fig. 28.1A–C).

Case 2: A 31-year-old man had a scaphoid fracture for 7 years during which he did not visit a hospital because it was less symptomatic. Radiographs revealed nonunion at the midthird of the scaphoid but no DISI deformity (Fig. 28.2A and B).

These two midthird scaphoid nonunions had remarkable differences in symptoms and natural histories. You are asked to present these two cases at the upcoming radiology meeting. How will you explain these differences?

IMPORTANCE OF THE PROBLEM

There is a wide variation in symptoms and radiographic patterns in the natural history of scaphoid nonunion. For example, Case 1 was symptomatic and quickly developed a humpback and dorsal intercalated segment instability (DISI) deformity over 6 months. Conversely, carpal collapse was not visible in Case 2 for 7 years during which it was less symptomatic. What is the difference between these two cases with midthird scaphoid nonunions? How do symptoms and deformity patterns affect the scaphoid nonunion? Although the midthird scaphoid fracture nonunion, as observed in Case 2, is common, a clear explanation for the abovementioned differences was lacking until three-dimensional (3D) analysis of scaphoid nonunion deformities was developed.

In Case 1, 3D bone models reconstructed from CT clearly demonstrated a scaphoid waist nonunion of Herbert type B2 fracture[1] (Fig. 28.3), with the fracture location distal to the apex of the dorsal scaphoid ridge (Fig. 28.4A). 3D CT also revealed that the humpback deformity of the scaphoid was accompanied with the dorsal rotation of the proximal scaphoid fragment and lunate, indicating large bone defects on the volar side of the scaphoid (Fig. 28.4B and C). In Case 2, 3D CT clearly demonstrated a scaphoid nonunion of Herbert type B1 fracture[1,2] (Fig. 28.3), with the fracture location proximal to the scaphoid apex at the dorsal side (Fig. 28.5A). However, 3D CT revealed no humpback deformity or dorsal rotation of the proximal scaphoid fragment and lunate (Fig. 28.5A and B).

Symptoms and natural histories of type B1 and B2 scaphoid nonunions are different.[3–8] The initial fracture types correlate with the deformity pattern of the scaphoid and other carpal bones. The mechanism of the development of different deformity patterns is explained as follows. Under normal conditions, the scaphoid is subjected to flexional force from the trapezium, trapezoid, and capitate, whereas the lunate and triquetrum are subjected to extensional force from the hamate.[9–11] The dorsal scapholunate interosseous ligament (DSLIL), which couples the scaphoid and lunate and is attached on the dorsal scaphoid apex, plays a role in stabilizing the scaphoid and lunate.[12] In type B2 (Case 1), the scaphoid and lunate complex is broken at the fracture site. The proximal fragment connected

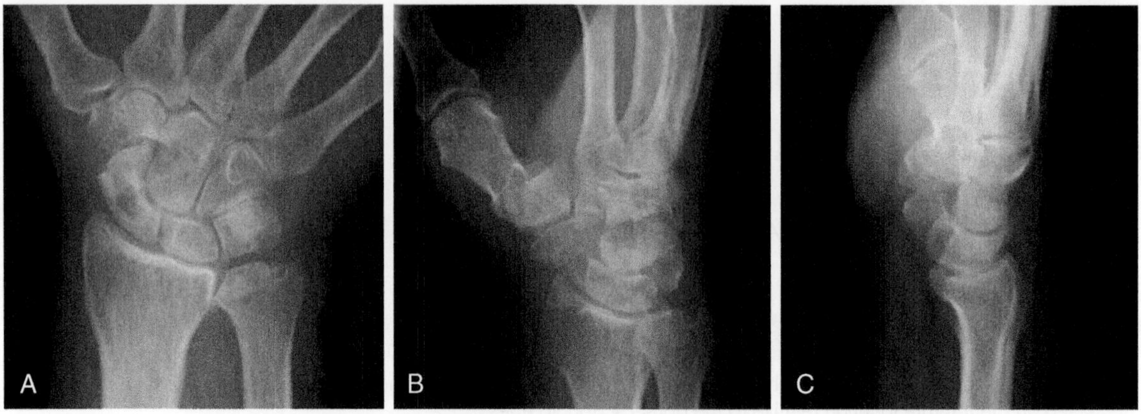

FIG. 28.1 Anteroposterior and pronated oblique radiographs demonstrate the scaphoid waist nonunion of type B2 fracture **(A** and **B)**. Lateral radiograph demonstrates the dorsal intercalated segment instability deformity **(C)**.

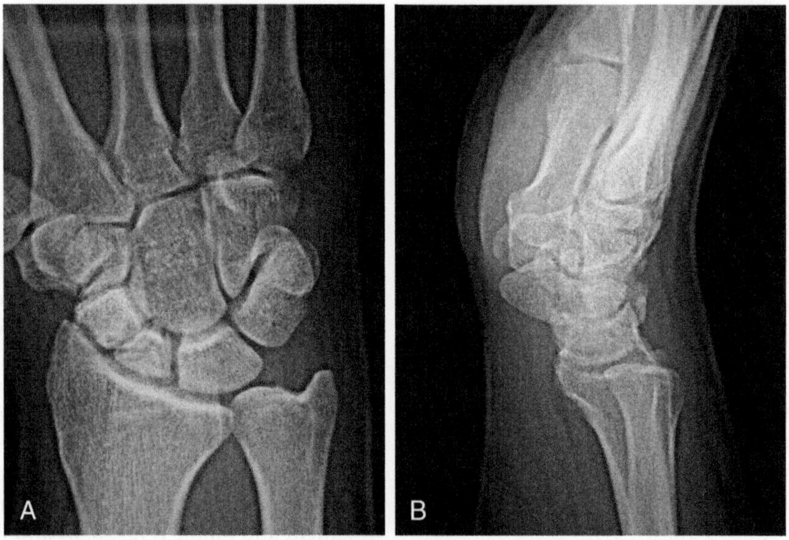

FIG. 28.2 Anteroposterior radiograph demonstrates the scaphoid waist nonunion of type B1 fracture **(A)**. Dorsal intercalated segment instability deformity is not visible in the lateral radiograph **(B)**.

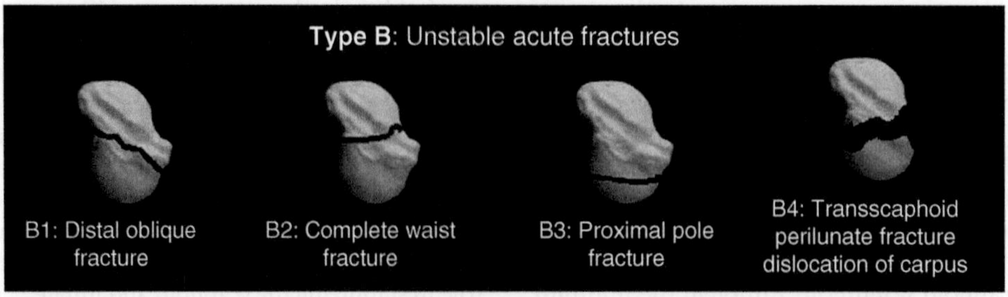

FIG. 28.3 The Herbert classification of unstable scaphoid fractures (types B1–B4). Distal oblique fracture (B1) is proximal to the apex, and complete waist fracture (B2) is distal to the apex. (From Haisman JM, et al. Acute fractures of the scaphoid. *J Bone Joint Surg Am*. 2006;88(12):2750–2758 with permission.)

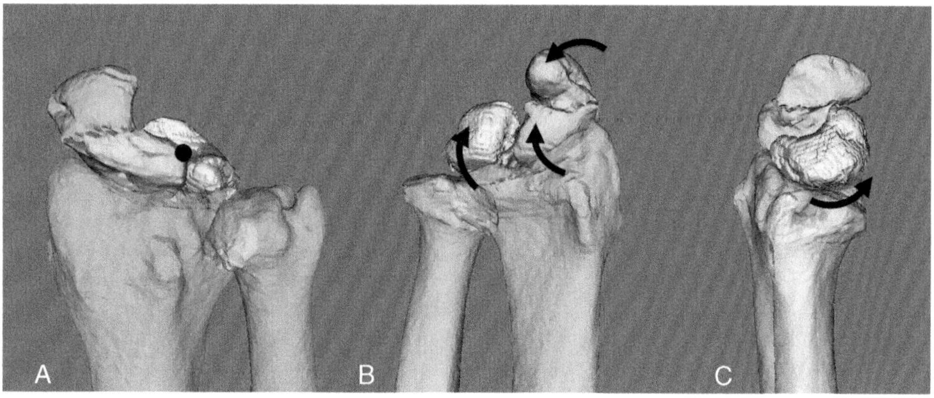

FIG. 28.4 *Black spot* indicates the dorsal scaphoid apex **(A)**. The humpback and dorsal intercalated segment instability deformities can be easily recognized in 3D reconstruction bone models **(B** and **C)**. Black arrows indicate the direction of subsequent deformity of each bone.

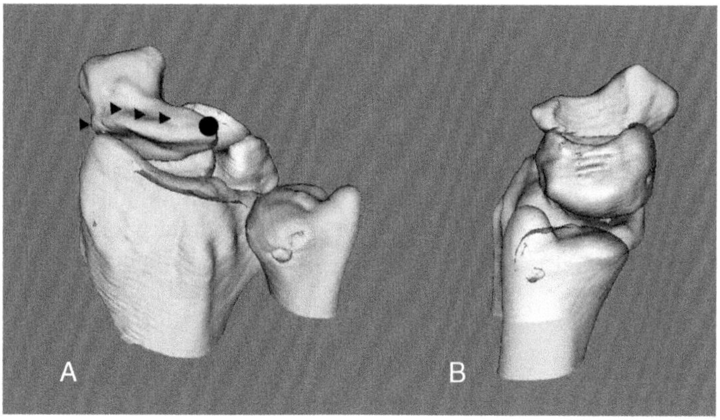

FIG. 28.5 *Black spot* indicates the dorsal scaphoid apex, and *black triangles* indicate the osteophyte formation on the scaphoid dorsal ridge **(A)**. Dorsal intercalated segment instability deformity is not visible **(B)**.

to the lunate via DSLIL extends, and the carpal collapse proceeds.[6,13] In type B1 (Case 2), the connection between the distal fragment and lunate is preserved via DSLIL so that the scaphoid and lunate complex remains stable and the carpal collapse is not prominent.[6,12] However, the differential diagnosis of each fracture type is not always easy using radiographs only. Moreover, the significance of a differential diagnosis of each type is not accurately recognized on a clinical basis.[7]

Untreated type B2 scaphoid fractures lead to a carpal collapse with large bone defects on the volar side of the scaphoid and subsequent degenerative arthritis of the wrist.[14–21] The dorsal translation and flexion of the distal fragment caused by the DISI deformity creates an impingement between the distal fragment and radial styloid, leading to osteophyte formation at the radial styloid. The surgery of type B2 scaphoid nonunion includes a rigid internal fixation with screws and wedge-shaped bone grafting via a volar approach.[22–25] Conversely, in long-standing type B1 scaphoid nonunion, as shown in Case 2, the carpal collapse and DISI deformity is not always visible, even with massive osteophyte formation along the dorsal ridge of scaphoid.[26,27] The bone defect is smaller, with a flat shape without humpback deformity.[3,28] The scaphoid nonunion is essentially stable, and the carpal alignment is preserved for a long time. Therefore, the scaphoid nonunion is less symptomatic and less likely to cause wrist impairment. However, the minor movement of the proximal fragment and impingement at the fracture site to the articular surface of the capitate and radius lead to gradual degeneration of the wrist. As for the surgery of type B1 scaphoid nonunion, the resection of the dorsal radial styloid process and of the osteophytes of the dorsal scaphoid ridge without fixation may be a viable option for low-demand patients.[27] If nonunion is treated with internal fixation, resection of the dorsal osteophyte and cancellous bone graft via the dorsal approach is recommended.[3,7]

MAIN QUESTION

What is the additional value of 3D analysis of scaphoid nonunion patterns?

Current Opinion

It is much easier to identify the scaphoid apex with 3D reconstruction images than 2D radiographs because the scaphoid apex overlaps the capitate head on radiographs.

3D analysis of the established scaphoid nonunion, which elucidates the relationship between the scaphoid apex and fracture location, is the key to predict subsequent carpal instability.

Finding the Evidence

- Pubmed (Medline): ("Scaphoid nonunion" [Mesh] OR scaphoid fracture*[tiab] OR scaphoid bone fracture*[tiab] OR scaphoid [tiab]) AND ("three-dimensional deformity" [Subheading] OR deformity*)
- Articles that were not in English were excluded

Quality of the Evidence

Level IV:

Case Series: 16

FINDINGS

Sixteen studies, including 2D and/or 3D evaluations, focused on the scaphoid nonunion deformity and all were retrospective case series (Level IV, 465 patients, range: 9–74). Of these 16 studies, 10 analyzed the wrist deformity in the scaphoid nonunion using 3D CT (277 patients, range: 9–74). Of these 10 studies, 7 investigated the patterns of scaphoid deformity, bone defects, osteophyte formation, and carpal malalignment according to the fracture location. The amount of bone defect was quantitatively analyzed in four studies.[3,26,27,29] Distal pole or type B2 waist fractures had significantly larger bone defects than proximal pole or type B1 fractures ($P \leq .01$). The relationship between the fracture location and DISI deformity was quantitatively investigated in six studies.[4,27,30–33] Analysis revealed that the extension rotations of the proximal fragment and lunate were significantly greater for type B2 than type B1 scaphoid nonunion ($P \leq .01$). Three studies investigated the scaphoid nonunion advanced collapse patterns based on the fracture location. In type B2 fractures, the osteophyte formation occurred between the radial styloid and scaphoid distal fragment. In type B1 or proximal third fractures, the osteophyte formation proceeded between the dorsal styloid process of the radius and scaphoid dorsal ridge.[6,27,34] One study classified type B2 into two types based on whether the fracture passes into the radial facet of the scaphoid (intraarticular fracture) or not (extraarticular fracture).[22] Significantly larger osteophyte formation at the radial styloid process was visible in type B2 intraarticular fractures than in extraarticular fractures ($P < .05$). One study analyzed the relationship between the fracture type and kinematic pattern. The interfragmentary motion of the scaphoid, which has the fracture line proximal to the scaphoid apex, was significantly smaller than that of the scaphoid that has the fracture line distal to the scaphoid apex ($P < .05$).[32]

RECOMMENDATION

- Evaluation with 3D CT is recommended to determine the initial fracture type, which helps to decide the best strategy for managing the scaphoid nonunion (overall quality: low).
- 3D CT can help determine whether the fracture line passes distally or proximally to the dorsal apex of the scaphoid, where the DSLIL is attached, and determines the subsequent carpal instability in nonunion (overall quality: moderate).

CONCLUSIONS

Whether the fracture line passes distally or proximally to the dorsal apex of the scaphoid, where the DSLIL is attached, determines the subsequent carpal instability if nonunion occurs:

- When the fracture line runs distally to the dorsal apex of the scaphoid (type B2), the stability between the distal fragment of scaphoid nonunion and lunate is disrupted at the fracture site. Scaphoid nonunion will progress quickly, resulting in humpback and DISI deformity patterns.
- When the fracture line runs proximally to the dorsal apex of the scaphoid (type B1), the distal fragment is connected to the lunate via the DSLIL so that the proximal row remains at equilibrium. The scaphoid nonunion is more stable, and the carpal collapse is less likely to occur.

PANEL 2
Authors' Preferred Technique

Nondisplaced acute scaphoid fractures are treated conservatively with cast immobilization. If the displacement of the fracture site is more than 2 mm, closed or open reduction and internal fixation with a double-threaded screw is recommended. The goals of surgery for scaphoid nonunion are to achieve union, correct the scaphoid deformity, and restore the carpal alignment. However, the natural history and deformity pattern that affect the therapeutic strategy are different between nonuniting type B1 and B2 fractures. Therefore, identifying the relationship between the fracture line and scaphoid apex with 3D CT is crucial to estimate the prognosis of scaphoid nonunion and to determine the treatment courses. Open reduction and internal fixation is recommended for nonunion of type B2 fractures because the risk of progressing to DISI deformity and scaphoid nonunion advanced collapse is considered to be high for these nonunions. Conversely, the conservative treatment of nonunion of type B1 fractures is considered an optional therapy for elderly patients or patients who cannot undergo surgery because of economic or social reasons because these fractures are less symptomatic; however, for these nonunions, open reduction and internal fixation remains the first choice as well.

Two types of approaches, volar or dorsal, are used for the open reduction and internal fixation of scaphoid nonunion. Classifying the patterns of bone defects, osteophyte formation, and carpal deformity into two types also helps the surgeon to select the best surgical approach between volar and dorsal. In nonunion of type B2 fractures, a wedge-shaped bone graft harvested from the iliac crest is required to correct the humpback deformity and to restore the scaphoid length. A volar approach is preferable to allow easy correction of the humpback deformity and implantation of the wedge-shaped bone graft. A rigid fixation is achieved by inserting the screw from the scaphoid tuberosity (Fig. 28.6A–C). In nonunion of type B1 fractures, the bone defect followed by the humpback deformity is minor and massive osteophytes develop on the dorsal ridge. A dorsal approach is recommended to remove dorsal osteophytes, and a small amount of cancellous bone graft into the nonunion site is adequate. Moreover, screw insertion from the dorsal side allows easier vertical penetration at the fracture site (Fig. 28.7A–C).

Even if 3D CT is not available for clinical use, radiographs can be useful in distinguishing stable nonunions (B1) from unstable ones (B2).[7,8] In the semipronated oblique view, the scaphoid apex can be observed as overlapping the capitate head. B1 and B2 types can be identified based on the fracture location relative to the apex (Fig. 28.8A and B). In the posteroanterior view with the wrist in the neutral position, obvious differences between type B1 and B2 types can be observed. In nonunion of type B1 fractures, the fracture line is evident because it is closely parallel to the posteroanterior direction of the wrist (Fig. 28.2A). Conversely, in nonunion of type B2 fractures, the fracture line is obscure because the fracture line, which is vertical to the scaphoid long axis, is oblique to the posteroanterior direction of the wrist (Fig. 28.1A). However, the diagnosis of the initial fracture types in scaphoid nonunion using radiographs has limited accuracy; therefore, evaluation using 3D CT is recommended.

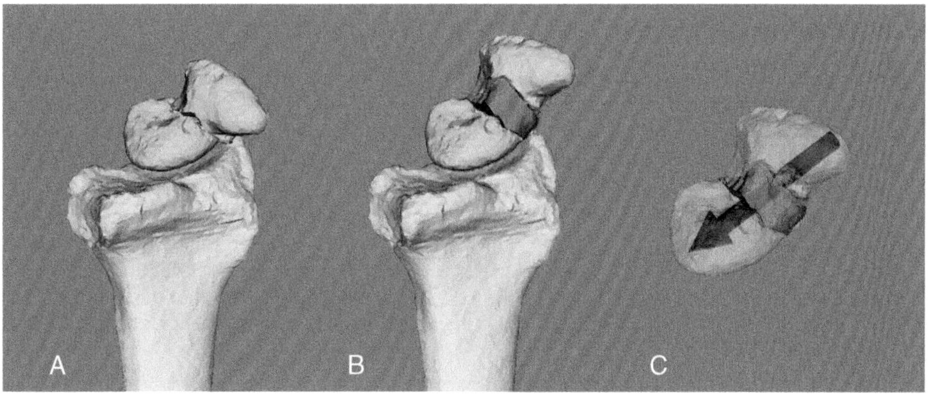

FIG. 28.6 Humpback deformity is corrected with a wedge-shaped bone from the volar aspect of scaphoid **(A** and **B)**. Screw insertion from the distal scaphoid (*black arrow*) allows for rigid fixation **(C)**.

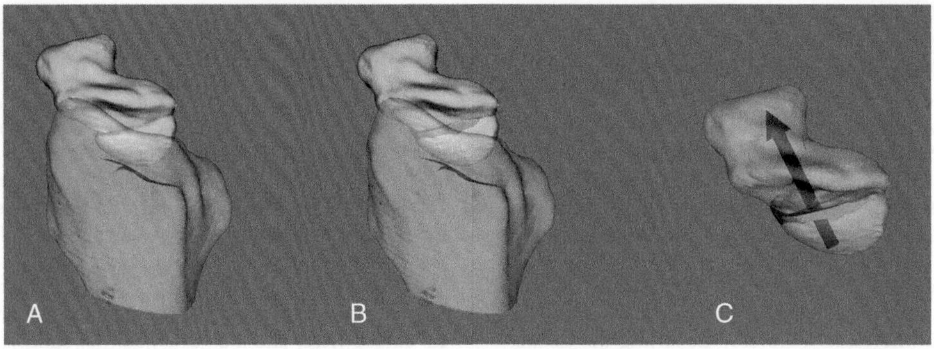

FIG. 28.7 A dorsal approach is adequate to remove osteophytes on the dorsal ridge and inserting an appropriate amount of cancellous bone graft **(A** and **B)**. Screw insertion from the dorsal side (*black arrow*) allows for easier vertical penetration at the fracture site **(C)**.

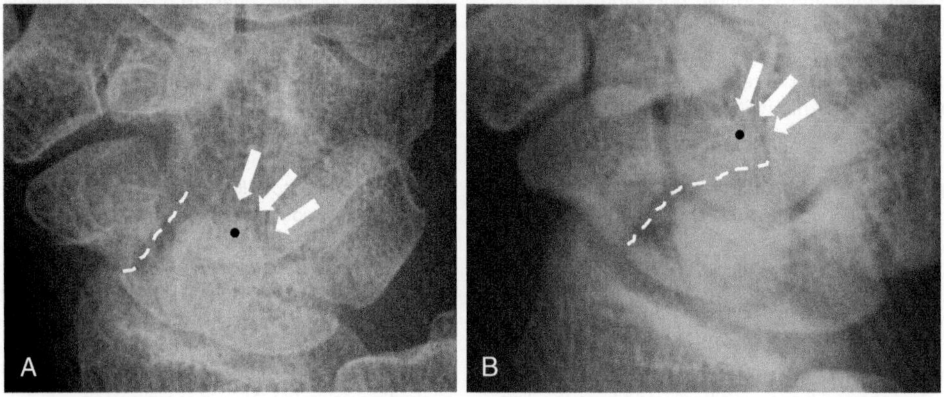

FIG. 28.8 *White arrows* indicate the scaphoid dorsal apex in semipronated oblique radiograph. The fracture line (*white dotted line*) is distal to the apex (*black spot*) in type B2 fracture **(A)** and proximal in type B1 fracture **(B)**.

PANEL 3
Pearls and Pitfalls

PEARLS

- Firstly, it is important to picture the 3D shape of scaphoid and to identify fracture location with respective to the scaphoid dorsal apex in plain radiographs.
- Then, the initial fracture type, 3D deformity pattern, osteophyte formation, and the amount of bone defect are confirmed with the use of 3D image of the scaphoid nonunion.

PITFALLS

- Dorsal intercalated segment instability (DISI) deformity and carpal instability occasionally occur in type B1 fractures accompanied with dorsal scapholunate interosseous ligament (DSLIL) tear. When the fracture location is close to the apex in type B1 fractures, the remaining DSLIL attached to the apex on the distal fragment can be damaged.
- It is essential not only to diagnose possible carpal instability by discerning fracture types (B1 or B2) but also to pay careful attention to the association of a latent DSLIL tear that can be diagnosed by the separation between the scaphoid apex and dorsal lunate horn.

REFERENCES

1. Herbert TJ, Fisher WE. Management of the fractured scaphoid using a new bone screw. *J Bone Joint Surg Br.* 1984;66(1):114–123.
2. Haisman JM, et al. Acute fractures of the scaphoid. *J Bone Joint Surg Am.* 2006;88(12):2750–2758.
3. Oka K, et al. Patterns of bone defect in scaphoid nonunion: a 3-dimensional and quantitative analysis. *J Hand Surg Am.* 2005;30(2):359–365.
4. Oka K, et al. Patterns of carpal deformity in scaphoid nonunion: a 3-dimensional and quantitative analysis. *J Hand Surg Am.* 2005;30(6):1136–1144.
5. Nakamura R, et al. Analysis of scaphoid fracture displacement by three-dimensional computed tomography. *J Hand Surg Am.* 1991;16(3):485–492.
6. Moritomo H, et al. Scaphoid nonunions: a 3-dimensional analysis of patterns of deformity. *J Hand Surg Am.* 2000;25(3):520–528.
7. Moritomo H. Radiographic clues for determining carpal instability and treatment protocol for scaphoid fractures. *J Orthop Sci.* 2014;19(3):379–383.
8. Inagaki H, et al. Differences in radiographic findings between scaphoid fracture patterns. *Hand Surg.* 2004;9(2):197–202.
9. Weber ER. Biomechanical implications of scaphoid waist fractures. *Clin Orthop Relat Res.* 1980;(149):83–89.
10. Kauer JM. Functional anatomy of the wrist. *Clin Orthop Relat Res.* 1980;(149):9–20.
11. Smith DK, et al. The effects of simulated unstable scaphoid fractures on carpal motion. *J Hand Surg Am.* 1989;14(2 Pt 1):283–291.
12. Garcia-Elias M. Kinetic analysis of carpal stability during grip. *Hand Clin.* 1997;13(1):151–158.
13. Garcia-Elias M, Lluch A. Partial excision of scaphoid: is it ever indicated? *Hand Clin.* 2001;17(4):687–695.
14. Ruby LK, Stinson J, Belsky MR. The natural history of scaphoid non-union. A review of fifty-five cases. *J Bone Joint Surg Am.* 1985;67(3):428–432.
15. Mack GR, et al. The natural history of scaphoid non-union. *J Bone Joint Surg Am.* 1984;66(4):504–509.
16. Kozin SH. Incidence, mechanism, and natural history of scaphoid fractures. *Hand Clin.* 2001;17(4):515–524.
17. Inoue G, Sakuma M. The natural history of scaphoid non-union. Radiographical and clinical analysis in 102 cases. *Arch Orthop Trauma Surg.* 1996;115(1):1–4.
18. Hidaka Y, Nakamura R. Progressive patterns of degenerative arthritis in scaphoid nonunion demonstrated by three-dimensional computed tomography. *J Hand Surg Br.* 1998;23(6):765–770.
19. Fisk GR. Osteo-arthrosis of the wrist. *Clin Rheum Dis.* 1984;10(3):571–588.
20. Fisk GR. An overview of injuries of the wrist. *Clin Orthop Relat Res.* 1980;(149):137–144.
21. Linscheid RL, et al. Instability patterns of the wrist. *J Hand Surg Am.* 1983;8(5 Pt 2):682–686.
22. Tsuyuguchi Y, et al. Anterior wedge-shaped bone graft for old scaphoid fractures or non-unions. An analysis of relevant carpal alignment. *J Hand Surg Br.* 1995;20(2):194–200.
23. Trumble TE, Clarke T, Kreder HJ. Non-union of the scaphoid. Treatment with cannulated screws compared with treatment with Herbert screws. *J Bone Joint Surg Am.* 1996;78(12):1829–1837.
24. Merrell GA, Wolfe SW, Slade 3rd JF. Treatment of scaphoid nonunions: quantitative meta-analysis of the literature. *J Hand Surg Am.* 2002;27(4):685–691.
25. Daly K, et al. Established nonunion of the scaphoid treated by volar wedge grafting and Herbert screw fixation. *J Bone Joint Surg Br.* 1996;78(4):530–534.
26. Ten Berg PW, et al. Analysis of deformity in scaphoid nonunions using two- and three-dimensional imaging. *J Hand Surg Eur Vol.* 2016;41(7):719–726.
27. Oura K, et al. Three-dimensional analysis of osteophyte formation on distal radius following scaphoid nonunion. *J Orthop Sci.* 2016;22(1):50–55.
28. Buijze GA, Ochtman L, Ring D. Management of scaphoid nonunion. *J Hand Surg Am.* 2012;37(5):1095–1100. quiz 1101.
29. Schweizer A, Furnstahl P, Nagy L. Three-dimensional computed tomographic analysis of 11 scaphoid waist nonunions. *J Hand Surg Am.* 2012;37(6):1151–1158.
30. Kim BJ, et al. The role of lunate morphology on scapholunate instability and fracture location in patients treated for scaphoid nonunion. *Clin Orthop Surg.* 2016;8(2):175–180.
31. ten Berg PW, et al. Quantifying scaphoid malalignment based upon height-to-length ratios obtained by 3-dimensional computed tomography. *J Hand Surg Am.* 2015;40(1):67–73.
32. Moritomo H, et al. Relationship between the fracture location and the kinematic pattern in scaphoid nonunion. *J Hand Surg Am.* 2008;33(9):1459–1468.
33. Belsole RJ, et al. Computed analyses of the pathomechanics of scaphoid waist nonunions. *J Hand Surg Am.* 1991;16(5):899–906.
34. Moritomo H, et al. The relationship between the site of nonunion of the scaphoid and scaphoid nonunion advanced collapse (SNAC). *J Bone Joint Surg Br.* 1999;81(5):871–876.

CHAPTER 29

Surgical Treatment for Fibrous-Delayed Scaphoid Nonunions

WILLIAM B. GEISSLER, MD • ALAN E. FREELAND

KEY POINTS

- Fibrous and delayed scaphoid nonunions may be addressed arthroscopically or open.
- Type I–III scaphoid nonunions may be addressed with a headless screw and no bone grafting. This may be done arthroscopically or open.
- Type IV scaphoid nonunions require some type of grafting, either cancellous bone or demineralized bone matrix (DBM). This may be performed arthroscopically under fluoroscope control or open.
- In small proximal pole fractures or when greater stability is desired, the midcarpal space may be temporarily locked up to provide additional stability to the fracture.

PANEL 1
Case Scenario

A 22-year-old major college football player presents to the clinic with approximately 2-month history of wrist pain following the football season. The patient did not report the pain to the trainers, as he was concerned he would not be allowed to continue to play. He presents with severe wrist pain with decreased range of motion to the wrist. He had a previous attempt at open reduction and distal radius bone grafting. What are your next options for this delayed union in a high-demand athlete?

IMPORTANCE OF THE PROBLEM

The failure of a scaphoid fracture to heal results in well-known predictable patterns of wrist arthritis.[1] To minimize the instances of arthrosis, the goal of management of scaphoid fractures should be consolidation of the fracture with the scaphoid in anatomic alignment.[2,3] Generally, scaphoid nonunions with severe collapse and humpback deformity must be approached volarly with intercalary bone graft and some type of internal fixation.[4,5] Proximal pole nonunions are generally approached from the dorsal aspect. Vascularized bone grafts are recommended to manage scaphoid nonunions with osteonecrosis.[6]

In an effort to match the healing potential of a scaphoid nonunion to a specific treatment algorithm, Slade and Geissler proposed a revised classification of scaphoid nonunions (Table 29.1).[7] In our classification, scaphoid nonunions can be divided into two groups. The classification comprises early scaphoid nonunions without substantial bone resorption and (2) chronic nonunions with substantial bone resorption. The classification is further subdivided based on the width of the devitalized scaphoid zone and the amount of bone loss, requiring the need of additional structural or biologic enhancements. The goal of the grading systems reflects the natural degradation that occurs at a scaphoid nonunion site over time and the difficulties that arise when these changes occur.

MAIN QUESTION

What is the preferred treatment for fibrous/delayed scaphoid unions?

Current Opinion

Fibrous and delayed scaphoid nonunions are mostly addressed arthroscopically or open, although there still seems a role for conservative treatment in selected cases. Type I–III scaphoid nonunions may be addressed with a headless screw and bone grafting. Type IV scaphoid nonunions require some type of grafting, either cancellous bone or DBM. These surgeries may be performed arthroscopically under fluoroscope control or open. There is a debate which is most

TABLE 29.1
Slade-Geissler Classification

Type	Description
I	Delayed presentation at 4–12 weeks
II	Fibrous union, minimal fracture line
III	Minimal sclerosis <1 mm
IV	Cystic formation, 1–5 mm
V	Humpback deformity with >5 mm cystic change
VI	With arthrosis

successful. It is the author's opinion that management with DBM is equal to cancellous grafting and is a lot easier to perform.

Finding the Evidence

- Cochrane search: Scaphoid Fracture
- Pubmed (Medline): ("Scaphoid Bone" [Mesh] OR scaphoid fracture*[tiab] OR scaphoid bone Fracture*[tiab] OR scaphoid[tiab]) AND (delay* OR fibrous)
- Bibliography of eligible articles
- Articles that were not in English were excluded

Quality of the Evidence

Level IV:
  Case series: 13
Level V:
  Expert opinion: 5

FINDINGS

Conservative Treatment

Because of extensive casting duration and unsatisfactory union rates, there seems to be a limited role for conservative treatment of delayed unions. Recently, Grewal et al. reported a series of isolated subacute scaphoid fractures (missed fractures) that presented between 6 weeks and 6 months from injury.[31] There were 20 males and 8 females, with a mean age of 30, treated with casting alone. There were 20 waist, 7 proximal, and 1 distal pole fracture. The mean casting time was 11 (waist) and 14 (proximal pole) weeks with a union rate of 82% (23/28). Diabetes, comminution, and a humpback deformity increased the nonunion risk in this cohort. Exclusion of these cases resulted in a 96% union rate (24/24). The expected time frame for union with cast treatment is shorter than previously reported. This would confirm the author's classification that if a humpback deformity is present, then operative fixation is indicated.

In an uncontrolled case study, Farkah et al. reviewed low-intensity pulsed ultrasound (LIPUS) as an alternative to surgery to improve scaphoid fracture healing.[32] In their study, 29 patients with a delayed union to the scaphoid were offered LIPUS treatment as an alternative to surgery. They noted 22 of 29 (76%) fractures healed. Patients diagnosed within 3 months had a 92% healing rate as compared with patients diagnosed greater than 3 months, which had only a 63% healing rate.

Scaphoid Unions Without Substantial Bone Loss

Grade 1 scaphoid nonunions without substantial bone loss require only rigid fixation to heal if there is adequate perfusion to the scaphoid. Grade 1 scaphoid nonunions are classified as delayed presentation at 4–12 weeks after injury. Stable subacute fractures of the scaphoid have already developed bone absorption at the fracture site from sharing forces that is not typically detected by a standard radiographs. These fractures may require 4–6 months of cast mobilization to heal. For that reason, most authors recommend internal fixation for delayed for presentation. Similarly, subacute proximal pole fractures have a high nonunion rate. Grade 1 nonunions may be managed with reduction and rigid fixation without bone grafting for successful healing. This can be accomplished either arthroscopically or by open techniques.

In Grade 2 fibrous nonunions presented with a minimal fracture line. Barton reviewed 10 symptomatic patients with radiographic nonunion of the scaphoid and for patients with the suspected nonunion.[8] Interoperatively all, 10 scaphoids appeared healed by visual inspections, but only 5 of them ultimately united radiographically. Another five patients appeared to have a partial union at surgery and all four of those fractures went on to unite. This study helps underscore the importance of CT scans to detail the extent of osseous healing following cast treatment or internal fixation. Visual radiograph expression is often insufficient compared with CT evaluation. Shah and Jones, reported on 50 scaphoid nonunions managed by open Herbert screw fixation in scaphoids that had an intact cartilages envelope or a stable fibrous nonunion.[9] All patients healed with screw fixation alone without any bone grafting. Based on these studies, rigid fixation is recommended in stable fibrous nonunions to prevent micromotion and allow bone healing.

Grade 3 scaphoid nonunions have minimal bone absorption of the anterior cortical bone and minimal fracture sclerosis less than 1 mm. These nonunions still have the potential for healing with rigid fixation without or bone grafting.

Slade and Geissler published their series of 15 patients with fibrous nonunion of the scaphoid less than 1 mm treated by arthroscopic-assisted fixation alone without bone grafting.[10] In their combined series, all 15 patients healed in this case series at an average of 14 weeks. CT scans documented bridging cortical bone. Nonunions treated less than 6 months after the injury healed faster than those treated later. Similarly, Ikeda et al. achieved successful union in 51 of 51 scaphoid nonunions with sclerosis less than 1 mm and displacement less than 2 mm by cannulated screw fixation alone without bone graft.[11]

Dorsal Percutaneous Approach

Joseph Slade was a pioneer in management of the fractures of scaphoid.[12–14] He and his coworkers published the dorsal percutaneous approach for fractures of the scaphoid. This technique became very popular because it involved limited surgical dissection and allowed arthroscopic evaluation and reduction of the scaphoid fracture. In Slade's technique, the patient is placed in a supine position on the hand table with the arm extended. Several towels are placed under the elbow with the forearm parallel to the floor. The wrist is pronated and flexed under fluoroscopic control until the proximal and distal poles of the scaphoid are aligned to form a perfect cylinder (Fig. 29.1). Slade recommended continuous fluoroscopy as the wrist is flexed to obtain the true ring sign as the proximal and distal pole are aligned.

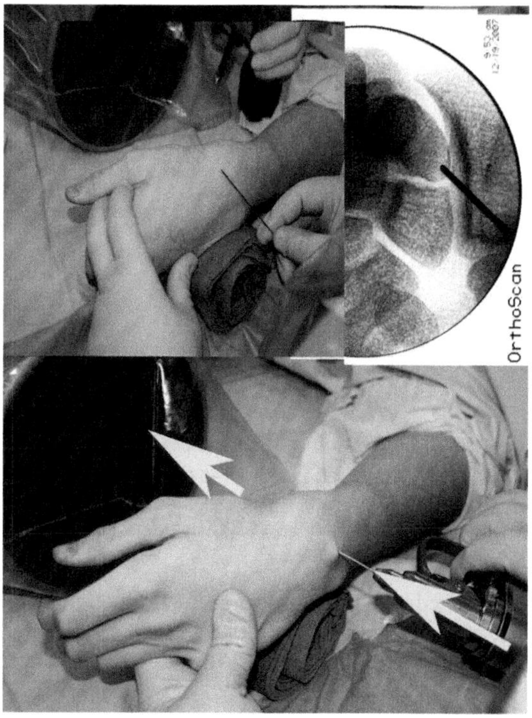

FIG. 29.1 In the Slade technique, the wrist is flexed and pronated to form a cylinder as the proximal and distal poles of the scaphoid align with each other (Angle of X-Ray beam).

Once a perfect ring is confirmed by fluoroscopy, a 14G needle is placed percutaneously in the center of the ring parallel to the fluoroscopic beam. A guide wire is inserted through the 14G needle and driven the across the central axis of scaphoid from a dorsal direction until the guide wire comes in contact with the distal pole of the scaphoid cortex (Fig. 29.2). The position of the guide wire is then evaluated under fluoroscopy in the posteroanterior, lateral, and oblique planes while the wrist is maintained in flexion (Fig. 29.3). It is vital to not extend the wrist at this point as this may bend the guide wire. A second guide wire is then placed parallel to the first so that it touches the proximal pole of the scaphoid to determine the screw length, or alternately a depth gauge may be utilized. The difference in length between the two guide wires is measured. It is of utmost vital importance that a screw at least 4 mm shorter is placed than when it is measured. There is nothing more frustrating, than when a headless cannulated screw is too long, and secure fixation will be lost when a shorter screw is placed. One option in that, for instance, is to use a screw one size up in diameter. If one is using headless screws, it is recommended to use the small-sized screw for this purpose. If the screw has

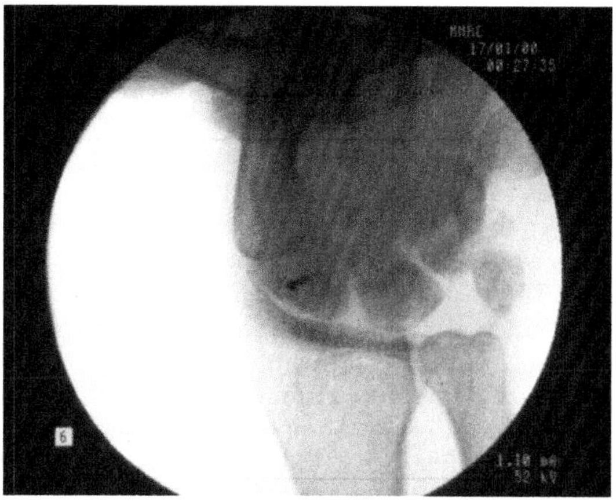

FIG. 29.2 Fluoroscopic view of the ring sign with the guide wire placed in central alignment.

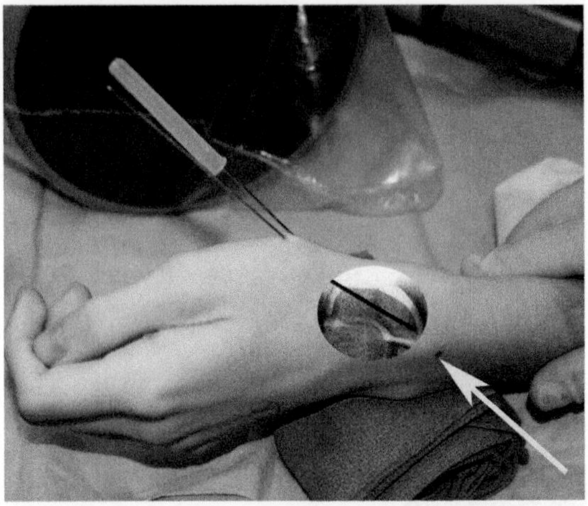

FIG. 29.3 Figure demonstrating the correct placement of the guide wire down the central axis of the scaphoid from the dorsal approach (Angle of X-Ray beam).

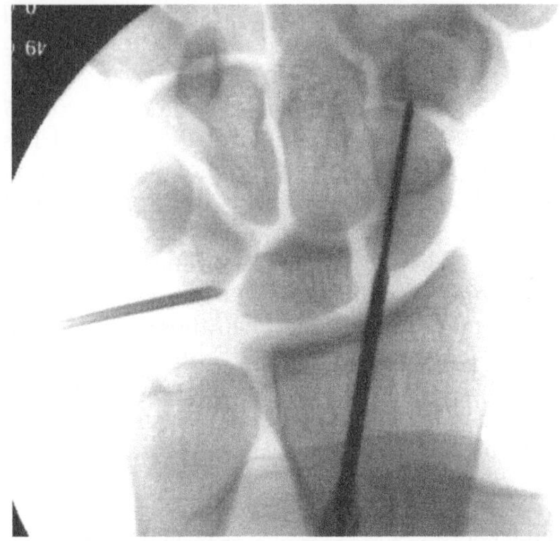

FIG. 29.4 Fluoroscopic view demonstrating central placement of the guide wire.

to be revised in the future, or the screwed measured was too long when inserted, then one can utilize to a larger diameter size screw without loss of secure fixation such as a standard screw.

Once the screw length is determined, the guide wire advanced distally to exit the skin on the volar aspect of the hand. The wire is continued to be advanced, until it is flush with the proximal pole of the scaphoid dorsally. The wrist may now be extended for arthroscopic evaluation.

The wrist is then suspended in a traction tower and the radiocarpal and midcarpal spaces are evaluated arthroscopically. The radiocarpal space is examined for any soft tissue injuries, particularly to the interosseous ligaments or the triangular fibrocartilage complex.[15,16] A fracture of the scaphoid cannot be seen with the arthroscope in the radiocarpal space. This is an opportunity to the see exact position of the guide wire in the proximal pole of the scaphoid (Fig. 29.4). The ideal entry point should be just radial to the insertion of the scapholunate interosseous ligament on the scaphoid. The arthroscope is then placed in the radial midcarpal portal to evaluate the fracture reduction. Fractures of the waist of the scaphoid are best seen with the arthroscope in the radial midcarpal portal.[17,18] Fractures of the proximal pole are best seen with the arthroscope in the ulnar midcarpal portal. If the reduction of the scaphoid fracture is not satisfactory, the guide wire can be advanced out volarly but still be maintained in the distal pole of the scaphoid. Joysticks may be placed in the proximal and distal poles of the scaphoid to facilitate reduction as viewed directly with the arthroscope in the midcarpal space. Once anatomic reduction has been achieved, the primary guide wire is advanced back proximately into the proximal pole of the scaphoid. Usually with flexion-extension and/or radial-ulnar deviation in the traction tower, the fracture can be reduced (Fig. 29.5).

Once anatomic restoration of the scaphoid is obtained as confirmed both arthroscopically and under fluoroscopy, the guide wire is advanced back out dorsally with the wrist flexed. It is important that blunt dissection is performed around the guide wire dorsally to minimize risk of any tendon injury by the guide wire as it exits back out dorsally. A portion of the guide wire is should still be left out on the volar aspect of the hand, so if it breaks or bends, easy access to the broken guide wire is possible. Through a soft tissue protector, the scaphoid is then reamed with the near and far reamers and a headless cannulated screw is then inserted.

The dorsal approach has several advantages the screw is inserted down the central axis of the scaphoid perpendicular to the fracture site compared with the volar approach. This allows compression directly across the fracture site compared with the more oblique orientation from the volar approach. The concern with the dorsal percutaneous approach by Slade is that, by hyperflexing the wrist to form a cylinder, it may displace the scaphoid fracture to create a humpback deformity. For this reason, the reduction of the scaphoid fracture should be evaluated with the arthroscope in

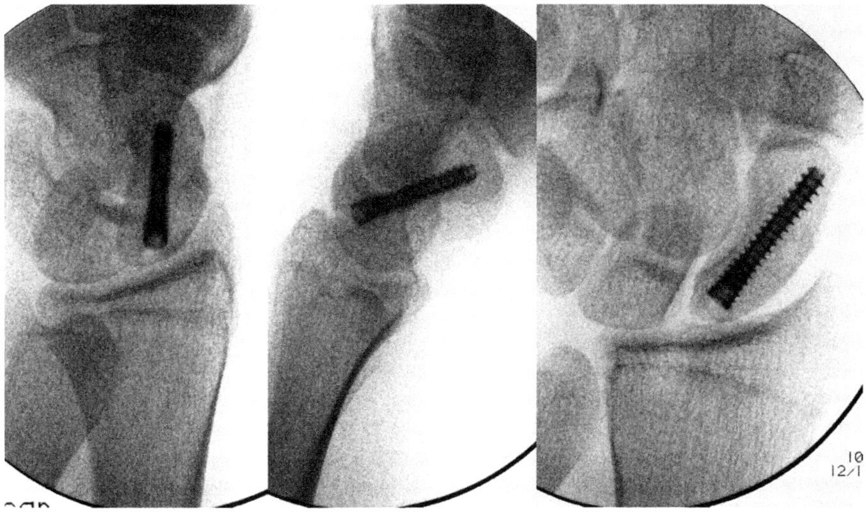

FIG. 29.5 Anterior posterior, oblique, and lateral radiographs demonstrating correct placement of the headless screw in the scaphoid.

the midcarpal space. Frequently, it takes a surgeon and a very capable surgical assistant to utilize the Slade dorsal technique.

Mini-open Technique

Many surgeons prefer a limited open technique for screw placement via the dorsal approach.[19–21] In addition, arthroscopic equipment my not be readily available. In those instances, a mini-open technique may be used. An approximate 2-cm skin incision is made centered over the traditional 3–4 wrist arthroscopic portal. This incision will be located approximately 1 cm distal to Lister's tubercle and centered between the third and fourth dorsal compartments. Blunt dissection is carried down to the extensor tendons where the extensor pollicis longus is released through the incision. A small dorsal arthrotomy is made where the dorsal aspect of the scaphoid is identified. Just like in arthroscopic reduction with the Slade technique, the ideal starting point is on the most dorsal aspect to the scaphoid just radial to the scapholunate interosseous ligament insertion. Once this landmark is identified, and guide wire is then passed down the central axis of the scaphoid in line with the thumb. The guide wire is checked under anteroposterior (AP), lateral, and oblique planes because it approaches the distal volar vortex of the scaphoid. Just as in Slade's technique, the screw length is measured and a screw of at least 4 mm shorter is inserted. It is important to advance the guide wire out the volar aspect before the screw is placed, so if the guide wire breaks, it is readily accessible. The joints capsule is closed and the extensor pollicis longus is left free.

Volar Percutaneous Approach

Haddad and Goddard popularized the volar percutaneous technique.[22] This technique is indicated for scaphoid nonunions with minimum sclerosis at the waist or distal to the waist. It is not indicated for proximal pole fractures. In their technique, they recommend suspending the thumb in a Chinese finger trap (Fig. 29.6). By placing the thumb under suspension with this technique allows ulnar deviation improving access to the distal pole of the scaphoid. An approximately 0.5-cm skin excision is made under fluoroscopic guidance over the most radial distal aspect of the scaphoid. Blunt dissection is carried down to expose the distal pole of the scaphoid to protect the cutaneous nerves as they pass over the surgical area.

They recommended using a large needle (14G), which is impaled into the distal pole of the scaphoid. Utilizing the needle in their technique, the bevel of the needle can help further correct the direction of the guide wire. They feel the advantage of their technique is that suspending the thumb in traction allows an almost 360-degree fluoroscopic view of the guide wire within the scaphoid as it is being inserted. They also emphasized that a screw 2- to 4-cm shorter than what was measured should be utilized in the volar approach. The guide wire is advanced to the proximal pole of the scaphoid and the screw length is measured. The drill is then inserted into a soft tissue protector and

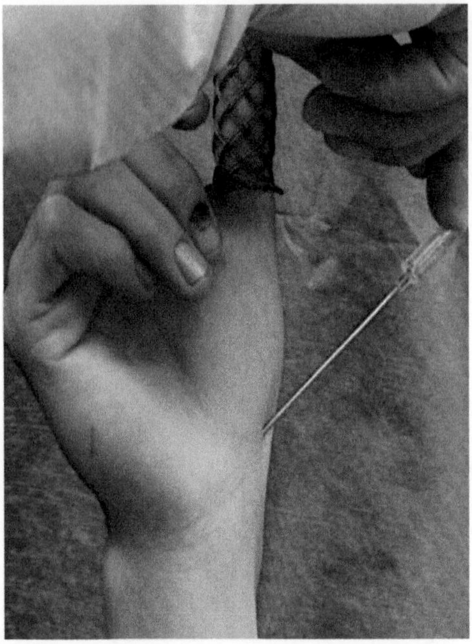

FIG. 29.6 Photograph demonstrating placement of the guide wire through the volar approach. Notice how the thumb is suspended, which permits it to rotate freely to allow fluoroscopic access in all planes to ensure the guide wire is in the ideal placement.

the scaphoid is reamed. A headless cannulated screw is inserted over the guide wire. They recommended using occasionally a second guide wire useful to prevent rotation of the fracture fragments while the screw is being inserted.

Haddad and Goddard reported their initial results in a pilot study of 15 patients with a fracture of the scaphoid.[22] Union was achieved all in patients in an average of 57 days (range 38–117 days). They found that the range of motion at union was equal to the contralateral limb and grip strength averaged 90% at 3 months. Patients were cleared to return to sedentary work within 4 days and manual work within 5 weeks.

The advantage of volar the technique is that it's relatively straight forward, simple, and requires minimal specialized equipment. The disadvantage of the volar approach is that the screw may be slightly oblique to the midwaist fracture line. The scaphoid is shaped like a cone with the widest part being distally and the smallest portion more proximally. It is easier to place a screw in the exact center of the scaphoid while starting at the narrower proximal pole dorsally than the wider distal pole of the scaphoid.

Correctly Aligned and Perfused Scaphoid Nonunion With Substantial Bone Loss Grade 4

When the scaphoid nonunion fragments are well perfused, and there is substantial bone loss without any flexion deformity, these fractures may still be able to heal with bone grafting or potentially DBM with rigid fixation.[23–26] Radiographically, the scaphoid appears with a cystic formation with a defect between 1 and 5 mm. In these instances, if the fracture of the scaphoid is treated by anatomic rigid fixation and bone grafting, the nonunion will be allowed to heal by vascular ingrowth by creeping substitution and bridging bone trabecula. Arthroscopic evaluation of the scaphoid nonunion is utilized to confirm the presence of a fibrous scare tissue at the scaphoid nonunion site. The peripheral fibrocartilaginous scar tissue acts as a net to prevent percutaneous graft at the nonunion site from leaking into the radiocarpal space.

Treatment of Grade IV Scaphoid Nonunion With Percutaneous Bone Grafting and Fixation

Slade and Gillon described their experience with percutaneous bones grafting in a series of 234 scaphoid fractures.[27] In their technique, bone graft is harvested from either the distal radius or the lilac crest utilizing several commercially available bone grafting devices. In their series, they preferred a 4-inch 8G bone biopsy needle to perform the bone biopsy. A guide wire is percutaneously inserted just proximal to Lister's tubercle (Fig. 29.7). A small incision and blunt dissection is carried down to the dorsal cortex and a hand reamer is used to penetrate it. The bone biopsy canula is inserted over the Kirschner wire, and the wire is removed. Several cancellous bone plugs are harvested (Figs. 29.8 and 29.9). Once the bone graft has been harvested, a guide wire is then inserted into the scaphoid through the previously described Slade technique utilizing the ring sign.

Following central wire axis placement, the scaphoid is then reamed from the proximal pole across the nonunion site to a point approximately 2 mm to the distal cortex of scaphoid. The reaming of the scaphoid establishes a conduit for fresh blood supply and removes some of the devitalized bone at the nonunion site. The arthroscope may be placed through the 3–4 portal and is inserted to the proximal pole of the drill hole to access vascularity of the scaphoid. A curette may be place through the 3–4 portal to further clear out the nonunion site. It is vital that the outer vortex fibrous tissue must not be violated as this tissue acts as a net holding the percutaneously introduced bone graft.

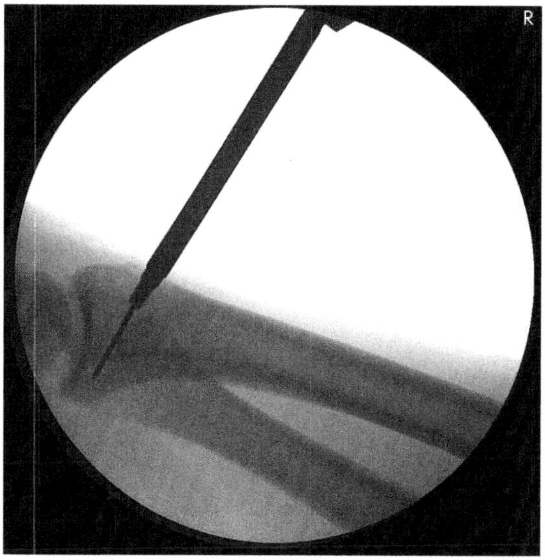

FIG. 29.7 Fluoroscopic view with bone biopsy needle being slid over the guide wire to harvest cancellous bone grafts in the distal radius.

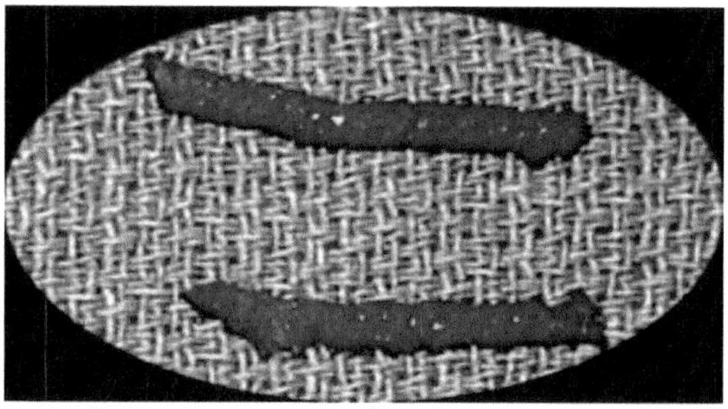

FIG. 29.8 As the cancellous bone is harvested, they are in a cylinder form.

Utilizing the previously placed 18G bone biopsy needle, the cannula is inserted over the guide wire into the nonunion site (Fig. 29.10). Bone plugs are implanted through the cannula to the nonunion site under fluoroscopic imaging (Fig. 29.11). The bone plugs are tapped into place. As previously described, screw length is determined and screw 4 mm shorter than measured is inserted. By doing this, permits 2 mm of clearance at each end of the scaphoid, thus ensuring complete implantation of the screw (Fig. 29.12). For small proximal pole fractures when there are concerns with the stability of the fixation, an additional fixation may be used to lock the midcarpal joint to the scaphoid and capitate (Fig. 29.13). Very rarely, with a small proximal pole,

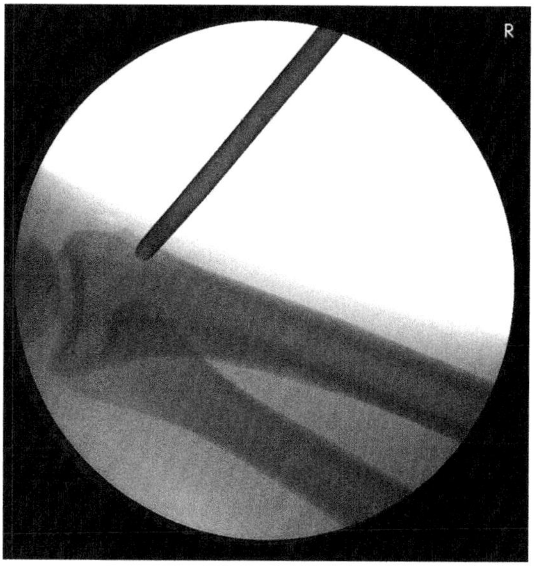

FIG. 29.9 Fluoroscopic view demonstrating harvesting of the cancellous bone graft.

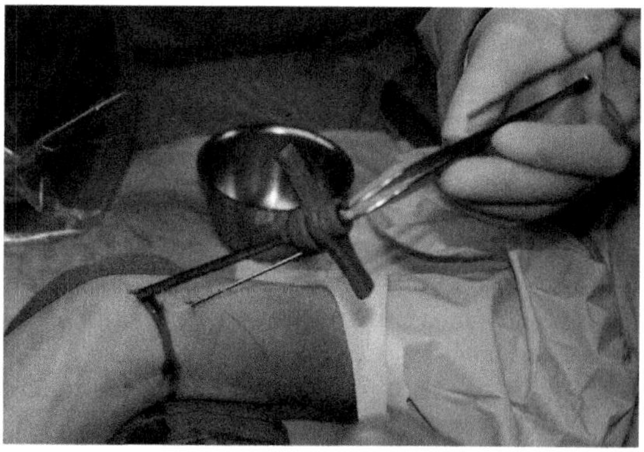

FIG. 29.10 Photograph demonstrating percutaneous placement of the cancellous bone at the scaphoid nonunion.

nonunion has been treated with a sandwiching technique with a screw from the scaphoid into the lunate as described by Slade.

Arthroscopic Reduction and Demoralizing Bone Matrix Grafting of Scaphoid Nonunions Grade IV (Geissler Technique)

Recently, Geissler described his arthroscopic technique for arthroscopic reduction and internal fixation of selective scaphoid nonunions[7,24,26] (Fig. 29.14). The advantage of this technique is that the starting point for the guide wire is viewed directly with the arthroscope

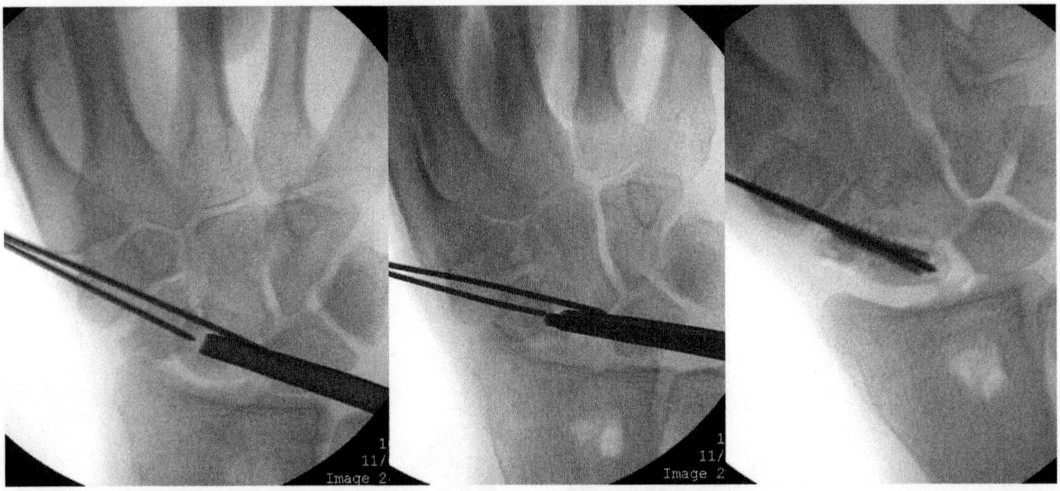

FIG. 29.11 Fluoroscopic view demonstrating the percutaneous cancellous bone grafting into the scaphoid nonunion site.

and graft material can be introduced into the nonunion site without an incision. The wrist is not hyperflexed, which could potentially cause a humpback deformity. It is also thought that traction with a tower helps brings the scaphoid out to length and corrects a humpback deformity.

In this technique, the wrist is suspended in the traction tower with an approximately 10 pounds of traction (Fig. 29.15). The arthroscope is introduced into the standard 3–4 arthroscopy portal to evaluate for any soft tissue injuries of the interosseous ligaments or the triangular fibrocartilage complex. Any soft tissue lesions identified are managed arthroscopically. A standard 6R portal is made and the arthroscope is transferred to 6R portal. It is important that the wrist is flexed approximately 30 degrees in the traction tower to allow easier access to the proximal pole of the scaphoid. A 14G needle is then inserted through the 3–4 portal and then the junction of the interosseous ligament to the proximal pole of the scaphoid is palpated (Fig. 29.16). It is important that as the 14G needle is inserted through the 3–4 portal, and it passes easily through the portal. A hemostat is useful to help the spread the portal while the 14G needle is being inserted. The junction of the scaphoid and the interosseous ligament is then palpated with the needle (Fig. 29.17). The most ideal starting point is at the junction is the scapholunate interosseous ligament and the scaphoid and at its midpoint in the AP direction.

Occasionally, dorsal capsular synovitis may block visualization of the ideal starting point with the arthroscope in the 6R portal. In this case the dorsal capsule is debrided to facilitate visualization. Wrist flexion is decreased to help visualization.

The proximal pole of the scaphoid is then impaled with the 14G needle (Figs. 29.18 and 29.19). The traction tower is then flexed to make it easier to access the starting point under fluoroscopy (Fig. 29.20). Once the starting point is confirmed, the needle is aimed toward the thumb and the guide wire is advanced through the needle and down the central axis of the scaphoid to the distal pole of the scaphoid (Fig. 29.21). The position of the guide wire is then evaluated under the posteroanterior, oblique, and lateral planes under fluoroscopy (Fig. 29.22). This is done by simply rotating the forearm in the traction tower. As the traction support beam is off to the side, the fluoroscopic beam is not hindered and blocks visualization (Fig. 29.23). Once the ideal position of the guide wire is confirmed under fluoroscopy, the length of the guide wire is measured as previously described. A screw length is 4 mm shorter is recommended. The reduction of the scaphoid is evaluated with the arthroscope both in the radiocarpal and midcarpal spaces. If further reduction is required, the guide wire is then advanced across the trapezium and out the volar aspect of the hand. Reduction of the fracture usually can be reduced by flexion/extension radial/ulnar deviation of the wrist in the traction tower. Once anatomic reduction of the fracture is confirmed under arthroscopy with the scope in the midcarpal portal, the guide wire is advanced into the proximal pole into the subchondral bone.

In selected fibrous nonunion, Slade-Geissler stage IV with cystic formation between 1 and <5 mm,

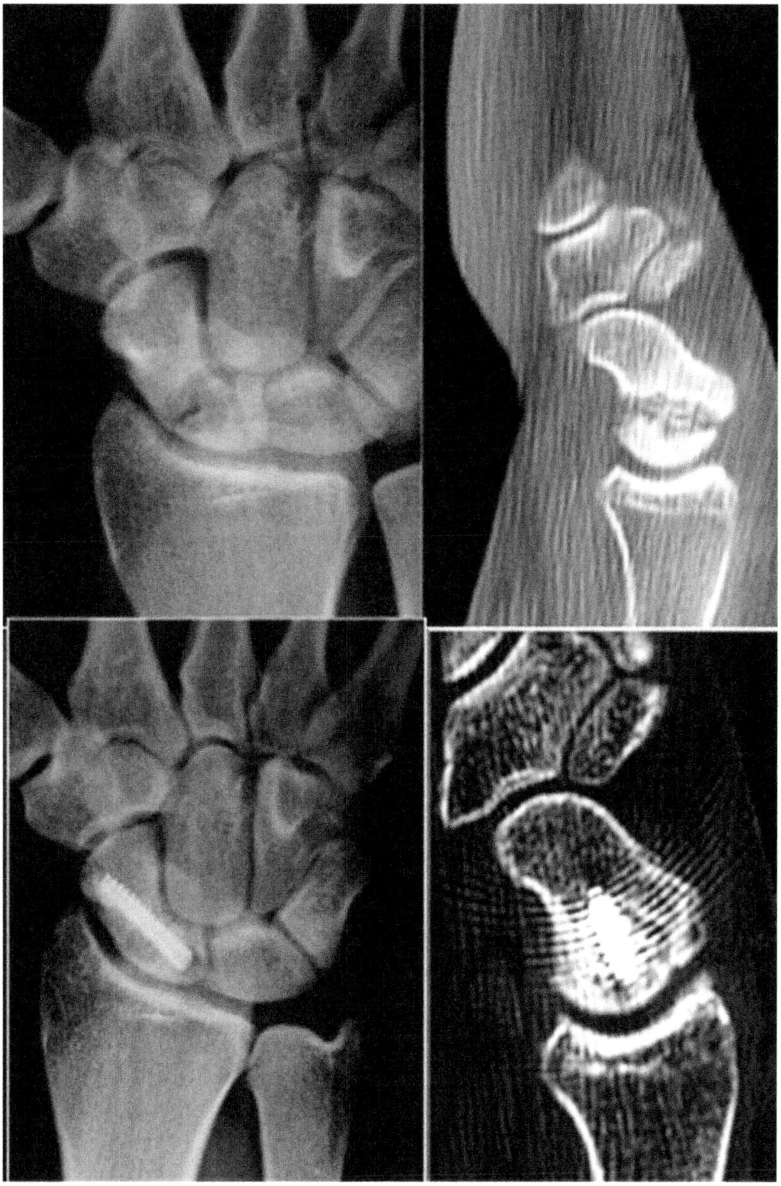

FIG. 29.12 Plain radiographs and CT evaluation demonstrating a healed scaphoid nonunion following percutaneous cancellous bone grafting.

percutaneous cancellous bone grafting or injection of DBM putty may be performed.[24,26] The scaphoid is reamed through a soft tissue protector with the near and far drills for preparation of the headless cannulated screw. A bone biopsy needle is filled with DBM (Fig. 29.24). The bone biopsy needle is then placed over the dorsally placed guide wire and inserted through the drill-hole in the proximal pole of the scaphoid directly into the nonunion site (Fig. 29.25). The guide wire is then retracted back into the distal pole of the scaphoid. The DBM is injected through the bone biopsy needle directly into the nonunion site (Fig. 29.26). The putty is advanced through the cannula until resistance is felt. Once the putty has been injected, the guide wire is advanced from distal to proximal through the bone biopsy needle and out the dorsal skin, so it keeps the

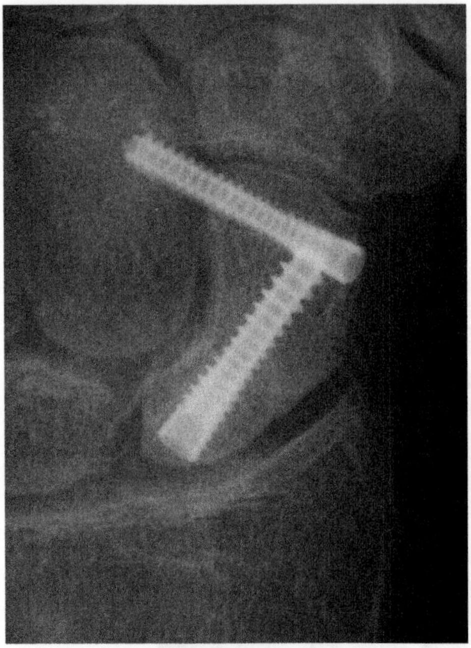

FIG. 29.13 A small proximal pole scaphoid nonunion can be further stabilized with nonunion additional stability by temporarily locking up the midcarpal joint with a headless screw to provide greater stability and decreasing micromotion at the fracture size.

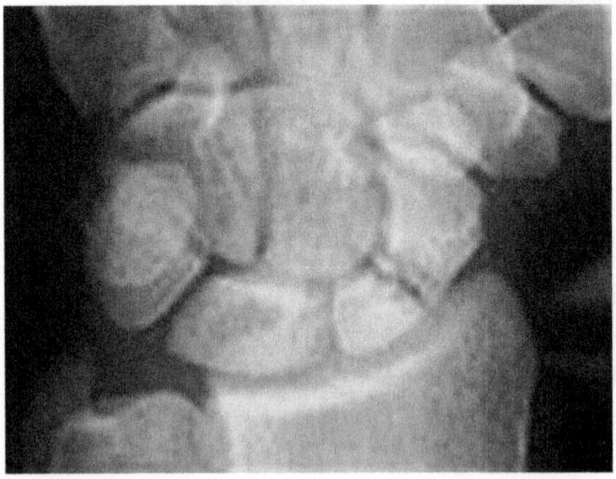

FIG. 29.14 Posteroanterior radio graft demonstrating a cystic nonunion.

same path and decreases the chance of any extensor tendon injury. The bone biopsy needle is then removed and the cannulated screw is inserted over the guide wire compressing the nonunion site (Fig. 29.27). Both the radiocarpal and midcarpal spaces are arthroscopically revaluated to confirm the reduction and compression

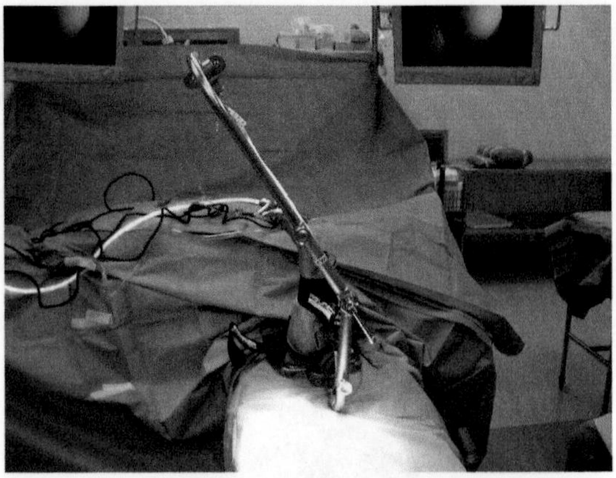

FIG. 29.15 Utilizing the Geissler technique, the wrist is suspended in about 30 degrees of flexion in the traction tower to allow easier access to the proximal pole of the scaphoid.

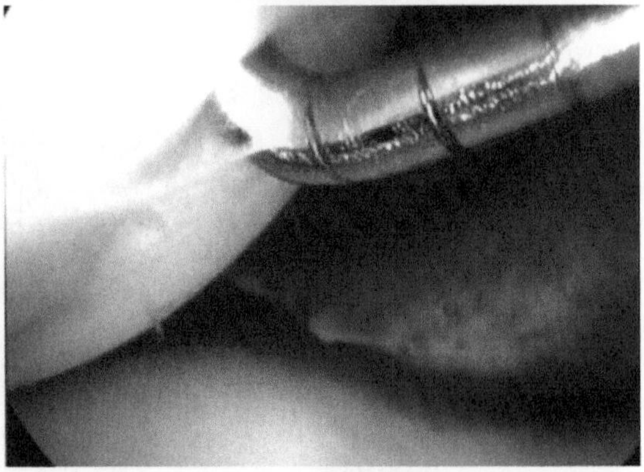

FIG. 29.16 Arthroscopic view with the arthroscope in the 6R portal. A probe is used to palpate the junction of the scapholunate interosseous ligament to the proximal pole of the scaphoid.

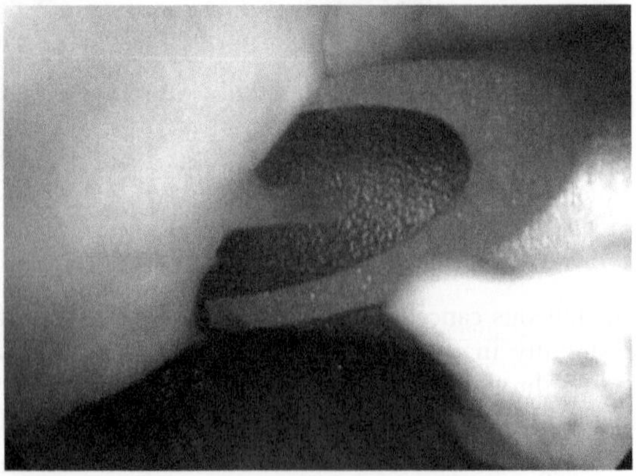

FIG. 29.17 Arthroscopic view demonstrating the 14G needle as it is about to be impaled into the proximal pole of the scaphoid just radial to the attachment of the scapholunate interosseous ligament.

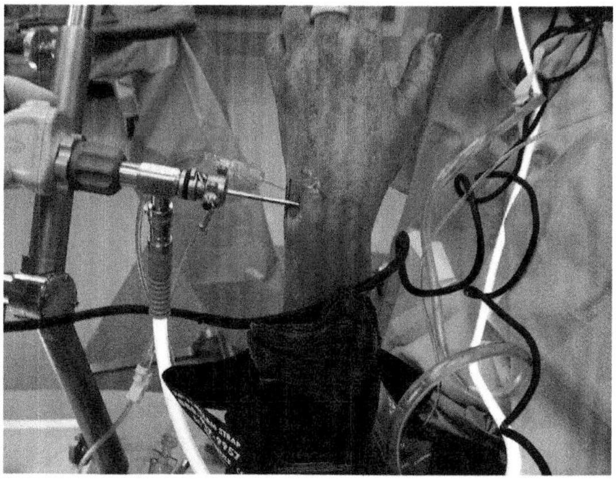

FIG. 29.18 Photograph showing the arthroscope in the 6R portal with the 14G needle being inserted into the 3–4 portal. It is vital not to impale the extensor tendon as the needle is being inserted into the 3–4 portal.

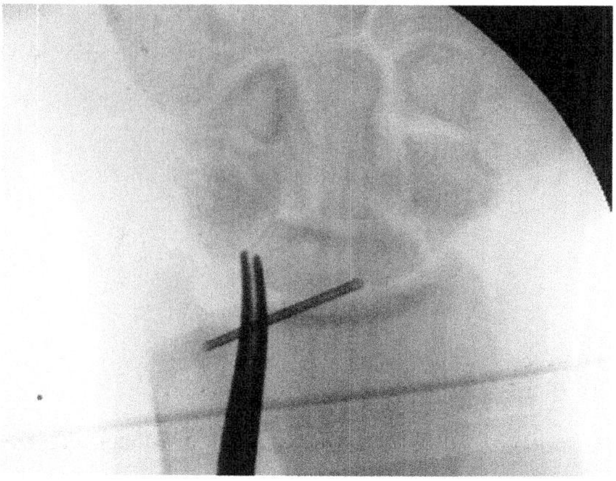

FIG. 29.19 Under fluoroscopic control, the ideal staring point is confirmed and the needle is then simply aimed toward the thumb for guide wire placement.

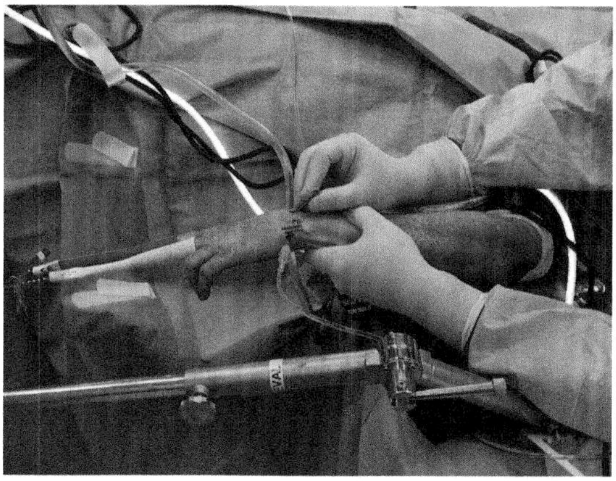

FIG. 29.20 Photograph demonstrating the aiming of the needle toward the thumb for guide wire placement.

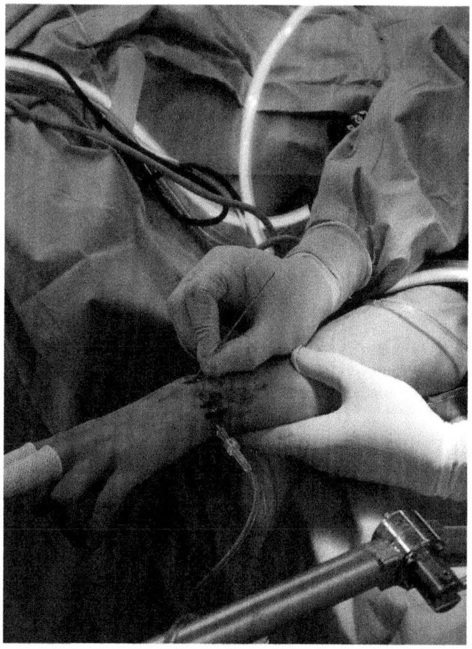

FIG. 29.21 The guide wire for the headless screw is inserted through the 14G needle. By inserting through the needle helps protects the extensor tendons and allows finer motor control to aim the guide wire down the central axis of the scaphoid.

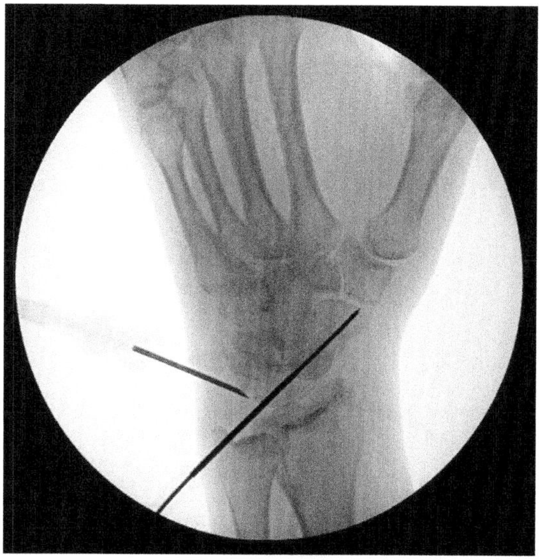

FIG. 29.22 Fluoroscopic view demonstrating central placement of the guide wire down the central axis of the scaphoid.

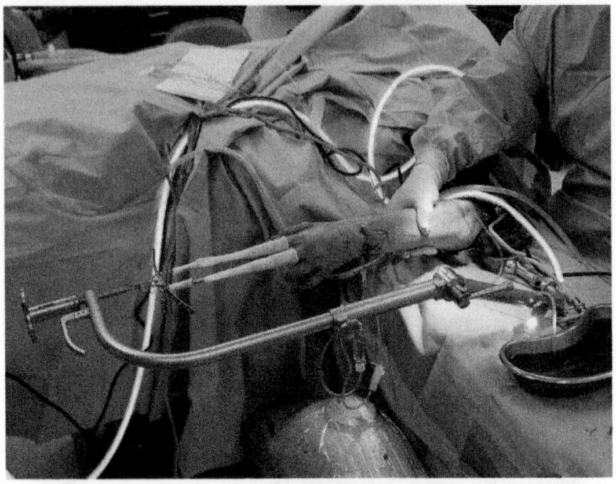

FIG. 29.23 Photograph demonstrating placement of the guide wire through the needle with the traction tower in a flexed position.

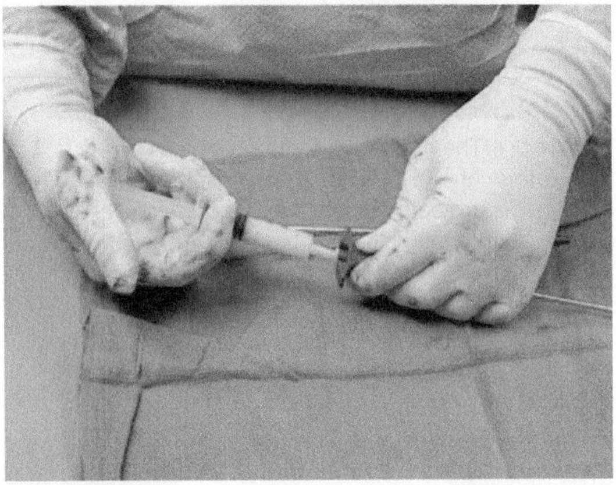

FIG. 29.24 A bone biopsy needle is filled with demineralized bone matrix.

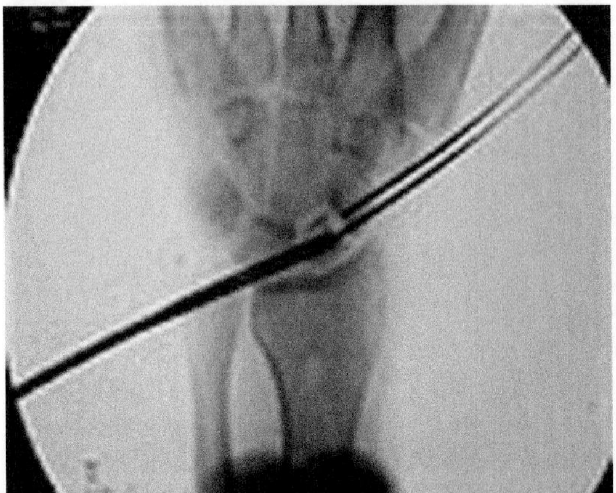

FIG. 29.25 A bone biopsy needle is placed over the guide wire into the nonunion site under fluoroscopic guidance.

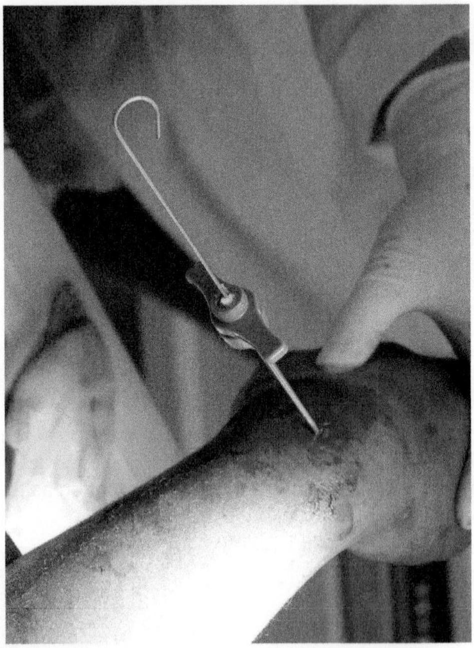

FIG. 29.26 The putty is then simply pushed with a plunger until resistance is felt.

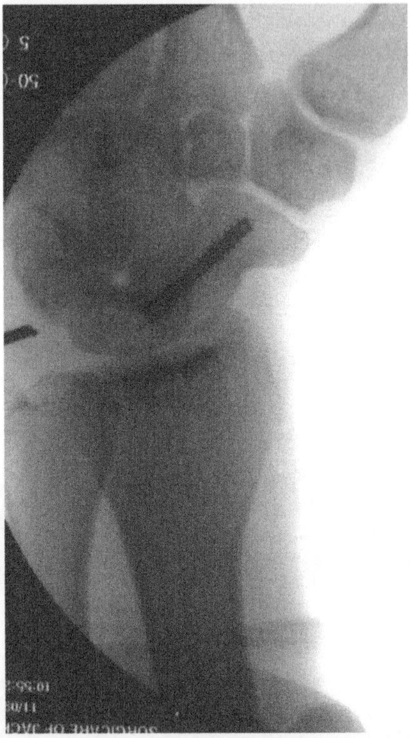

FIG. 29.27 Fluoroscopic view confirms ideal placement of the headless screw into the scaphoid following putty injection.

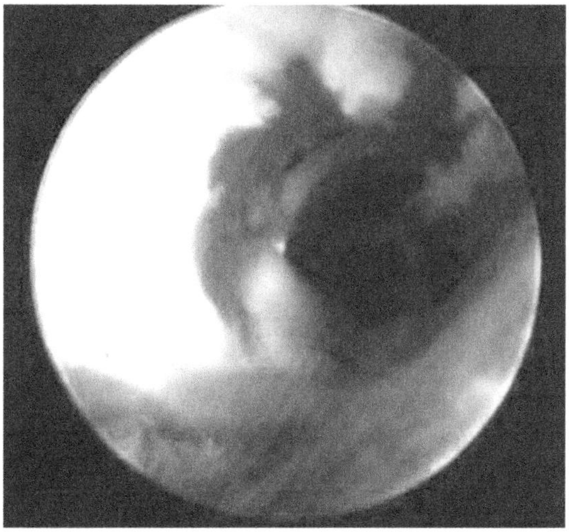

FIG. 29.28 It's important that the position of screw is checked under arthroscopically following screw placement. In this manner, ensure that the screw is well up into the scaphoid and not prominent to affect the articular cartilage of scaphoid facet of the distal radius.

of the fracture. Evaluation of the midcarpal space ensures complete containment of the DBM and evaluation of the radiocarpal space and ensures that the screw is inserted well up into the scaphoid (Fig. 29.28). It is important that the screw is not prominent proximally to affect the articular cartilage of the scaphoid facet of the distal radius.

Postoperative Care

Digital range of motion exercises are initiated immediately. Wrist range of motion exercises are started approximately 2 weeks from surgery, and strengthening exercises are initiated at approximately 6 weeks postoperatively.

Scaphoid Nonunions

Geissler and Slade described their results utilizing Slade's dorsal percutaneous technique in 15 patients with stable fibrous nonunion of the scaphoid (Grades I–III).[27] There were 12 horizontal oblique, 1 transverse fracture, and 2 proximal pole fractures. The average time till presentation to surgery was 8 months. All patients underwent percutaneous dorsal fixation with headless cannulated screw fixation with no bone grafting. Of the 15 patients, 8 underwent CT evaluation postoperatively to evaluate healing. All patients healed their fractures in an average time of 3 months. Patients demonstrated excellent range of motion at the final

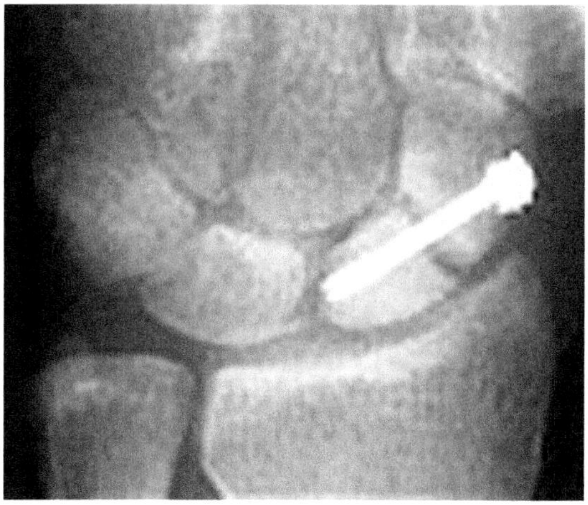

FIG. 29.29 Radiograph showing a scaphoid nonunion with attempt at open reduction and internal fixation with bone grafting. The patients fracture had not healed. It was felt that the screw placement was not ideal.

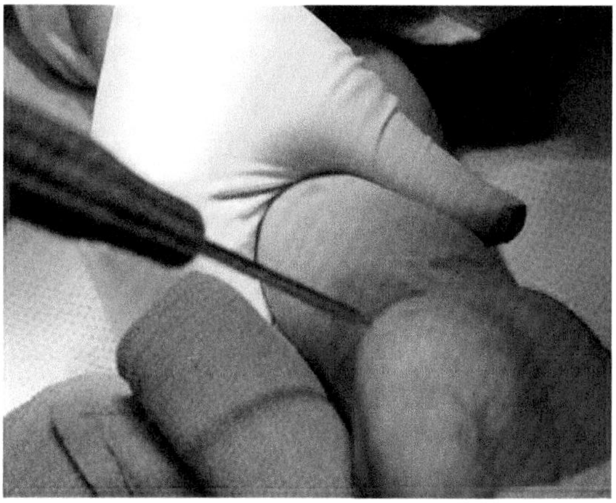

FIG. 29.30 Percutaneously the screw is removed.

follow-up because of limited surgical dissection. Utilizing the Modified Mayo Score, 12 of the 15 patients had excellent results. Dorsal percutaneous fixation without bone grafting was recommended in patients who have a stable fibrous nonunion with no signs of a humpback deformity. In patients of a cystic scaphoid nonunion without a humpback deformity or rotated lunate, percutaneous cancellous bone grafting or injection DBM may be used. Geissler reported his results using 1 cc of DBM putty for cystic nonunions of the scaphoid.[26,28] There were 15 patients in his series that were classified by the Slade and Geissler classification as type IV. Of 15 patients, 14 healed their scaphoid nonunions utilizing this technique (Figs. 29.29–29.34). The average time

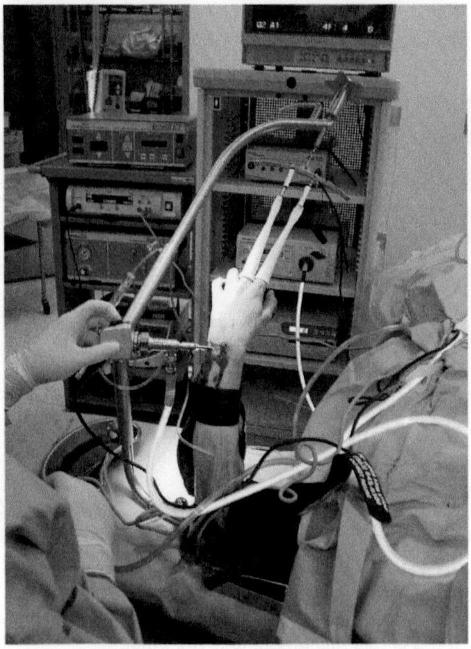

FIG. 29.31 The wrist is set up in the traction tower with the arthroscope in the 6R portal and the guide wire to be placed down the central axis of the scaphoid. The scaphoid is then reamed and demineralized bone matrix is inserted.

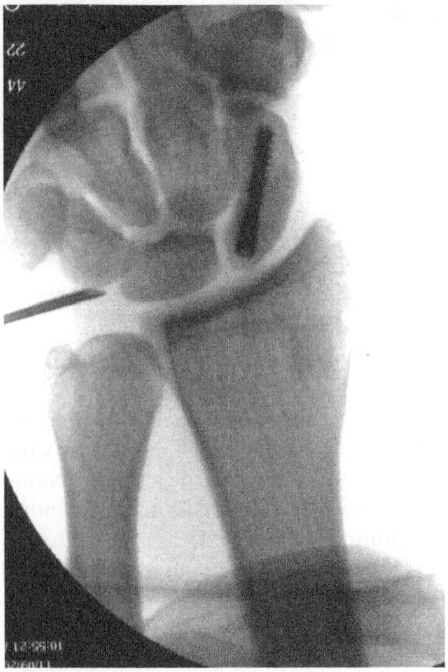

FIG. 29.32 Fluoroscopic image showing ideal placement of the headless screw in the scaphoid following injection of the bone matrix.

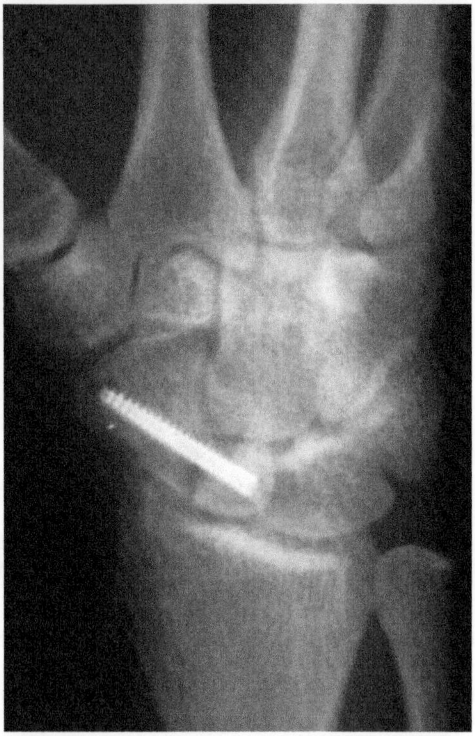

FIG. 29.33 Initial postoperative radiograph showing the persistent scaphoid nonunion.

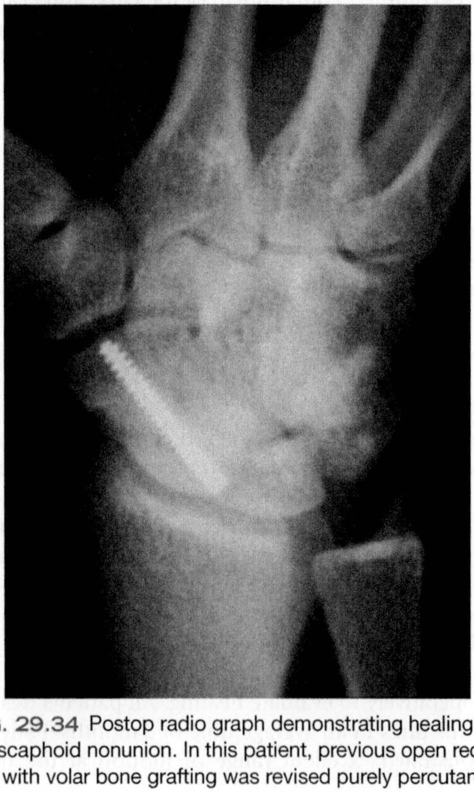

FIG. 29.34 Postop radio graph demonstrating healing of the scaphoid nonunion. In this patient, previous open reduction with volar bone grafting was revised purely percutaneously with demineralized bone matrix to achieve healing.

for union was 16 weeks (range 8–24 weeks). Utilizing the Mayo Modified Wrist Score, there were 12 excellent and 3 good results.

Somerson et al. reviewed their results in 14 patients who presented with scaphoid nonunions, managed by compression screw fixation alone without bone grafting.[30] Of the 14 patients, 12 healed successfully (86%), whereas 2 patients required secondary vascularized bone grafting.

Chu and Shih treated 15 consecutive patients with minimal sclerosis with arthroscopically assisted fixation combined with injected DBM.[23] Of 15 patients, 14 healed (93%) with a mean of 15 weeks. Functional outcome was excellent in 10 patients and good in 4.

Wong and Ho presented 68 patients with a scaphoid nonunion managed by an arthroscopic technique.[21] Average follow-up was 10 months and the overall union rate was 92%. The average time till union was only 12 weeks.

Kim et al. reviewed 36 patients who underwent arthroscopic fixation for chronic scaphoid nonunion with bone loss. Union was achieved in 31 (86%).[29]

Of the five union failures, four did not have bone grafting. This would suggest that, in scaphoid nonunion with bone loss (Grade 4), some type of bone grafting should be used.

RECOMMENDATION

In patients with fibrous/delayed scaphoid unions, evidence suggests the following:

- Subacute scaphoid fractures (presenting within 6 months from injury) can be expected to successfully heal with casting alone, even if the initial diagnoses is delayed (overall quality: low).
- Types I–III may be addressed by screw fixation alone (overall quality: low).
- Type IV scaphoid nonunions are recommended to be treated by any type of bone grafting (overall quality: low).

CONCLUSION

In conclusion, fibrous scaphoid nonunions are mostly treated arthroscopically or through open techniques. When utilizing the Slade-Geissler classification, types I–III may be addressed by screw fixation alone. Type IV scaphoid nonunions require some type of grafting, either cancellous bone on DBM.

PANEL 2
Case Scenario (Continued)

In the case initially presented, the patient presented with a Slade-Geissler Stage IV nonunion. The previous cannulated screw was removed percutaneously. The wrist was then suspended in the traction tower and underwent arthroscopic stabilization and percutaneous demineralized bone grafting. The patient revision of open surgery arthroscopy and healed at 4 months to return to play (Figs. 29.29–29.34).

REFERENCES

1. Linschied RL, Dobyns JH, Beabout JW, Bryan RS. Traumatic instability of the wrist: diagnosis, classification and pathmechanics. *J Bone Joint Surg Am*. 1972;54:1612–1632.
2. Cooney WP, Dobyns JH, Linscheid RL. Fractures of the scaphoid: a rational approach to management. *Clin Orthop*. 1980;149:90–97.
3. Gelberman RH, Wolock BS, Siegel DB. Current concepts review: fractures and nonunions of the carpal scaphoid. *J Bone Joint Surg*. 1989;71A:1560–1565.
4. Fernandez DL. Anterior bone grafting and conventional lag screw fixation to treat scaphoid nonunions. *J Hand Surg*. 1990;15A:140–147.
5. Garcia-Elias M, Vall A, Salo JM, et al. Carpal alignment after different surgical approaches to the scaphoid: a comparative study. *J Hand Surg*. 1988;13:604–612.
6. Gelberman RH, Menon J. The vascularity of the scaphoid bone. *J Hand Surg*. 1980;5:508–513.
7. Geissler WB. *Wrist Arthroscopy*. New York: Springer; 2005.
8. Barton NJ. Experience with the scaphoid grating. *J Hand Surg Br*. 1997;22:153–160.
9. Shah J, Jares WA. Fractures affecting the outcome in 50 cases of scaphoid nonunion treated with Herbert screw fixation. *J Hand Surg Br*. 1998;23:680–685.
10. Slade 3rd JF, Geissler WB, Gutow AP, Merrell GAGA. Percutaneous internal fixation of selected scaphoid nonunions with an arthroscopically assisted dorsal approach. *J Bone Joint Surg Am*. 2003;85-A(suppl 4):20–32.
11. Fkeda K, Osamuna N. Tomitak, percutaneous screw fixation without bone grafting for cystic type schopid fractures. *J Trauma*. 2008;65:1453–1458.
12. Slade III JF, Grauer JN. Dorsal percutaneous repair of scaphoid fractures with arthroscopic guidance. *Atlas Hand Clin*. 2001;6:307–323.
13. Slade III JF, Grauer JN, Mahoney JD. Arthroscopic reduction and percutaneous fixation of scaphoid fractures with a novel dorsal technique. *Orthop Clin N Am*. 2000;30:247–261.
14. Slade III JF, Jaskwhich J. Percutaneous fixation of scaphoid fractures. *Hand Clin*. 2001;17:553–574.
15. Geissler WB, Freeland AE, Savoie FH, et al. Intracarpal soft tissue lesions associated with intraarticular fracture of the distal end of the radius. *J Bone Joint Surg*. 1996;78:357–365.

16. Geissler WB. Arthroscopic Management of Scaphoid Fractures and Non-unions. In: Geissler WB ed. *Wrist and Elbow Arthroscopy*. New Talk: Springer: 2015:251–260. 29: Vol. 31: 460–469.
17. Geissler WB. Arthroscopic assisted fixation of fractures of the scaphoid. *Atlas Hand Clin*. 2003;8:37–56.
18. Geissler WB, Hammit MD. Arthroscopic aided fixation of scaphoid fractures. *Hand Clin*. 2001;17:575–588.
19. Adams BD, Blair WF, Regan DS, et al. Technical factors related to Herbert screw fixation. *J Bone Joint Surg*. 1988;13:893–899.
20. O'Brien L, Herbert TJ. Internal fixation of acute scaphoid fractures: a new approach to treatment. *Aust NZ J Surg*. 1985;55:387–389.
21. Wong WY, Ho PC. Minimal invasive management of scaphoid fractures: from fresh to nonunion. *Hand Clin*. 2011;27:291–307.
22. Haddad FS, Goddard NJ. Acute percutaneous scaphoid fixation: a pilot study. *J Bone Joint Surg*. 1998;80:95–99.
23. Chu PJ, Shih JT. Arthroscopically assisted use of injectable bone graft substitutes for management of scaphoid nonunions. *Arthroscopy*. 2011;27:31–37.
24. Geissler WB. Arthroscopic management fractures and non-unions. In: Geissler WB, ed. *Wrist and Elbow Arthroscopy/ A Practical Surgical Guide to Techniques*. 2nd ed. New York City, NY: Springer Science+Business Media; 2015:251–259.
25. Slade JF, Merrell GA, Geissler WB. Fixation of acute and selected nonunion scaphoid fractures. In: Geissler WB, ed. *Wrist Arthroscopy*. New York: Springer; 2005:112–124.
26. Geissler WB, Slade JF. *Green's Operative Hand Surgery 6th Edition, Fractures of the Carpal Bones*. Philadelphia, PA: Elsevier Churchill Livingstone; 2011:639–741.
27. Slade JF, Gillon T. Retrospective review of 234 scaphoid fractures and nonunions treated with arthroscopy for union and complications. *Scand J Surg*. 2008;97: 280–289.
28. Geissler WB. *Arthroscopic Fixation of Cystic Scaphoid Nonunions with DBM*. Tucson, AZ: American Association Hand Surgery; January 2006.
29. Kim JP, Seo JB, Yoo JY. Arthroscopic management of chronic unstable scaphoid nonunions: effects on restorations of carpal alignment and recovery of wrist function. *Arthroscopy*. 2014.
30. Somerson JS, Fletcher DJ, Srinivasan RC, Green DP. Compression screw fixation without bone grafting for scaphoid fibrous nonunion. *Hand (NY)*. 2015;10(3):450–453.
31. Grewal R, Suh N, MacDermid JC. The missed scaphoid fracture-outcomes of delayed cast treatment. *J Wrist Surg*. 2015;4:278–283.
32. Farkah U, Bain O, Gam A, Nyska M, Sagiv P. Low-intensity pulsed ultrasound for treated delayed scaphoid fractures: case series. *J Orthop Surg Res*. 2015;10:72. http://dx.doi.org/10.1186/s13018-015-0221-9. 1–7.

CHAPTER 30

Scaphoid Plating

ARTHUR TUROW, MBBS • GREGORY I. BAIN, MBBS, FRACS, PHD

KEY POINTS

- Scaphoid plating is evolving and should be reserved for cases where stability is paramount.
- An angular-stable plate can provide a more rotationally stable construct than a single compression screw can.
- Plate fixation can yield high union rates in select patients.
- Scaphoid plate positioning depends on the fracture configuration and surgeon preference.

PANEL 1
Case Scenario

A 30-year-old male fell onto his outstretched hand after tripping over, presented to his local practitioner, and was treated for a soft-tissue injury. His pain settled with conservative treatment. A recurrent fall 7 months later exacerbated his pain and prompted a presentation to the orthopedic outpatient department where radiographs of his wrist showed a nonunited scaphoid waist fracture (Fig. 30.1). Given the delayed presentation and the paramount stability issue, a senior consultant suggests scaphoid plating. Would this be a good indication for plate fixation, and if so, how is best performed?

IMPORTANCE OF THE PROBLEM

Overview

A single headless compression screw has been the mainstay of scaphoid fracture treatment, since it became available in the 1980s.[1] A single screw provides only limited stability and is especially poor with rotation. There are alternatives to screw fixation, which include using multiple screws, staples, plates, and potentially external fixators.[2]

Two screws[3] can be used to reduced interfragmentary rotation. Increased fixation can also be achieved with an antirotation wire[4–6] instead. Accomplishing rotational stability and accurate screw positioning with two screws across a usually narrow scaphoid waist can be very challenging, though.

The scaphoid staple is an alternative to screw fixation. Since its introduction in 1980, only a few authors have reported on clinical outcomes, with described union rates of 92% for nonunions.[7]

Nonunion remains an important complication of scaphoid fractures. Scaphoid waist fractures have a reported nonunion rate of 5%–15%,[8,9] irrespective of treatment. Internal fixation was previously reserved for unstable fracture patterns but can also include high-demand patients with simple, transverse fractures.

Plating Rationale

The concept of plating of the scaphoid has been first introduced in the middle of last century with compression plates by Ender and Vespasiani[10] (Fig. 30.3). These beaked plates were designed to allow for compression across the scaphoid and prevented escape of the bone graft from the fracture site, something that other fixation methods at that time were not able to provide. These hooked plates saw some use in the late 1980s and early 1990s, but their use rapidly declined with the clinical introduction of the Herbert screw in 1984.[1]

Scaphoid plating has been reintroduced recently with both volar (Fig. 30.4) and dorsal techniques. The need for plating has arisen from concerns regarding mechanical stability of a single screw across scaphoid fractures with an unstable fracture pattern[2,11,12] and the assumption that a plate would provide a more stable construct than a compression screw. Plate fixation of the scaphoid has been pursued with the theoretical benefit of a multiple divergent screw fixation that lends stability in multiple vectors. The potential advantages of stable plate fixation are likely to be greater in unstable fractures, where greater stability is required to obtain stability, such as fractures that are oblique, with comminution or nonunions with bone loss.

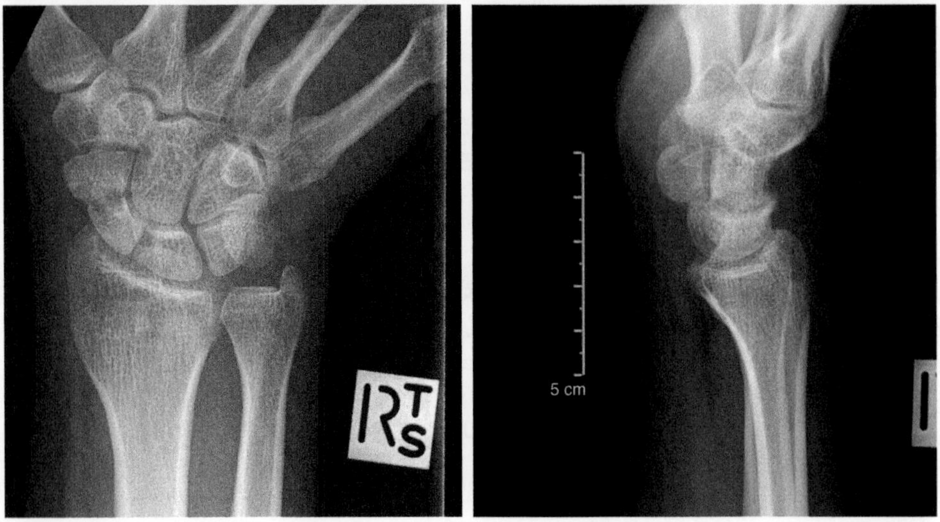

FIG. 30.1 Radiographs of 30-year-old man with right wrist pain after a repeat fall onto his outstretched hand.

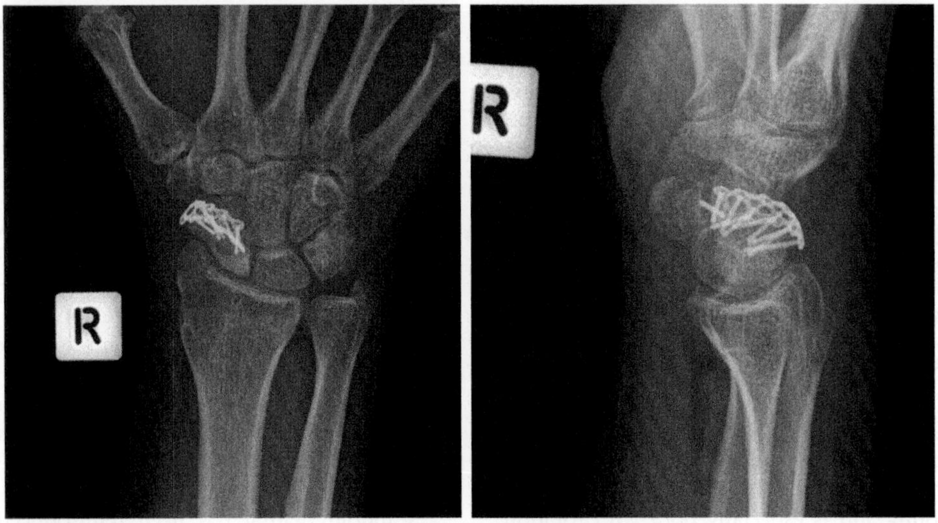

FIG. 30.2 Dorsal scaphoid plating—postoperative radiographs of the patient from Fig. 30.1.

MAIN QUESTION

What are the indications and techniques for plate fixation of acute scaphoid fractures and scaphoid nonunions?

Current Opinion

Scaphoid plating is evolving and should be reserved for cases where stability is paramount. This could include patients with high-energy injuries with associated scaphoid fracture, nonunion where previous treatment has failed, or in high-demand patients who require early return to activities.

Finding the Evidence

Pubmed (Medline): (scaphoid bone[MeSH Terms]) OR scaphoid fracture) AND plate*[Title/Abstract])) OR plating* [Title/Abstract]) AND (Humans[Mesh] AND (English[lang] OR French[lang] OR German[lang]) NOT fusion[Title/Abstract]) AND (Humans[Mesh] AND (English[lang] OR French[lang] OR German[lang])))) NOT four-corner[Title/Abstract]) NOT humerus[Title/Abstract]) NOT radius[Title/Abstract]) NOT ulna*[Title/Abstract]) AND (Humans[Mesh] AND (English[lang] OR French[lang] OR German[lang])))) NOT arthrodesis[Title/

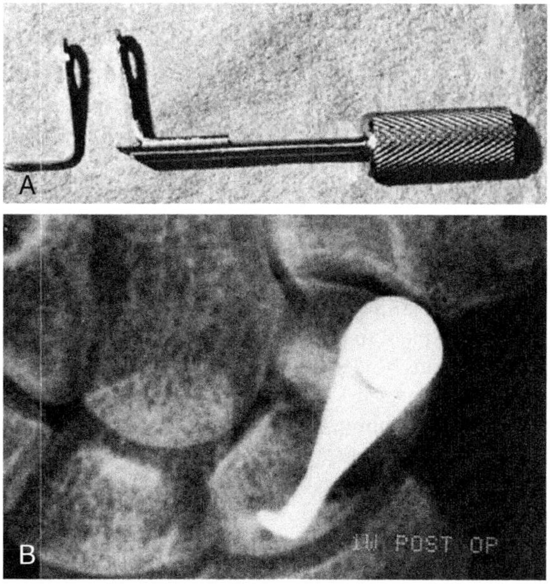

FIG. 30.3 **(A)** Hooked Ender compression plate with a drill guide for the hook. **(B)** Ender plate in a nonunited scaphoid. (From Huene DR, Huene DS. Treatment of nonunions of the scaphoid with the Ender compression blade plate system. *J Hand Surg*. 1991;16(5):913–922, with permission.)

Abstract]) NOT knee[Title/Abstract] Sort by: Relevance Filters: Humans; English; French; German.

Quality of the Evidence

Level IV:

Case series: 9

Biomechanical studies: 9

FINDINGS

Biomechanics

When placed perpendicular to the fracture line, the Herbert screw is able to achieve interfragmentary compression. It is capable of resisting bending forces but is unable to withstand cyclical multiaxis loading or rotation.[13–17] Previous biomechanical work has focused predominantly on pull-apart and compression strengths as well as bending resistance.[17–19] Torsional resistance has been evaluated among different screw designs in scaphoid models,[13,19] but the lack of in vivo studies leaves a large gap between such models and the complex kinematics[20] and torsional forces and scaphoid experiences.

A recent in vitro study[21] compared rotational stability of a single compression screw to two screws and to an angular stable plate. The authors found superior

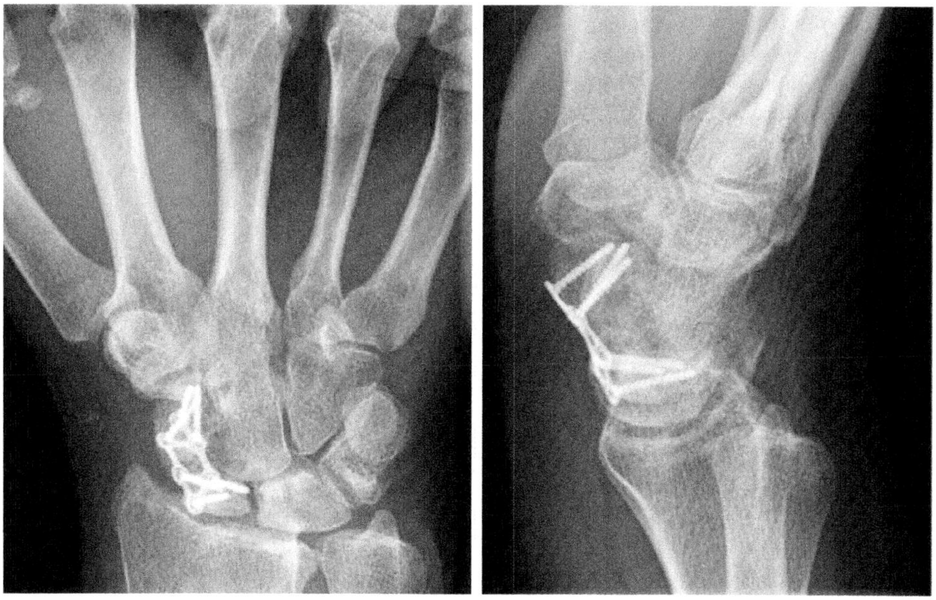
FIG. 30.4 Volar scaphoid plating of a previously nonunited scaphoid waist fracture. (From Leixnering M, Pezzei C, Weninger P, et al. First experiences with a new adjustable plate for osteosynthesis of scaphoid nonunions. *J Trauma*. 2011;71(4):933–938, with permission.)

rotational stability for two screws and for the locking plate construct ($P < .05$). There were no statistically significant differences between two screws and the plate.

More than 80% of the surface area of the scaphoid is articular surface with small nonarticular areas on the volar and dorsal aspects.[22] Consequently, plate placement depends on those bare areas. Dorsal placement of the plate has been hypothesized to be biomechanically superior to a volar position, as a dorsal plate occupies the tension side of the scaphoid. Thereby, a dorsal plate is thought to act as a tension band plate during wrist mobilization, achieving dynamic compression.[2,23] In fact, some research indicates that kinematics of various scaphoids differ substantially depending on their dorsal ligamentous arrangement. Fogg[20] examined 100 scaphoids and divided them based on their dorsal morphology. In type I scaphoids, the dorsal intercarpal ligament (DIC) does not attach to the dorsal bare area and the scapho-trapezio-trapezoid (STT) ligament complex has a V-shaped configuration. In contrast, type II scaphoids receive a DIC slip and the STT ligament has an inverted-V attachment (Fig. 30.5). Fogg[20] hypothesized type I scaphoids to be rotating and type II scaphoids to undergo flexion and extension through wrist palmar and dorsiflexion.

Indications

Scaphoid plating has been used in a variety of circumstances. Broadly, plating is indicated where greater stability is sought. This may be the case in unstable fracture patterns, following high-energy injury with associated carpal dislocations or in cases of nonunion. High-demand patients might also be a potential cohort where early return to activity is critical.

In the acute setting, a plate can be used for unstable fracture patterns (Herbert type B). An angle stable plate can buttress bone graft, prevent fracture collapse, and provide rotational stability. Consequently, a scaphoid plate can be used to bridge comminution and to neutralize shear forces across an oblique scaphoid fracture. The ideal indication for a dorsal plate is a comminuted scaphoid fracture.

Scaphoid nonunion is challenging to treat and requires a rigid fixation for a longer period than acute fractures. Biomechanically, plating provides greater stability than screw fixation.[21] The plate can also be used as a buttress for bone graft to avoid graft escape. Graft options include cancellous, corticocancellous, or vascularized[24] bone grafts. Cancellous autologous bone graft can be obtained from the ipsilateral distal radius[2] or iliac crest.[12] Corticocancellous grafts have been advocated by some authors[11,25] to restore volar cortical loss.

Contraindications

Plating of the scaphoid invites a new set of challenges. The scaphoid is a small bone, with a large articular surface. Therefore, there are some situations where plating will be difficult or contraindicated.

Scaphoid fractures of the proximal or distal pole usually prevent adequate fragmentary screw purchase and, consequently, are not suitable to plate fixation. Volar cortical loss and severe humpback deformity require osseous reconstruction and significant implant support. A volar plate with bone graft is one option.

A dorsal plate may still be considered with concurrent cancellous bone grafting. Some studies have shown union rates up to 96% in nonunited scaphoid fractures with associated humpback deformity that were treated with cancellous bone grafting.[26–29]

Scaphoid fractures with advanced carpal arthritis are better managed with a salvage procedure. Patients with mild radiocarpal arthritis can still be considered for internal fixation, when a radial styloidectomy is performed in conjunction with the scaphoid fixation.

Clinical Data

The majority of the available outcome data on scaphoid plating are on the Ender plate.[30–35] Union rates are reported between 89%[32] and 99%.[35] The Ender plate has been used for both the volar and dorsal approaches. Huene and Huene,[36] for example, report on 20 scaphoid nonunion cases treated with plating. Eleven patients underwent dorsal plating and nine volar plating. Only one patient had persistent nonunion patient with subsequent hardware removal. Despite promising results and wide use in Europe in the late 1980s and early 1990s, the Ender plate has all but vanished from the scaphoid literature. The decline of the Ender plate is likely a consequence of the clinical introduction and rapid uptake of the Herbert screw in 1984.

Outcomes for volar locking plating have been equally promising.[11,12,24] Cumulative union for volar plating is 93%[11,12] at approximately 4 months. For dorsal plating, recent preliminary published data on 10 scaphoid fractures show 90% union rate.[2]

RECOMMENDATIONS

In patients with (1) high-energy injuries with associated scaphoid fractures, (2) nonunion where previous treatment has failed, or (3) in high-demand patients:

- An angle-stable plate can provide a more rotationally stable construct than a single compression screw (overall quality: moderate)

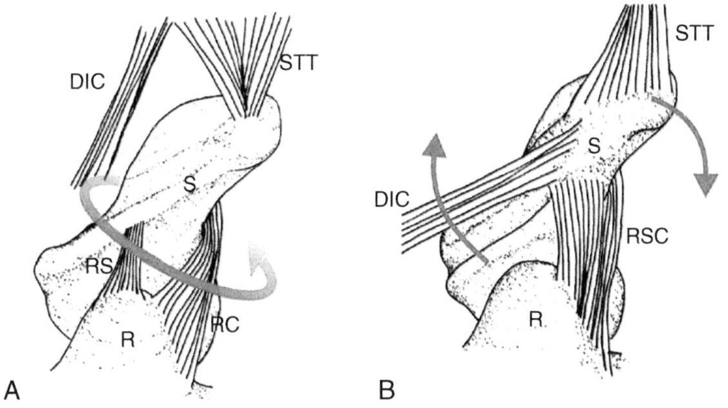

FIG. 30.5 **(A)** Rotating-type scaphoid: arrangements of dorsal intercarpal (DIC) and radiocapitate (RC) ligaments predispose the scaphoid to rotation. **(B)** Flexing/extending-type scaphoid: direct attachment of DIC and a radioscaphocapitate (RSC) ligament limit rotation; *R*, radius; *RS*, radioscaphoid; *S*, scaphoid; *STT*, scapho-trapezio-trapezoid. (From Fogg QA. *Scaphoid Variation and an Anatomical Basis for Variable Carpal Mechanics* [Ph.D. thesis]. Adelaide: Department of Anatomical Sciences, The University of Adelaide; 2004, with permission.)

- Plate fixation can yield high union rates in select patients (overall quality: low)
- Scaphoid plate positioning depends on the fracture configuration and surgeon preference (overall quality: low)

CONCLUSION

Scaphoid plating has been used since the 1970s, and its use has recently seen some renewed interest. Plating of the scaphoid remains an area of ongoing research and is currently reserved for challenging high-energy injuries, nonunions with previously failed nonoperative or surgical management, and for patients who have high wrist demands. Adequate screw fixation into both fracture fragments remains an important part of fixation. Volar or dorsal plate placement depends on fracture configuration and stability. Operative and radiologic assessment for impingement is imperative for scaphoid plating..

PANEL 2
Author's Preferred Technique

The case scenario (Figs. 30.1 and 30.2) shows a relatively young patient with a nonunited scaphoid fracture due to delayed union. The preferred method is as follows:

- Bony evaluation with a preoperative CT to assess fracture configuration and bone stock
- A dorsal plate was chosen in this case due to the delayed presentation and the obliquity of the fracture rendering unsuitable for single screw fixation
- Postoperatively the patient was followed up with serial radiographs and a CT to assess for union

SURGICAL TECHNIQUE

Volar

An incision overlying the flexor carpi radialis (FCR) is commenced 2 cm proximal to the scaphoid tubercle and carried toward the base of the thumb. The superficial palmar branch of the radial artery may be ligated if required. The FCR sheath is incised and the tendon retracted ulnar to expose the wrist capsule. Pronator quadratus is exposed through a longitudinal incision of the floor of the FCR sheath. Radial artery and volar carpal branch to the distal pronator quadratus are identified and protected. Incision of the radioscaphocapitate ligament exposes the volar scaphoid.

The fracture is prepared by debriding the fibrous tissue and sclerotic bone. Preservation of the dorsal fibrous nonunion tissue can aid in preventing extrusion of bone graft from the dorsal scaphoid. K-wires in each fracture fragment are used as joysticks to facilitate manipulation and reduction. In some instances, a scaphocapitate K-wire can aid in provisional fixation during bone grafting. The fracture site and bone defects are packed with cancellous bone graft from the iliac crest or the distal radius.

Continued

PANEL 2
Author's Preferred Technique—cont'd

A titanium, precontoured volar scaphoid 1.5-mm miniplate (Medartis AG, Austrasse, Basel, Switzerland) is placed on the volar bare area. In some instances, it might be required to recontour the plate or to remove some of the screw holes to avoid impingement. The plate acts a bridging plate and buttresses any bone graft. At least three screws are then placed into each fracture fragment. Screws are aimed away from the fracture plane and positioned in a divergent configuration to increase angular fixation. Fluoroscopy is then used to ensure that the plate and screws do not impinge in any wrist position and that they do not protrude dorsally.

Dorsal

A longitudinal incision is made halfway between the radial and ulnar styloid. The extensor retinaculum is released over the second compartment, and the extensor tendons retracted. The joint capsule is incised longitudinally and the dorsal bare area of the scaphoid exposed. For plate fixation the soft tissue attachment over the dorsal ridge needs to be released; unfortunately, this includes the dorsal vessels. For this reason, the main indication is complex wrist injuries with scaphoid comminution. The scapholunate ligament should not be disturbed.

The fracture site is debrided and reduced, with either K-wire joysticks or point-to-point reduction clamps. Cancellous bone from the distal radius can be harvested and impacted into the fracture site. The humpback deformity can represent a challenge for dorsal plating. In acute fractures, volar cortical loss is usually minimal and the deformity can be corrected with anatomic fracture reduction and cancellous bone grafting. Nonunion with volar cortical loss requires bone grafting and stable internal fixation.

A titanium, trapezoidal 8- to 10-hole locking 1.5-mm miniplate (Medartis AG, Austrasse, Basel, Switzerland) is contoured to conform to the dorsal shape of the scaphoid. Similar to volar plating, one of the proximal and/or distal screw holes may need to be cut from the plate to prevent plate impingement. For fractures that extend into the distal waist, plate position over the increasing convex scaphoid requires careful evaluation. Plate insetting may be required to avoid impingement into the STT joint and to ensure adequate fracture spanning.

Principles of screw placement are similar to volar plating. Following fracture compression, at least three screws are placed into each fracture fragment. Screws are aimed away from the fracture site to maximize angular fixation and rigidity. Once fixation is complete, the wrist is closely examined clinically and under fluoroscopy to ensure that the plate and screws do not impinge in any wrist position. This includes identifying if (1) the plate impinges on the dorsal radius in wrist extension, (2) if the screws violate the articulations including the STT and midcarpal joints, and (3) if the screws protrude excessively through the volar cortex.

PANEL 3
Pearls and Pitfalls

PEARLS

- Preoperative CT and 3D reconstruction to plan for most suitable fixation.
- Use K-wires as joysticks or a laminar spreader to allow debridement of scar tissue and impaction of bone graft into the fracture site.
- Image the proposed plate position early to allow for trimming of prominent screws holes and for consideration of plate insetting to avoid impingement.

PITFALLS

- If the plate is too prominent or screws protrude in the neighboring joints, impingement and secondary joint degeneration will require revision surgery or early removal of the plate.
- If the fracture is too distal or too proximal preventing at least three screws to be placed into each fragment, consider alternative fixation options.

REFERENCES

1. Herbert TJ, Fisher WE. Management of the fractured scaphoid using a new bone screw. *J Bone Joint Surg Br Vol.* 1984;66(1):114–123.
2. Bain GI, Turow A, Phadnis J. Dorsal plating of unstable scaphoid fractures and nonunions. *Tech Hand Up Extrem Surg.* 2015;19(3):95–100.
3. Garcia RM, Leversedge FJ, Aldridge JM, Richard MJ, Ruch DS. Scaphoid nonunions treated with 2 headless compression screws and bone grafting. *J Hand Surg.* 2014;39(7):1301–1307.
4. Adolfsson L, Lindau T, Arner M. Acutrak screw fixation versus cast immobilisation for undisplaced scaphoid waist fractures. *J Hand Surg.* 2001;26(3):192–195.
5. Bond CD, Shin AY, McBride MT, Dao KD. Percutaneous screw fixation or cast immobilization for nondisplaced scaphoid fractures. *J Bone Joint Surg Am Vol.* 2001;83-A(4):483–488.
6. Soubeyrand M, Thomsen L, Doursounian L, Gagey O, Nourissat G. Percutaneous retrograde screw fixation of non-displaced fractures of the scaphoid waist: an anti-rotation wire may not be necessary. *J Hand Surg Eur Vol.* 2010;35(3):209–213.

7. Dunn J, Kusnezov N, Fares A, Mitchell J, Pirela-Cruz M. The scaphoid staple a systematic review. *Hand*. 2016. http://dx.doi.org/10.1177/1558944716658747.
8. Prosser GH, Isbister ES. The presentation of scaphoid non-union. *Injury*. 2003;34(1):65–67.
9. Langhoff O, Andersen JL. Consequences of late immobilization of scaphoid fractures. *J Hand Surg*. 1988;13(1): 77–79.
10. Saffar P, SpringerLink (Online service). *Carpal Injuries Anatomy, Radiology, Current Treatment*. Paris: Springer; 1990. http://dx.doi.org/10.1007/978-2-8178-0777-5.
11. Ghoneim A. The unstable nonunited scaphoid waist fracture: results of treatment by open reduction, anterior wedge grafting, and internal fixation by volar buttress plate. *J Hand Surg*. 2011;36(1):17–24.
12. Leixnering M, Pezzei C, Weninger P, et al. First experiences with a new adjustable plate for osteosynthesis of scaphoid nonunions. *J Trauma*. 2011;71(4):933–938.
13. Wheeler DL, McLoughlin SW. Biomechanical assessment of compression screws. *Clin Orthop Relat Res*. 1998;(350):237–245.
14. Luria S, Hoch S, Liebergall M, Mosheiff R, Peleg E. Optimal fixation of acute scaphoid fractures: finite element analysis. *J Hand Surg*. 2010;35(8):1246–1250.
15. Rankin G, Kuschner SH, Orlando C, McKellop H, Brien WW, Sherman R. A biomechanical evaluation of a cannulated compressive screw for use in fractures of the scaphoid. *J Hand Surg*. 1991;16(6):1002–1010.
16. Shaw JA. A biomechanical comparison of scaphoid screws. *J Hand Surg*. 1987;12(3):347–353.
17. Toby EB, Butler TE, McCormack TJ, Jayaraman G. A comparison of fixation screws for the scaphoid during application of cyclical bending loads. *J Bone Joint Surg Am Vol*. 1997;79(8):1190–1197.
18. Hart A, Harvey EJ, Rabiei R, Barthelat F, Martineau PA. Fixation strength of four headless compression screws. *Med Eng Phys*. 2016;38(10):1037–1043.
19. Newport ML, Williams CD, Bradley WD. Mechanical strength of scaphoid fixation. *J Hand Surg*. 1996;21(1): 99–102.
20. Fogg QA. *Scaphoid Variation and an Anatomical Basis for Variable Carpal Mechanics* [Ph.D. thesis]. Adelaide: Department of Anatomical Sciences, The University of Adelaide; 2004.
21. Jurkowitsch J, Dall'Ara E, Quadlbauer S, et al. Rotational stability in screw-fixed scaphoid fractures compared to plate-fixed scaphoid fractures. *Arch Orthop Trauma Surg*. 2016;136(11):1623–1628.
22. Schmidt H-M, Lanz U. *Surgical Anatomy of the Hand*. Stuttgart, New York: Thieme; 2004.
23. Müller ME, Allgöwer M, Schneider R, Willenegger H, Allgöwer M, SpringerLink (Online service). *Manual of INTERNAL FIXATION Techniques Recommended by the AO-ASIF Group*. Berlin, Heidelberg: Springer Berlin Heidelberg; 1992.
24. Dodds SD, Patterson JT, Halim A. Volar plate fixation of recalcitrant scaphoid nonunions with volar carpal artery vascularized bone graft. *Tech Hand Up Extrem Surg*. 2014;18(1):2–7.
25. Merrell GA, Wolfe SW, Slade 3rd JF. Treatment of scaphoid nonunions: quantitative meta-analysis of the literature. *J Hand Surg*. 2002;27(4):685–691.
26. Finsen V, Hofstad M, Haugan H. Most scaphoid nonunions heal with bone chip grafting and Kirschner-wire fixation. Thirty-nine patients reviewed 10 years after operation. *Injury*. 2006;37(9):854–859.
27. Kirkham SG, Millar MJ. Cancellous bone graft and Kirschner wire fixation as a treatment for cavitary-type scaphoid nonunions exhibiting DISI. *Hand*. 2012;7(1):86–93.
28. Park HY, Yoon JO, Jeon IH, Chung HW, Kim JS. A comparison of the rates of union after cancellous iliac crest bone graft and Kirschner-wire fixation in the treatment of stable and unstable scaphoid nonunion. *Bone Joint J*. 2013;95-B(6):809–814.
29. Slade 3rd JF, Geissler WB, Gutow AP, Merrell GA. Percutaneous internal fixation of selected scaphoid nonunions with an arthroscopically assisted dorsal approach. *J Bone Joint Surg Am Vol*. 2003;85-A(suppl 4):20–32.
30. Braun C, Gross G, Buhren V. Osteosynthesis using a buttress plate–a new principle for stabilizing scaphoid pseudarthroses. *Unfallchirurg*. 1993;96(1):9–11.
31. Stankovic P, Burchhardt H. Experience with the Ender hooked plate in the management of 42 scaphoid pseudarthroses. *Handchir Mikrochir Plast Chir*. 1993;25(4): 217–222.
32. Geisl H, Puhringer A. Chronic fractures and pseudarthroses of the scaphoid bone of the hand. Experiences with the Ender scaphoid bone plate. *Aktuelle Traumatol*. 1986;16(4):149–152.
33. Ender HG. A new method of treating traumatic cysts and pseudoarthrosis of the scaphoid (author's transl). *Unfallheilkunde*. 1977;80(12):509–513.
34. Mirrer J, Yeung J, Sapienza A. Anatomic locking plate fixation for scaphoid nonunion. *Case Rep Orthop*. 2016; 2016:7374101.
35. Bohler J, Ender HG. Pseudarthrosis of the scaphoid. *Orthopade*. 1986;15(2):109–120.
36. Huene DR, Huene DS. Treatment of nonunions of the scaphoid with the Ender compression blade plate system. *J Hand Surg*. 1991;16(5):913–922.

CHAPTER 31

Vascularized Versus Nonvascularized Bone Grafts

ROHIT ARORA, MD • MARKUS GABL, MD • TOBIAS KASTENBERGER, MD • GERNOT SCHMIDLE, MD

KEY POINTS

- Vascularized and nonvascularized bone grafts for scaphoid nonunion surgery can be taken from different locations with specific donor-site morbidities.
- Risk factors for failed scaphoid nonunion surgery (dislocation, carpal instability, impaired vascularity, long-standing nonunion, smoking, and previous surgeries) influence bone graft selection.
- Bone grafts bring viable tissue to the nonunion site, structural bone grafts increase stability, and vascularized bone grafts add vascularity to otherwise impaired bone.
- Both vascularized and nonvascularized bone grafts can lead to good healing rates if preoperative diagnosis, risk factor assessment, and selection of type of nonunion are performed diligently.

IMPORTANCE OF THE PROBLEM

Scaphoid fractures are sometimes unrecognized, but even when primarily recognized and treated appropriately, nonunion may occur in 5%–15%.[1] Scaphoid nonunion is highly related to an interruption of the tenuous blood supply, either by the fracture itself, where the fracture remains displaced preventing new capillary blood formation across the fracture or excessive interfragmentary fracture motion also preventing neovascularization with a nonunion risk of up to 55%.[2] Other risk factors include a combination of a long-standing nonunion, previous failed surgery, avascularity of the proximal fragment or proximal fracture location.[3] Observations on the natural history of scaphoid nonunion reveal that osteoarthritis is time dependent and may become progressively worse in association with long-standing nonunion and finally will lead to scaphoid nonunion advanced collapse of the wrist. Therefore, most surgeons involved in scaphoid nonunion treatment would recommend surgical treatment of symptomatic nonunion.[4]

There are various types of scaphoid nonunions that can be treated with bone grafts:

1. Very early nonunion in the waist with no scaphoid deformity.
2. Nonunion with humpback deformity and manifested dorsal intercalated segment instability (DISI) deformity (volar-type nonunion)
3. Nonunion without humpback deformity (dorsal-type nonunion)
4. Long-standing pseudarthrosis with cysts and bone loss and fragmented proximal pole
5. Long-standing pseudarthrosis with several previous surgeries and loosened screw
6. Nonunion with avascular necrosis (AVN) of the proximal pole

In our opinion, it is very important to have a preoperative diagnosis of the bony configuration of the nonunion and the vascular status of the nonunited proximal pole to plan the surgery and inform the patient. Phrases such as "we will decide intraoperatively about the source of bone graft or if we need vascularized bone graft and if yes may be from the wrist or hip or knee" should be avoided because they lead to decreased patient compliance and intraoperative setting.

Especially the postoperative rehabilitation time and the time to return to work and sport activities that depends to the treatment option has a significant impact for patients. Therefore postoperative care should be discussed with the settled preoperatively.

MAIN QUESTION

Where are the limits of conventional bone grafting for scaphoid nonunions and are there any evidence-based indications for the use of vascularized versus nonvascularized bone grafts?

Current Opinion

Nonvascularized bone grafts are used for simple, minimally displaced nonunions as standard treatment. Vascularized bone grafts should be considered in cases of AVN, long-standing proximal pole pseudarthrosis, or failed previous surgery. In long-standing pseudarthrosis with proximal pole fragmentation and bone loss osteochondral grafts from the medial femoral condyle are most favorable.

PANEL 1
Case Scenarios

CASE 1

A 27-year-old male patient presented with wrist pain and restriction of active range of motion. Especially wrist extension was limited and patient was unable to perform sport activities. X-ray (Fig. 31.1A) and CT scan (Fig. 31.1B and 31.1C) showed scaphoid waist nonunion with humpback deformity. Patient remembered a wrist injury almost 3 years back. He never visited a physician.

Which of the following treatment options can be considered optimal evidence-based management?

1. Use a volar incision and perform a conventional nonvascularized bone graft from the distal radius and retrograde screw fixation.
2. Use a volar incision and perform a conventional nonvascularized bone graft from the iliac crest and retrograde screw fixation.
3. Use a dorsal incision and perform a pedicled vascularized bone graft from the distal radius 1,2 intercompartmental supraretinacular artery (1,2 ICSRA) and antegrade screw fixation.
4. Use a volar incision and perform a free vascularized bone graft from the medial femoral condyle (MFC) and retrograde screw fixation.

CASE 2

A 17-year-old male patient sustained a proximal pole fracture that was treated with antegrade screw fixation. Because of delayed nonunion, conventional bone grafting from the distal radius and repeated screw fixation was performed 6 months after the primary surgery. In total 16 months after antegrade screw fixation the patient presented with persistent symptomatic nonunion and screw loosening (Fig. 31.2).

Which of the following treatment options can be considered optimal evidence-based management?

1. Use the dorsal incision, remove the screw, conventional bone grafting from the iliac crest, and antegrade screw fixation.
2. Use the dorsal incision, remove the screw, pedicled vascularized bone grafting from the distal radius (1,2 ICSRA) with antegrade screw fixation of the graft.
3. Use the dorsal incision, remove the screw, and perform a second volar incision with free vascularized MFC bone grafting with retrograde K-wire fixation.

CASE 3

A 25-year-old male patient complained pain during manual work and restricted wrist extension and flexion (Figs. 31.3 and 31.4).

Which of the following treatment options can be considered optimal evidence-based management?

1. Use a dorsal incision and perform a conventional nonvascularized bone graft from the dorsal radius and antegrade screw fixation.
2. Use a dorsal incision and perform a conventional nonvascularized bone graft from the iliac crest and antegrade screw fixation.
3. Use a dorsal incision and perform a pedicled vascularized bone graft from the distal radius (1,2 ICSRA) and antegrade screw fixation.
4. Use a volar incision and perform a free vascularized osteochondral bone graft from the MFC to replace the entire fragmented proximal pole. To protect the harvested cartilage, use a plate fixation.

CASE 4

A 42-year-old man had an X-ray done by his general physician 2 weeks before. A scaphoid nonunion was diagnosed and the patient referred to our department. He could remember a hyperextension injury around 2 years ago but did not visit a physician. Patient complained about wrist pain in extreme wrist extension. There were no restrictions of active range of motion (Figs. 31.5 and 31.6).

Which of the following treatment options can be considered optimal evidence-based management?

1. Use a volar incision and perform a conventional nonvascularized bone graft from the distal radius and retrograde screw fixation.
2. Use a volar incision and perform a conventional nonvascularized bone graft from the iliac crest and retrograde screw fixation.
3. Use a dorsal incision and perform a pedicled vascularized bone graft from the distal radius (1,2 ICSRA) and antegrade screw fixation.
4. Use a volar incision and perform a free vascularized bone graft from the MFC and retrograde K-wire fixation.

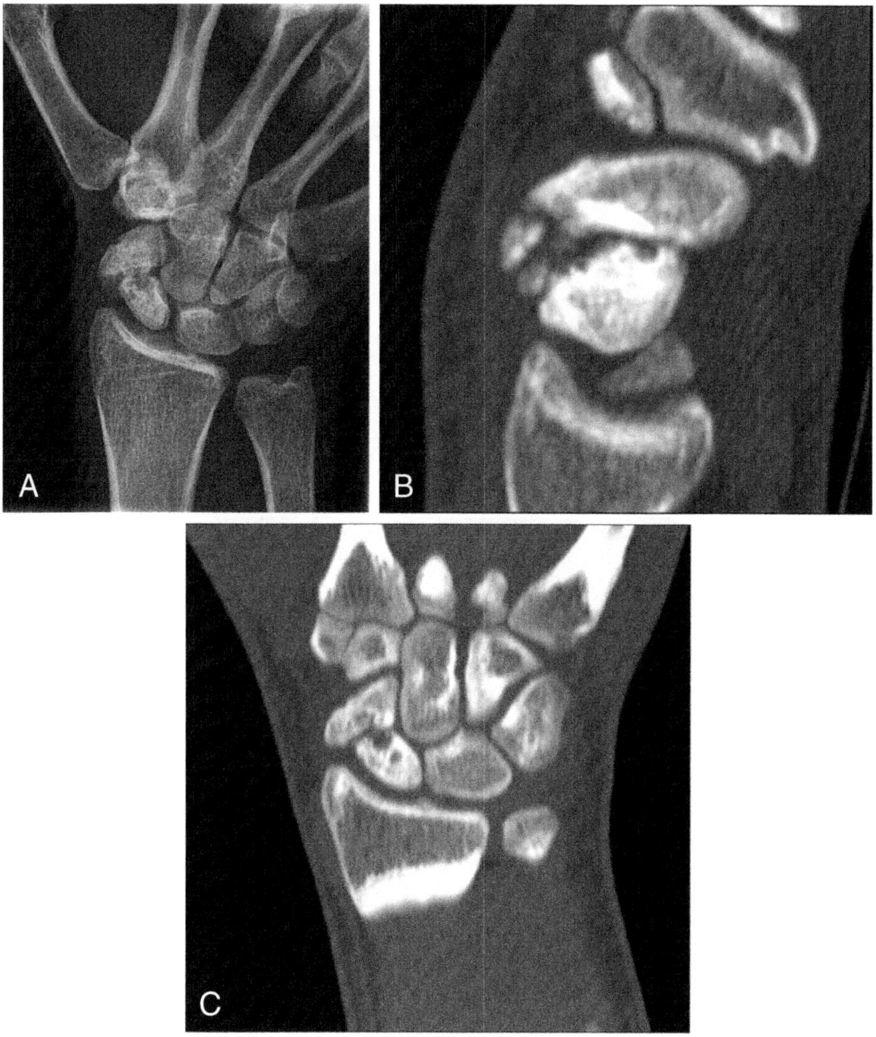

FIG. 31.1 X-ray **(A)** and CT scan **(B** and **C)** showed scaphoid waist nonunion with humpback deformity.

Finding the Evidence

- Cochrane search: Scaphoid Nonunion Bone Graft, Scaphoid Graft
- Pubmed (clinical queries): (systematic[sb] OR Therapy/Broad[filter]) AND Scaphoid Nonunion Bone Graft
- Pubmed (Medline): (("scaphoid bone"[MeSH Terms] OR ("scaphoid"[All Fields] AND "bone"[All Fields]) OR "scaphoid bone"[All Fields] OR "scaphoid"[All Fields]) AND nonunion[All Fields] AND ("bone transplantation"[MeSH Terms] OR ("bone"[All Fields] AND "transplantation"[All Fields]) OR "bone transplantation"[All Fields] OR ("bone"[All Fields] AND "graft"[All Fields]) OR "bone graft"[All Fields])) AND (Review[ptyp] AND (English[lang] OR French[lang] OR German[lang]))
- Bibliography of eligible articles
- Articles that were not in English, French, or German were excluded.

Quality of the Evidence

Level I:

Randomized trials: 1

Level II:

Randomized trials with methodological limitations: 1

Level III:

Systematic reviews of case series and retrospective comparative studies: 5

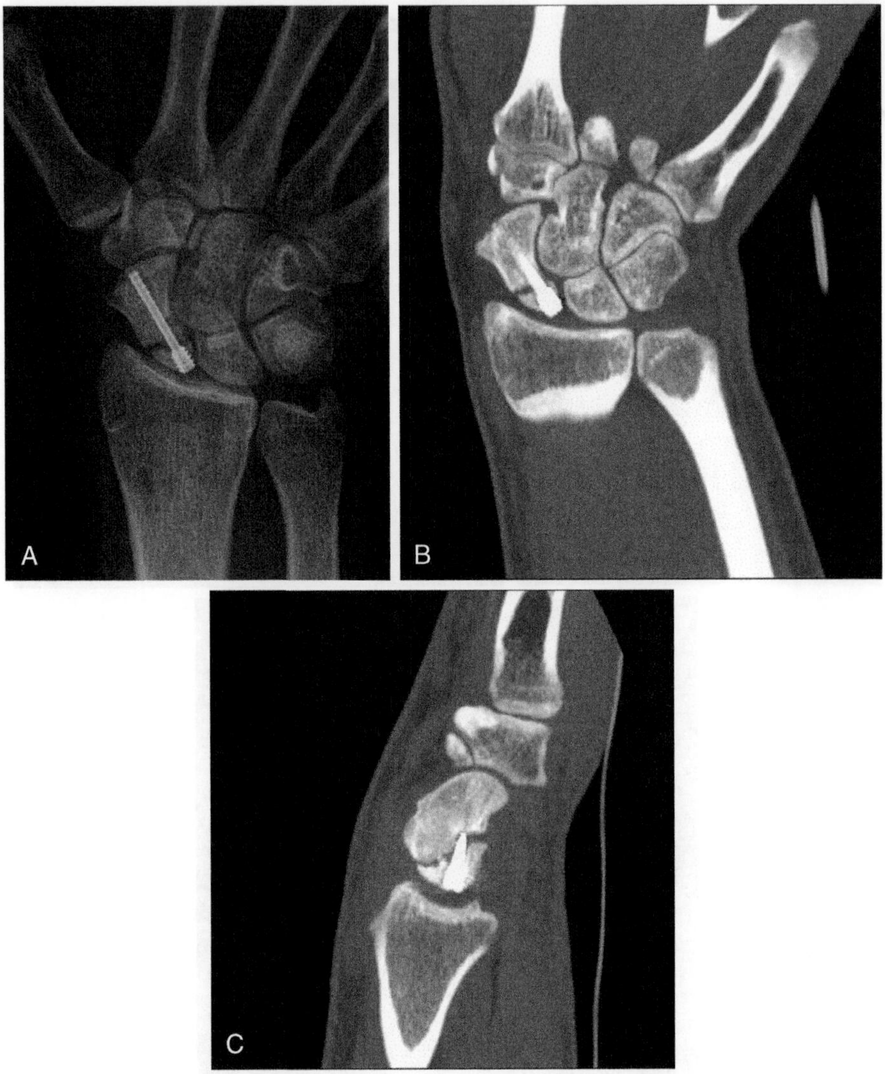

FIG. 31.2 **(A)** X-ray, **(B)** AP, and **(C)** lateral CT scan.

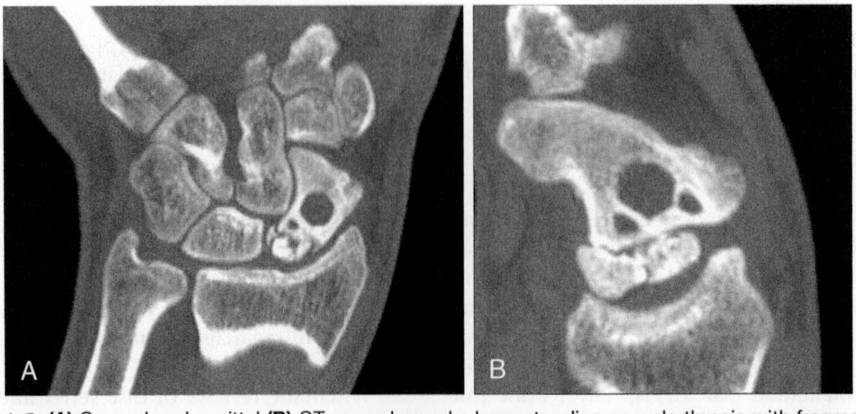

FIG. 31.3 **(A)** Coronal and sagittal **(B)** CT scan showed a long-standing pseudarthrosis with fragmented proximal pole and cystic bone loss in the scaphoid waist. The patient did not know the date of injury. To assess the cartilage status, we performed a diagnostic arthroscopy.

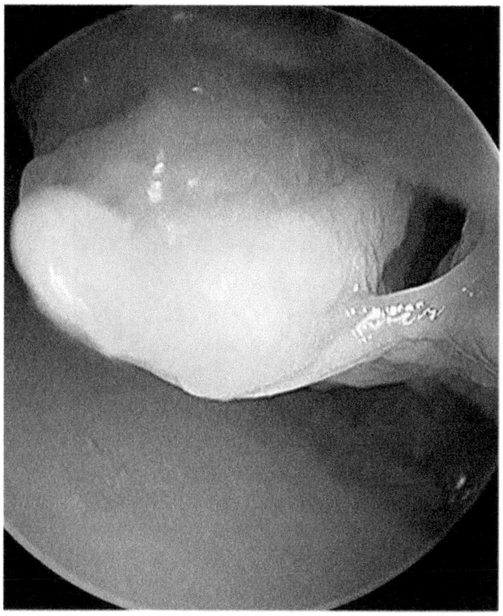

FIG. 31.4 The completely separated proximal pole protruding into the radiocarpal joint.

Level V:

Expert opinion and summary of current concepts: 2

FINDINGS

Scaphoid nonunions are not quite so amenable to true randomized trials with enough statistical power because of their relative infrequency and the multitude of variables reported to influence the outcome. In such circumstances, information from quantitative analysis of case series is preferable to treatment decisions merely based on conjecture or unassessed personal experience. Therefore our article selection focused on the few available randomized controlled trials and systematic reviews (Table 31.1).

Ribak et al.[5] conducted a prospective randomized study comparing the results of 46 vascularized and 40 nonvascularized bone grafts from the distal radius in the treatment of scaphoid nonunion. Preoperative imaging consisted in conventional radiographs and vascularity of the proximal pole was assessed by intraoperative punctate bleeding. 30 patients in the vascularized group (65.2%) and 20 patients in the nonvascularized group (50%) showed no intraoperative bleeding and were sclerotic. In sclerotic, poorly vascularized proximal pole nonunions vascularized bone grafts were even more superior with healing rates of 83.3% as opposed to 55% for nonvascularized bone grafts. Patients with well-vascularized fragments yielded favorable consolidation rates irrespective of the technique (100% vs. 90%).

In another randomized controlled study Braga-Silva et al.[6] compared 35 vascularized bone grafts from the distal radius and 45 nonvascularized bone grafts from the iliac crest. Preoperative work-up was limited to standard radiographs and cases with AVN were not differentiated. In addition, no information on scaphoid angles and presence or correction of DISI deformity was given. All nonvascularized bone grafts healed, whereas three patients with vascularized bone grafts failed to heal, all of which were related to technical difficulties.

Al-Jabri et al.[7] collected the evidence for free vascularized bone grafting in scaphoid nonunion in a systematic review. They included 12 retrospective case series with a total of 245 patients. In 188 patients the bone graft was taken from the iliac crest with a union rate of 87.7%. The early results for medial femoral condyle grafts were presented in 56 patients with a significantly higher union rate of 100% ($P<.05$). A single united case of free vascularized rib graft was also described. A significantly higher donor-site morbidity was found in patients with bone grafts from the iliac crest ($P<.05$).

In their review Sayegh et Strauch[8] focused on nonvascularized bone grafts in unstable scaphoid nonunions. They compared procedures with corticocancellous (CC) bone grafts and cancellous-only (C-only) bone grafts. A total of 23 retrospective case series with 604 patients were included. There was no statistical difference in union rate (CC 92% vs. C-only 95%). C-only grafts showed a significantly shorter interval to union (11.1 ± 4.3 vs. 16.2 ± 4.6 weeks, $P<.001$), whereas CC grafting led to superior improvement of carpal geometry ($P<.001$).

Merrell et al.[9] performed a systematic quantitative metareview of literature on scaphoid nonunion treatment. They included 36 studies (case series) with 1827 patients. Patients with AVN, assessed by intraoperative punctate bleeding, benefited from vascularized grafts with union rates of 88% versus 47% ($P<.01$) in nonvascularized wedge grafts with screw fixation. In patients with previous surgery, there was a trend toward better healing rates with vascularized grafts (94% union vs. 81% union), but there was not enough statistical power to reach statistical significance. Patients with a delay of less than 12 months between injury and surgery had a significantly better healing rate than those with a delay of more than 12 months (90% vs. 80%, $P<.01$). The location of the nonunion had a significant impact on healing rates (distal 100%, waist 85%, proximal 67%, $P<.01$).

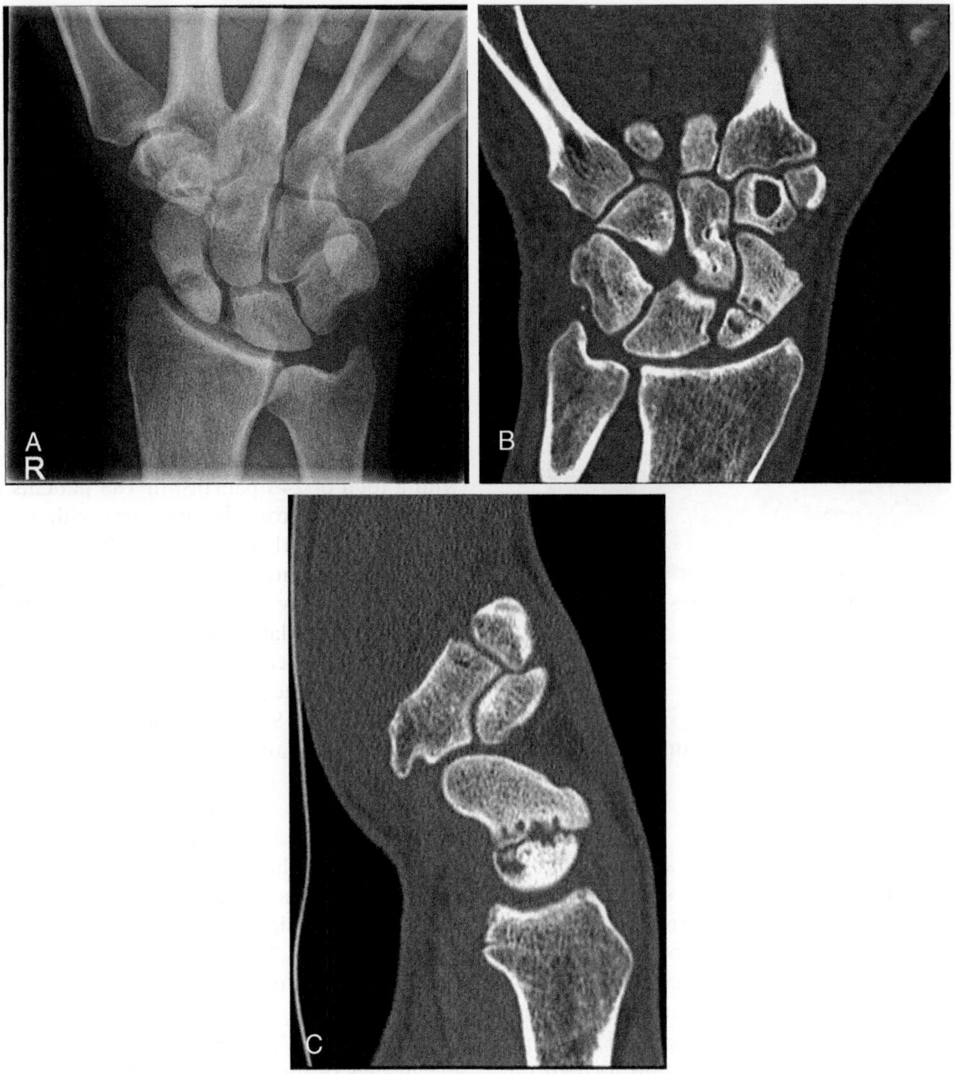

FIG. 31.5 **(A)** X-ray and **(B** and **C)** CT-scan showed scaphoid nonunion with cystic changes and sclerotic proximal pole. Because of the proximal pole sclerosis, we decided to perform an MRI with gadolinium contrast to assess the vascularity of the proximal pole.

The systematic review conducted by Munk et al.[10] compared union rates and immobilization time for three groups of patients: patients treated with nonvascularized bone grafts with and without internal fixation and those treated with vascularized bone grafts. Union rates of 80% with a mean postoperative immobilization period of 15 weeks were reported for nonvascularized bone grafts without internal fixation. Patients treated with nonvascularized bone grafts with internal fixation achieved union in 84% with an average immobilization of 7 weeks. Scaphoid nonunions treated with vascularized bone grafts healed in 91% of the cases with a mean immobilization of 10 weeks.

In the systematic review by Pinder et al.[11] vascularized bone grafts showed union in 95%–100% of cases with AVN. Overall, there was no significant difference in reported union rates for vascularized and nonvascularized grafts (92% vs. 88%) with comparable time to union (13.8 vs. 13.6 weeks). As vascularized grafts were more often used for nonunions that are more likely to fail (proximal pole/AVN/humpback deformities), this result may be skewed in favor of nonvascularized grafts.

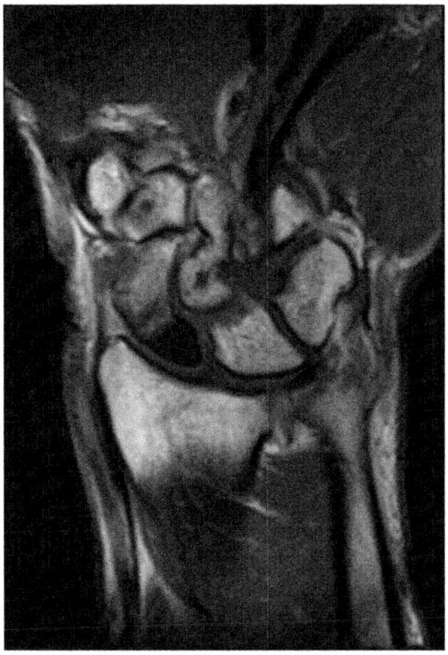

FIG. 31.6 Preoperative MRI with gadolinium contrast showing avascular proximal pole.

In a current opinion symposium on scaphoid fractures, Hovius and de Jong[12] provided an overview on the most commonly used bone grafts in scaphoid nonunion surgery. In their opinion free vascularized bone grafts should, as major surgery, be reserved for therapy resistant cases and for small proximal pole reconstruction. Nonvascularized bone grafts are less technically demanding and mostly used in simple, nondislocated nonunions. Pedicled bone grafts are increasingly used and originate most often from the distal radius. Free vascularized bone grafts are used after failed surgery, AVN, or if a large wedge to correct a humpback deformity is indicated.

Buijze et al.[13] present... their current study concepts of scaphoid nonunion management. Nonvascularized wedge grafting from the iliac crest following the Fisk-Fernandez technique allows for superior restoration of alignment compared to the classical Matti-Russe procedure. There are different sources for nonvascularized bone grafting with latest results, showing similar union rates from dorsal distal radius and iliac crest. The role of nonvascularized grafts in AVN is still debated. There are several

TABLE 31.1
Findings

Author	LoE	Study Design	Objective	Patients/ Studies	Healing Rate	Comments
Ribak[5]	IB	Prospective randomized controlled trial	Comparison vascularized versus nonvascularized bone grafts from the distal radius	86/1	All cases: NVBG 72.5%, VBG 89.1% Proximal pole: NVBG 68.9%, VBG 90.5% AVN: NVBG 55%, VBG 83.3%	VBG better in sclerotic, poorly vascularized proximal pole nonunions
Braga-Silva[6]	IIB	Prospective randomized controlled trial with methodological limitations	Comparison vascularized bone grafts from the distal radius and nonvascularized bone grafts from the iliac crest	80/1	NVBG 100% VBG 91.4%	No information on vascularity of the fragments VBG mainly fixed with K-wires (30/35) All NVBG fixed with screws
Al-Jabri[7]	IIIA	Systematic review of case series	Evidence for free vascularized bone grafts	245/12	IC 87.7% MFC 100%	MFC less donor-site morbidity
Sayegh[8]	IIIA	Systematic review of case series	Comparison corticocancellous (CC) versus cancellous-only (C-only) bone grafts for unstable scaphoid nonunions	604/23	CC 92% C-only 95%	CC superior in deformity correction

Continued

TABLE 31.1
Findings—cont'd

Author	LoE	Study Design	Objective	Patients/ Studies	Healing Rate	Comments
Merrell[9]	IIIA	Systematic review of case series	Evidence based suggestions for treatment	1827/36	AVN: NVBG 47%, VBG 88% Previous surgery: NVBG 81%, VBG 94%	Trend toward improved union rate with VBG in patients with previous surgery (NVBG 81% vs. VBG 94%)
Munk[10]	IIIA	Systematic review of case series and retrospective comparative studies	Union rate and postoperative immobilization period of the different scaphoid bone grafting procedures	5246/147	NVBG without IF 80%, with IF 84% VBG 91%	Immobilization period: NVBG without IF 15 weeks NVBG with IF 7 weeks VBG 10 weeks
Pinder[11]	IIIA	Metaanalysis of proportions	Determine by systematic review the optimal treatment of scaphoid nonunion	1602/48	NVBG 88% VBG 92%	Vascularized grafts are more often used for nonunions that are more likely to fail (proximal pole/AVN/humpback)
Hovius[12]	V	Current opinion symposium on scaphoid fracture	Overview and indications of most used bone grafts	5330/144	NVBG: without IF 80%, with IF 84% VBG: 1,2 ICSRA 78%, volar carpal artery 97%, MFC 93%	Absence of high-level evidence Expert opinion: VBG for cases of avascular necrosis, proximal pole nonunion, long standing pseudarthrosis, or failed prior surgery
Buijze[13]	V	Current concepts	Overview on scaphoid nonunion management	?/57	Not presented in detail	NVBG: Wedge grafting provides superior alignment Healing rate of grafts from different locations equivalent VBG: distal radius inconsistent union rates IC and MFC similar union rates MFC superior to distal radius grafts

1,2 ICSRA, 1,2 Intercompartmental supraretinacular artery; *AVN*, avascular necrosis; *CC*, corticocancellous; *C-only*, cancellous-only; *IC*, Iliac crest; *IF*, internal fixation; *LoE*, Level of evidence; *MFC*, medial femoral condyle; *NVBG*, nonvascularized bone graft; *VBG*, vascularized bone graft.

locations vascularized grafts can be derived from with pedicle grafts from the distal radius being the most commonly used. The reports on distal radius grafts vary greatly with union rates ranging from 27% to 100%. Free vascularized bone grafts from the iliac crest and the medial femoral condyle lead to similar union rates. There exists some evidence that nonunions treated with the medial femoral condyle graft show higher union rate and shorter time to healing compared with dorsal distal radius pedicle grafts.

There is still a lack of series that are truly comparable. The main problem is that the preoperative work-up of patients varies to a great extent. Fracture characteristics are not reported consistently and are often poorly documented or not examined in the results. Especially the assessment of vascularity of the proximal pole, a supposedly relevant prognostic factor, is not standardized, making it difficult to compare similar groups and hence to arrive at clear conclusions.

The current available evidence does not demonstrate a significantly superior method for treating scaphoid nonunions.

A large multicenter randomized trial would be the best option to obtain high-level evidence. However, this would require very large numbers to gain enough statistical power, making it very unrealistic. The evidence created with case series is therefore still valuable but has to be optimized by reporting standardized information making future comparison easier.[11]

RECOMMENDATION

In patients with unstable nonunion and DISI, evidence suggests the following:

- Nonvascularized CC wedge grafts implanted from volar provide a better restoration of carpal geometry (overall quality: moderate).

Concerning donor-site-related complications, evidence suggests the following:

- Bone grafts (vascularized and nonvascularized) from the distal radius and the medial femoral condyle result in less donor-site morbidity (overall quality: high).

In patients with AVN of the proximal pole, evidence suggests the following:

- Vascularized bone grafts provide a higher rate of union (overall quality: moderate).

In patients with AVN of the proximal pole and carpal collapse, evidence suggests the following:

- Vascularized bone grafts from the medial femoral condyle show a higher union rate and faster union time than distal radial pedicle vascularized grafts (overall quality: low to moderate).

PANEL 2
Case Scenarios: Used Treatment Option and Final Results

CASE 1

There was no history of previous surgery. The nonunion site was localized at the scaphoid waist and the proximal pole was viable; there was no need for a vascularized bone graft. To correct the humpback deformity, a volar approach was done and a wedge-type corticocancellous iliac crest bone grafting was done and fixed with retrograde screw fixation. Additional K-wire was used to increase the instability on the radial side (Fig. 31.7). At 6 months a CT-scan was done to confirm the bone union (Fig. 31.8A and B), showing union with correction of the humpback deformity.

CASE 2

A history of previous surgery is one of the main causes of an unsatisfactory result after a second attempted grafting. As a primary dorsal incision, bone graft from the dorsal distal radius with antegrade screw fixation has already been performed; we assumed that the two operations on the scaphoid might have damaged the surrounding soft tissues, including the 1,2 ICSRA, and that any further excision of fibrous tissue after screw removal at the nonunion site worsens the scaphoid blood supply. Therefore we decided to use a free vascularized MFC bone graft (Figs. 31.9 and 31.10).

CASE 3

In this patient the proximal pole was fragmented, separated from the waist, and bone loss in the waist was evident. Using a conventional nonvascularized bone graft either from the distal radius or from the iliac crest, we would not have been able to achieve stable bony reconstruction apart from reestablishing the vascularity of the entire proximal pole. Considering these technical limitations, we decided to replace the entire proximal pole using a free osteochondral MFC bone graft. We didn't want to perforate the cartilage of the harvested osteochondral bone graft using K-wire or screw and therefore used a volar locking plate fixation of the graft (Figs. 31.11–31.14).

Continued

CASE 4

The preoperative MRI with gadolinium contrast showed an avascular proximal pole. Possible options were either a pedicled 1,2 ICSRA for the distal radius or a free vascularized MFC bone graft. As there was some additional cystic bone loss at the nonunion site, we believed that the amount of bone that could be harvested from the distal radius pedicled on the 1,2 ICSRA would not be sufficient to fill the defect. Harvesting bigger amount of bone would weaken the distal radius and increase the risk of fracture.

The second reason for our decision was that the existing evidence reports that vascularized bone grafts from the medial femoral condyle show a higher union rate and faster union time than distal radial pedicle vascularized grafts (Fig. 31.15).

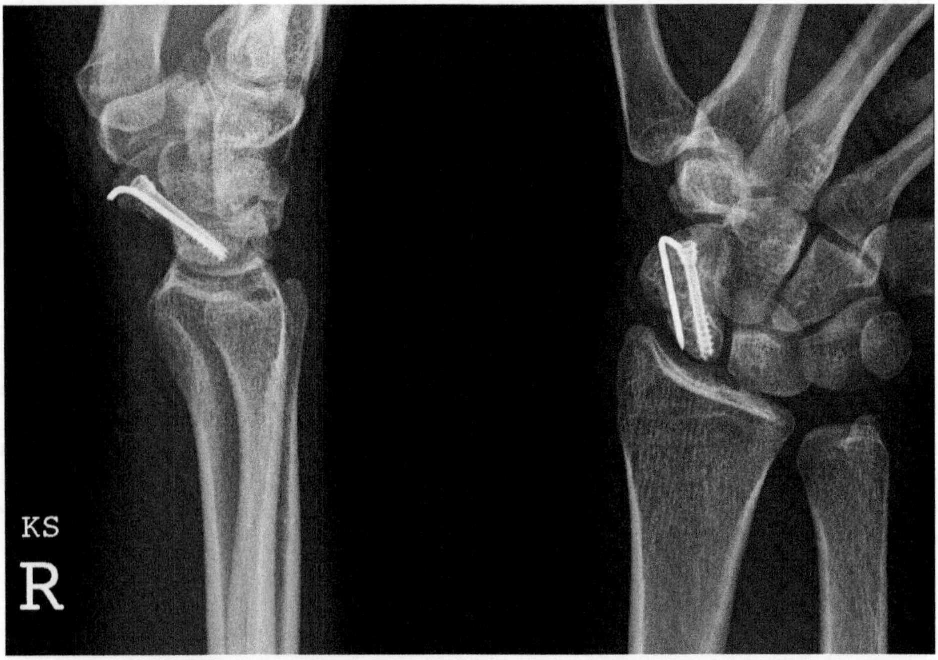

FIG. 31.7 Additional K-wire was used to increase the instability on the radial side.

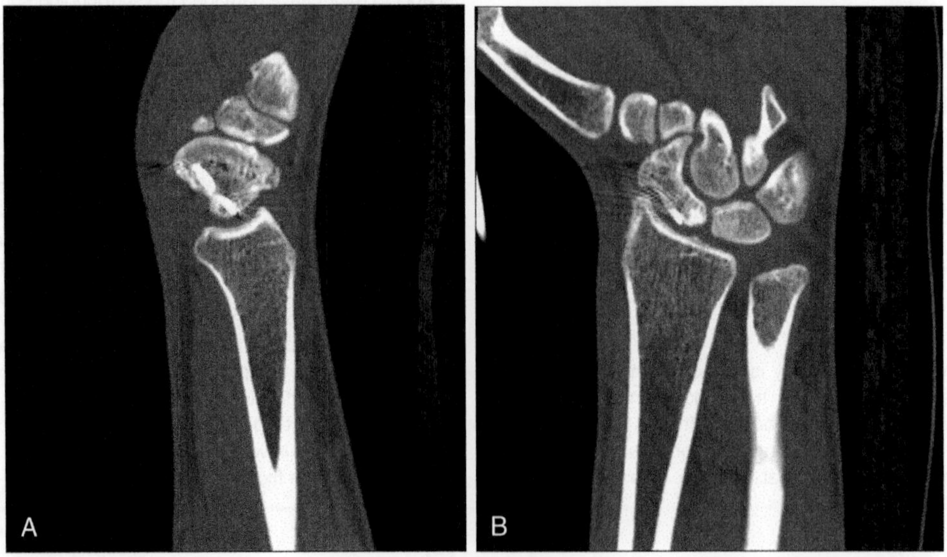

FIG. 31.8 Image of union with correction of the humpback deformity CT imaging (A: sagittal and B: coronal) of union with correction of the humpback deformity.

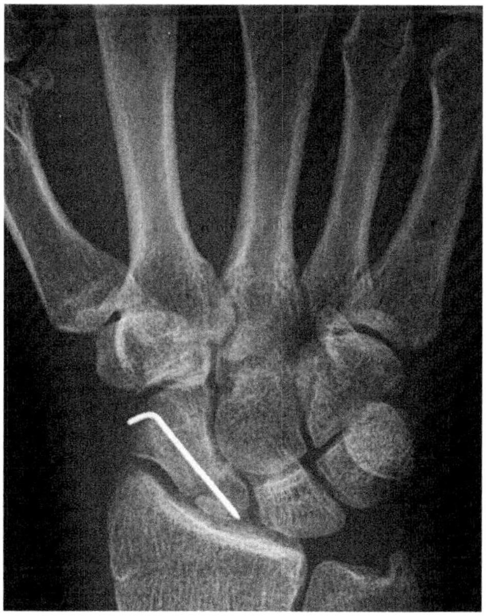

FIG. 31.9 Postoperative X-ray after free vascularized medial femoral condyle bone graft with K-wire fixation.

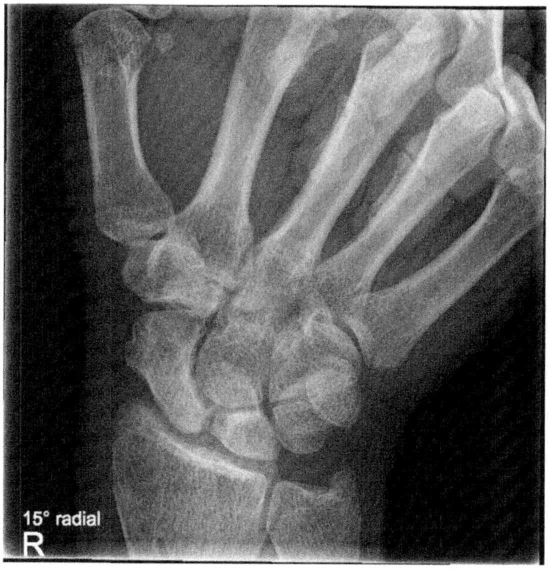

FIG. 31.10 X-ray at 3-year follow up showing bony union.

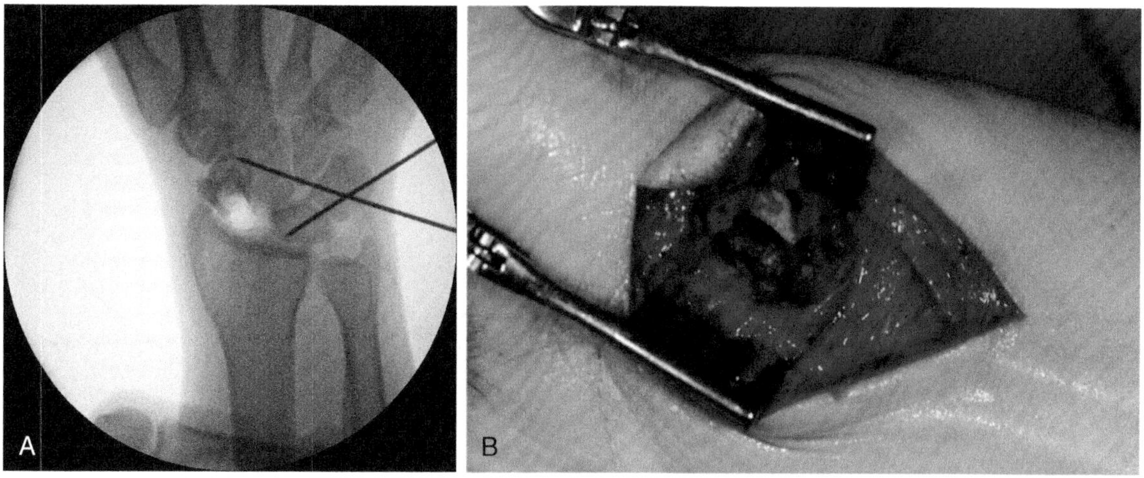

FIG. 31.11 **(A)** Intraoperative intensifier X-ray showing resection of the fragmented proximal pole. **(B)** Scaphoid defect after resection proximal pole.

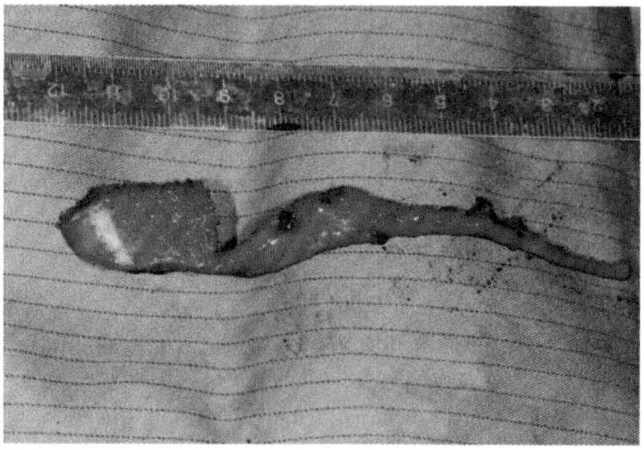

FIG. 31.12 Free vascularized osteochondral medial femoral condyle with pedicle.

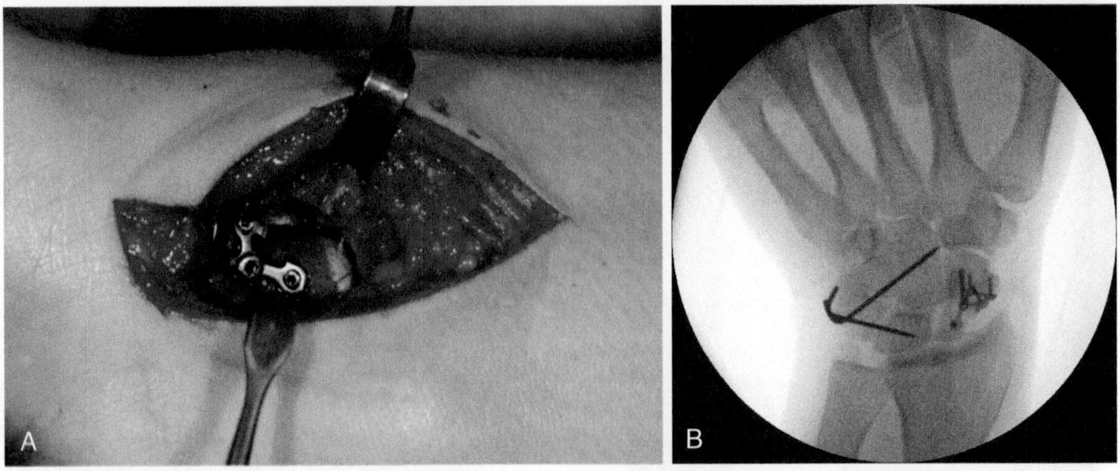

FIG. 31.13 **(A)** Plate fixation of free vascularized osteochondral medial femoral condyle. **(B)** Intraoperative intensifier X-ray showing plate fixation.

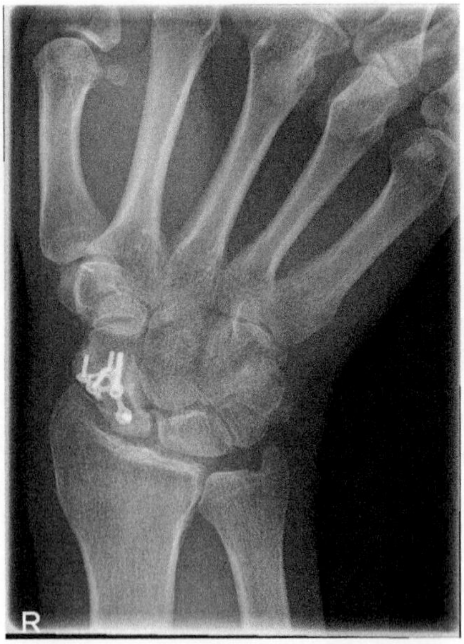

FIG. 31.14 X-ray at 3-year follow-up showing bony union of free vascularized osteochondral medial femoral condyle without any signs of scapholunate instability.

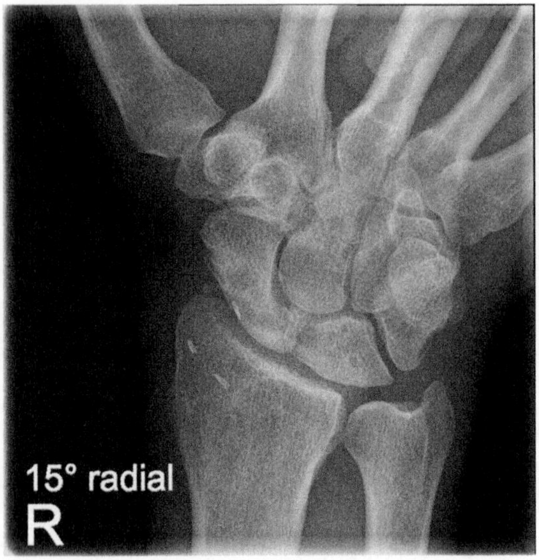

FIG. 31.15 X-ray at 18-month follow-up showing bony union of the proximal pole.

PANEL 3
Author's Preferred Treatment Algorithm

NONVASCULARIZED BONE GRAFTS (ILIAC CREST/DISTAL RADIUS)	
Early waist nonunion without deformity	Cancellous bone with retrograde screw fixation/ K-wire fixation
Early waist nonunion with humpback deformity	Volar corticocancellous bone grafting with retrograde screw fixation
Early proximal pole nonunion without deformity	Cancellous bone with antegrade screw fixation/ K-wire fixation
VASCULARIZED BONE GRAFTS	
Avascular necrosis (AVN) proximal pole without humpback deformity	Pedicled bone grafts volar carpal artery/1,2 intercompartmental supraretinacular artery with antegrade/ retrograde screw fixation
Long-standing AVN proximal pole with humpback deformity	Free medial femoral condyle (MFC) bone graft with K-wire fixation
Long-standing pseudarthrosis with previous failed surgery	Free MFC bone graft with K-wire fixation
Long-standing pseudarthrosis with cysts, bone loss, fragmented proximal pole	Free osteochondral MFC bone graft with K-wire fixation

CONCLUSION

There is a lack of high-level evidence comparing vascularized and nonvascularized bone grafts for the treatment of scaphoid nonunion. Further studies should report standardized specific assessments and outcome measures to optimize future comparison. To obtain evidence for the indication of vascularized bone grafts, a consensus on diagnosing preoperative vascularity of the proximal pole is deemed mandatory.

Nonvascularized bone grafts are used for simple, minimally displaced nonunions as standard treatment. Nonvascularized bone grafts heal by creeping substitution, involving gradual resorption of the graft followed by callus formation, whereas vascularized bone grafts heal without extensive resorption, callus formation, or remodeling. Therefore, bone viability and mechanical strength are preserved during bone healing. By providing osteoinductive and conductive stimuli, union appears to be faster in vascularized bone grafts.

Vascularized bone grafts should be considered in cases of AVN, long-standing proximal pole pseudarthrosis, or failed previous surgery. In long-standing pseudarthrosis with proximal pole fragmentation and bone loss, osteochondral grafts from the medial femoral condyle are most favorable.

REFERENCES

1. Cooney WP, Linscheid RL, Dobyns JH. Scaphoid fractures: problems associated with nonunion and avascular necrosis. *Orthop Clin North Am*. 1984;15:381–391.
2. Szabo RM, Manske D. Displaced fractures of the scaphoid. *Clin Orthop Relat Res*. 1988;230:30–38.
3. Osterman AL, Mikulics M. Scaphoid nonunion. *Hand Clin*. 1988;4:437–455.
4. Mack GR, Bosse MJ, Gelberman RH, Yu E. The natural history of scaphoid nonunion. *J Bone Joint Surg Am*. 1984;66-A:504–509.
5. Ribak S, Medina CE, Mattar Jr R, et al. Treatment of scaphoid nonunion with vascularised and nonvascularised dorsal bone grafting from the distal radius. *Int Orthop*. 2010;34:683–688.
6. Braga-Silva J, Peruchi FM, Moschen GM, et al. A comparison of the use of distal radius vascularised bone graft and non-vascularised iliac crest bone graft in the treatment of non-union of scaphoid fractures. *J Hand Surg Eur Vol*. 2008;33:636–640.
7. Al-Jabri T, Mannan A, Giannoudis P. The use of the free vascularised bone graft for nonunion of the scaphoid: a systematic review. *J Orthop Surg Res*. 2014;9:21.
8. Sayegh ET, Strauch RJ. Graft choice in the management of unstable scaphoid nonunion: a systematic review. *J Hand Surg Am*. 2014;39:1500–1506 e7.
9. Merrell GA, Wolfe SW, Slade 3rd JF. Treatment of scaphoid nonunions: quantitative meta-analysis of the literature. *J Hand Surg Am*. 2002;27:685–691.
10. Munk B, Larsen CF. Bone grafting the scaphoid nonunion: a systematic review of 147 publications including 5,246 cases of scaphoid nonunion. *Acta Orthop Scand*. 2004;75:618–629.
11. Pinder RM, Brkljac M, Rix L, et al. Treatment of scaphoid nonunion: a systematic review of the existing evidence. *J Hand Surg Am*. 2015;40:1797–1805 e3.
12. Hovius SE, de Jong T. Bone grafts for scaphoid nonunion: an overview. *Hand Surg*. 2015;20:222–227.
13. Buijze GA, Ochtman L, Ring D. Management of scaphoid nonunion. *J Hand Surg Am*. 2012;37:1095–1100.

CHAPTER 32

Vascularized Bone Grafts

CHRISTOPHE L. MATHOULIN, MD • MATHILDE GRAS, MD

KEY POINTS

- Using a vascularized bone graft for the treatment of scaphoid nonunion has revolutionized the treatment of this problem in the last decade.
- Adding vascularization allows for obtaining high rate of union for a bone with classically poorly vascularized proximal part.

PANEL 1
Case Scenario

A 22-year-old young man consults for wrist pain after a recent motorcycle injury. The radiologic assessment shows nonunion of the scaphoid with a significant bone loss, D2 stage according to Herbert's classification. Lateral view of radiologic assessment shows an adaptive dorsal intercalated segment instability, and CT scan shows the proximal pole bent on the distal tubercle (Figs. 32.1 and 32.2). The initial scaphoid fracture cause is unknown. This young patient presents with a scaphoid nonunion with significant bone loss. There is a breakdown of the general architecture of his carpus by reducing the height of the scaphoid; osteoarthritic changes are inevitable with decreased mobility of the wrist. The aim is to restore the high of carpus. Because of unknown date of primary fracture, large bone loss, and doubt regarding the quality of vascularization, a vascularized bone graft could be advantageous. What are the preferred techniques for a vascularized bone graft?

The Herbert classification may be particularly helpful when determining treatment options. The type A Herbert classification fracture is a stable acute fracture, and a type B is an unstable acute fracture. Stable fractures include fractures of the tubercle (A1) and an incomplete fracture of the waist (A2). These fractures can potentially be treated nonoperatively. The other types of fracture in the Herbert classification usually require surgical treatment. Type B (acute unstable fractures) include subtypes B1 (oblique fractures of the distal third), B2 (displaced or mobile fractures of the waist), B3 (proximal pole fractures), B4 (fracture dislocations), and B5 (comminuted fractures). Type C fractures are those that demonstrate delayed union after >6 weeks of plaster immobilization, and type D fractures are established nonunions, either fibrous (D1) or sclerotic (D2).

IMPORTANCE OF THE PROBLEM

As fractures may disturb the scaphoid's tenuous blood supply, the healing process may be compromised. Osteonecrosis is said to occur in 13%–50% of cases of fracture of the scaphoid, and the incidence of osteonecrosis is even higher in those with involvement of the proximal one-fifth of the scaphoid.[1-4]

The proximal pole, therefore, is dependent entirely on intraosseous blood flow. This tenuous blood supply can result in a protracted healing process after fracture, with the average time to healing of an acute proximal pole fracture averaging 3–6 months.

Nonunion may occur (in 5%–10% of all cases, with an even higher incidence in displaced fractures), and numerous series document progression of nonunion to collapse and arthritis.[4-6] Scaphoid nonunion is a significant problem. Around 5%–15% of all scaphoid fractures will progress to nonunion, with the incidence as high as 30% in fractures of the proximal pole.[7] Even after nonvascularized bone grafting, the overall rate of persistent nonunion remains at around 30%.[8,9] Untreated scaphoid nonunions are likely to progress to periscaphoid arthritis and carpal collapse.[5,10]

Treatment of scaphoid nonunion with vascularized bone grafting is associated with improved rates of consolidation in the context of avascular necrosis (AVN) of the proximal pole or secondary scaphoid nonunion, where the initial surgical failure is likely to be related to a poorly vascularized distal fragment. The simpler pedicled techniques are usually preferred to free bone transfer, unless there is a very large bone deficiency. A recent metaanalysis investigating vascularized bone grafting for AVN has shown union rates of 88%, versus 47% with nonvascularized wedge grafting.[9]

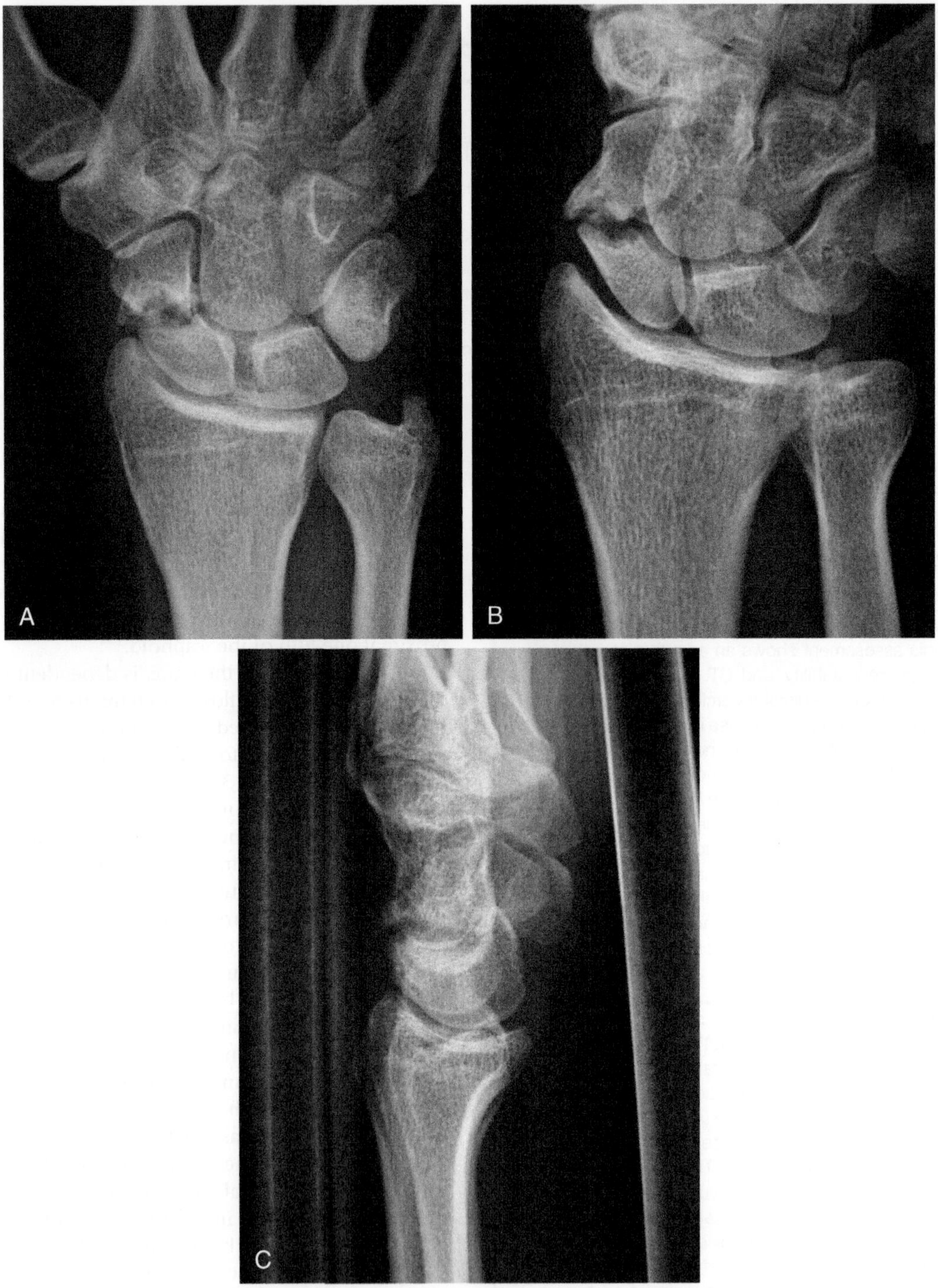

FIG. 32.1 **(A)** Frontal X-ray showing large volar bone loss of waist of scaphoid. **(B)** Schneck 1 X-rays, showing the importance of defect. **(C)** Lateral X-rays showing an adaptive dorsal intercalated segment instability with humpback deformity of scaphoid.

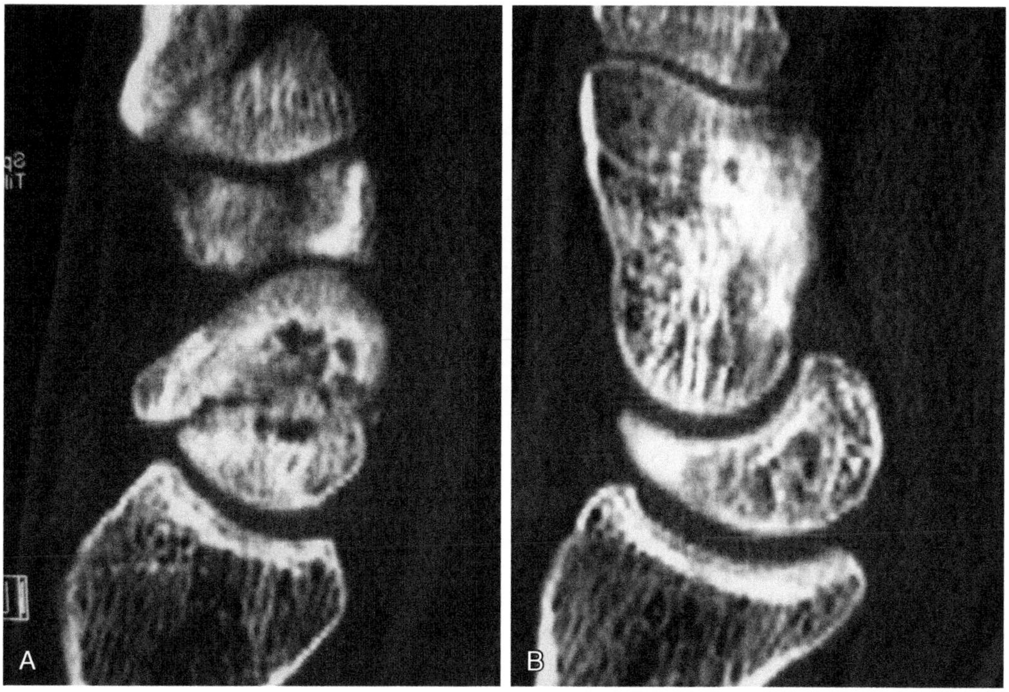

FIG. 32.2 **(A)** CT-scan cut passing through the scaphoid showing the proximal pole bent on the distal tubercle. **(B)** CT-scan cut passing through the lunate showing the dorsiflexion of lunate because it follows the proximal pole bent on the distal tubercle.

MAIN QUESTION

What are the preferred techniques for a vascularized bone graft?

Current Opinion

In lack of consensus for a preferred technique, several vascularized grafts have been described,[11-20] including a graft pedicled on the palmar carpal artery.[21] The authors prefer a graft harvested from the volar radius vascularized by the volar carpal artery with an anastomosis between the radial and ulnar arteries, following a cadaver study.[22,23]

Finding the Evidence

- Cochrane search: scaphoid nonunion
- Pubmed (Medline): ("scaphoid bone" [Mesh] OR scaphoid fracture*[tiab] OR scaphoid bone fracture*[tiab] OR scaphoid[tiab]) AND ("nonunion" [subheading] OR nonunite* OR non-union OR non-unite*) AND vascular*
- Bibliography of eligible articles
- Articles that were not in English, French, or German were excluded

Quality of the Evidence

Level IV: Systematic reviews of case series: 3
  Case series: 16
Level V: Anatomic studies: 6
  Expert opinion: 5

FINDINGS

Part 1: The Variety of Techniques

The chosen source of pedicled vascularized bone is varied,[24] and each graft has its advantages and limitations without clear superiority of any specific graft, based on a recent comparative metaanalysis of 54 (mostly retrospective) case series.[24] Considering its important methodological limitations, it showed that the early reports of the medial femoral condyle free flap showed the most successful results with no failures in 38 cases described to that date in the literature, despite the complexity of the operation. However, when looking at more recent studies such as the one from Chaudhry et al. (17 of 19 patients, 88.5% union), there clearly is no superiority from this graft in terms of union rates.[31]

Most reports concern the dorsal radius bone graft, which is pedicled on the 1,2 intracompartmental supra-retinacular artery (ICSRA) as described by Zaidemberg.[15] It can be performed through the same dorsal incision as that used for the scaphoid exposure, with a proximal extension. The artery raises 5 cm above the radiocarpal joint and goes distally superficially to the extensor retinaculum in-between the first and second compartment, going under the flexor pollicis brevis and the abductor pollicis longus until an anastomosis with the radial artery or the dorsal radiocarpal arch. The artery branches come from this artery and go into the bone 2 cm above the radiocarpal joint; the graft is raised at this location, with a distal rotation on the pedicle. Sheetz[25] recommended to include the proximal branch.

Other donor sites include the first or second metacarpal: Brunelli[18,26] proposed a graft raised from the head of the second metacarpal with a palmar and dorsal approach, depending on the first web space artery, which come from the radial artery. The graft is used in retrograde from the origin of the artery at the first web to fill the bone loss. Bertelli[27] harvested the graft from the metacarpal head of the thumb, centered on the first dorsal metacarpal artery. Two facial incisions were made ulnarly and radially to the artery. The fascia and pedicle are dissected from the trapeziometacarpal joint back to the radial artery. The graft is pushed palmarly down to the tendons of the first compartment. Sawaizumi[28] harvested the graft from the base of the second metacarpal. The dorsal intercarpal arch and the second dorsal metacarpal artery, which originates from the radial artery, are identified and dissected to the level of the shaft of the second metacarpal. The pedicle is dissected proximally, and the graft is raised from the base of the second metacarpal bone. The graft is then inserted dorsally in the scaphoid nonunion. In case of dorsal intercalated segment instability (DISI), a curved incision over the scaphoid from the volar side is performed and the graft is rotated distally to correct the DISI.

In 1965 Judet and Roy-Camille suggested using bone graft from the palmar radius, pivoted on the pronator quadratus muscle to repair scaphoid nonunions.[11] In 1987 Kuhlmann et al. were the first to describe the branch of the radial artery supplying the bone.[13] With this knowledge the muscular pedicle could be narrowed, allowing harvest of a larger graft with an improved arc of rotation that simplified transposition. The reduced bulk of the pedicle also facilitated repair of the radioscaphocapitate ligament over the scaphoid.

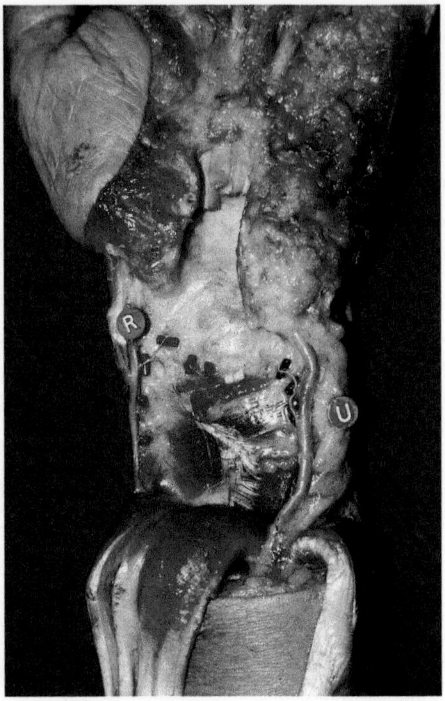

FIG. 32.3 Cadaveric dissection showing the volar carpal artery running along the distal edge of the pronator quadratus before anastomosing with the anterior interosseous artery and a branch of the ulnar artery (*R*, radial artery; *U*, ulnar artery).

Kuhlmann's report stimulated us to confirm the anatomy and the reliability of the flap by performing our own anatomic study.[22] We injected the arterial system of 40 fresh upper limb specimens with colored latex. The distal volar vascular network was then dissected, revealing the radial, ulnar, and anterior interosseous arteries. The volar carpal artery was identified in 100% of the specimens dissected. It was found that the vessel originates from the radial artery at the level of the radial styloid, traversing the palmar aspect of the distal radius in a plane between the periosteum and the distal edge of pronator quadratus. The vessel travels along the radial third of the distal radius, sends branches to penetrate the radius at the level of the distal epiphysis, then continues laterally to form a "T"-shaped anastomosis with the anterior interosseous artery superficial to the distal radioulnar joint[21] (Fig. 32.3).

Part 2: Author's Preferred Technique and Findings

The volar carpal artery bone graft has several advantages over other sources of pedicled vascularized bone. The defect created by correction of the humpback deformity is volar and can be difficult to reach using the 1,2 ICSRA bone graft due to limitations of pedicle length and difficulties accessing the defect from a dorsal approach.[29] In contrast, a volar approach allows excellent access for debridement of devitalized bone and insertion of a volar wedge shaped graft to restore the anterior defect apparent after restoration of scaphoid height. A volar approach is also less likely to disrupt the important dorsal vascular supply of the scaphoid bone. Compared with the classic Matti-Russe grafting for primary nonunion, the technique of volar carpal artery bone grafting is advantageous because it avoids the iliac crest donor site, allowing a single incision, regional anesthesia, and minimal discomfort for the patient, who may be treated on an outpatient basis. The harvest technique is similar to that used in nonvascularized volar radial bone harvest, and the additional dissection required to mobilize the pedicle is minimal so that the procedure is rapid, technically straightforward, and does not increase morbidity. For these reasons, the authors prefer to use the volar vascularized bone graft to treat not only cases of AVN or secondary nonunion after previously failed surgery but also all cases of primary scaphoid nonunion (Fig. 32.4A and B).

The authors reported a retrospective single-surgeon series included patients operated on for scaphoid nonunion between January 1994 and September 2008. Nonunions of grade 1 or 3B or grade 4 with necrosis were excluded. Two homogeneous groups of vascularized bone graft from the volar radius were identified.[30] Group 1 comprised 73 patients with primary vascularized graft for nonunion and group 2 comprised 38 patients with secondary vascularized graft (Table 32.1). None of the patients were lost to follow-up. Mean follow-up was 25.5 months (10–65 months) in group 1 and 33 months (10–63 months) in group 2. In group 2, there was clear improvement in pain; these results were less satisfactory than for first-line treatment (Table 32.2). In group 1, the functional results on the Mayo Wrist Score were excellent or good in 94.5% of cases. 98.5% of patients were completely satisfied or had only minor reservations. In group 1, radiologic consolidation was achieved in 70 cases, i.e., 96% Proximal Pole (PP), 89.5%, Waist (W), 98.2%) at a mean 9.7 weeks (PP 11.3 weeks; W 9.2 weeks). In group 2, radiologic consolidation was achieved in 34 cases, i.e., 89.5% (PP, 80%, W, 91%) at a mean 10.8 weeks (PP, 17 weeks, W, 10 weeks).

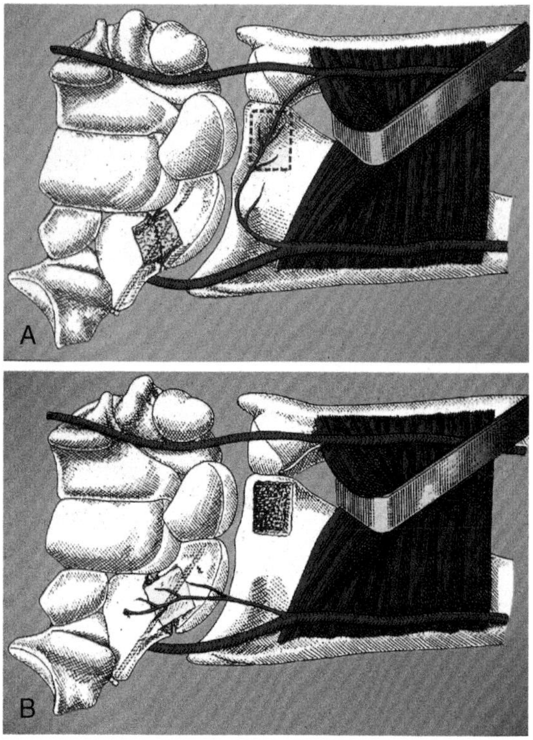

FIG. 32.4 Drawing summarizing the principle of volar vascularized bone grafting; **(A)** the graft is harvested on the distal volar medial aspect of the radius, vascularized by volar carpal artery; **(B)** after freshening of scaphoid nonunion area, the volar vascularized bone graft is put into the volar bone loss.

RECOMMENDATION

For patients with scaphoid nonunion after failed primary repair or in presence of proximal pole necrosis:

- Vascularized grafts may yield high rates of union (overall quality: moderate).
- Treatment of humpback deformity requires restoration of scaphoid height (overall quality: low).
- Vascularized bone graft harvested from the volar aspect of radius is a good solution to treat the volar bone loss defect (overall quality: low).

CONCLUSION

Numerous vascularized grafts have shown successful and reproducible results for avascular scaphoid nonunion. In the absence of any evidence-based vascular graft superiority, volar vascularized bone grafting is the authors' preferred technique for treatment of all scaphoid nonunion because it has advantages over other vascularized grafts in terms of approach, humpback correction, and comorbidity.

TABLE 32.1
Demographics and Injury Characteristics

	Primary Treatment Patients N = 73	Secondary Treatment Patients N = 38
Sex	89% ♂ (65) 11% ♀ (8)	87% ♂ (33) 13% ♀ (5)
Mean age (years)	30.41 ± 11.2 (15–61)	31.16 ± 8.6 (19–47)
Dominant involvement	64% (47)	66% (25)
Occupation	26% manual workers (19) 74% sedentary (54)	71% manual workers (27) 29% sedentary (11)
Fracture-surgery interval (months)	20.51 (4–120)	23.38 (10–72)
Initial treatment	55% nondiagnosed 45% (33) conservative treatment (10.3 weeks immobilization)	92% (35) immobilization (15.4 weeks)
Type of fracture	26% proximal pole (19) 74% waist (54)	13% proximal pole (5) 87% waist (33)
Type of nonunion (Alnot classification)	2A: 67% (49) 2B: 30% (22) 3A: 3% (2)	2A: 39.5% (15) 2B: 52.5% (20) 3A: 8% (3)

TABLE 32.2
Clinical and Radiologic Results per Group

	Primary Treatment Patients N = 73		Secondary Treatment Patients N = 38	
Follow-up (months)	25.5 ± 14.5 (10–65)		33 ± 18.3 (10–63)	
Radiologic consolidation	96%		89.5%	
Mean time to consolidation (weeks)	9.7 ± 4.9 (6–24)		10.8 ± 4.2 (6–24)	
Flexion (degrees)	+10.6 ± 13.7 (–30 to 40)		+11.3 ± 12.2 (–10 to 40)	
Extension (degrees)	+7.8 ± 10.4 (–5 to 40)		+16.3 ± 14.6 (0–50)	
Radial deviation (degrees)	+5.3 ± 5.5 (–8 to 20)		+6.3 ± 6.3 (–5 to 15)	
Ulnar deviation (degrees)	+5.6 ± 5.9 (–5 to 20)		+7.4 ± 6.8 (0–20)	
Muscle force (kg)	+16.4 ± 9.5 (0–35)		+18.2 ± 12 (–6 to 45)	
Pain	Preop	Postop	Preop	Postop
Severe	8% (6)	0%	60.5% (23)	2.5% (1)
Moderate	92% (67)	4% (3)	39.5% (15)	42% (16)
None	0%	96% (70)	0%	55.5% (21)
Complications				
Nonunion	4%		10.5%	
Stiffness	4%		2.5%	
CRPS	0%		8%	

TABLE 32.2
Clinical and Radiologic Results per Group—Cont'd

	Primary Treatment Patients N=73	Secondary Treatment Patients N=38
Functional results (Mayo Wrist Score)		
Excellent	83.5% (61)	42% (16)
Good	11% (8)	31.5% (12)
Moderate	4% (3)	16% (6)
Poor	1.5% (1)	10.5% (4)
Overall satisfaction		
Completely satisfied	85% (62)	44.5% (17)
Minor reservations	13.5% (10)	31.5% (12)
Major reservations	0%	16% (6)
Dissatisfied	1.5% (1)	8% (3)

CRPS: Complex Regional Pain Syndrm

PANEL 2
Authors' Preferred Technique

The volar approach allows graft harvesting and treatment of the nonunion to be performed as a single procedure. The surgery is performed under locoregional anesthesia through a single incision with reduced surgery time as a day case, thus reducing hospital stay and overall costs. It was first described for failure of classical techniques. However, the authors recommend it as primary treatment of scaphoid nonunion.

We perform the volar carpal artery bone graft under local regional anesthesia on an outpatient basis. The patient is placed in a supine position with the arm supported by a hand table and the wrist is placed in extension and ulnar deviation. Under tourniquet control, the scaphoid bone is accessed in the usual manner between the radial artery and the flexor carpi radialis tendon. The inferior aspect of the incision is extended 2 cm proximally to allow exposure of the distal radius (Fig. 32.5).

The anterior capsule is reflected, exposing the distal radial margin and the scaphoid. Fibrous scar tissue is debrided and necrotic bone at the fracture site is curetted until healthy bone is reached and punctate bleeding can be demonstrated. The scaphoid fragments are pulled out to length through thumb distraction and a narrow osteotome is used to separate them. Intraoperative imaging is used to confirm the scaphoid reduction and the bony defect is measured.

The bone graft is then harvested. The wrist is flexed to allow ulnar retraction of the flexor carpi radialis and finger flexor tendons and the pronator quadratus muscle is exposed. Parallel incisions are then made, the first 1 cm proximal to the distal border of the pronator quadratus and the second a few millimeters distal to it. These incisions are made ulnar to the radial artery over the distal radius, but radial to the bone graft site. A scalpel and periosteal elevator are then used to detach the strip of muscle and periosteum containing the volar carpal artery, thus mobilizing the pedicle (Fig. 32.6). The bone graft, attached to the ulnar end of the pedicle, is then harvested. The dimensions of the required graft are marked on the bone. The lateral borders of the bone graft are osteotomized first using a 10-mm osteotome. The proximal and distal borders of the bone graft are then osteotomized in an oblique direction to form a wedge shape followed by the medial border (Fig. 32.7). The bone graft is levered from the distal radius with a 5-mm osteotome with care to protect the pedicle. The radial fibers of the pronator quadratus muscle may be dissected as far laterally as the radial vessels to allow maximum mobilization and a pedicle length of up to 5 cm (Fig. 32.8A and B). The scaphoid fragments are then stabilized with a Herbert screw, which is inserted volarly in a distal to proximal direction and placed as posteriorly as possible to allow placement of the graft. The graft is positioned within the scaphoid defect (Fig. 32.9A and B), and if required can be secured through further screw tightening. Alternatively, a K-wire can be inserted through the scaphoid fragments and graft, in a direction parallel to the screw to avoid damaging the pedicle. Any bone gaps may be filled with additional cancellous bone graft harvested from the distal radius,

Continued

PANEL 2
Authors' Preferred Technique—Cont'd

although this is usually not required with careful graft shaping. The position of the screw and fragments is checked with intraoperative imaging (Fig. 32.10). The joint capsule and ligaments are then repaired, with particular care to reconstitute the radioscaphocapitate ligament while protecting the pedicle. The pronator quadratus muscle is sutured back into position and a suction drain is placed over the distal radius.

The wrist is immobilized until radiologic and clinical union, which is generally achieved after a minimum of 6 weeks and an average of 10 weeks (Figs. 32.11 and 32.12A,B). Mobilization is then gradually increased under a physiotherapy exercise program.

The indication for the procedure is a scaphoid nonunion without periscaphoid arthritis. Patients with radiologic or clinical evidence of early radioscaphoid arthritis may require arthroscopy or MRI of the joint surface before proceeding. Radioscaphoid arthritis involving the styloid and distal scaphoid only, i.e., scaphoid nonunion advanced collapse (SNAC) wrist grade I, may be managed with a radial styloidectomy in addition to vascularized bone grafting. Most patients with scaphoid nonunion present in their fourth decade; however, there are no age limitations for the repair and the senior author has performed the procedure in patients ranging from 15 to 61 years of age. A recent metaanalysis of treatment of scaphoid nonunion found that patient age had little effect on union rates, but that the chance of secondary nonunion increases with delay to surgery of more than 12 months from injury. The authors have performed volar vascularized bone grafting on patients presenting up to 10 years after the initial injury; however, early surgery is likely to improve union rates, thereby avoiding further degenerative changes and allowing an earlier return to normal activity for a greater number of patients.

Absolute contraindications to volar vascularized bone grafting for scaphoid reconstruction include periscaphoid degeneration involving the entire scaphoid fossa, the scaphocapitate joint (i.e., SNAC stage II or III), and previous surgery or injury to the distal radius or radial artery, resulting in disruption of the blood supply at the volar radius graft site.

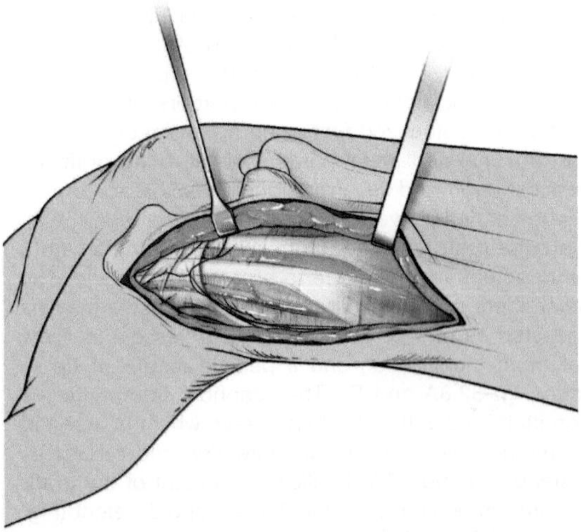

FIG. 32.5 Drawing showing the volar "Henry" approach, merely extended toward the distal tubercle of scaphoid. The passage is between the flexor carpi radialis and the radial pedicle.

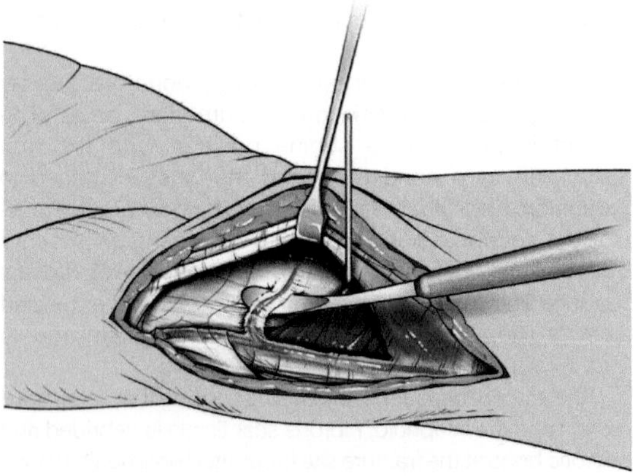

FIG. 32.6 Drawing showing the subperiosteal dissection of the lateral part of the pedicle. The wrist is in flexion with retraction of flexor pollicis longus and flexor carpi radialis tendons. The volar carpal artery is located in front of the superficial aponeurosis of pronator quadratus, running along the distal edge of the pronator quadratus.

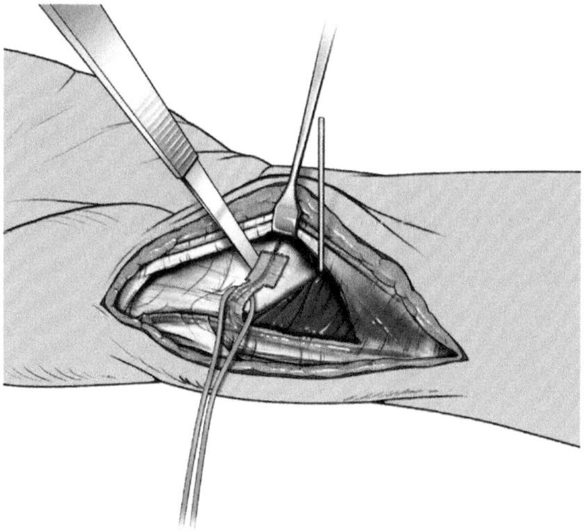

FIG. 32.7 Drawing showing the harvesting of the graft, using osteotome in oblique way, to avoid periosteal detachment from the graft and because the volar bone loss is classically in a pyramidal shape.

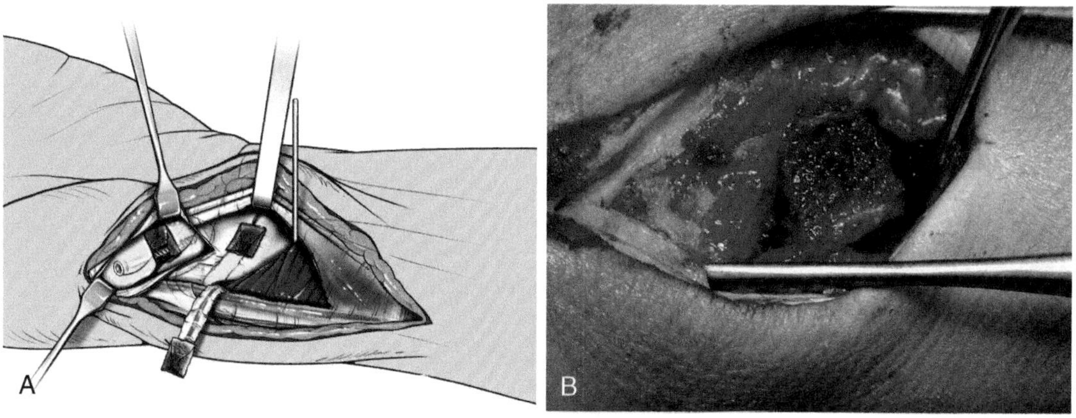

FIG. 32.8 **(A)** Drawing showing the graft harvested, with complete lateral dissection of the pedicle, to have a sufficient length. **(B)** Operating view showing in our presentation case, the important size of vascularized bone graft.

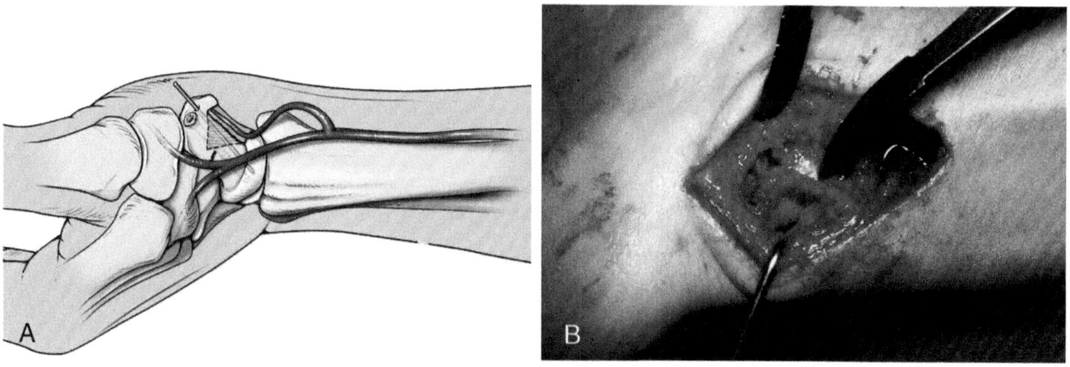

FIG. 32.9 **(A)** Drawing showing the vascularized bone graft put inside the volar bone defect of scaphoid. The scaphoid is fixed with a screw, and the graft is temporarily stabilized with a volar K-wire. **(B)** Operating view showing in our presentation case, the scaphoid filled by the volar vascularized bone graft.

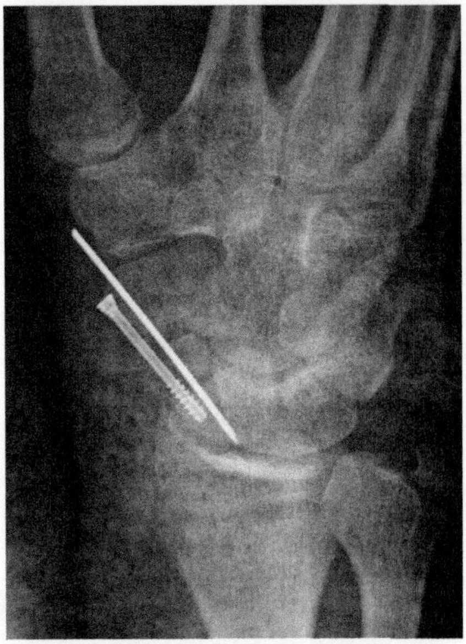

FIG. 32.10 Immediate postoperative frontal X-ray of our presentation case, with the graft perfectly in place into the scaphoid. We can check that the scaphoid humpback deformity is reduced and carpal height restored.

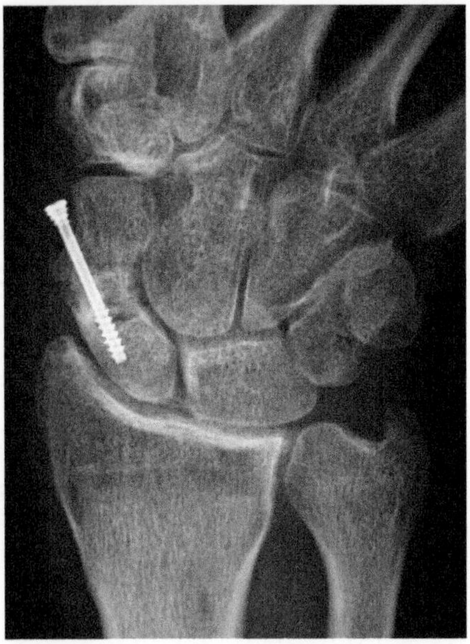

FIG. 32.11 Frontal X-ray of our case presentation showing a good union after only 45 days. It is noted that the pin has been removed. In this case the screw was placed laterally depending on the intraoperative risks, but easily to remove.

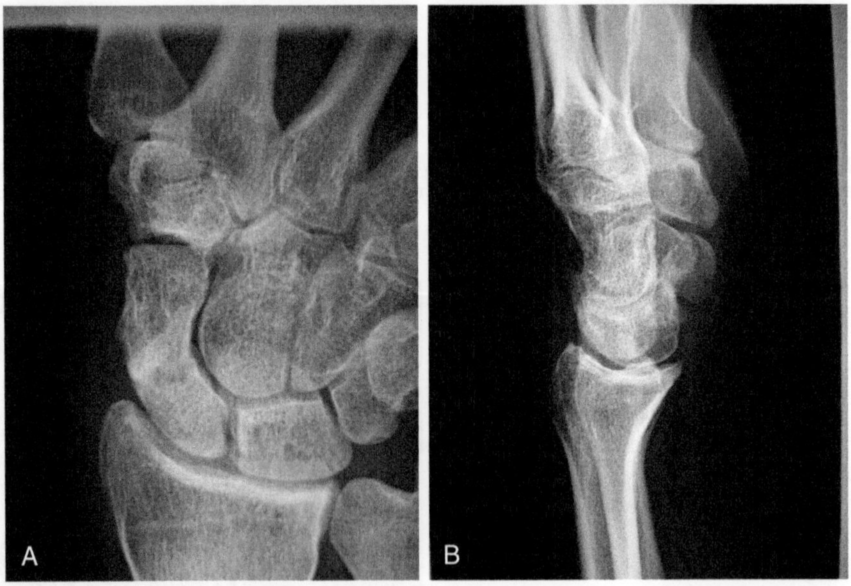

FIG. 32.12 **(A)** Frontal X-ray of our case presentation showing a perfect union at 6 months. **(B)** Lateral X-ray of our presentation case showing good reduction of preoperative adaptive dorsal intercalated segment instability.

PANEL 3
Pearls and Pitfalls

PEARLS

- During scaphoid reduction, a transverse K-wire from the scaphoid fragments to the lunate and capitate can be used to temporarily maintain the reduction. In the presence of dorsal intercalated segment instability deformity, the lunate may first require stabilization to the radius using an additional dorsal K-wire.
- To release tension of flexor tendons, the wrist is flexed before harvesting the graft.
- The pronator quadratus could be retracted proximally and temporarily fixed with vertical 1.5-mm K-wire.
- The volar carpal artery is located in front of the superficial aponeurosis of pronator quadratus and up to periosteum of volar aspect of radius.
- The proximal and distal borders of the bone graft should be osteotomized in an oblique direction to form a wedge shape followed by the medial border because the shape of bone loss into the scaphoid is regularly pyramidal and to avoid detachment of periosteum from the graft.
- The radial fibers of the pronator quadratus muscle may be dissected as far as laterally on lateral aspect of radius, to allow maximum length of pedicle.
- If necessary a temporary K-wire, which is removed after 3 weeks, can be inserted through the distal fragment but volar to the graft to prevent graft extrusion.

PITFALLS

- If the screw is placed too volar in case of comminution, it may compress the fracture back into its volar angulation and could expulse the volar graft.
- Take care not to separate the periosteum from the graft, to avoid nonvascularization of the graft.
- Postoperative wrist instability may occur if the height of the scaphoid is inadequately restored or if the radioscaphocapitate ligament is not carefully repaired.
- Wrist pain may be related to damage to the scapho-trapezio-trapezoid joint during the screw fixation procedure.
- Fracture of the articular surface of the distal radius during bone graft harvest has been reported and should be avoided by oblique direction of osteotome during harvesting.

REFERENCES

1. Herbert TJ, Fisher WE. Management of the fractured scaphoid using a new bone screw. *J Bone Joint Surg Br*. 1984;66(1):114–123.
2. Cooney WP, Dobyns JH, Linscheid RL. Fractures of the scaphoid: a rational approach to management. *Clin Orthop Relat Res*. 1980;(149):90–97.
3. Freedman DM, Botte MJ, Gelberman RH. Vascularity of the carpus. *Clin Orthop Relat Res*. 2001;(383):47–59.
4. Szabo RM, Manske D. Displaced fractures of the scaphoid. *Clin Orthop Relat Res*. 1988;(230):30–38.
5. Mack GR, Bosse MJ, Gelberman RH, Yu E. The natural history of scaphoid non-union. *J Bone Joint Surg Am*. 1984;66(4):504–509.
6. Ruby LK, Leslie BM. Wrist arthritis associated with scaphoid nonunion. *Hand Clin*. 1987;3(4):529–539.
7. Kuschner SH, Lane CS, Brien WW, Gellman H. Scaphoid fractures and scaphoid nonunion. Diagnosis and treatment. *Orthop Rev*. 1994;23(11):861–871.
8. Megerle K, Keutgen X, Muller M, Germann G, Sauerbier M. Treatment of scaphoid non-unions of the proximal third with conventional bone grafting and mini-Herbert screws: an analysis of clinical and radiological results. *J Hand Surg Eur Vol*. 2008;33(2):179–185.
9. Merrell GA, Wolfe SW, Slade 3rd JF. Treatment of scaphoid nonunions: quantitative meta-analysis of the literature. *J Hand Surg Am*. 2002;27(4):685–691.
10. Ruby LK, Stinson J, Belsky MR. The natural history of scaphoid non-union. A review of fifty-five cases. *J Bone Joint Surg Am*. 1985;67(3):428–432.
11. Roy-Camille Jr R. Fractures et pseudarthroses du scaphoïde carpien. Utilisation d'un greffon pédiculé. *Actual Chir Orthop*. 1965;4:197–214.
12. Kawai H, Yamamoto K. Pronator quadratus pedicled bone graft for old scaphoid fractures. *J Bone Joint Surg Br*. 1988;70(5):829–831.
13. Kuhlmann JN, Mimoun M, Boabighi A, Baux S. Vascularized bone graft pedicled on the volar carpal artery for non-union of the scaphoid. *J Hand Surg Br*. 1987;12(2):203–210.
14. Guimberteau JC, Panconi B. Recalcitrant non-union of the scaphoid treated with a vascularized bone graft based on the ulnar artery. *J Bone Joint Surg Am*. 1990;72(1):88–97.
15. Zaidemberg C, Siebert JW, Angrigiani C. A new vascularized bone graft for scaphoid nonunion. *J Hand Surg Am*. 1991;16(3):474–478.
16. Mathoulin C, Haerle M, Vandeputte G. Vascularized bone graft in carpal bone reconstruction. *Ann Chir Plast Esthet*. 2005;50(1):43–48.
17. Yuceturk A, Isiklar ZU, Tuncay C, Tandogan R. Treatment of scaphoid nonunions with a vascularized bone graft based on the first dorsal metacarpal artery. *J Hand Surg Br*. 1997;22(3):425–427.

18. Brunelli F, Mathoulin C, Saffar P. Description of a vascularized bone graft taken from the head of the 2nd metacarpal bone. *Ann Chir Main Memb Super.* 1992;11(1):40–45.
19. Pistre V, Reau AF, Pelissier P, Martin D, Baudet J. Vascularized bone pedicle grafts of the hand and wrist: literature review and new donor sites. *Chir Main.* 2001;20(4): 263–271.
20. Arora R, Lutz M, Zimmermann R, Krappinger D, Niederwanger C, Gabl M. Free vascularised iliac bone graft for recalcitrant avascular nonunion of the scaphoid. *J Bone Joint Surg Br.* 2010;92(2):224–229.
21. Mathoulin C, Haerle M. Vascularized bone graft from the palmar carpal artery for treatment of scaphoid nonunion. *J Hand Surg Br.* 1998;23(3):318–323.
22. Haerle M, Schaller HE, Mathoulin C. Vascular anatomy of the palmar surfaces of the distal radius and ulna: its relevance to pedicled bone grafts at the distal palmar forearm. *J Hand Surg Br.* 2003;28(2):131–136.
23. Technique CM. Vascularized bone grafts from the volar distal radius to treat scaphoid nonunion. *J Am Soc Surg Hand.* 2004;4(1).
24. Ditsios K, Konstantinidis I, Agas K, Christodoulou A. Comparative meta-analysis on the various vascularized bone flaps used for the treatment of scaphoid nonunion. *J Orthop Res.* 2017;35(5):1076–1085.
25. Sheetz KK, Bishop AT, Berger RA. The arterial blood supply of the distal radius and ulna and its potential use in vascularized pedicled bone grafts. *J Hand Surg Am.* 1995;20(6):902–914.
26. Mathoulin C, Brunelli F. Further experience with the index metacarpal vascularized bone graft. *J Hand Surg Br.* 1998;23(3):311–317.
27. Bertelli JA, Peruchi FM, Rost JR, Tacca CP. Treatment of scaphoid non-unions by a palmar approach with vascularised bone graft harvested from the thumb. *J Hand Surg Eur Vol.* 2007;32(2):217–223.
28. Sawaizumi T, Nanno M, Nanbu A, Ito H. Vascularised bone graft from the base of the second metacarpal for refractory nonunion of the scaphoid. *J Bone Joint Surg Br.* 2004;86(7):1007–1012.
29. Henry M. Collapsed scaphoid non-union with dorsal intercalated segment instability and avascular necrosis treated by vascularised wedge-shaped bone graft and fixation. *J Hand Surg Eur Vol.* 2007;32(2):148–154.
30. Gras M, Mathoulin C. Vascularized bone graft pedicled on the volar carpal artery from the volar distal radius as primary procedure for scaphoid non-union. *Orthop Traumatol Surg Res.* 2011;97(8):800–806.
31. Chaudhry T, Uppal L, Power D, Craigen M, Tan S. Scaphoid nonunion with poor prognostic factors: the role of the free medial femoral condyle vascularized bone graft. *Hand (NY).* 2017;12(2):135–139 (Epub ahead of print).

CHAPTER 33

Nonvascularized Bone Grafts

DIEGO L. FERNANDEZ, MD • SANJEEV KAKAR, MD • GEERT A. BUIJZE, MD, PHD

KEY POINTS

- Both structural (wedge) and nonstructural grafts are reproducible techniques with good long-term outcomes.
- Structural (wedge) grafts allow for better correction of deformity (scapholunate and radiolunate angles) more than nonstructural grafts.
- Improved functional outcome after accurate restoration of alignment slightly favors structural interpositional wedge grafting.
- Long-term radiographic findings suggest that neither grafting technique prevents osteoarthritis but both types may postpone or diminish it.

PANEL 1
Case Scenario

This 17-year-old male student was treated for a wrist sprain after a fall onto his outstretched hand with an elastic bandage for 2 weeks. No radiographs were made. One year after injury, he complains of progressive wrist pain with strenuous activities. Plain radiographs reveal an unstable nonunion of the left scaphoid, without avascular changes on MRI (Fig. 33.1). Comparative radiographs and CT scans reveal a shortened scaphoid and a mild dorsal intercalated segment instability (DISI) malalignment of the carpus (Fig. 33.2). What nonvascularized bone grafting technique is preferably used to restore malalignment and get this nonunion healed?

IMPORTANCE OF THE PROBLEM

It seems that untreated scaphoid nonunion will lead to degenerative wrist arthritis—the so-called SNAC wrist (scaphoid nonunion advanced collapse). Nonunion of the scaphoid has a known natural history,[1,2] not all are symptomatic,[3] not all destabilize the carpus, and symptoms are accelerated by strenuous use of the hand. The two most important factors affecting the success in gaining union are the time elapsed between initial injury and treatment, and the presence of avascular necrosis of the proximal fragment.[4,5] These parameters, as well as the presence of periscaphoid degenerative changes, must be carefully evaluated, as they represent major impediments to achieve a successful outcome with bone grafting and internal fixation.

Scaphoid nonunion often results in deformity.[6–10] Mobile (cystic) nonunions are unstable, have early collapse patterns (dorsal intercalated segment instability [DISI]), have a good prognosis, and have been classically treated with anterior interpositional wedge grafting to correct deformity. Sclerotic nonunions have advanced deformity, marked collapse, and early degenerative changes, ischemic proximal poles, and therefore carry a fair prognosis. A reconstruction trial is recommended according to age, occupation, and symptoms. Vascularized bone grafts may be indicated in this category, if there is impaired perfusion of the proximal fragment.

The standard surgical procedure for unstable scaphoid nonunion is internal fixation and bone grafting. Interpositional grafting can be performed with structural (corticocancellous) wedge grafts or nonstructural (cancellous) grafts. Many techniques have been described and any preferred graft or technique still remains the topic of debate.

MAIN QUESTION

What are the preferred techniques for a nonvascularized bone graft for scaphoid nonunion?

Current Opinion

Nonstructural grafts were the original treatment for scaphoid nonunion but do not allow for accurate

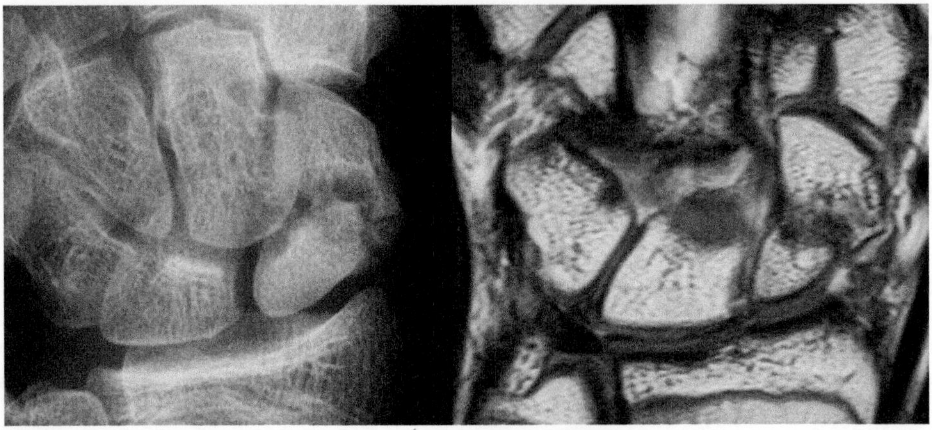

FIG. 33.1 Radiographs and MRI.

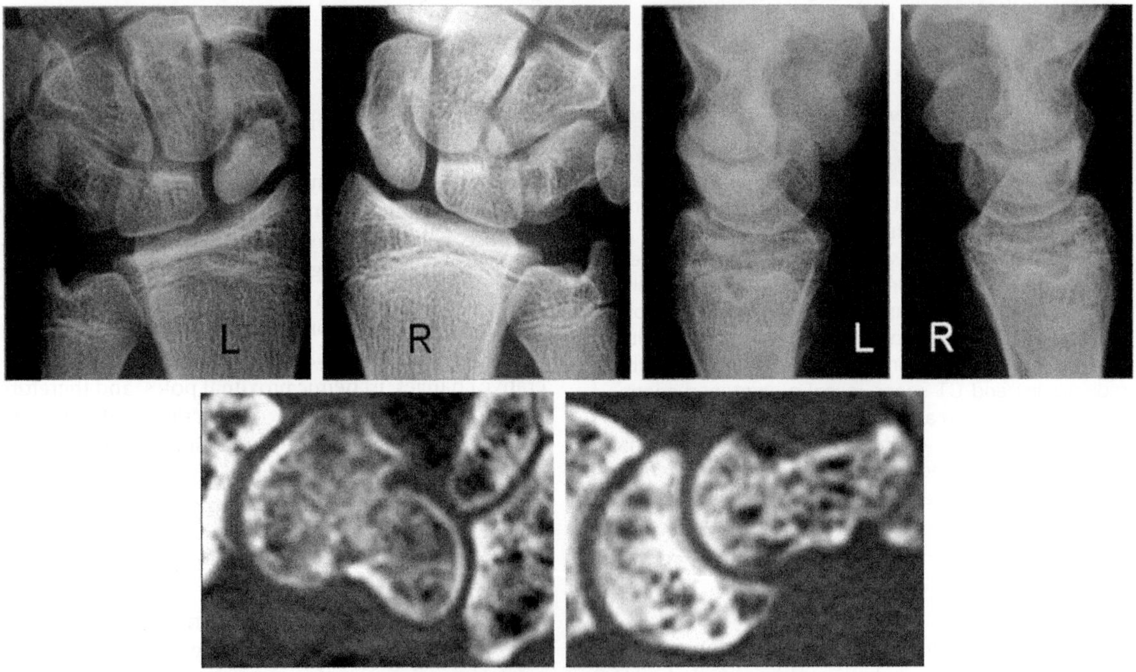

FIG. 33.2 Comparative radiographs and CT scans.

restoration of alignment. Nonunions with deformity are preferably treated using interpositional wedge grafting with structural (corticocancellous) grafts.

Finding the Evidence

- Cochrane search: scaphoid nonunion
- Pubmed (Medline): ("scaphoid bone" [Mesh] OR scaphoid fracture*[tiab] OR scaphoid bone fracture*[tiab] OR scaphoid[tiab]) AND ("nonunion" [subheading] OR nonunite* OR non-union OR non-unite*)
- Bibliography of eligible articles
- Articles that were not in English, French, or German were excluded

Quality of the Evidence

Level III:

Case-controlled study: 2

Level IV:
Systematic review of case series: 1
Case series: 26

FINDINGS

Both the structured and nonstructured grafting techniques have similar indications and emphasize the need to resect substantial portions of the scaphoid fracture surfaces to encourage healing, under the rationale that the sclerotic fracture ends will not support healing.

Nonstructured Grafts

Nonstructured grafting is the longest established and reproducible technique for scaphoid nonunion. It was first described by Matti in 1937 and modified by Russe in the 1960s.[11,12] Hence, the Matti-Russe procedure is the traditional treatment for scaphoid nonunion and some series suggest that the results correlate only with union and not with alignment.[13] The Matti-Russe technique consists of a volar approach in which the nonunion is excavated with either hand- or power-driven instruments, and the defect is packed with cortical struts and cancellous bone. Fixation with Kirschner wires (K-wires) is recommended only when the scaphoid does not move as a unit after placement of the graft, otherwise it is optional. Union rates are generally good to excellent, varying between 85% and 100%.[14–19] The main criticism to this procedure is that it does not allow for accurate restoration of alignment.

Structured Grafts

Structured (wedge) grafting was popularized in the 1970s and was intended to improve the restoration of length and angulation of the scaphoid. Although union rates were comparable to nonstructured grafts (between 85% and 100%), early advocates of this technique were confident that it would yield to better functional outcomes. The procedure highly depends on preoperative assessment of deformity. The flexion deformity of the scaphoid associated with DISI carpal instability was described by Fisk in 1970 and recommended the correction with a triangular anterior bone graft taken from the osteotomized radial styloid (Fig. 33.3).[20–22] Restoration of scaphoid length was strongly recommended by Segmüller who used an interpositional corticocancellous iliac graft introduced through a radial approach.[23] Internal fixation with a 4.0-mm cancellous screw was also performed (Fig. 33.4). One of the authors (DLF) modified Fisk's procedure emphasizing the use of a preoperative planning based on comparative radiographs of both wrists to calculate the resection zone and the size of the graft.[24] To assess the scaphoid length in millimeters, anteroposterior views of both wrists in maximal ulnar deviation were used. A volar approach was performed, the graft was taken from the iliac crest, and K-wires were inserted for fixation.

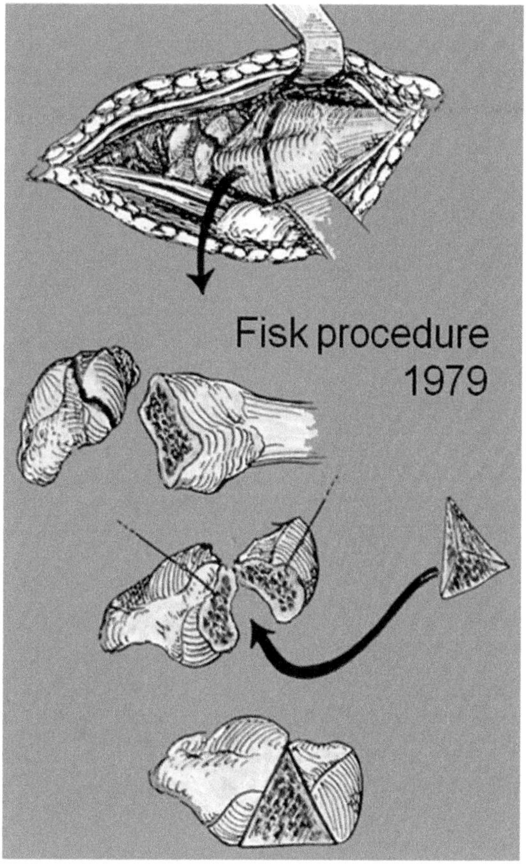

FIG. 33.3 Original drawing of the structured wedge grafting. (From Fisk GR. In: Bentley G, ed. *Operative Orthopaedics Part III*. Butterworth; 1979, with permission.)

Three-Dimensional Reconstruction

With the advent of computed tomography and three-dimensional reconstruction, accurate imaging of normal scaphoid anatomy and deformity in both nonunions and malunions was obtained. Planning with CT scans and the use of the intrascaphoid angles to measure angular deformity were suggested by Cooney[25] and Amadio[26] (Fig. 33.5). Bain et al.[27,28] refined the lateral intrascaphoid angle measurement using longitudinal CT scans[29] and described the dorsal scaphoid angle and the height to length ratio as further measurement techniques. It was concluded that fractures distal to the apex of the dorsal ridge usually develop a palmar type of late deformity (flexion and overhang of the distal fragment), whereas fractures of the proximal third develop a dorsal type of late deformity with dorsal "slipping" of the distal fragment without carpal malalignment (Fig. 33.6).[30–32] The defect following reduction of the scaphoid fragments to match the contralateral side was studied by Oka et al.[33] The palmar type of deformity (distal) resulted in larger triangular defects, while proximal nonunions exhibited a flat "crescent"-like smaller defect. Schweizer et al. described a dorsal or dorsoradial overlapping of the fragments following virtual reduction (Fig. 33.7).[34] Failure to remove excess bone dorsally would shift the center of rotation dorsally, create a larger gap, and therefore result in an overcorrection of scaphoid length and limited radial deviation.[18,35] Resection of dorsal new bone or "callus" formation was however not recommended to prevent damage to the dorsal ridge nourishing vessels.

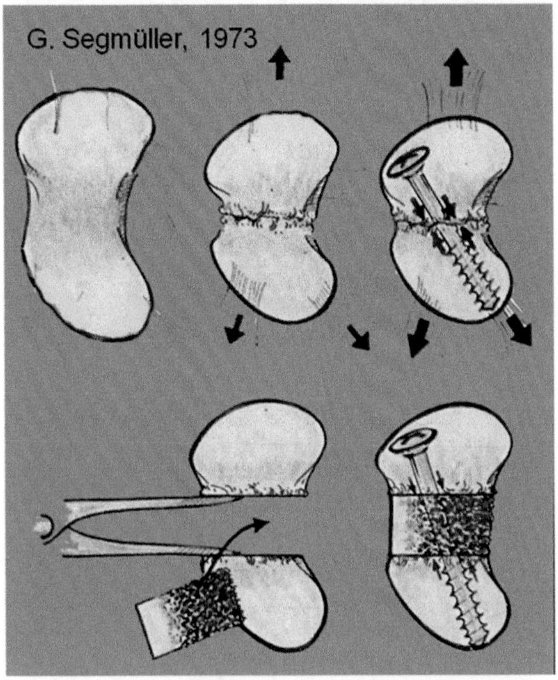

FIG. 33.4 Original drawing of the modified structured wedge grafting. (From Segmüller G. *Operative Stabilisierung am Handskelett*. Bern, Stuttgart, Wien: Hans Huber Verlag; 1973, with permission.)

Multiplanar Deformity

Summarizing the findings of the abovementioned studies, unstable nonunions of the waist of the scaphoid exhibit the following multiplanar deformity (according to the position of the distal fragment): (1) flexion ("humpback deformity"), (2) ulnar deviation (radial angulation), (3) pronation (rotatory malalignment), (4) shortening, and (5) translation (step offs in radial, ulnar, dorsal, palmar direction).

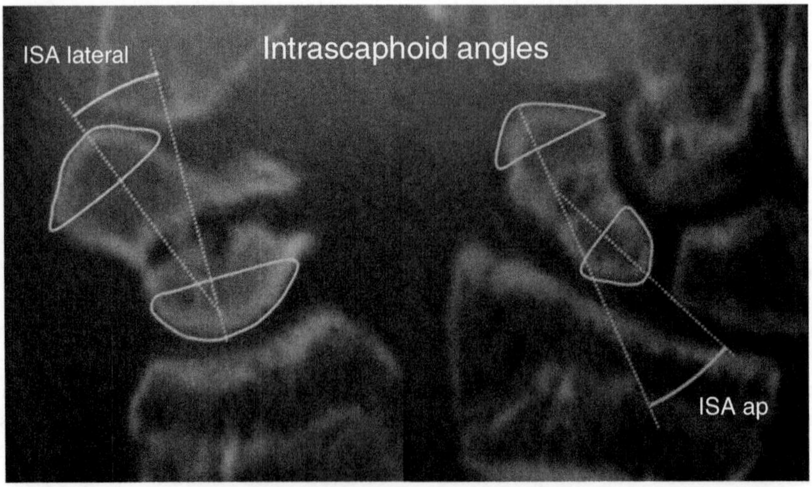

FIG. 33.5 Assessment of intrascaphoid angles on sagittal and coronal CT scans.

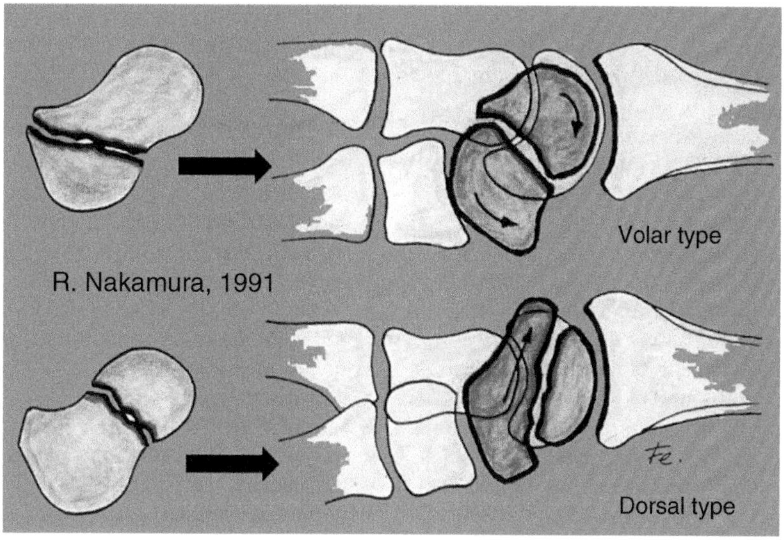

FIG. 33.6 Volar and dorsal patterns of scaphoid nonunion. (From Nakamura R, Imaeda T, Horii E, et al. Analysis of scaphoid fracture displacement by three-dimensional computed tomography. *J Hand Surg*. 1991;16A:485–492, with permission.)

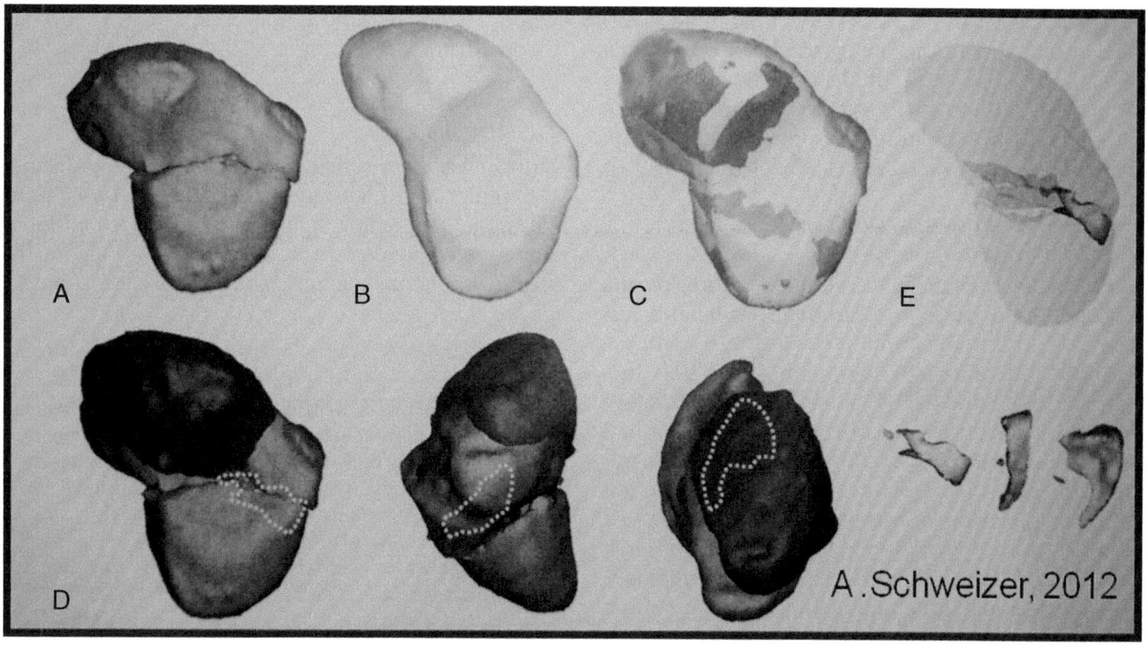

FIG. 33.7 Dorsal or dorsoradial overlapping of the fragments following virtual reduction. (From Schweizer A, Fürnstahl P, Nagy L. Three-dimensional computed tomographic analysis of 11 scaphoid waist nonunions. *J Hand Surg*. 2012;37A:1151–1158, with permission.)

Patient-Specific Developments

Recent developments include reconstruction techniques using three-dimensional printed patient-specific drill guides, where the contralateral side serves as a model.[36,37] These techniques are discussed in Chapter 25.

Preferred Techniques

There was one systematic review on the graft choice for unstable scaphoid nonunions analyzing 604 patients in 23 retrospective studies from the beginning of 1987 and the end of 2013. It primarily compared nonstructured (cancellous) grafts to structured (corticocancellous) grafts and it showed equivalent union rates. Taking in account the highly limited quality of evidence inherent to uncontrolled designs in heterogeneous series, nonstructured grafts provided the shortest interval to union (11 vs. 16 weeks), whereas structured wedge grafts were associated with consistent deformity correction and superior Mayo Wrist Scores (86 vs. 80 points).[38] The difference in time to union is likely due to the fact that corticocancellous grafts have a higher compression resistance than cancellous grafts. With regard to graft origin, a retrospective comparative study by Tambe et al. showed that the union rate of scaphoid nonunions treated with iliac bone or distal radius grafts was comparable, although the quality of the iliac bone was superior.[39] The main disadvantage is donor site pain over the iliac crest, which was present in 9 of the 44 patients.

Long-Term Results

Reestablishment of normal scaphoid anatomy results in a majority of good and excellent results and cessation of scaphoid nonunion advanced collapse deformity. In mid- and long-term series of structural grafting, none of the patients developed severe degenerative changes at the wrist, but 81% had radiographic evidence of mild or moderate degenerative changes on latest follow-up.[40,41] In the longest follow-up series on nonstructural grafts, at 28 years postoperatively, 78% had a pain free range of wrist motion and slow progression of osteoarthritis.[15] These late radiographic findings suggest that neither grafting technique prevents osteoarthritis but may postpone or diminish it.

RECOMMENDATION

In patients with an unstable scaphoid nonunion, evidence suggests the following:

- Both structural (wedge) and nonstructural grafts are reproducible techniques with good long-term outcomes (overall quality: moderate).
- There is no difference in union rate between structural (wedge) and nonstructural grafts (overall quality: moderate).
- Structural (wedge) grafts allow for better correction of deformity (scapholunate and radiolunate angles) more than nonstructural grafts (overall quality: moderate).
- Structural (wedge) grafts have been associated with slightly better functional outcome (based on Mayo Wrist Score), whereas nonstructural grafts have been associated with a greater improvement of wrist flexion (overall quality: low).
- Long-term radiographic findings suggest that neither grafting technique prevents osteoarthritis, but both types may postpone or diminish it (overall quality: moderate).

CONCLUSION

Structural and nonstructural grafts are both reproducible techniques with high union rates and good long-term functional and radiographic outcomes. Improved functional outcome after accurate restoration of alignment slightly favors structural interpositional wedge grafting.

PANEL 2
Case Scenario (Continued)

In this case, a structured iliac crest interpositional anterior wedge graft was preferred. Internal fixation was achieved with a cannulated headless screw and an additional K-wire (Fig. 33.8). Notice the restoration of scaphoid anatomy and correction of the DISI deformity. Follow-up radiographs show a well-healed scaphoid and anatomic carpal alignment and well-preserved wrist motion (Fig. 33.9).

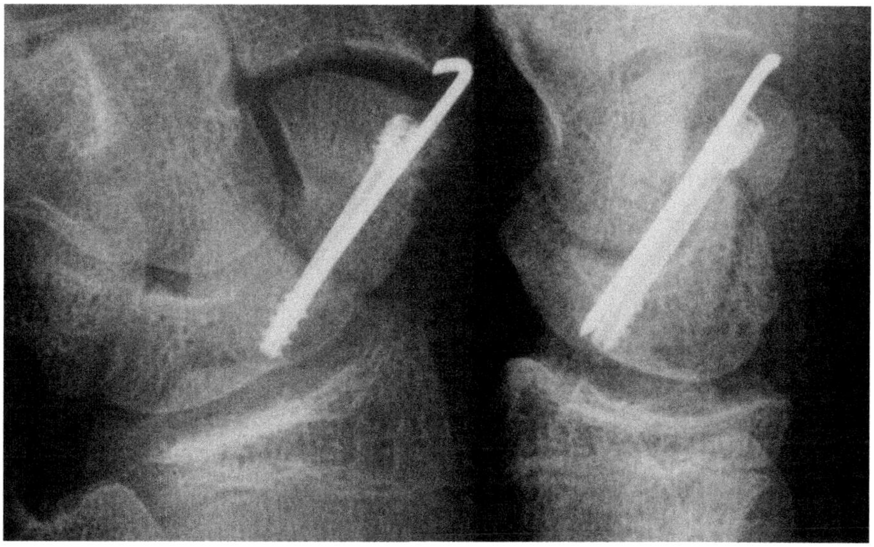

FIG. 33.8 Immediate postoperative radiographs of the case.

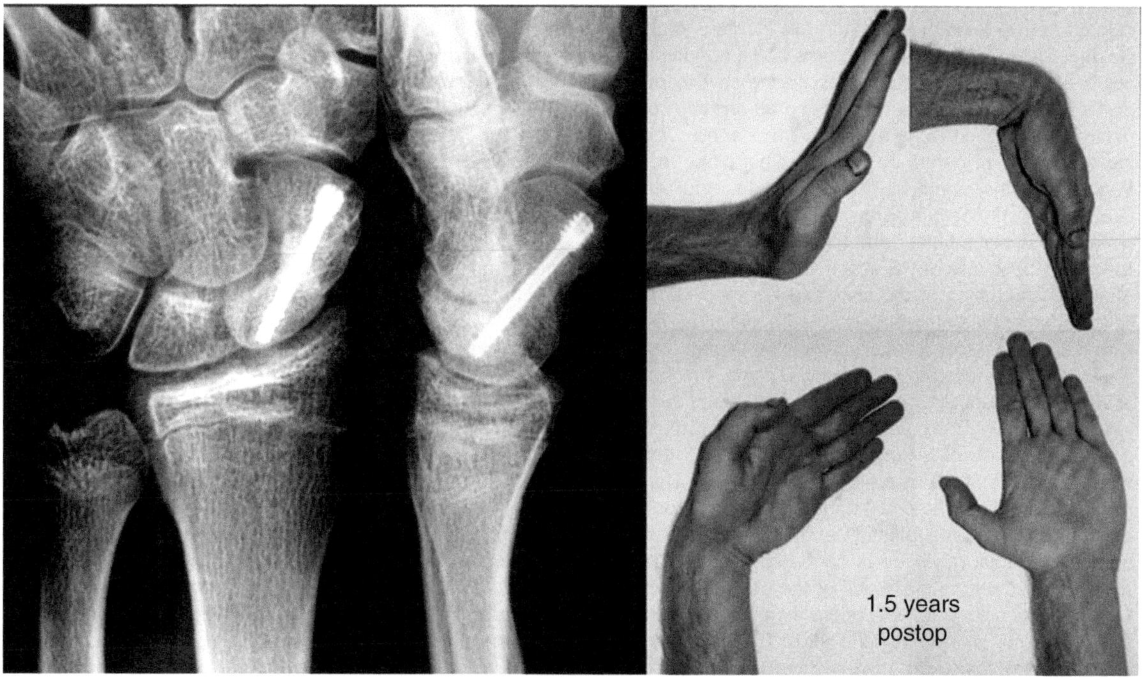

FIG. 33.9 Follow-up radiographs at 1.5 years.

PANEL 3
Author's Preferred Technique

PREOPERATIVE PLANNING

The only component of the deformity that can be approximately calculated with plain X-rays is the scaphoid length using maximally ulnar deviated AP views. The amount of resection and size of the graft needed in millimeters are calculated preoperatively by carefully tracing the radiographic findings of the affected and normal scaphoids in the frontal plane (Fig. 33.10).[42] Using CT scan cuts in the long axis of the scaphoid,[29] the AP and lateral intrascaphoid angles, the dorsal cortical angle, and the height to length ratio can be measured.[28] The amount of correction is given by the difference of the values of the deformed and the contralateral normal scaphoid. Accordingly Kirschner wires (K-wires) can be inserted in the scaphoid fragments subtending the correction angles in both nonunions and malunions.[43,44] The size and form of the defect to be grafted is given by the virtual correction with three-dimensional reconstructions.

SURGICAL TECHNIQUE

An extended volar Russe approach is used. The capsule is incised in line with the skin incision. The capsular flaps that contain the strong radioscaphocapitate ligament are held on both sides with stay sutures to facilitate anatomic closure. Sclerotic or irregular borders of the nonunion site are then resected with a small oscillating saw to offer a perfect surface contact between the graft and the scaphoid fragments. Then 1.2-mm K-wires are inserted subtending the angles of deformity in the sagittal plane in each fragment of the scaphoid (Fig. 33.11). In order not to interfere with the central screw track for final fixation, the distal wire is placed ulnar and the proximal wire radial to the central long axis of the scaphoid.[43] The flexion deformity and shortening of the scaphoid are then corrected by distracting the osteotomy on the palmar ulnar aspect with a small spreader clamp or simply by hyperextending the wrist over a rolled towel. As this is done, the surgical assistant simultaneously corrects the dorsal rotation of the lunate by pushing the palmar pole toward the radius with a fine bone spike or by using a K-wire inserted through the palmar pole of the lunate to control rotation. The pronatory deformity of the distal fragment usually spontaneously derotates into supination as the distal fragment is extended. Radial deviation is corrected by opening the nonunion gap on the ulnar side of the osteotomized surfaces. Additional cystic defects are then curetted out and filled with small cancellous bone chips. The corticocancellous graft is obtained from the iliac crest[41,42] or the distal radius,[45] shaped according to the intraoperative dimensions of the bone defect, and is inserted with the cortical part of the graft being oriented palmarly.

Stable fixation is then performed with a cannulated Herbert screw. Alternatively, following correction of the deformity and having accomplished extension translation, radial deviation, and supination of the distal fragment, a provisional guide pin for cannulated screw fixation can be inserted along the long axis of the scaphoid. Following fluoroscopic control of the corrected deformity and carpal alignment, the bone defect is filled with compressed cancellous bone graft taken from the distal radius as proposed by Cohen et al.[18] Then internal fixation is performed with a headless screw. If access to the central axis of the scaphoid is difficult, the anterior border of the trapezium is removed to facilitate the correct point of entry of the guide wire. The latter subtends an angle of 45 degrees with the long axis of the forearm in the frontal and sagittal planes. Usually the headless screw is 4 mm shorter than the length of the guide wire within the scaphoid. During screw insertion, an additional radially placed K-wire may be useful to control rotation and stability of the graft. If a long-standing fixed dorsal intercalated segment instability deformity is present with a radiolunate angle greater than 20 degrees, usually additional pinning of the lunate to the radius for 6–8 weeks is advisable to prevent recurrence of carpal malalignment.[2,46] Through the volar approach, lunate derotation from the extended to a neutral position (radiolunate angle 0 degree) is performed either by using a 1.6-mm K-wire inserted into the lunate through the palmar pole as a joystick, or by simply flexing the wrist as suggested by Linscheid.[46] Occasionally radiocarpal adhesions in the radiolunate joint have to be released with a dissector through the volar approach. Having verified correct lunate rotation, a 1.2-mm K-wire is driven through the distal radius across the radiocarpal joint into the body of the lunate. Then scaphoid reduction, grafting, and screw fixation are performed. Careful closure of the palmar capsule with fine nonresorbable sutures completes the operation.

POSTOPERATIVE MANAGEMENT

A radial plaster splint that includes the thumb is applied postoperatively for 2 weeks. Following suture removal, a thumb spica cast is applied for 6 weeks. At 8 weeks the cast is removed and healing is radiographically assessed with scaphoid views and CT scans (Fig. 33.12). The criteria to establish healing are (1) the absence of pain, (2) the radiographic evidence of bridging bony trabeculae on both sides of the interposed graft, (3) disappearance of the osteotomy lines in conventional X-rays, and (4) no signs of screw loosening. If there is any doubt regarding radiographic healing, cast immobilization is continued for another 4–5 weeks.

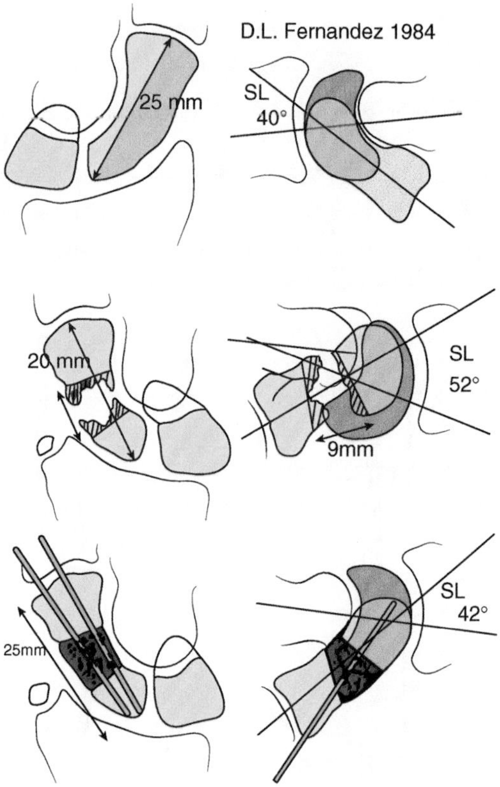

FIG. 33.10 Calculating the amount of resection and size of the graft preoperatively. (From Fernandez DL. A technique for anterior wedge-shaped grafts for scaphoid nonunions with carpal instability. *J Hand Surg*. 1984;9A:733–737, with permission.)

PANEL 4
Pearls and Pitfalls

PEARLS

- It may be advisable to use a temporary K-wire to stabilize the interposed graft during drilling and screw insertion
- Screw placement in the central axis of the scaphoid is mandatory. Careful fluoroscopic control of the guide wire position in all planes is necessary.
- If a dorsal intercalated segment instability (DISI) is present, temporary dorsal 1.6-mm K-wire fixation of the radiolunate joint (in full volar flexion) can be used to correct the DISI deformity temporarily fixating the lunate, while grafting and fixation of the scaphoid is performed.

PITFALLS

- Failure to shape the graft correctly to fill the defect after resection of the sclerotic nonunion site
- Failure to recognize a nonvascularized proximal pole (presence of bleeding points)
- Bad screw placement, unrecognized joint penetration

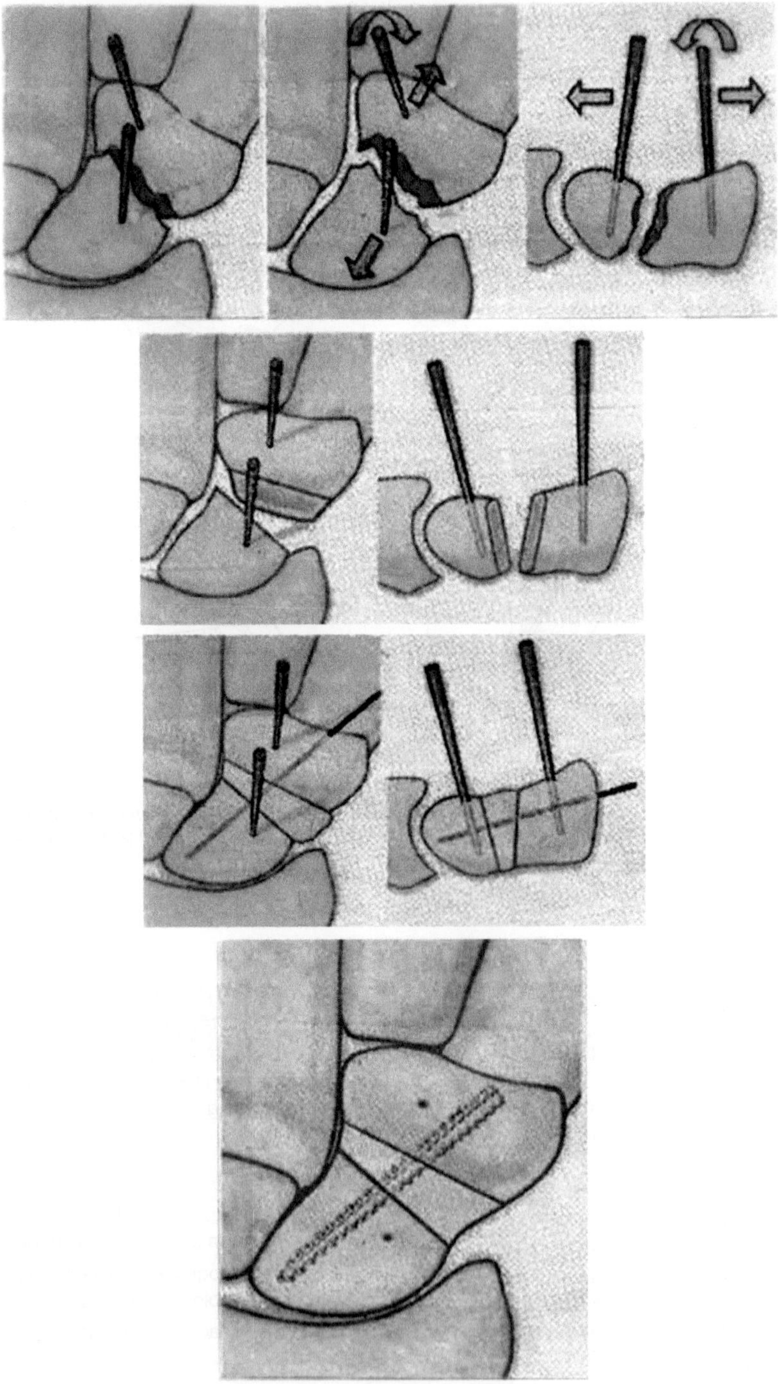

FIG. 33.11 Surgical technique. (Redrawn from Bindra R, Bednar M, Light T. Volar wedge grafting for scaphoid non-union with collapse. *J Hand Surg*. 2008;33A:974–979.)

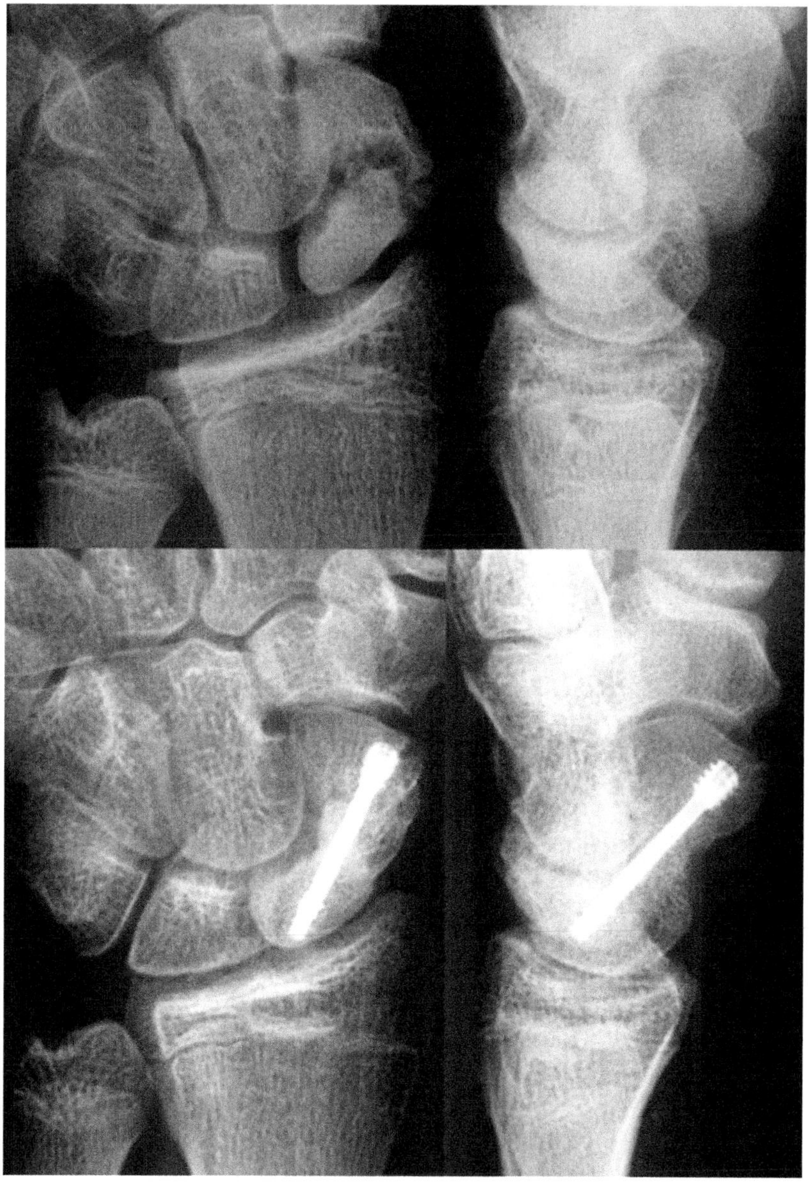

FIG. 33.12 Radiographs following reconstruction.

PANEL 5
Innovative Techniques: Iliac Peg With Arc de Triomphe Graft

This personal technique is indicated for viable scaphoid nonunions with failed screw fixation. Usually the loose screw produces an additional longitudinal bone defect in both the proximal and distal fragments. For these cases, after having checked the vascularity of the proximal pole (at least two bleeding points), an iliac peg corticocancellous strut placed in the screw channel is combined with an anterior wedge graft. To fit over the longitudinal peg, a notch is created in the center of the wedge by removing enough cancellous bone with a fine rongeur. Shaped like an arch we call it "Arc de Triomphe" graft (Fig. 33.13).

A volar extended Russe approach is used. The loose screw is removed and scar tissue is curetted out of the screw channel. Resection of the nonunion site is carried out

Continued

PANEL 5
Innovative Techniques: Iliac Peg With Arc de Triomphe Graft—Cont'd

with a mini-oscillating saw. To facilitate the placement of the peg, graft I recommends to remove the bone directly over the screw channel on the distal fragment volarly. Therefore the peg is an inlay graft distally and intramedullary on the proximal fragment. If attempts are done to force the peg from distal to proximal in the old screw channel, more often the peg may fracture. However, if it goes in loosely, it could be done, but most probably the graft will not have a snug fit. Before inserting the interpositional graft on top of the peg, be sure and fill all spaces with free cancellous bone chips. Then the wedge graft is fitted and impacted being careful not to damage the underlying peg graft.

Internal fixation is performed with two or three 1.25-mm K-wires inserted from distal to proximal. Screw fixation is contraindicated because there is very little bone left in the proximal fragment to guarantee solid screw purchase.

Postoperatively a dorsoradial splint is applied for 2 weeks. Following suture removal, a forearm cast including the base of the thumb is applied for 8 weeks.

Scaphoid views and CT scans are done between 8 and 10 weeks following surgery. If bridging trabeculae is confirmed on both sides of the interposed graft, immobilization is discontinued and wrist rehabilitation begun. Often the K-wire ends in the thenar region may disturb and need to be removed in local anesthesia.

PEARLS

- Be sure the proximal fragment has adequate irrigation.
- Careful manual shaping of both grafts to adapt into the bone defect is mandatory.
- Remove the volar bone over the distal screw channel to facilitate insertion and snug fit of the axial peg graft.

PITFALLS

- Fracture of the peg graft due to forceful insertion in the old screw channel
- Failure to obtain adequate K-wire placement in the proximal fragment
- Early migration of K-wire and skin irritation
- Case immobilization shorter than 8 weeks

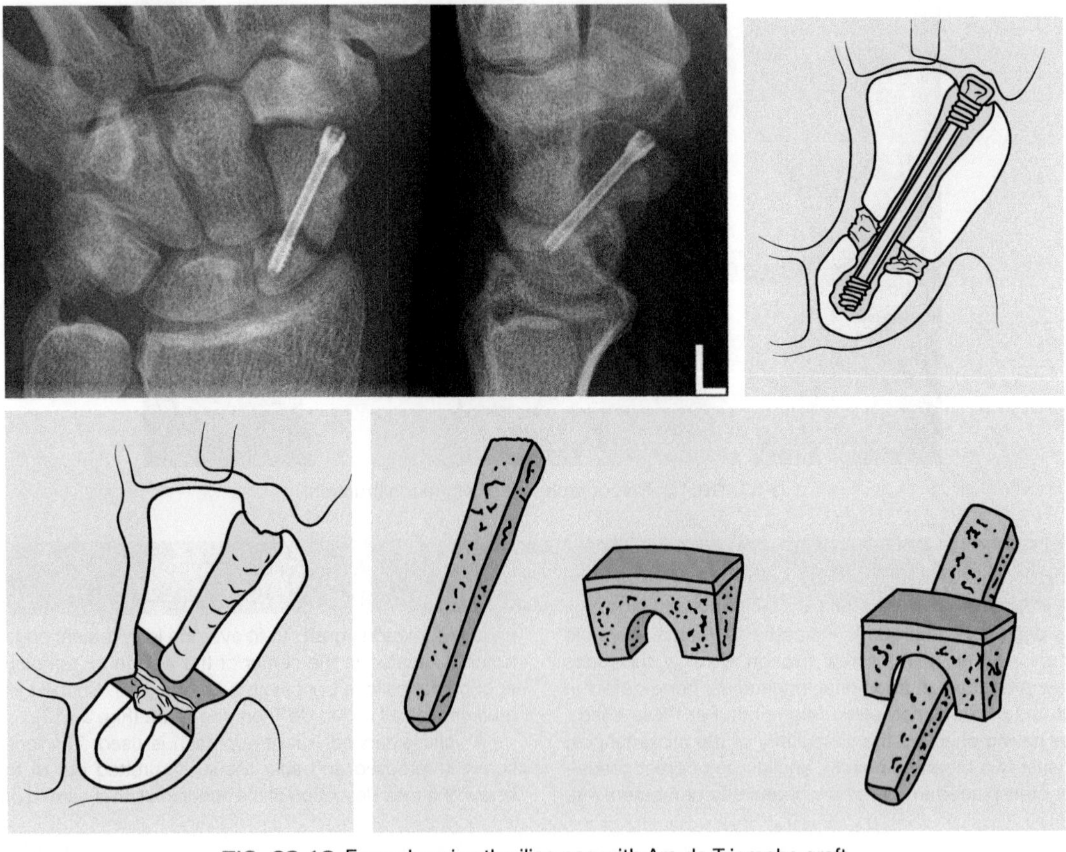

FIG. 33.13 Example using the iliac peg with Arc de Triomphe graft.

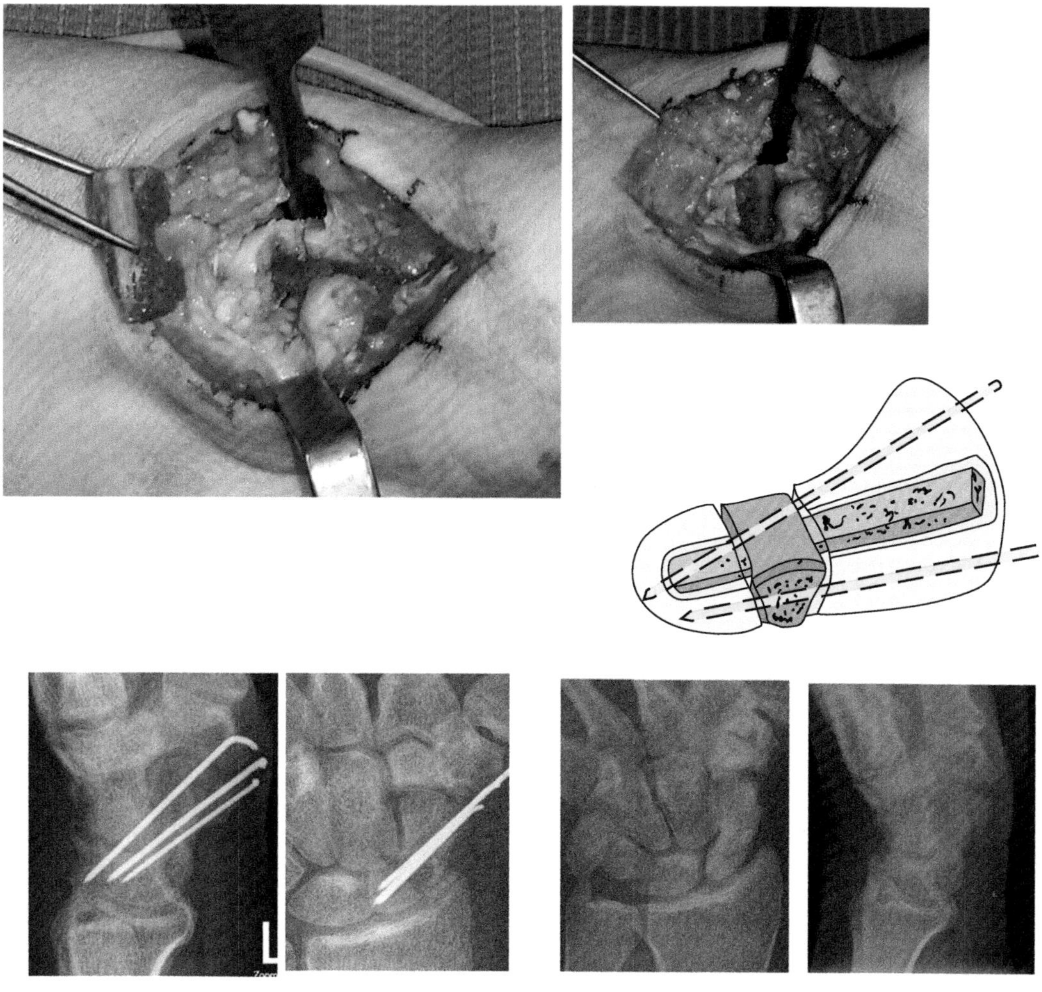

FIG. 33.13, cont'd

PANEL 6
Innovative Techniques: The Hamate Graft

Proximal pole scaphoid fracture nonunions can be difficult to treat.[47] Factors that may contribute to this include their small size, propensity for avascular necrosis, and secondary comminution and fragmentation.[47,48] Multiple techniques have been devised to address this problem including partial scaphoid excision, nonvascularized and vascularized bone grafts, rib autografts, and, more recently, the use of free vascularized osteochondral grafts.[49,51–53,55–57] Sandow reported favorable results using rib autograft. In a series of 47 patients, at a median follow-up of 15 months, all patients demonstrated improved functional outcomes. Donor-site morbidities were primarily related to rib harvest and included pneumothorax and lung injury. Burger and colleagues detailed the use of a free vascularized medial femoral osteochondral graft to treat 16 patients with proximal pole scaphoid nonunions. Of 16 patients, 12 reported resolution of their symptoms at a mean follow-up of 14 months. Despite these promising results, the long-term sequelae, as it pertains to the donor site, is not known.

Recently, Elhassan, Noureldin, and Kakar[54] reported on the successful reconstruction of a proximal pole scaphoid nonunion with avascular necrosis using the ipsilateral proximal hamate (Fig. 33.14). At 3.5 years of follow-up, the patient was asymptomatic, working as a carpenter with a Mayo Wrist Score of 90 (excellent).

Continued

PANEL 6
Innovative Techniques: The Hamate Graft—Cont'd

This technique is attractive, as the donor site is limited to the operative site and allows for simultaneous repair of the scapholunate ligament. In brief, a dorsal approach to the wrist is performed utilizing a ligament sparing capsulotomy.[50] The avascular proximal pole is excised with care to protect the scapholunate ligament insertion onto the lunate for later repair. The size of the defect is measured and matched to the ipsilateral proximal hamate (Fig. 33.15). An osteotomy is performed to ensure sufficient proximal hamate is obtained that matches the scaphoid defect. Care is taken when harvesting the graft to ensure the underlying flexor tendons and ulnar neurovascular bundle are not injured (Fig. 33.16). In addition, meticulous technique is needed to protect the volar capitohamate ligament by placing a retractor between the triquetrum and hamate. In this way, as the proximal hamate is turned 180 degrees, the volar capitohamate ligament lies dorsal to be repaired to the native scapholunate ligament (Fig. 33.17) and the capitohamate articular surface articulates with the lunate. The graft is inserted into the scaphoid defect to assess its match before any contouring is performed (Figs. 33.18 and 33.19). During this process, it is important to assess the graft's match to the scaphoid, scapholunate, and scaphocapitate joints, and the scaphoid facet of the distal radius. Once it is contoured to meet these surfaces, the graft is secured to the scaphoid with compression screw fixation. Prior to scapholunate ligament repair to the volar capitohamate ligament (which now lies dorsal on the insetted proximal hamate), the lunate is reduced into neutral alignment and the ligaments repaired using a 2-0 nonabsorbable suture. To further augment the scapholunate ligament repair, a distally based strip of the dorsal intercarpal ligament can be used as a capsulodesis reconstruction. The dorsal capsule and extensor retinaculum are closed and the patient placed into a thumb spica splint for 2 weeks followed by a short-arm thumb spica cast until radiographic confirmation of union (Figs. 33.20 and 33.21).

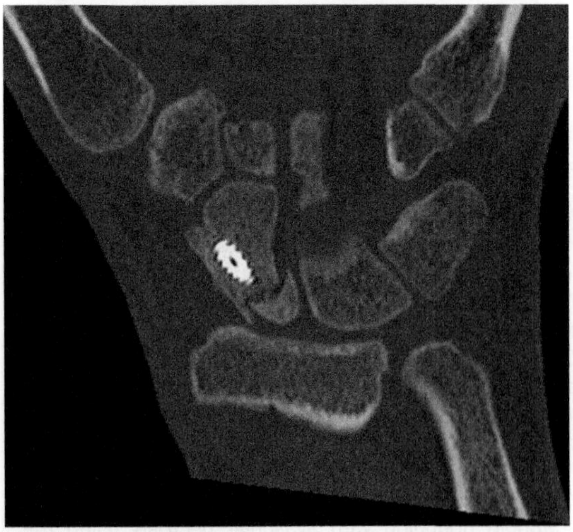

FIG. 33.14 Preoperative CT scan of a proximal pole scaphoid nonunion in a patient who had undergone previous attempted scaphoid fixation. Note the small size of the proximal pole of the scaphoid.

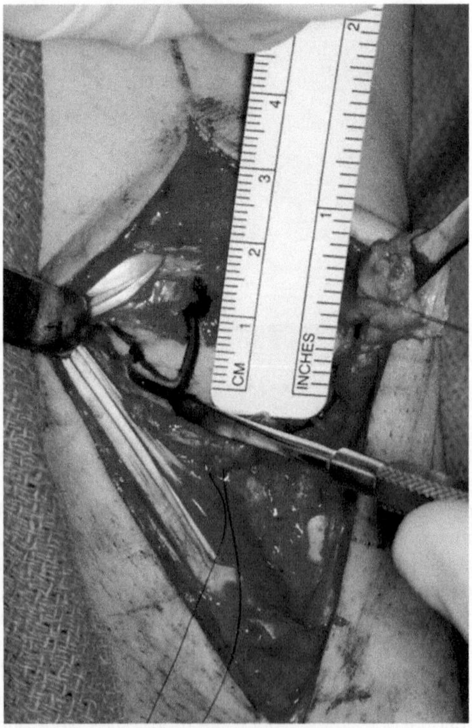

FIG. 33.15 Templating the proximal hamate to match the size of the proximal pole of the scaphoid that was excised.

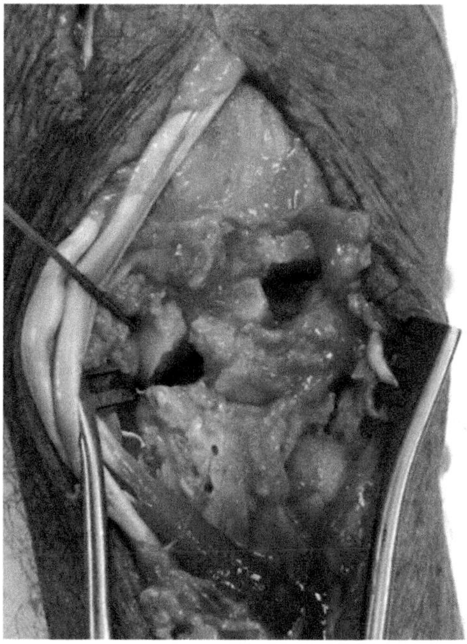

FIG. 33.16 Note the proximal scaphoid and hamate after respective osteotomy.

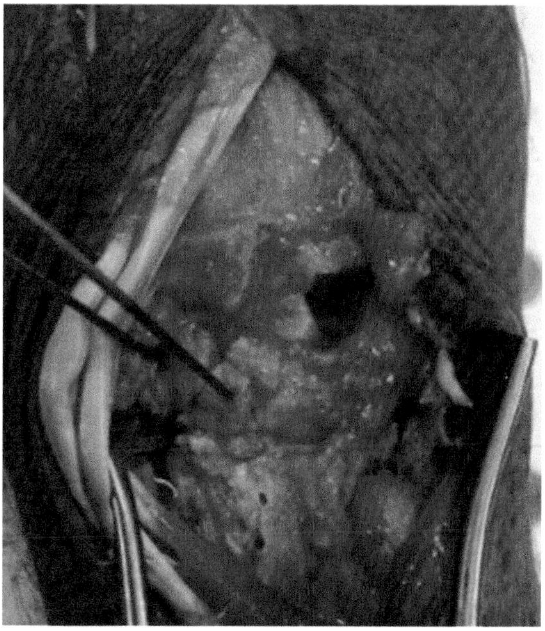

FIG. 33.18 Provisional insetting of the hamate into the proximal scaphoid to assess its match to the scaphoid, scaphocapitate, scapholunate, and radiocarpal joints.

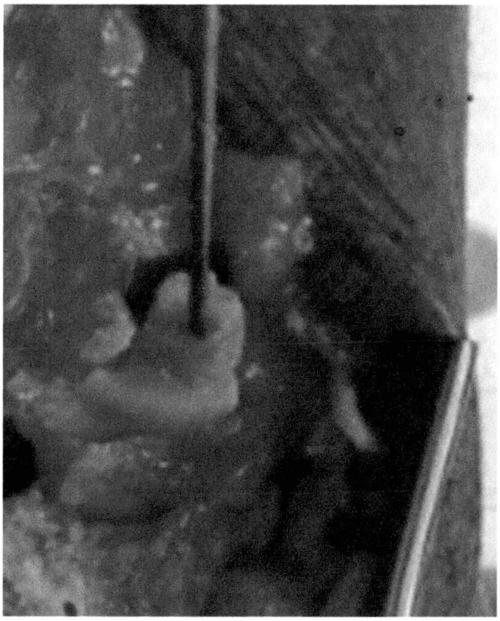

FIG. 33.17 Proximal hamate rotated 180degrees such that the volar capitohamate ligament lies dorsal.

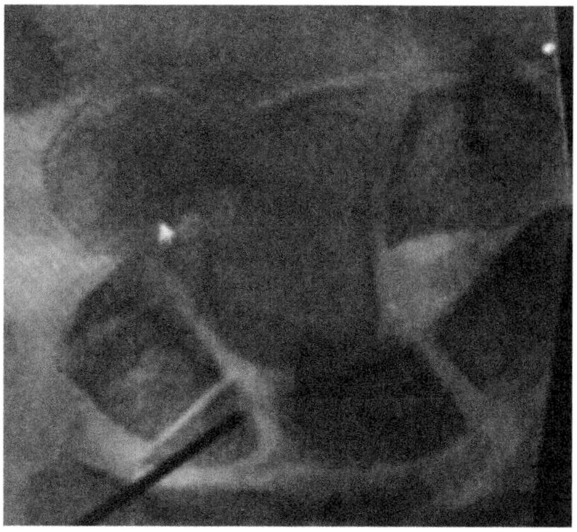

FIG. 33.19 Fluoroscopic image showing the near perfect match of the proximal pole of the hamate to the proximal scaphoid without any contouring.

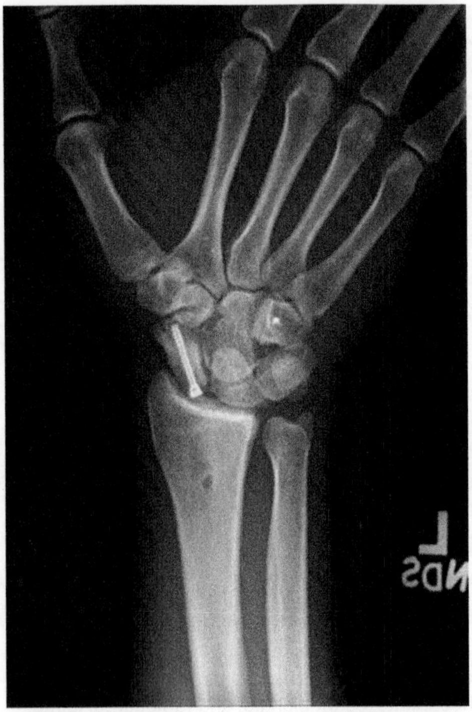

FIG. 33.20 Anteroposterior radiograph demonstrating union of the proximal hamate to the scaphoid.

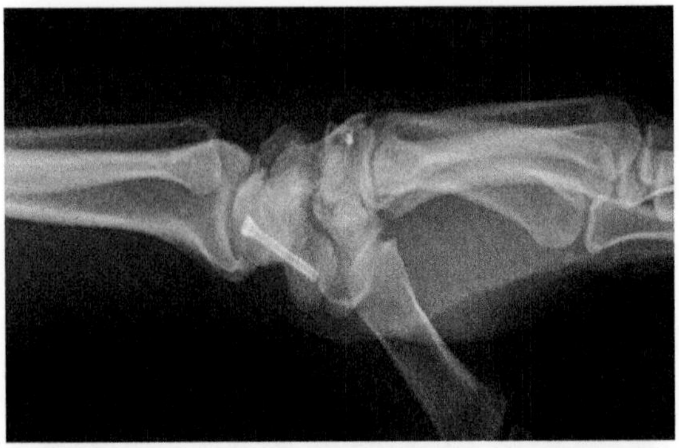

FIG. 33.21 Lateral radiograph demonstrating union of the proximal hamate to the scaphoid.

REFERENCES

1. Mack GR, Bosse MJ, Gelberman RH, et al. The natural history of scaphoid non-union. *J Bone Joint Surg.* 1984;66A:504–509.
2. Tomaino MM, King J, Pizillo M. Correction of lunate malalignment when bone grafting scaphoid nonunion with humpback deformity: rationale and results of a technique revisited. *J Hand Surg.* 2000;25A:322–329.
3. Lindström G, Nyström A. Natural history of scaphoid non-union with special reference to "asymptomatic" cases. *J Hand Surg.* 1992;17B:697–700.
4. Green DP. The effect of avascular necrosis on Russe bone grafting for scaphoid nonunion. *J Hand Surg.* 1985;10A:597–605.
5. Schuind F, Haentjens P, Van Innis F, et al. Prognostic factors in the treatment of carpal scaphoid nonunions. *J Hand Surg.* 1999;24A:761–776.
6. Herbert TJ, Fisher WE. Management of the fractured scaphoid using a new bone screw. *J Bone Joint Surg.* 1984;66B:114–123.
7. Herbert TJ. *The Fractured Scaphoid.* St. Louis: Quality Medical Publishing; 1990.
8. Merrell G, Slade J. Technique for percutaneous fixation of displaced and nondisplaced acute scaphoid fractures and select non-unions. *J Hand Surg.* 2008;33A:966–973.
9. Slade JF, Geissler WB, Gutow AP, Merell GA. Percutaneous internal fixation of selected scaphoid non-unions with an arthroscopically assisted dorsal approach. *J Bone Joint Surg.* 2003;85A(suppl 4):20–32.
10. Slade JF, Dodds SD. Percutaneous fixation of scaphoid fibrous/nonunion with and without percutaneous bone graft. In: Slutsky DJ, Slade JF, eds. *The Scaphoid.* New York, Stuttgart: Thieme; 2011:175–187.
11. Matti H. Über die Behandlung der Navicularefraktur und der Refractura patellae dutch Plombierung mit Spongiosa. *Zentralbl Chir.* 1937;64:2353–2359.
12. Russe O. Fracture of the carpal navicular. Diagnosis, nonoperative treatment, and operative treatment. *J Bone Joint Surg Am.* 1960;42-A:759–768.
13. Jiranek WA, Ruby LK, Millender LB, Bankoff MS, Newberg AH. Long-term results after Russe bone-grafting: the effect of malunion of the scaphoid. *J Bone Joint Surg Am.* 1992;74:1217–1228.
14. Zarezadeh A, Moezi M, Rastegar S, Motififard M, Foladi A, Daneshpajouhnejad P. Scaphoid nonunion fracture and results of the modified Matti-Russe technique. *Adv Biomed Res.* 2015;4:39.
15. Hooning van Duyvenbode JF, Keijser LC, Hauet EJ, Obermann WR, Rozing PM. Pseudarthrosis of the scaphoid treated by the Matti-Russe operation. A long-term review of 77 cases. *J Bone Joint Surg Br.* 1991;73:603–606.
16. Stark HH, Rickard TA, Zemel NP, et al. Treatment of ununited fractures of the scaphoid by iliac bone grafts and Kirschner-wire fixation. *J Bone Joint Surg.* 1988;70A:982–991.
17. Stark A, Brostrom LA, Svartengren G. Scaphoid nonunion treated with the Matti-Russe technique. Long-term results. *Clin Orthop Relat Res.* 1987;214:175–180.
18. Cohen MS, Jupiter JB, Fallahi K, Shukla K. Scaphoid waist nonunion with humpback deformity treated without structural bone graft. *J Hand Surg.* 2013;38A:701–705.
19. Tsuyuguchi Y, Murase T, Hidaka N, Ohno H, Kawai H. Anterior wedge-shaped bone graft for old scaphoid fractures or non-unions. An analysis of relevant carpal alignment. *J Hand Surg Br.* 1995;20:194–200.

20. Fisk GR. Carpal instability and the fractured scaphoid. *Ann R Coll Surg Engl*. 1970;46:63–76.
21. Fisk GR. In: Bentley G, ed. *Operative Orthopaedics Part III*. Butterworth; 1979.
22. Fisk GR. An overview of injuries of the wrist. *Clin Orthop*. 1980;149:137–144.
23. Segmüller G. *Operative Stabilisierung am Handskelett*. Bern, Stuttgart, Wien: Hans Huber Verlag; 1973.
24. Fernandez DL, Eggli S. Scaphoid nonunion and malunion: how to correct deformity. *Hand Clin*. 2001;17(4):631–646.
25. Cooney WP, Linscheid RL, Dobyns JH, et al. Scaphoid nonunion: role of anterior interpositional bone grafts. *J Hand Surg*. 1988;13A:635–650.
26. Amadio PC, Berquist TH, Smith DK, et al. Scaphoid malunion. *J Hand Surg*. 1989;14A:679–687.
27. Bain GI, Bennett JD, Richard RS, et al. Longitudinal computed tomography of the scaphoid: a new technique. *Skeletal Radiol*. 1995;24:271–273.
28. Bain GI, Bennett JD, MacDermid JC, et al. Measurement of the scaphoid humpback deformity using longitudinal computed tomography: intra and interobserver variability using various measurement techniques. *J Hand Surg*. 1998;23A:76–81.
29. Sanders WE. Evaluation of the humpback scaphoid by computed tomography in the longitudinal axial plane of the scaphoid. *J Hand Surg*. 1988;13A:182–187.
30. Moritomo H, Viegas SF, Elder KW, et al. Scaphoid nonunions: a 3-dimensional analysis of patterns of deformity. *J Hand Surg*. 2000;25A:520–528.
31. Nakamura R, Imaeda T, Horii E, et al. Analysis of scaphoid fracture displacement by three-dimensional computed tomography. *J Hand Surg*. 1991;16A:485–492.
32. Nakamura R, Imaeda T, Miura T. Scaphoid malunion. *J Bone Joint Surg*. 1991;73B:134–137.
33. Oka K, Murase T, Moritomo H, et al. Patterns of bone defect in scaphoid nonunion: a 3-dimensional and quantitative analysis. *J Hand Surg*. 2005;30A:359–365.
34. Andreas S, Fürnstahl P, Nagy L. Three-dimensional computed tomographic analysis of 11 scaphoid waist nonunions. *J Hand Surg*. 2012;37A:1151–1158.
35. Rajagopalan BM, Squire DS, Samuels LO. Results of Herbert-screw fixation with bone-grafting for the treatment of nonunion of the scaphoid. *J Bone Joint Surg*. 1999;81A:48–51.
36. Haefeli M, Schaefer DJ, Schumacher R, et al. Titanium template for scaphoid reconstruction. *J Hand Surg*. 2015;40E:526–533.
37. Schweizer A, Mauler F, Vlachopoulos L, Nagy L, Fürnstahl P. Computer-assisted 3-dimensional reconstructions of scaphoid fractures and nonunions with and without the use of patient-specific guides: early clinical outcomes and postoperative assessments of reconstruction accuracy. *J Hand Surg Am*. 2016;41:59–69.
38. Sayegh ET, Strauch RJ. Graft choice in the management of unstable scaphoid nonunion: a systematic review. *J Hand Surg*. 2014;39A:1500–1506.
39. Tambe AD, Cutler L, Murali SR, et al. In scaphoid nonunion, does the source of graft affect outcome? Iliac crest versus distal end of radius bone graft. *J Hand Surg*. 2006;31B:47–51.
40. Eggli S, Fernandez DL, Beck T. Unstable scaphoid nonunion: a medium-term study of anterior wedge grafting procedures. *J Hand Surg*. 2002;27B:36–41.
41. Fernandez DL. Anterior bone grafting and conventional lag screw fixation to treat scaphoid non-unions. *J Hand Surg*. 1990;15A:140–147.
42. Fernandez DL. A technique for anterior wedge-shaped grafts for scaphoid nonunions with carpal instability. *J Hand Surg*. 1984;9A:733–737.
43. Bindra R, Bednar M, Light T. Volar wedge grafting for scaphoid non-union with collapse. *J Hand Surg*. 2008;33A:974–979.
44. Fernandez DL, Martin CL, Gonzalez del Pino J. Scaphoid malunion: the significance of rotational malalignment. *J Hand Surg*. 1998;23B:771–775.
45. Aguilella L, Garcia-Elias M. The anterolateral corner of the radial metaphysic as a source of bone graft for the treatment of scaphoid non-union. *J Hand Surg*. 2012;37A:1258–1262.
46. Linscheid RL, Dobyns JB, Cooney WP. Volar wedge grafting of the carpal scaphoid in non-union associated with dorsal instability patterns. *J Bone Joint Surg*. 1982;64B:632–633.
47. Gelberman RH, Menon J. The vascularity of the scaphoid bone. *J Hand Surg Am*. 1980;5(5):508–513.
48. Trumble TE. Avascular necrosis after scaphoid fracture: a correlation of magnetic resonance imaging and histology. *J Hand Surg Am*. 1990;15(4):557–564.
49. Boyer MI, von Schroeder HP, Axelrod TS. Scaphoid nonunion with avascular necrosis of the proximal pole. Treatment with a vascularized bone graft from the dorsum of the distal radius. *J Hand Surg Am*. 1998;23(5):686–690.
50. Berger RA, Bishop AT, Bettinger PC. New dorsal capsulotomy for the surgical exposure of the wrist. *Ann Plast Surg*. 1995;35(1):54–59.
51. Burger HK, Windhofer C, Gaggl AJ, Higgins JP. Vascularized medial femoral trochlea osteocartilaginous flap reconstruction of proximal pole scaphoid nonunions. *J Hand Surg Am*. 2013;38(4):690–700.
52. Chang MA, Bishop AT, Moran SL, Shin AY. The outcomes and complications of 1,2-intercompartmental supraretinacular artery pedicled vascularized bone grafting of scaphoid nonunions. *J Hand Surg Am*. 2006;31(3):387–396.
53. Garcia-Elias M, Lluch A. Partial excision of scaphoid: is it ever indicated? *Hand Clin*. 2001;17(4):687–695.
54. Elhassan BT, Noureldin M, Kakar S. Proximal scaphoid pole reconstruction utilizing ipsilateral proximal hamate autograft. *Hand*. 2017. [in print].
55. Sandow MJ. Costo-osteochondral grafts in the wrist. *Tech Hand Up Extrem Surg*. 2001;5(3):165–172.
56. Shah J, Jones WA. Factors affecting the outcome in 50 cases of scaphoid nonunion treated with Herbert screw fixation. *J Hand Surg Am*. 1998;23(5):680–685.

57. Yao J, Read B, Hentz VR. The fragmented proximal pole scaphoid nonunion treated with rib autograft: case series and review of the literature. *J Hand Surg Am*. 2013;38(11):2188–2192.

FURTHER READING

1. Belsole RJ, Hilbelink DR, Llewellyn JA, et al. Computed analysis of the pathomechanics of scaphoid waist nonunions. *J Hand Surg*. 1991;16A:899–906.
2. Filan SL, Herbert TJ. Herbert screw fixation of scaphoid fractures. *J Bone Joint Surg*. 1996;78B:519–529.
3. Huang YC, Liu Y, Chen T. Long-term results of scaphoid non-union treated by intercalated bone grafting and Herbert's screw fixation – a study of 49 patients for at least five years. *Int Orthop*. 2009;33:1295–1300.
4. Ruby LK, Stinson J, Belsky MR. The natural history of scaphoid non-union: a review of fifty-five cases. *J Bone Joint Surg*. 1985;67A:428–432.
5. Watanabe K. Analysis of carpal malalignment caused by scaphoid nonunion and evaluation of corrective bone graft on carpal alignment. *J Hand Surg*. 2011;36A:10–16.

CHAPTER 34

Bone Morphogenetic Proteins for Scaphoid Nonunion

MICHEL CHAMMAS, MD, PHD • EMMANUELLA PERAUT, MD •
GEERT A. BUIJZE, MD, PHD • PIERRE E. CHAMMAS

KEY POINTS

- Application of recombinant human bone morphogenetic protein (rhBMP) in case of scaphoid nonunion is an off-label use.
- Use of rhBMP has not shown a reproducible superior rate of union in patients with scaphoid nonunion.
- Patients should be counseled that, when rhBMP is used for the treatment of scaphoid nonunion, there are risks of heterotopic ossification and reoperation.

PANEL 1
Case Scenario

A 34-year-old male right-handed manual worker without medical history—other than heavy smoking—presented with a scaphoid fracture of his left wrist with a delay of 6 months after a fall. Clinical examination showed mechanical pain in the dorsal aspect of the wrist and decreased range of motion. Radiographs showed nonunion of the proximal pole of the scaphoid with limited resorption at the fracture site (Fig. 34.1A and B). There was an early dorsal intercalated segment instability deformity and limited bone loss on CT (Fig. 34.2A and B). MRI confirmed the diagnosis and did not show any sign of osteonecrosis of the proximal pole (Fig. 34.3A and B). You are considering a nonvascularized bone graft with additional biologics. Will adding rhBMP increase the likelihood of union?

IMPORTANCE OF THE PROBLEM

Five to thirty percent of all scaphoid fractures involve the proximal pole (proximal fifth of the scaphoid).[2] The proximal pole has a tenuous blood supply and mechanical disadvantage that places it at greater risk of delayed or failed union. Treatment of nonunion of the proximal pole scaphoid without avascular necrosis and without osteoarthritis is preferentially operative. It aims to reduce painful symptoms, restore the height and angulation of the scaphoid and achieve bone healing, and reduce the risk of degenerative changes such as a scaphoid nonunion advanced collapse wrist. Autologous bone graft (vascularized or nonvascularized) with or without osteosynthesis is the most used technique.[3] Simple screw fixation is optional in case of an early nonunion stage.[4,5] Recent studies, including a metaanalysis, do not reveal a substantial difference in union rates between different sources of bone graft and types of fixation.[6] Vascularized bone grafting has not shown more successful union rates than nonvascularized graft in all but nonunions with avascular necrosis of the proximal pole.[6] However, controversy remains. Despite attempts to advance the surgical management of scaphoid nonunion, approximately 10% of recalcitrant nonunion persists after treatment.[3,7]

MAIN QUESTION

Does the use of rhBMP and internal fixation improve functional outcome, fracture healing, and complication rates in the management of scaphoid proximal pole nonunion?

Current Opinion

Clinical trials investigating long bone applications have provided supportive evidence for the use of rhBMP—especially rhBMP-2 and rhBMP-7—in the treatment of open tibial fractures, distal tibial fractures, tibial nonunions, atrophic long bone nonunions, and posterolateral lumbar models.[8] Studies utilizing rhBMP-2 or rhBMP-7 in hand and wrist surgery are rare, and controversy exists regarding rate of bone healing and complications.

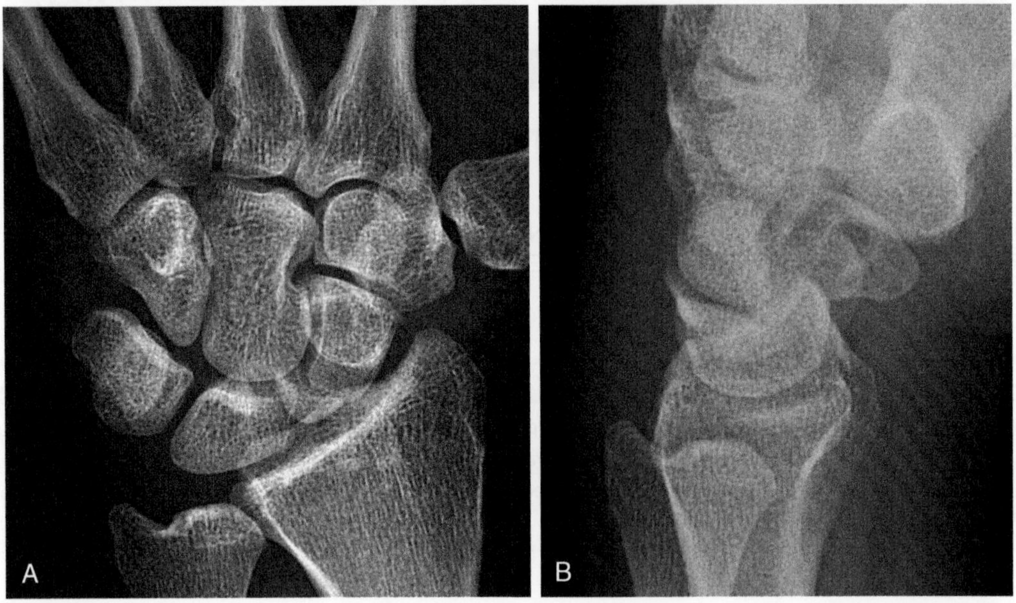

FIG. 34.1 (A and B) A 34-year-old man with a delayed union of a scaphoid proximal pole fracture.

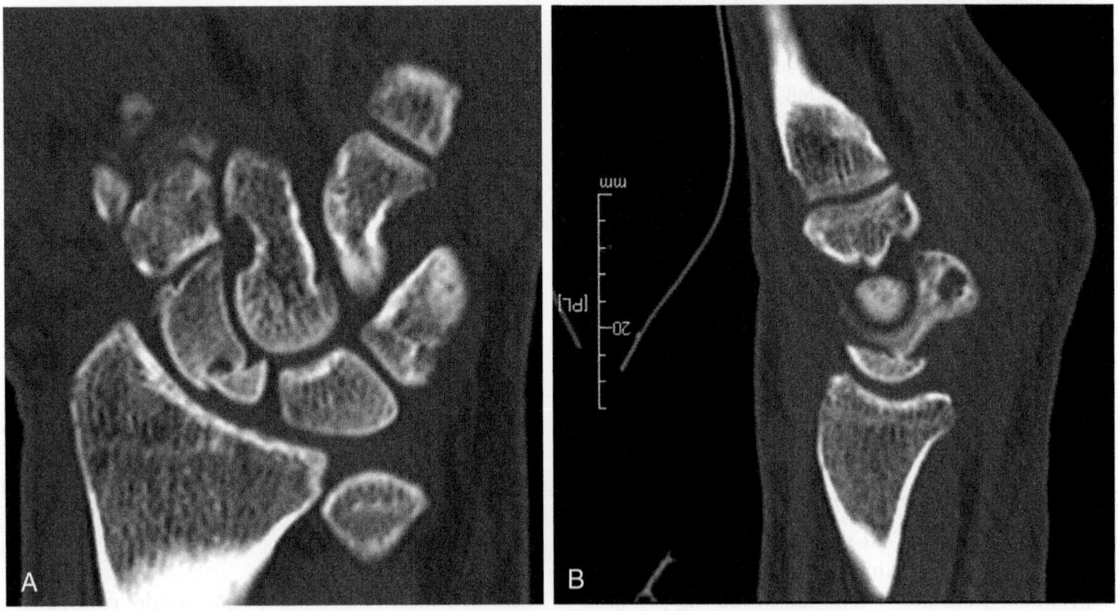

FIG. 34.2 (A and B) Very proximal displaced nonunion on CT with limited bone loss.

Finding the Evidence

- Cochrane search: scaphoid nonunion, bone morphogenetic protein
- Pubmed (Medline): ("scaphoid bone"[MeSH Terms] OR ("scaphoid"[All Fields] AND "bone"[All Fields]) OR "scaphoid bone"[All Fields] OR "scaphoid"[All Fields]) AND nonunion[All Fields] AND bmp[All Fields]
- Bibliography of eligible articles
- Articles that were not in English, French, or German were excluded

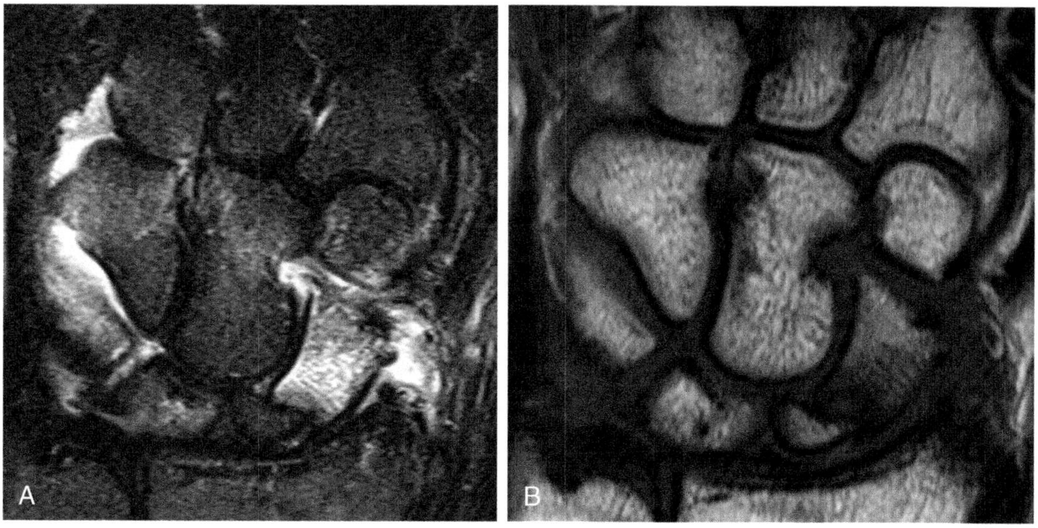

FIG. 34.3 (A and B) MRI showed no sign of osteonecrosis of the proximal pole.

Quality of the Evidence

Level II:

Randomized controlled trial with methodological limitations: 1

Level IV:

Case series: 3

FINDINGS

In the Level II study,[9] 17 patients with scaphoid nonunion of the proximal pole were randomly assigned to three treatment groups: (1) autologous iliac graft (n = 6), (2) autologous iliac graft + osteogenic protein-1 (rhBMP-7; n = 6), and (3) allogenic iliac graft + rhBMP-7 (n = 5). In groups 2 and 3, the rhBMP-7 implant (rhBMP-7 and collagen as a carrier) was applied to both scaphoid fragments and subsequently autogenous or allogenic bone implants were positioned using the Matti-Russe technique.

At 8 weeks of follow-up, 90%–100% of bone showed trabecular bridging on radiographs in the patients of group 2 compared with 75%–90% of bone in patients from both group 3 and group 1. At 24 months of follow-up, union assessed by conventional radiography and CT was confirmed in all 17 patients. Helical CT scans and bone scintigraphy showed that, in the 11 patients treated with rhBMP-7, the sclerotic bone was replaced by well-vascularized bone. Despite the opinion of the authors, no evidence of reduction of the healing time in group 2 was demonstrated. The addition of rhBMP-7 to allogenic bone implant seemed to result in equal clinical outcome compared with the autologous graft procedure. No complications were reported. These results should be interpreted with caution in light of important methodological limitations. Although the percent of radiographic bone bridging is presented as the main outcome in this study, the authors did not report on a primary outcome and the study was not powered. The authors draw a firm conclusion based on this outcome that is subject to high imprecision and may be spurious. It has been well demonstrated by Dias et al.[10] and recognized by others that the assessment of radiographic signs of union of scaphoid fractures has poor interobserver reliability and reproducibility.

In the three case series (with a total of 19 patients), rhBMP-2 was used.[1,11,12]

Rice and Lubahn[12] reported on 9 scaphoid nonunions in 27 patients with various types of nonunion of the hand and wrist. Sites of nonunion included the phalanx (7), carpus (9), distal radius (5), and distal ulna (6). Radiographic union was consistent with published rates of scaphoid nonunion repair without complications. rhBMP-2 did not produce superior rates of union in the patients with wrist and hand nonunion.

A retrospective review by Above and Abrams[11] analyzed the outcome of four patients in whom initial open reduction and internal fixation (ORIF) of a scaphoid fracture (three at the waist and one at the proximal pole) had failed. All patients underwent screw exchange and application of a rhBMP-2 sponge at the nonunion site without additional bone grafting. Data on the delay between the two procedures were lacking.

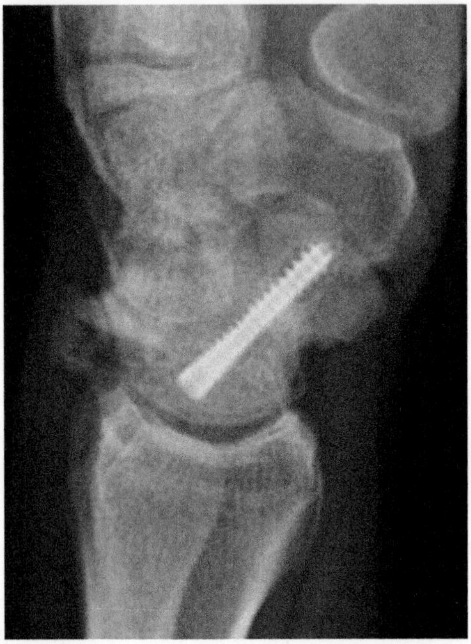

FIG. 34.4 Heterotopic ossification following revision fixation, bone grafting, and application of rhBMP-2 for persistent nonunion of the proximal pole of the scaphoid. (From Brannan PS, Gaston RG, Loeffler BJ, Lewis DR. Complications with the use of BMP-2 in scaphoid nonunion surgery. *J Hand Surg Am*. 2016;41(5):602–608, with permission.)

Union occurred in all patients at an average of 53 days from surgery without complication.

Brannan et al.[1] retrospectively reviewed six cases of scaphoid nonunion revision surgery. All patients had failed an initial attempt at ORIF after delayed union or nonunion. All patients were treated with revision screw fixation, nonvascularized bone grafting, and application of rhBMP-2. The donor site of the autologous bone grafts included the iliac crest (three cases) and distal radius (one case); in the other two cases, an allograft was used. Revision surgery with rhBMP-2 was performed at an average of 6 months from the index ORIF. Of the six cases, two resulted in a persistent nonunion (one allograft, one cancellous distal radius). Several complications were reported. Four cases developed notable heterotopic ossification (one of which required revision surgery, Fig. 34.4). One patient had a notable decreased range of wrist motion after the revision surgery. There were no cases of delayed wound healing. Only one of the six patients healed without complications.

Our limited experience does not confirm the positive influence of rhBMP-7 in case of proximal pole nonunion of the scaphoid. Both of our cases treated with autologous bone grafting combined with rhBMP-7 were complicated in terms of early osteolysis at the nonunion site, necessitating salvage procedures (unpublished data).

RECOMMENDATION

- Application of rhBMP for scaphoid nonunion has not shown a reproducible superior rate of union in patients (overall quality: moderate).
- Shared decision-making is recommended for application of rhBMP in the treatment of scaphoid nonunion—including informed consent of performing off-label use and the considerable risks of heterotopic ossification and reoperation[1] (overall quality: low).

PANEL 2
Author's Preferred Technique

- In case of a very proximal displaced nonunion without osteonecrosis (like the present case), an open reduction via dorsal approach is preferred to provide for anatomic reduction and fixation with direct visualization.
- Fibrous union and sclerotic bone are debrided at the nonunion site.
- Cancellous bone graft is preferred in case of limited bone loss.
- Definitive fixation is achieved by placement of an anterograde cannulated headless compression screw.
- Generally, cast immobilization is recommended until union. A CT may be used to evaluate final consolidation.

CONCLUSION

There is a paucity of data on the use of rhBMP in scaphoid nonunion healing. The most significant study limitations are the small sample size, the retrospective design (three of four studies) and the lack of controls potentially introducing bias. Surgeons performing the off-label use of rhBMP should be aware of the potential for complications including heterotopic ossification and a considerable reoperation rate. Randomized controlled trials of high methodological rigor and economic evaluations are warranted to allow conclusions to be drawn regarding the clinical effectiveness and cost-effectiveness of rhBMP for scaphoid nonunion. Further investigation is also required to investigate clinical differences between rhBMP-2 and rhBMP-7.

PANEL 3
Pearls and Pitfalls

PEARLS

- Avascular necrosis may be evaluated by observing the presence or absence of punctate bleeding intraoperatively.
- Dorsal intercalated segment instability deformity is corrected.
- A dorsal approach also allows for harvesting bone graft at the distal radius.

PITFALLS

- If rhBMP is considered, it is applied using a technique of alternating layers of the collagen carrier and bone graft throughout the nonunion site.[1] This limits the application of rhBMP to the nonunion site.

REFERENCES

1. Brannan PS, Gaston RG, Loeffler BJ, Lewis DR. Complications with the use of BMP-2 in scaphoid nonunion surgery. *J Hand Surg Am*. 2016;41(5):602–608.
2. Kozin SH. Incidence, mechanism, and natural history of scaphoid fractures. *Hand Clin*. 2001;17(4):515–524.
3. Pinder RM, Brkljac M, Rix L, Muir L, Brewster M. Treatment of scaphoid nonunion: a systematic review of the existing evidence. *J Hand Surg Am*. 2015;40(9):1797–1805. e1793.
4. Alnot JY, Bellan N, Oberlin C, De Cheveigne C. Fractures and non unions of the proximal pole of the carpal scaphoid bone. Internal fixation by a proximal to distal screw. *Ann Chir Main*. 1988;7(2):101–108.
5. Slade 3rd JF, Geissler WB, Gutow AP, Merrell GA. Percutaneous internal fixation of selected scaphoid nonunions with an arthroscopically assisted dorsal approach. *J Bone Joint Surg Am*. 2003;85-A(suppl 4):20–32.
6. Janowski J, Coady C, Catalano 3rd LW. Scaphoid fractures: nonunion and malunion. *J Hand Surg Am*. 2016; 41(11):1087–1092.
7. Braga-Silva J, Peruchi FM, Moschen GM, Gehlen D, Padoin AV. A comparison of the use of distal radius vascularised bone graft and non-vascularised iliac crest bone graft in the treatment of non-union of scaphoid fractures. *J Hand Surg Eur Vol*. 2008;33(5):636–640.
8. White AP, Vaccaro AR, Hall JA, Whang PG, Friel BC, McKee MD. Clinical applications of BMP-7/OP-1 in fractures, nonunions and spinal fusion. *Int Orthop*. 2007; 31(6):735–741.
9. Bilic R, Simic P, Jelic M, et al. Osteogenic protein-1 (BMP-7) accelerates healing of scaphoid non-union with proximal pole sclerosis. *Int Orthop*. 2006;30(2):128–134.
10. Dias JJ, Taylor M, Thompson J, Brenkel IJ, Gregg PJ. Radiographic signs of union of scaphoid fractures. An analysis of inter-observer agreement and reproducibility. *J Bone Joint Surg Br*. 1988;70(2):299–301.
11. Ablove RH, Abrams SS. The use of BMP-2 and screw exchange in the treatment of scaphoid fracture non-union. *Hand Surg*. 2015;20(1):167–171.
12. Rice I, Lubahn JD. Use of bone morphogenetic protein-2 (rh-BMP-2) in treatment of wrist and hand nonunion with comparison to historical control groups. *J Surg Orthop Adv*. 2013;22(4):256–262.

CHAPTER 35

Arthroscopic Bone Grafting for Scaphoid Nonunion

PAK-CHEONG HO, MBBS, FRCS, FHKAM (ORTHOPAEDIC SURGERY), FHKCOS • WING-YEE C. WONG, MBCHB, MRCS, FRCSED (ORTH), FHKAM (ORTHOPAEDIC SURGERY), FHKCOS • WING-LIM TSE, MBCHB, MRCS, FRCSED (ORTH), FHKAM (ORTHOPAEDIC SURGERY), FHKCOS

KEY POINTS

- Arthroscopic bone graft (ABG) and percutaneous fixation is a highly effective minimally invasive technique to achieve high union rate in scaphoid delay union and nonunion.
- Preservation of the blood supply and soft tissue envelop around the scaphoid is the key to success, providing a biologically favorable environment to enhance healing.
- In contrast to the conventional open surgery, the more proximal the nonunion site is, the more technically appealing the procedure is.
- The presence of proximal fragment ischemia and humpback and DISI deformities are not contraindications, although nonunion with poor blood supply of the proximal pole has higher tendency of persistent nonunion.
- The use of multiple K-wires to fix the nonunion is technically less demanding and does not compromise the outcome comparing the use of compression screws.

PANEL 1
Case Scenario 1

A 43-year-old male right-handed salesman, a non-smoker, presented with acute left radial sided wrist pain after a fall during a football match. Examination revealed swelling and tenderness over the anatomical snuffbox region of the left wrist. Radiographs showed a chronic nonunion of the left scaphoid at the proximal third region. There was marked sclerosis at the nonunion site with minimal cystic change. The scaphoid appeared shortened without sclerotic change of the proximal pole. There was minimal arthritic change at the radiocarpal and midcarpal joint. The patient recalled a history of significant fall on his left outstretched hand 25 years ago during another football match, although he had been asymptomatic all along. Magnetic resonance imaging showed no evidence of avascular necrosis. There was mild dorsal intercalated segment instability (DISI) deformity, generalized cartilage thinning, and synovitis compatible with early scaphoid nonunion advanced collapse wrist change (Fig. 35.1). He was treated with a wrist splint for 3 months but without significant improvement in pain. He was keen on surgical reconstruction. What is the additional value of arthroscopy for the diagnostic work-up or treatment of this scaphoid nonunion?

IMPORTANCE OF THE PROBLEM

Scaphoid nonunion continues to present a unique clinical challenge. Natural history studies by Mark,[1] Ruby,[2] and Linstrom and Nystrom[3] et al. demonstrated an almost 100% incidence of radiographic wrist arthritis between 5 and 20 years after scaphoid nonunion in symptomatic patients. As most scaphoid nonunions happen in young and active individuals, the development of SNAC (scaphoid nonunion advanced collapse) changes poses a significant threat to their normal wrist and upper limb function. Timely surgical intervention, by anatomic restoration of a stable scaphoid architecture and its linkage to adjacent bones, is the goal before arthritis sets in.

Conventional Bone Grafting

Numerous techniques have been reported to heal a scaphoid nonunion. Nagle[4] summarized the essence of surgical principles: correction of scaphoid malalignment, debridement of necrotic bone and scar tissue, exposure of healthy, well-vascularized cancellous scaphoid bone (if available), bone grafting (either cancellous or corticocancellous), and stabilization of the scaphoid with internal fixation or an intrinsically stable

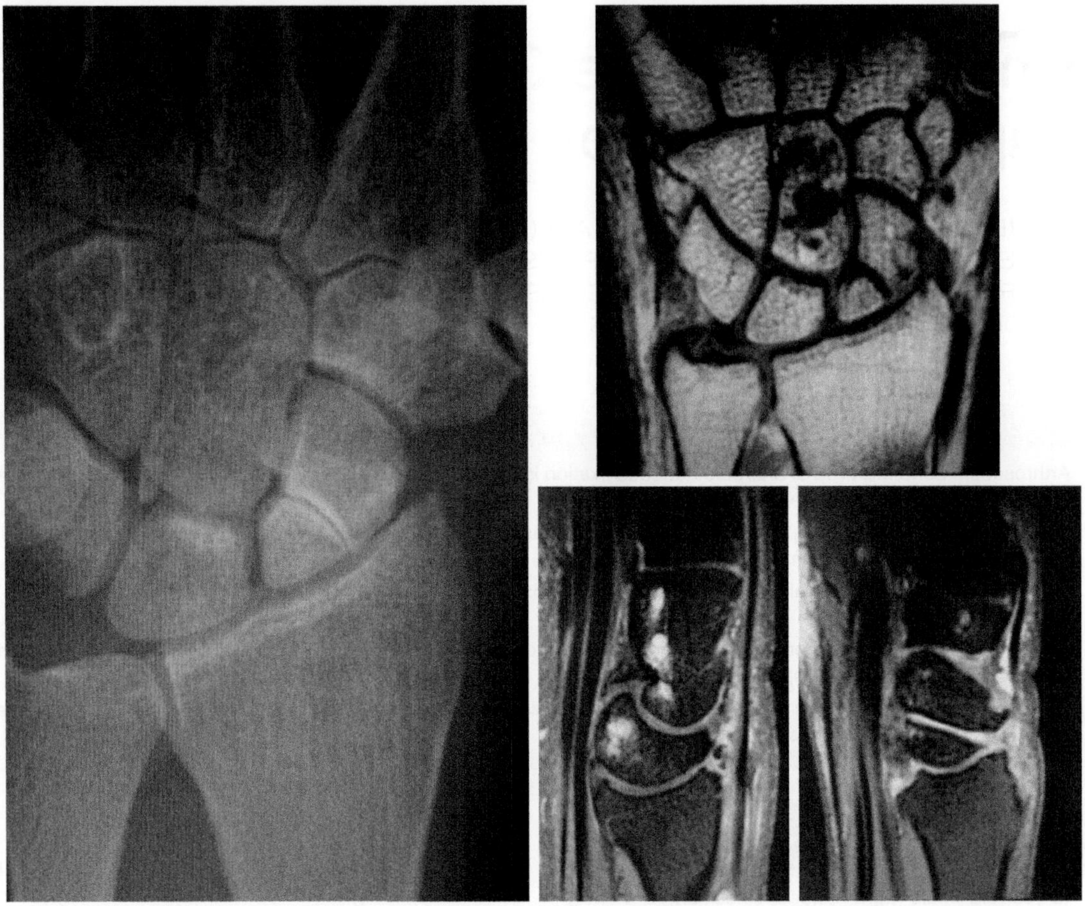

FIG. 35.1 Radiographs and MRI images showed a chronic nonunion of the left scaphoid at the proximal third region, with mild dorsal intercalated segment instability deformity, generalized cartilage thinning, and synovitis compatible with early scaphoid nonunion advanced collapse wrist change.

corticocancellous bone graft. Conventional techniques utilize either corticocancellous[5] or cancellous bone graft such as the inlay grafting by Russe[6] for scaphoid nonunion. In the last decades, various techniques of vascularized bone grafting were also introduced and mainly reserved for salvage procedure of failed surgical treatment of scaphoid nonunion. Although the literature has reported variable but somewhat good results on open grafting procedure with union rate ranging from 55% to 95%,[7–9] potential problems do exist.

The wrist joint has complicated ligamentous structures and bony architecture with precarious blood supply. Surgical dissection in such limited joint space would potentially create damage to the capsular structures and hence lead to increased stiffness of wrist and hand. Additional surgical trauma may also jeopardize the blood supply to the carpal bones. In 2004, Munk & Larsen et al. conducted a systematic review on bone grafting for scaphoid nonunion in 147 publications including 5246 cases.[10] They reviewed the literature from 1928 to 2003 for union rates, postoperative immobilization periods, and complications of the different bone grafting procedures. The outcomes were evaluated in three treatment groups. In the first group involving nonvascularized bone grafting without internal fixation, they found a union rate of 80% (95% confidence interval [CI]: 78–82) after an average immobilization period of 15 weeks. In the second group involving nonvascularized bone grafting with internal fixation, the figures were 84% (CI: 82–85) and 7 weeks, respectively. In the last group involving vascularized bone grafting with or without internal fixation, the figures were 91%

(CI: 87–94) and 10 weeks, respectively. There was no prospective randomized study comparing different treatment options. They concluded that there still was a need for improvement in the treatment of scaphoid nonunion.

Arthroscopic Bone Graft—A Novel Concept and Technique

The accumulated experience on wrist arthroscopy over the past 30 years has shed light on a possible alternative surgical approach to the diseased scaphoid. The scaphoid is well covered with articular cartilage in over 50% of its surface area. Its entire intraarticular location allows an arthroscopic approach for both evaluation and therapeutic intervention with maximal preservation of the blood supply and ligamentous architecture and thus potentially favors union and functional restoration. In the midcarpal joint, the gentle curvature of the waist and proximal portion of the scaphoid enables a fairly stable and spacious platform for the surgeon to carry out the necessary bone works in fixing a scaphoid nonunion.

MAIN QUESTION

What is the additional value of arthroscopic bone grafting for scaphoid nonunion?

Current Opinion

Arthroscopic approach can reduce potential morbidity associated with an open arthrotomy, such as pain and stiffness, maximally preserve blood supply to carpal bone for improved healing, and create minimal disturbance to the ligamentous structures. A comprehensive assessment of the wrist joint and evaluation of any concomitant intraarticular pathology and associated degenerative changes can also be carried out prior to the definitive treatment of the nonunion at the same setting. The latter changes can significantly affect the logical choice of treatment for the nonunion, its prognosis, and the surgical outcome. Moreover, arthroscopic surgery differs from the conventional open surgery that tourniquet and bloodless field is often not necessary during most parts of the surgical procedure. It thus renders the assessment of the vascularity of the scaphoid nonunion fragments more accurate and reliable. The fracture can be fixed with minimally invasive surgical methods such as percutaneous screw or multiple K-wires. Based on these sound surgical principles and the potential advantages, the senior author (Pak-cheong Ho) has developed a novel technique of arthroscopic bone grafting and percutaneous fixation of the fracture since 1997. It has become the authors' standard primary treatment in all scaphoid delayed union and nonunion.

PANEL 2
Case Scenario 1 (Continued)

A diagnostic wrist arthroscopy under wide-awake portal site local anesthesia was performed to evaluate the wrist condition. At the radiocarpal joint, the fracture was seen communicating with the midcarpal joint with a positive drive-through sign. Eburnation of cartilage was noted in the radial styloid (Fig. 35.2). The rest of the scaphoid fossa was good. The cartilage surface of both proximal and distal fragment of the scaphoid was healthy looking. There was a 2-mm central perforation of the TFCC. At the midcarpal joint, a complete nonunion of the scaphoid with markedly sclerotic surfaces was noted at the proximal third (Fig. 35.3). The nonunion was mobile with no fibrous tissue interposition. All cartilage surfaces were well maintained except a stable chondral fragment adhering to the lunotriquetral junction indicating an old injury. Thus a SNAC wrist of stage I was diagnosed and confirmed. The patient was offered the treatment of arthroscopic bone graft, percutaneous fixation, and arthroscopic radial styloidectomy.

The operation was performed under general anesthesia on June 13, 2012. The arm tourniquet was not inflated. Wrist arthroscopy was performed with a 2.7-mm arthroscope. Synovectomy and joint debridement was performed at the radiocarpal joint. The sclerotic surfaces of the nonunion were debrided at the midcarpal joint using a 2.9-mm arthroscopic burr until the healthy cancellous bone was exposed. Vascularity of the distal fragment was good with profuse bleeding. Bleeding from the proximal fragment was fair and punctate looking (Fig. 35.4). A size 6 Foley catheter was inserted into the radioscaphoid joint through the 3–4 portal, being inflated to occupy the space to prevent subsequent spillage of the bone graft (Fig. 35.5). The hand was brought down to the hand table. Under an image intensifier, reduction of the DISI deformity was then carried out using the Linscheid maneuver. The radiolunate joint was transfixed with a 1.6-mm K-wire inserted percutaneously from dorsal distal radius through a mini-incision. In this regard, the proximal scaphoid was then well aligned with the distal radius. Traction and manipulation by gentle passive ulnar deviation, hypersupination, and extension of the wrist was carried out to realign the distal fragment with the proximal one and to restore the length and alignment of the scaphoid. The fracture was then transfixed with a single 1.1-mm K-wire inserted percutaneously at the scaphoid tubercle. The arthroscope was reinserted into the midcarpal ulnar (MCU) portal to perform the arthroscopic bone grafting. Cancellous chip graft harvested from the iliac crest was delivered and

Continued

PANEL 2
Case Scenario 1 (Continued)—cont'd

densely packed into the fracture site through a 4.5-mm arthroscopic cannula inserted at the midcarpal radial (MCR) portal. The graft was directed to fill up all the dead spaces in between the fracture fragments (Fig. 35.6). Fibrin glue was injected at the end to stabilize the bone graft and to protect the articular surface. Fixation was completed by inserting two additional K-wires (Fig. 35.7). Wounds were apposed with steristrips and the wrist was protected with a below-elbow plaster slab (Fig. 35.8).

Early active mobilization was initiated 2 weeks after the procedure when the radiolunate pin was removed at clinic follow-up. He resumed his work at 4 weeks postoperation. At 7 weeks, he attained 50 degrees of extension, 40 degrees of flexion, 10 degrees of radial deviation, and 30 degrees of ulnar deviation of his left wrist (Fig. 35.9). At 10 weeks, bone union was apparent at CT scan and fluoroscopic assessment. The buried K-wires were removed under local anesthesia (Fig. 35.10). He received physiotherapy to enhance the wrist mobility and strength. On the latest follow-up at 2 years 3 months, he had no pain and had resumed his football hobby. Wrist performance score was 40 of 40 and pain score at 0 over 20. The wrist flexion extension arc was 85.2% and radioulnar deviation was 107.5% of the unaffected side (Fig. 35.11). Grip power was 95% of the opposite hand. The surgical scars were inconspicuous. X-ray and CT scan showed complete consolidation of the nonunion. Radiocarpal and midcarpal joint space were normal. The scaphoid alignment was good with anteroposterior intrascaphoid angle at 35 degrees and the scapholunate angle at 60 degrees (Fig. 35.12). The patient was very satisfied with the outcome.

Finding the Evidence

- Cochrane search: Scaphoid Fracture
- Pubmed (Medline): ("Scaphoid Bone" [Mesh] OR scaphoid fracture*[tiab] OR scaphoid bone Fracture*[tiab] OR scaphoid[tiab]) AND (arthroscop*)
- Bibliography of eligible articles
- Articles that were not in English were excluded

Quality of the Evidence

Level II:

Prospective cohort: 1

Level IV:

Case series: 7

FINDINGS

As arthroscopic bone grafting is a recent breakthrough in the history of arthroscopic surgery, the evidence is limited to a few small case series, all consistent in their good outcomes and high rates of union. While reviewing and discussing all reported series, the authors have opted to focus mainly on their personal series (and technical experience) for its originality and it is the largest to date.

Authors' Case Series

This series included 58 established symptomatic nonunion and 11 delayed union cases treated from April 1997 to November 2009. Nonunion was defined as failure of sign of healing in 4 months or more postinjury, whereas delayed union was defined as poor healing in fracture of less than 4 months of duration with or without cystic change and bony resorption at the fracture site. There were 65 male and 4 female patients, with an average age of 27.6 years (range 14–53 years) at the time of surgery. All patients presented with wrist pain, stiffness, and disturbance to their daily activities and works. Sixty-five patients were right hand dominant. The affected side was left wrist in 32 patients and right wrist in 37 patients. The median duration of the pathology was 10 months (range 4–276 months) in the nonunion group and 1.5 months (range 1–3 months) in the delayed union group. 41 patients were manual workers and 28 were sedentary workers. In 42 patients (60.9%), the original injury was sport related. Thirteen patients (18.8%) were injured on duty. Twenty-eight (40.6%) patients were chronic smokers. There were 10 distal third, 31 midthird, and 28 proximal third fractures. Seven cases had received previous surgeries for scaphoid fracture or nonunion but the fractures refused to heal. These included three cases of open reduction and screw fixation and four cases of closed reduction and percutaneous screw fixation for an acute fracture. Sixteen cases (23.2%) had evidence of avascular necrosis demonstrated on radiographs, CT scan or MRI, among which seven were proximal and nine were midwaist. Twenty cases (29%), including nine proximal, nine midwaist, and two distal third nonunion showed DISI deformity radiologically. Two patients had secondary arthritic changes, including one stage I and one stage II SNAC wrist changes on radiographs.

All patients were assessed by an occupational therapist before the index procedures, during, and at the final follow-up. The range of motion of the wrist, grip power, wrist functional performance score, pain score, and return to work status were charted. The wrist functional performance score developed by our hospital was modeled on the findings of D.L. Nelson.[11] It consists of 10 common standardized tasks of activities of daily living (ADL) to be performed by the patient under the scrutiny of an occupational therapist[12,13] (Table 35.1). The performance on each task was rated by the therapist according to a four-point scale, giving a maximum

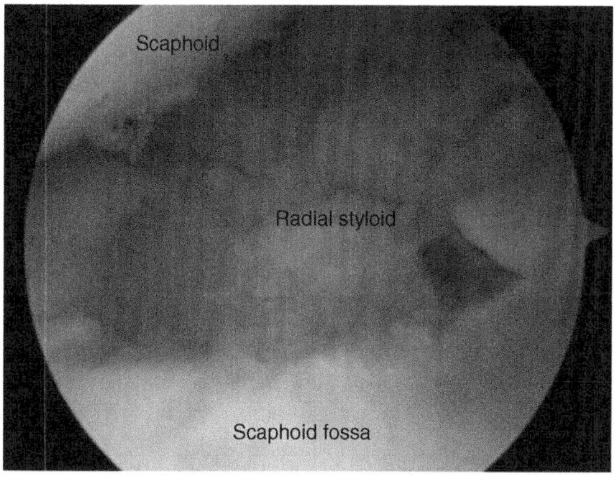

FIG. 35.2 Radiocarpal joint arthroscopy showing eburnation of cartilage at the radial styloid.

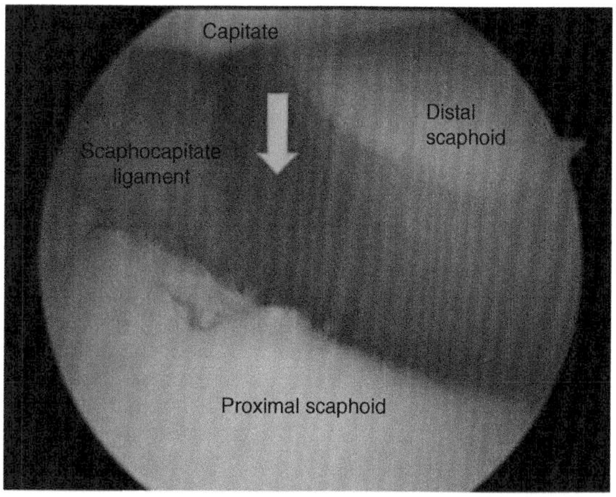

FIG. 35.3 Midcarpal arthroscopy showing a complete nonunion of the scaphoid with markedly sclerotic surface noted at the proximal third.

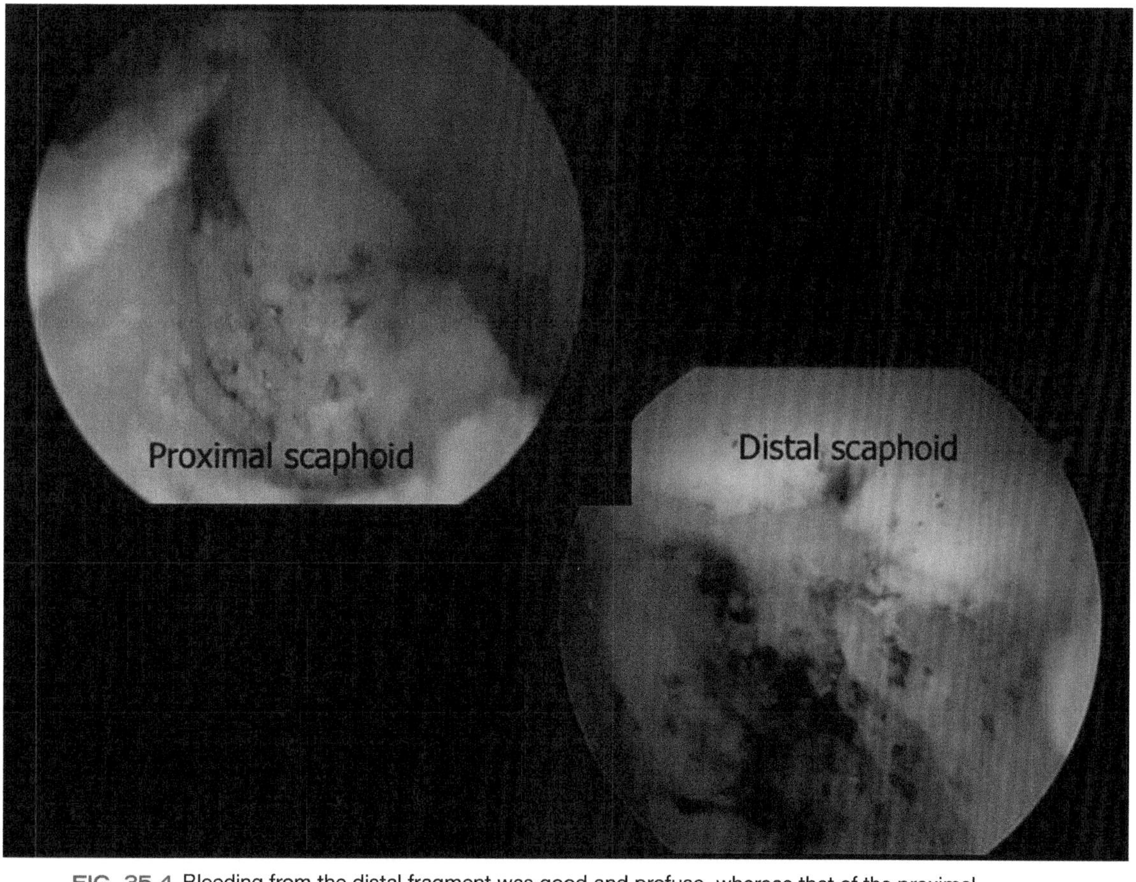

FIG. 35.4 Bleeding from the distal fragment was good and profuse, whereas that of the proximal fragment was fair and punctate looking.

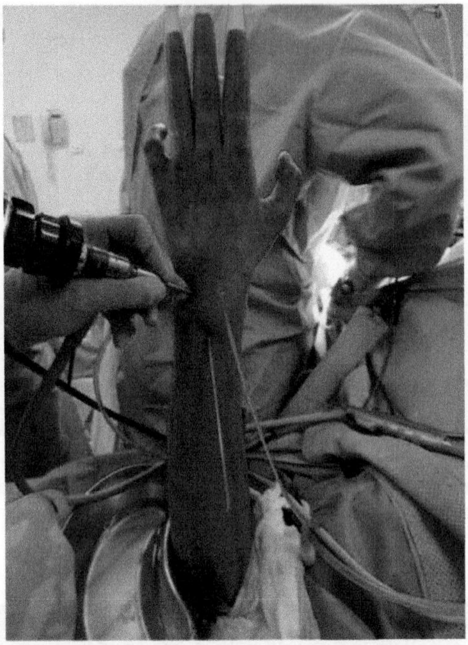

FIG. 35.5 A Foley catheter was inserted into the radioscaphoid joint through the 3–4 portal for blocking of bone graft migration.

total of 40 for a normal performance of the complete test (Table 35.2). A pain score of a three-point scale was rated by the patient according to the pain level perceived during the performance of each ADL task. The total score ranged from zero to a maximum pain level of 20 points (Table 35.3). Postoperative radiographs and CT scan were used at intervals to monitor bony union, degenerative changes and to measure the alignment of scaphoid, including scapholunate (SL) angle and anteroposterior intrascaphoid angle.

Surgical Technique

The patient is put in supine position while the operated arm is supported on a hand table. Either side of the iliac crest region is draped for bone graft harvesting depending on the patient's preference. An arm tourniquet is applied but need not be inflated unless necessary. Vertical traction of 4–6 kg force is applied through plastic finger trap devices to the middle three fingers for joint distraction. This can be achieved by using either wrist traction tower or overhead boom with balanced pulley system. We employ continuous saline irrigation and distension of the joint by using 3-L bag of normal saline solution instilled with aid of gravity. Infusion pump is not necessarily and potentially harmful in causing extravasation of fluid.

Arthroscopic Surveillance

Adrenaline 1 in 200,000 dilution is injected in the portal site skin and capsule to reduce bleeding. We perform a routine inspection of both the radiocarpal joint through the 3–4 portal and the midcarpal joint through the MCR portal using a 1.9-mm arthroscope. Any accompanying chondral lesion related to SNAC wrist changes should be documented because it may affect the prognosis and choice of procedure. The dorsal rim of the radial styloid is a common site of occurrence of early SNAC wrist changes and should be assessed in all cases, best observed with the arthroscope inserted from the 4–5 portal. Frequently the associated synovitis in this area may obscure the observation of the cartilage condition. This synovial growth needs to be eliminated by using a 2.0-mm shavers or radiofrequency probe inserted from 3–4 portal. Typically the fracture site cannot be seen from the radiocarpal joint unless it is very proximal. It is frequently embedded within the reflection of radiocarpal joint capsule. This capsular reflection helps to contain the bone graft, which is implanted through the midcarpal joint from a distal to proximal direction. We perform bone grafting through the midcarpal joint portals in all cases because it provides the most convenient and direct approach to the nonunion site.

Takedown of Nonunion

At the midcarpal joint, we generally select MCU portal as the entry portal and MCR as the working portal. The MCR portal can be more narrow and tight as a result of capsular contracture secondary to scaphoid nonunion. The MCU portal is the one that is more easy to approach initially as the ulnar side of the midcarpal joint is usually more normal. The MCR portal is however the best portal to takedown the fibrosis around the nonunion in the proximal and waist portion. In distal third nonunion, the scapho-trapezio-trapezoid (STT) portal is frequently required to provide a more direct access. The nonunion site is located by the presence of cleavage line in the scaphoid articular surface or with frank articular cartilage disruption and fibrous tissue interposition (Fig. 35.13).

The firmness of the fibrous interposition should be assessed carefully by direct palpation with a small probe inserted from the MCR portal. A stable firm fibrous fixation explains the relative lack of symptoms in some patients with radiologic nonunion. In delayed union, the fibrous tissue may cover the bridging callus, which usually forms in the central part of the fracture. If stable bony tissue is encountered after initial debridement of the overlying fibrous tissue, one may

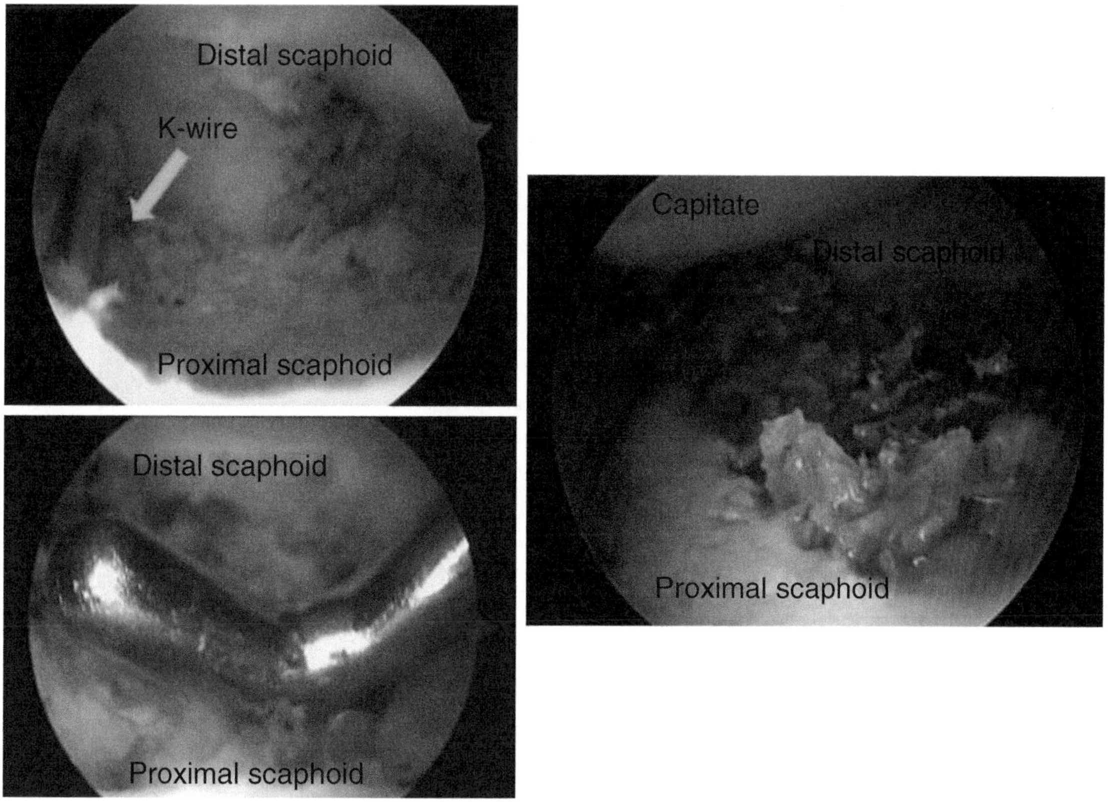

FIG. 35.6 Cancellous bone graft was being directed through a cannula to fill up the dead spaces in between the fracture fragments. The green arrow indicates the K wire transfixing the two bony fragments.

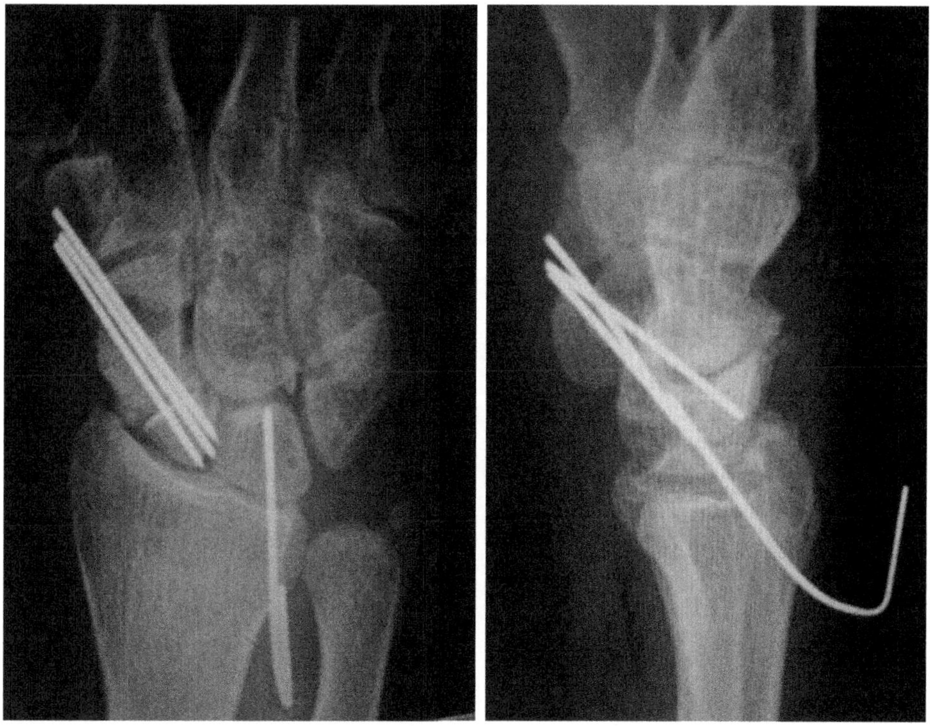

FIG. 35.7 Fracture fixation was achieved with three K-wires of 1.1 mm. Noted the radiolunate pin was being used to correct the dorsal intercalated segment instability deformity.

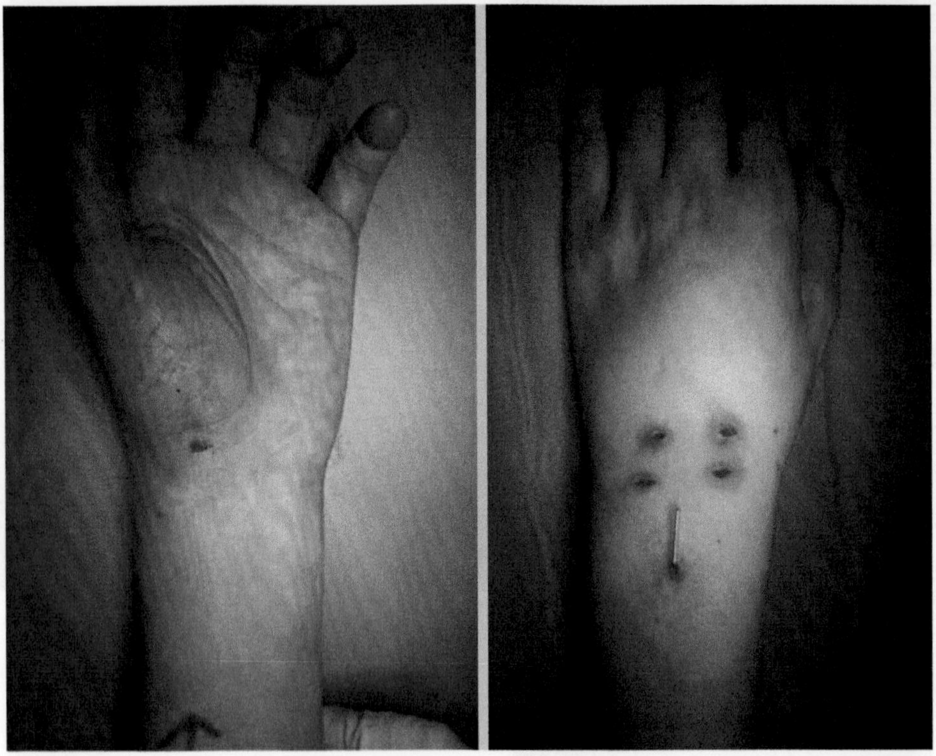

FIG. 35.8 The typical small incisions of the surgery. The radiolunate pin was exposed to be removed at 2 weeks postop at clinic.

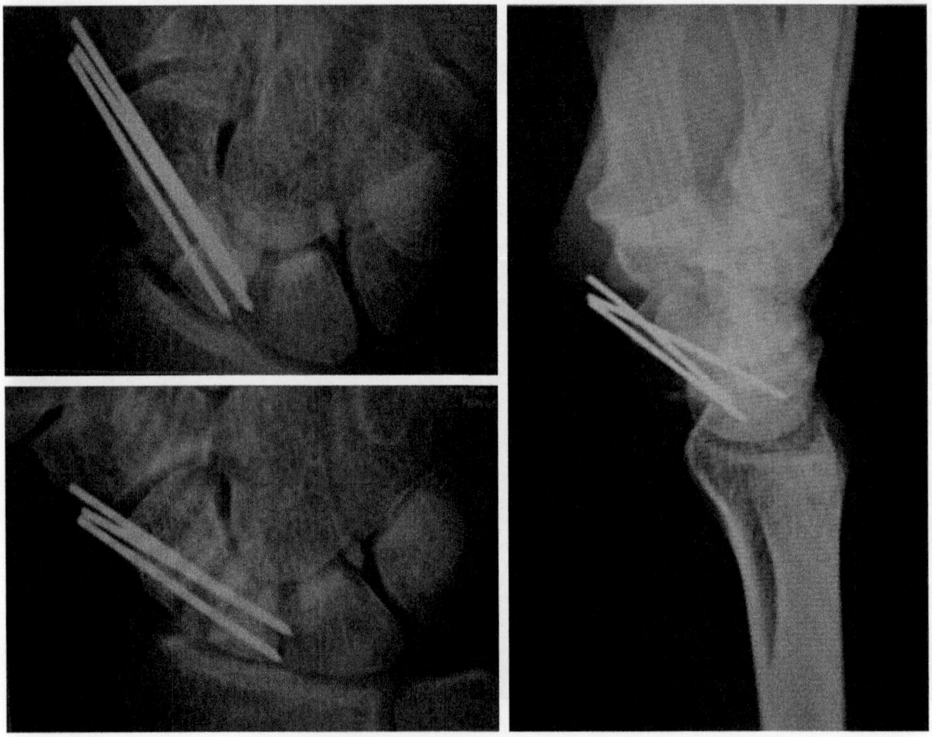

FIG. 35.9 Radiographs at 7 weeks postop.

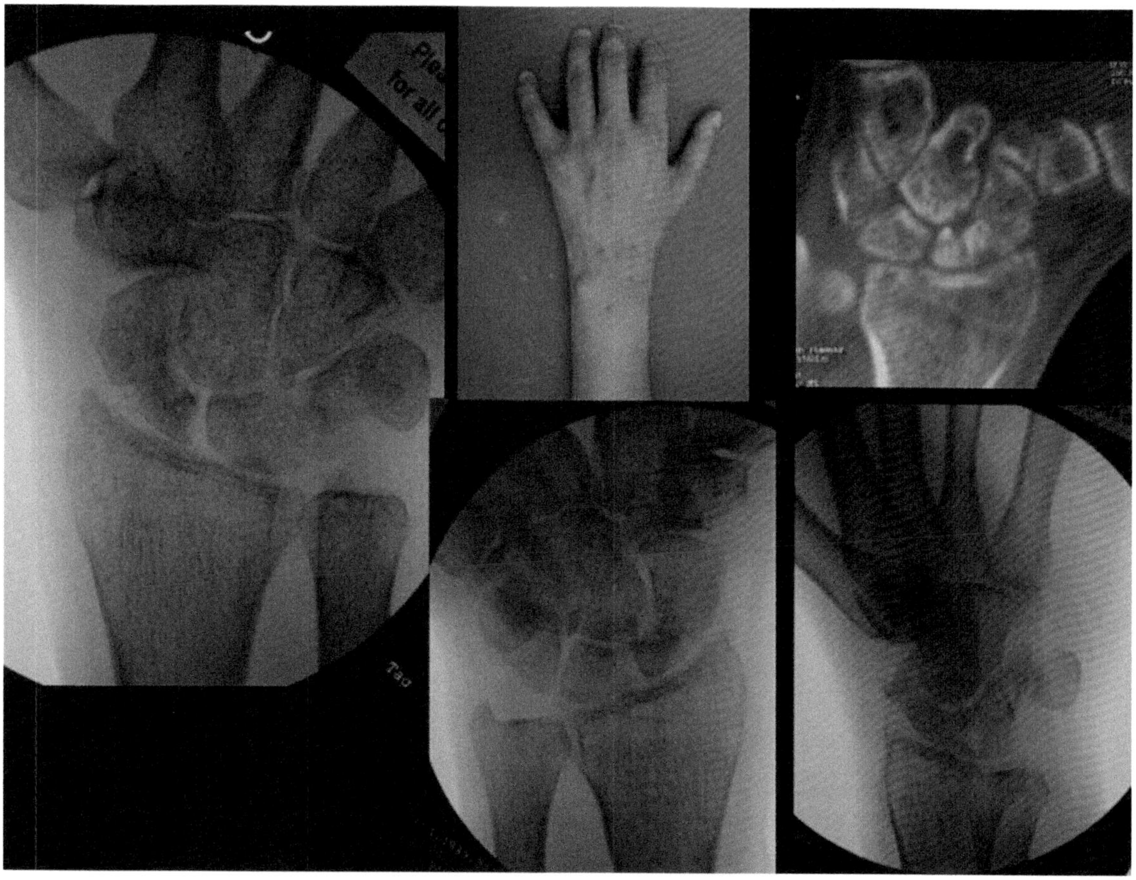

FIG. 35.10 Clinical and radiologic union obtained at 10 weeks postop.

reconsider whether bone grafting is needed, as this may represent an ongoing healing process. A simple screw fixation or even casting may suffice. If a frank bony defect is encountered, curettage of the nonunion site can be performed with a fine-angled curette, motorized 2.0- or 2.9-mm shaver, and 2.9-mm burr until all the fibrous scar tissue and sclerotic bone are removed. A loosened screw should be removed at this junction to facilitate a thorough debridement of the nonunion site. The frequently intact cartilage over the proximal side of the nonunion or any pseudocapsule formed should be preserved as much as possible to avoid subsequent graft spillage to the radiocarpal joint. Both ends of the nonunion are burred until cancellous bone with or without punctate bleeding is reached (Fig. 35.14). We find it unnecessary to inflate the tourniquet during this procedure, which helps to determine the vascularity of the remaining bone fragments more accurately. A better view of the proximal fragment can be obtained by changing the entry portal to MCR. Further curettage of the proximal fragment can be performed by switching the instrument to the STT portal if necessary. If bleeding is not obvious or uncertain, the saline irrigation can be stopped temporarily to reduce the hydrostatic pressure inside the joint to encourage bleeding from the flimsy blood vessels.

Correction of Humpback Deformity

After adequate debridement and curettage, the two fragments of the nonunion should be mobile enough for subsequent reduction. Any humpback or DISI deformity should be identified and corrected (Fig. 35.15).

1. Correction of the deformity can be facilitated by using the Linscheid maneuver. In the presence of intact SL ligament, dorsiflexion deformity of the proximal pole of scaphoid is corrected by firstly passive wrist flexion to realign the extended lunate with the radius (i.e., to restore the normal radiolunate [RL] angle).

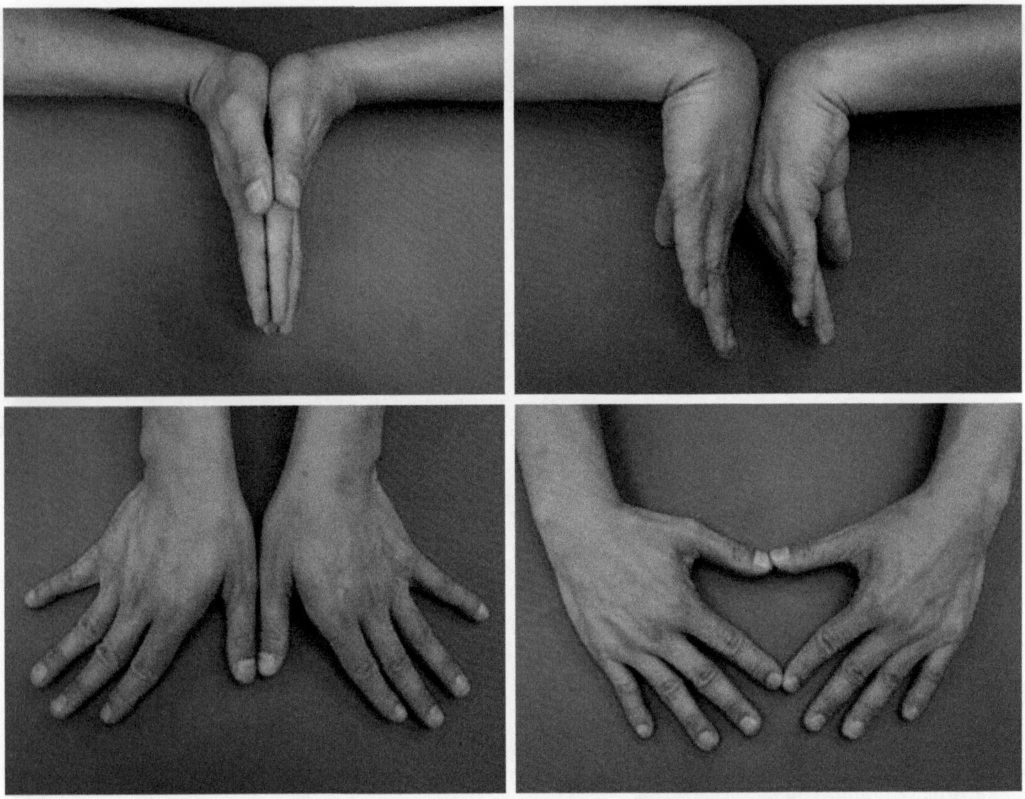

FIG. 35.11 Satisfactory clinical outcome at 2 years 3 months postop.

The RL joint is then temporarily transfixed with a percutaneous 1.6-mm K-wire inserted from dorsal distal radius through a small stab wound (Fig. 35.16). To minimize the risk of entrapping the extensor tendons, we adjust the pneumatic drill to an oscillating mode. Correcting the lunate alignment indirectly improves the extension deformity of the proximal part of scaphoid, provided that the SL ligament is intact.

2. Traction and manipulation by gentle passive ulnar deviation, hypersupination, and extension of the wrist is carried out to realign the distal fragment with the proximal one. A surgical towel row can be placed underneath the operated forearm. With the patient's forearm in full supination, the surgeon can rest his first web space on the patient's first web space. He then grasps and pulls on the patient's thumb and thenar area (Fig. 35.17). This maneuver helps to maintain the wrist in an extended, ulnarly deviated and slightly hypersupinated position, which favors restoration of the normal scaphoid length and alignment.
3. In distal third nonunion where manipulation of the distal fragment is more difficult, a 1.6-mm K-wire can be inserted into the distal fragment of scaphoid as a joystick for a better manipulation.
4. Manipulation of fragment can also be done from within the joint using a probe.

Percutaneous fixation and ABG should only be proceeded when the humpback and DISI deformities can be corrected by a closed technique after appropriate arthroscopic debridement of the nonunion site and an acceptable alignment confirmed with intraoperative fluoroscopy. In any case if the correction of deformity cannot be satisfactorily achieved, one should consider an open reduction and open bone grafting technique.

Once the fracture fragments are well aligned and the humpback deformity corrected, the fragments are provisionally transfixed with a 1.1-mm K-wire inserted percutaneously from the scaphoid tubercle region under image intensifier control. A 3-mm transverse skin incision is made along the skin crease 5 mm distal to the scaphoid tubercle. A small pointed-tip scissor is used to perforate the STT joint, release a hemarthrosis, and dilate

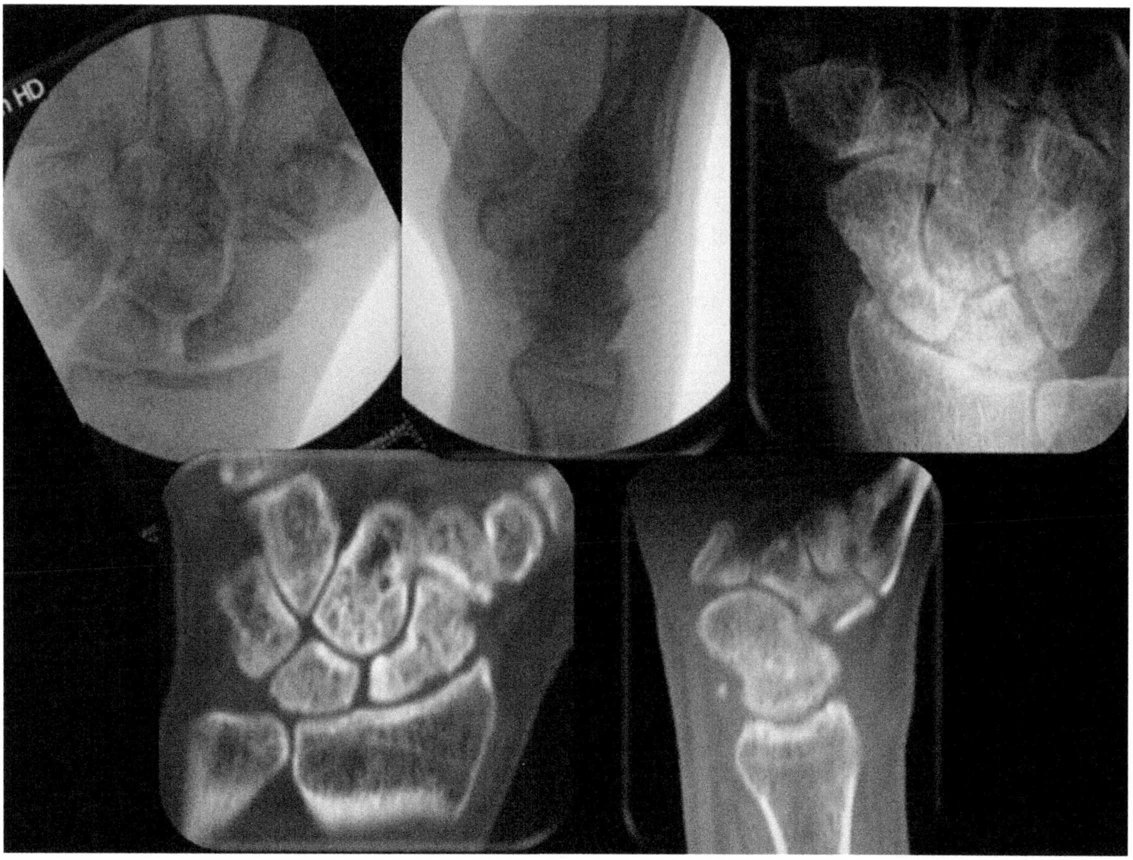

FIG. 35.12 Radiographs and CT scan images showed complete consolidation of the nonunion, good scaphoid alignment, and no arthrosis.

TABLE 35.1
Wrist Functional Performance Score

Tasks	Wrist Motion and Grip Required
Wash back	F, S, Rd, Ud, pinch
Pour water from a full water pot	F, Ud
Open gate	E, S
Open jar lid	Ud, Rd, grasp
Hold a wok	E, S, Ud, grasp
Wring towel	F, E, P, S, Ud, Rd, grasp
Pull out drawer of 7 lbs	S, grasp
Lift weight of 5 lbs	E, Ud, grasp
Write name	E, Ud, pinch
Turn door knob	P, S

E, extension; *F*, flexion; *P*, pronation; *Rd*, radial deviation; *S*, supination; *Ud*, ulnar deviation.

TABLE 35.2
Performance Score

PERFORMANCE SCORE (MAXIMAL TOTAL SCORE = 40)	
4	Can do without difficulty
3	Can do with minimum difficulty or frustration and with satisfactory outcome
2	Can do only with some modification of activity; it is awkward and frustrating
1	Frustrating to do and quality is poor; would stop doing it most of the time
0	Cannot do

TABLE 35.3
Pain Score

PAIN SCORE (MAXIMAL TOTAL SCORE = 20)	
2	Intolerable pain in doing
1	Tolerable pain in doing
0	Pain free in doing

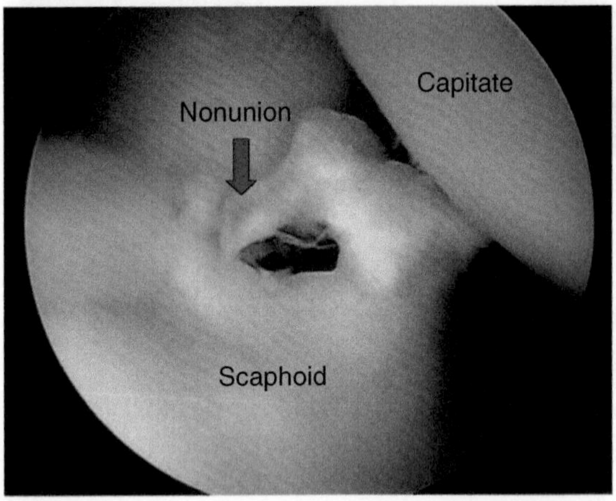

FIG. 35.13 Nonunion site of scaphoid over the waist position as viewed through the midcarpal ulnar portal.

the tract to the starting point on the scaphoid tubercle, which is located along the long axis of scaphoid on the semisupination view and between the middle and radial third of scaphoid tubercle in the AP (anteroposterior) view. A small trough is made with tip of the scissors on the scaphoid tubercle. The K-wire should aim eccentrically at a more radial and proximal location across the nonunion site so that the pin will not interfere with the subsequent procedure of insertion of bone graft

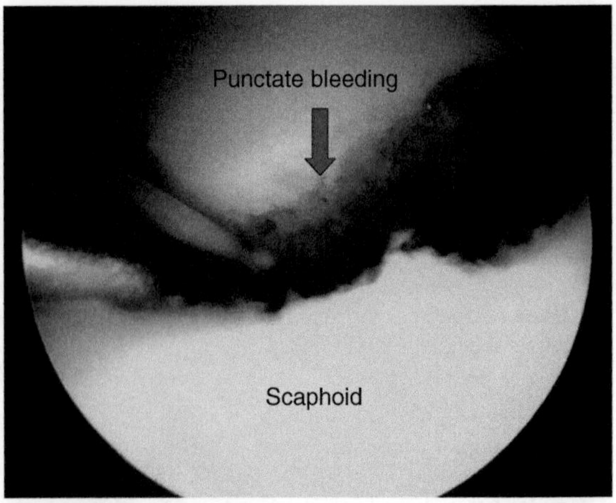

FIG. 35.14 Clear gap at nonunion site and punctate bleeding from cancellous bone over the distal part of the nonunion after initial burring and curettage.

arthroscopically (Fig. 35.18). With the arthroscope viewing from the midcarpal joint, the pin will be situated in a deeper and basal position inside the defect. If the pin is inserted centrally or in a more ulnar and distal manner, the pin will appear more superficial at the midcarpal joint and may block the trocar from pushing the bone graft into the deeper area. When the fixation is complete, the hand can be put back to the traction tower to begin the bone grafting procedure.

Bone Grafting at Midcarpal Joint

An arthroscopic cannula is introduced through an appropriate portal directly opposing the fracture defect. For fractures located at the proximal two-thirds of the scaphoid, the MCR portal is most direct. For distal one-third fractures, the STT portal can be considered. A 3.2-mm cannula can be inserted initially, which is then replaced by a 4.5-mm cannula when the joint space is considerably widened. Cancellous bone graft is harvested from the iliac crest using either a trephine or an open technique through a small incision. The volume of the bone graft obtained has to be at least three to five times that of the defect because the graft needs to be compressed tightly in the defect to increase its compaction and strength. The bone graft is cut into small chips using scissors and delivered through the cannula with a slightly undersized trocar with a flat end such as a bone biopsy trocar (Fig. 35.19). The arm tourniquet can be inflated to enhance the visibility of the graft impaction process.

The most proximal and dorsal parts of the defect need to be meticulously filled up first so as to reduce

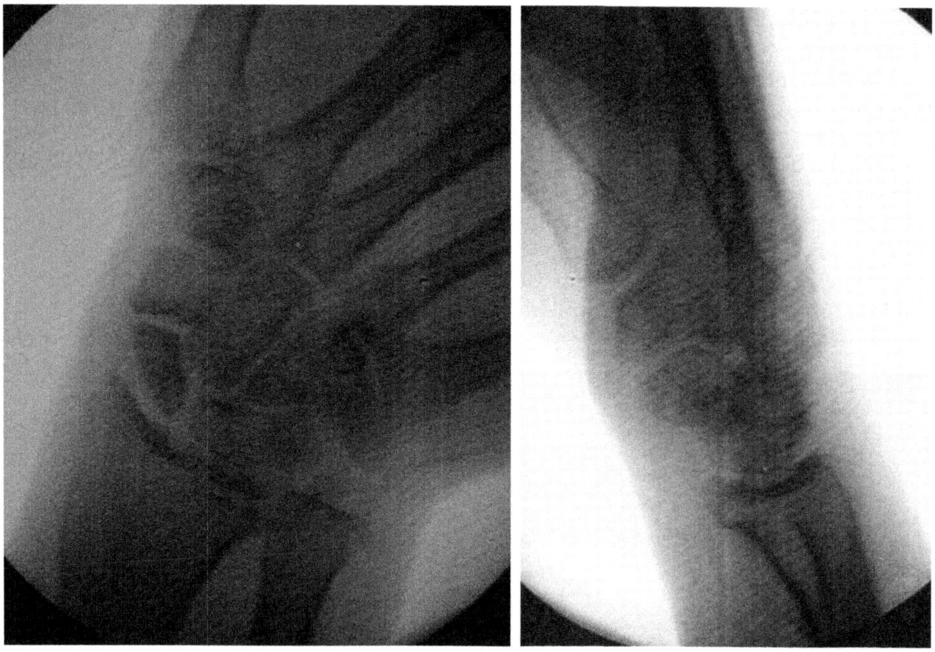

FIG. 35.15 A typical case of scaphoid nonunion with humpback and dorsal intercalated segment instability deformities indicated by the abnormal capitolunate angle.

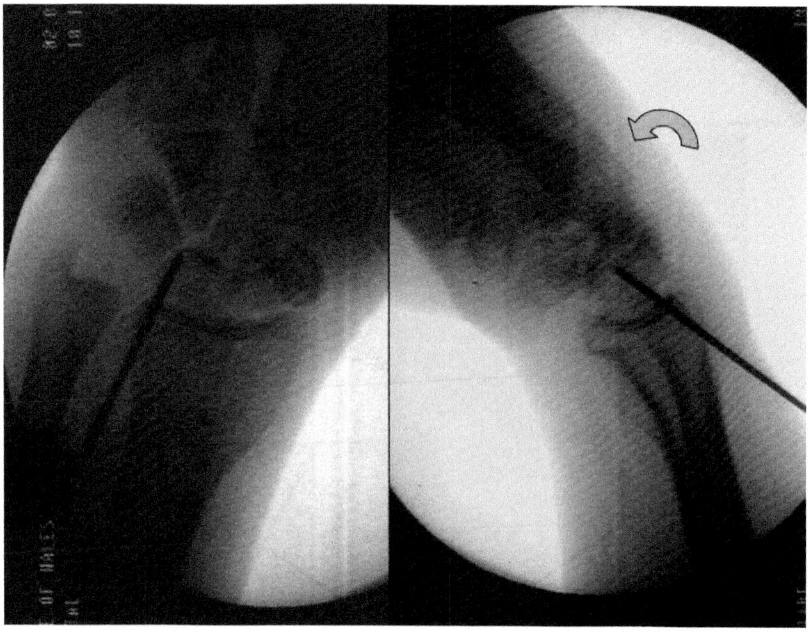

FIG. 35.16 Linscheid maneuver to correct the radiolunate angle and transfixation of the radiolunate joint with one 1.6-mm K-wire. The green arrow indicates that the wrist is flexed passively before the K wire is being inserted across the radiolunate joint.

subsequent void formation (Fig. 35.20). Similarly the empty space previously occupied by a loosen screw should also be filled in first in the process to avoid undergrafting.

In case of very proximal fracture, the nonunion cleavage site is directly communicating with the radiocarpal joint. Filing of the defect with bone graft from the midcarpal joint can result in significant spillage of the graft into the radiocarpal joint. To avoid this undesirable outcome, a pediatric size 6 urinary catheter can be inserted into the radiocarpal joint from the 3–4 portal and insufflated with saline, thereby producing a mechanical block right over the nonunion site to allow the graft to be contained within the bone defect. If the RL joint needs to be transfixed with a K-wire following the Linscheid maneuver for correction of the DISI deformity, the balloon should be inserted first to occupy the radioscaphoid space before the RL joint is reduced and transfixed. Nevertheless, significant humpback and DISI deformities are uncommon in the very proximal nonunion situation.

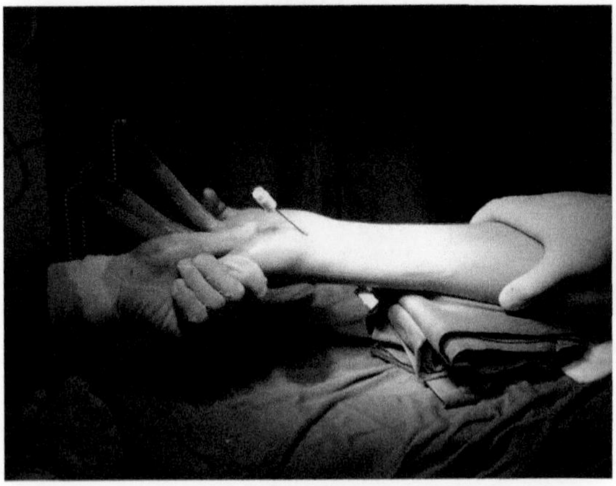

FIG. 35.17 The typical manual reduction maneuver to correctly align the scaphoid fragments before the fixation procedure.

Fluoroscopy is helpful to confirm the completeness and adequacy of the graft filling. A small depressor can be employed at intervals to mold and contour the graft to the articular surface of the scaphoid (Fig. 35.21).

Complete filling of the defect and satisfactory scaphoid alignment is then confirmed fluoroscopically (Fig. 35.22).

At the end of the procedure, we routinely inject 1 mL of fibrin glue on the surface of the graft substance after sucking out any excess fluid to contain the graft in place and to prevent adhesion of the graft to the capitate articular surface, which in some cases may lead to loss of motion at the midcarpal joint.

Routine surveillance of the joint is then carried out to remove any spilled out bone graft material and debris left behind in the midcarpal joint and sometimes in the radiocarpal joint. Release of traction would allow the natural compression effect of the capitate to stabilize the graft and keep it in situ.

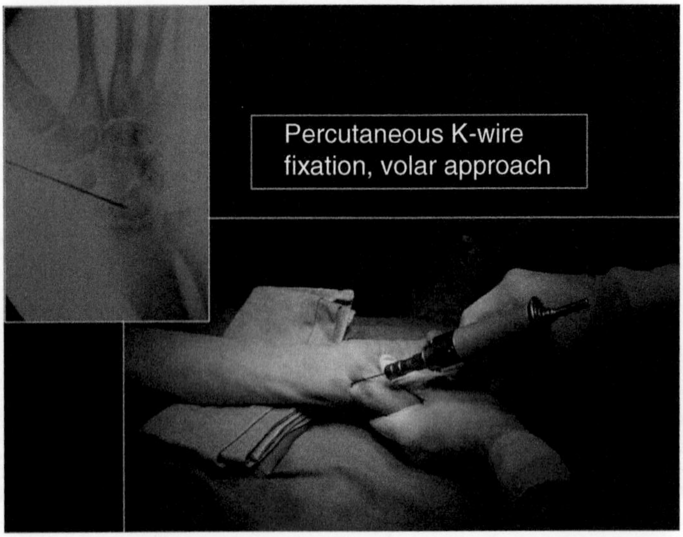

FIG. 35.18 The eccentric position of the first K-wire off the central axis of the scaphoid to align the two fragments.

Definitive fixation can be completed with either a compression screw or additional K-wires as described in the session below.

Percutaneous Screw Fixation

Percutaneous screw fixation is indicated when the nonunion has relatively small bony defect and is located at midwaist when both sides of the nonunion are sizable enough. The patient is placed supine; the arm is abducted 70 degrees and placed on the arm board. Excessive shoulder abduction may cause difficulty in passively pronating the forearm for proper evaluation of the implant position.

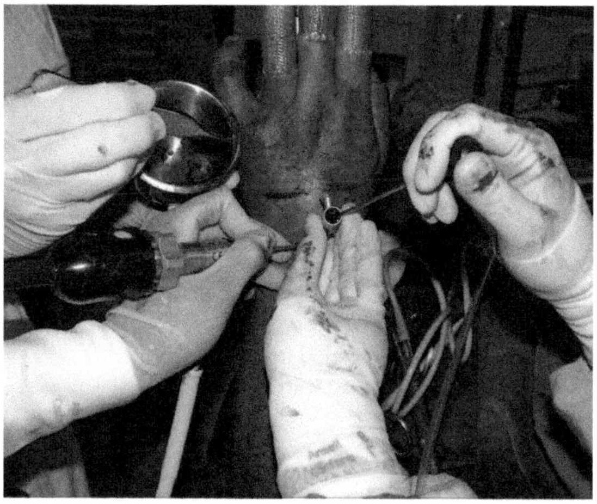

FIG. 35.19 Chip cancellous bone graft was delivered through arthroscopic cannula at the midcarpal radial portal into the nonunion site. The arthroscope was inserted through the midcarpal ulnar portal.

A good-quality fluoroscopy is essential to confirm the fracture alignment and hardware position. Five views are mandatory during the procedure to assess the fracture alignment, guide pin, and screw position. It includes an AP view, lateral view, scaphoid view (AP ulnar deviation), semisupination view, and semipronation view. The semisupination view is used to assess the correct position of the guide pin because this view gives the best spatial relationship of the guide pin with the proximal pole, distal pole, and dorsal and volar border of the scaphoid. For a normal scaphoid, it appears as a bean shape in the semisupination view. We name this the "bean view."[14] The midportion of the "bean" is the sharp turn between the proximal and distal part of scaphoid. The semipronation view demonstrates the longest axis of the scaphoid and the concave inner articulating surface of the scaphoid with capitate.

We routinely used the volar or retrograde approach for percutaneous screw fixation. The correct position of the guide pin determines the screw position. There are several landmarks to guide the entry point and direction of the guide pin.

1. The "bean view" is the most important view to ensure optimal placement of the guide pin, which should pass through the interval between the middle and volar one-third of the bean along its volar border (Fig. 35.23). If the guide pin does not appear to cut out of the scaphoid on the other views, this represents the longest scaphoid length with maximum bone purchase.

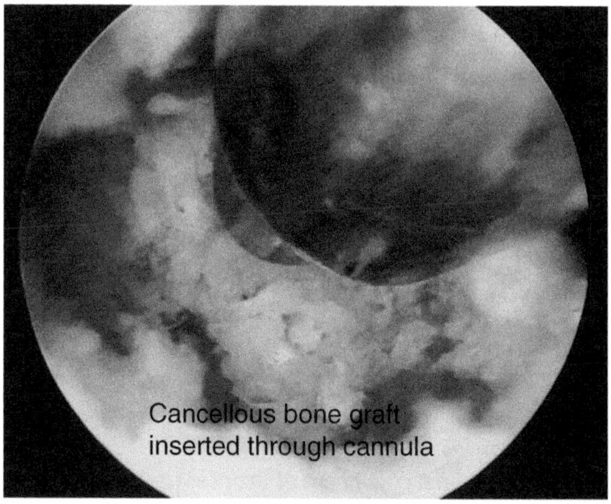

FIG. 35.20 Arthroscopic view of the cancellous graft being delivered into the joint through the cannula.

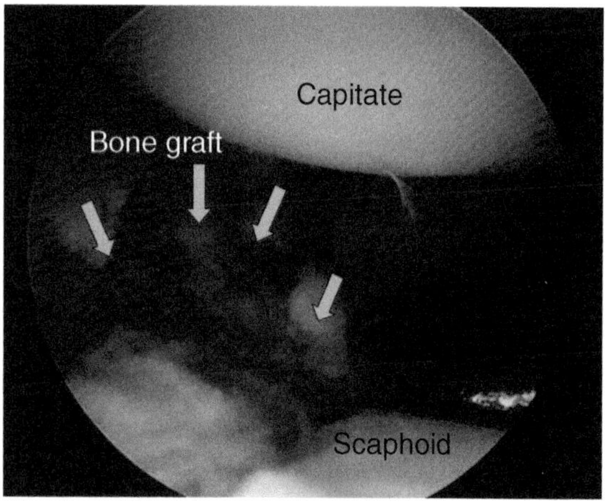

FIG. 35.21 Bone graft was packed and molded to the shape of a scaphoid using a small depressor. The green arrows indicate the bone graft at the nonunion site.

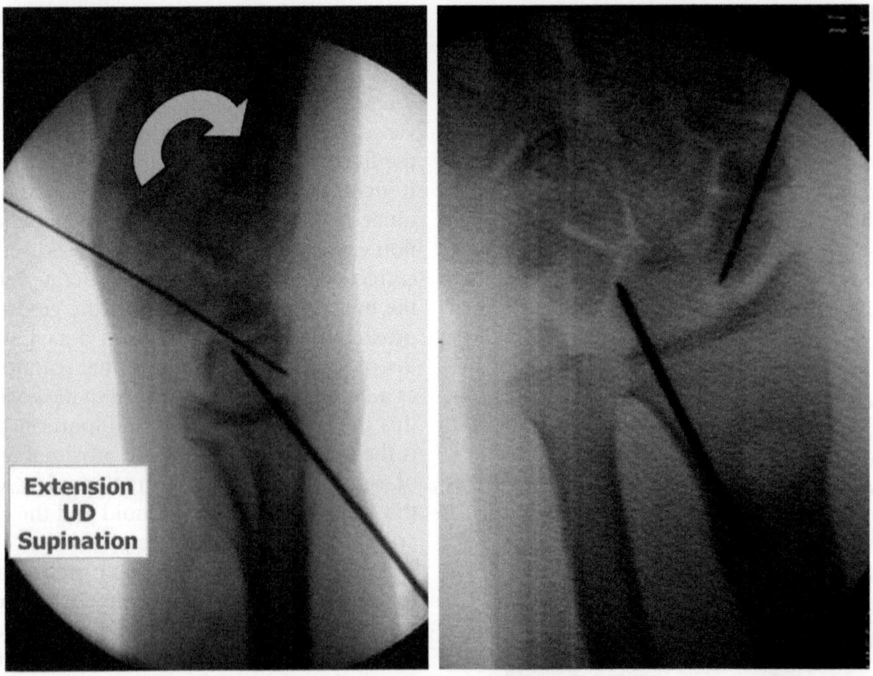

FIG. 35.22 Complete filling of the defect and satisfactory scaphoid alignment. *UD*, ulnar deviation. The green arrow indicates that the wrist is extended passively to realign the distal scaphoid fragment to the proximal one to achieve a good alignment before the fragments are being transfixed with a K wire.

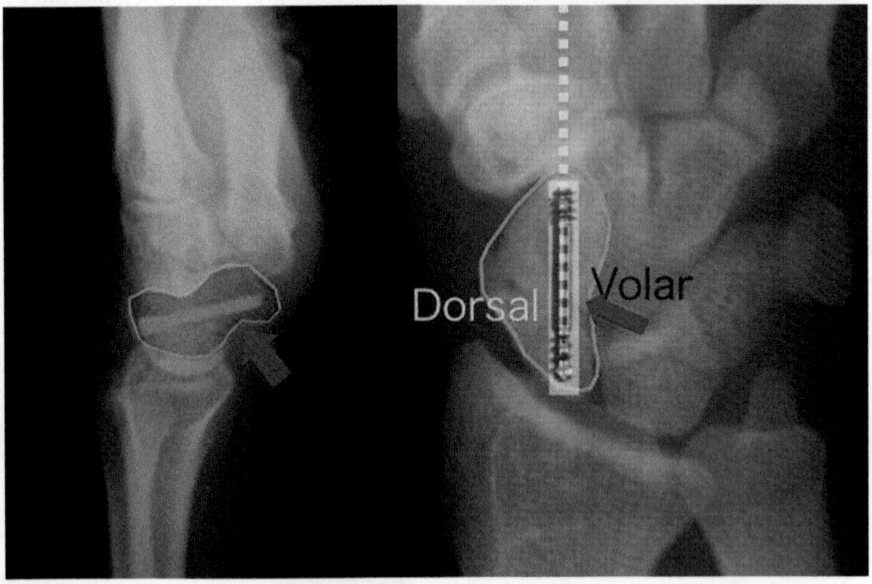

FIG. 35.23 The "bean view" as the most important view to ensure optimal placement of the guide pin. The red arrows indicate the position of the screw in different radiological views of the scaphoid.

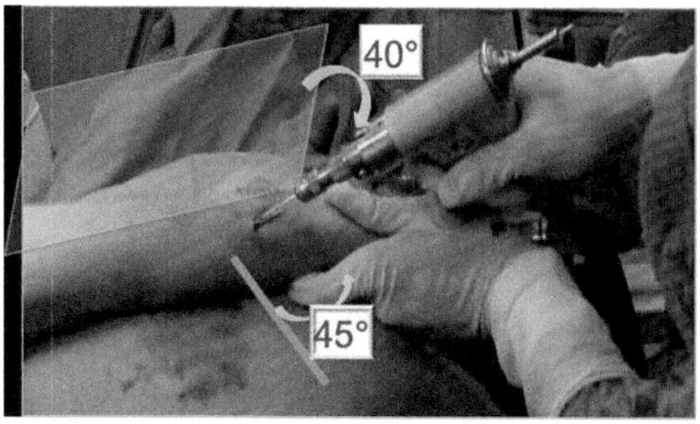

FIG. 35.24 The best angle of insertion of guide pin was 40 degrees to the sagittal plane and 45 degrees to the coronal plane.

2. Hung L.K. advocated tracing the direction of the K-wire on the skin with a marker.[15,16] In the AP view, a K-wire is placed over the skin to produce an overlap image on the scaphoid. A true lateral radiograph is then obtained. The K-wire is again placed over the skin and the position is again marked on the skin. These two lines provide references as to the direction of the guide pin.
3. The best angle of insertion of guide pin is 40 degrees to the sagittal plane and 45 degrees to the coronal plane. The entry point should be between the middle of the scaphoid tubercle, and the exit point should be around the distal half of the proximal pole of the scaphoid (Fig. 35.24). This provides the maximum purchase of the screw but may be modified according to the fracture type and pattern.[15–17]

We employed the same incision used for the provisional fixation to enter the guide pin. The guide pin is aiming 40 degrees in the sagittal plane and 45 degrees in the coronal plane. We find it is easier by aiming the guide pin toward the Lister's tubercle located with the index finger of surgeon's hand. The position should be checked with all five views.

Bone resistance is normally felt when the guide pin approaches the cortex at the exit point. When the guide wire is in a foreshortened position, the exit point is too close to the entry point. This indicates that the pin is directed too dorsally, hitting the dorsal cortex, and away from the long axis of the scaphoid. This erroneous position can easily be judged using the bean's view. This will not provide adequate fracture fixation and should be readjusted.

With the tip of the guide pin at the opposite cortex, the length of the inserted part is measured. The actual screw length should be 4 mm subtracted from this measured pin length to allow for subsequent fracture compression and "sinking" of the screw head at the entry point. The guide pin is advanced further after measurement through the opposite cortex and out of skin and secured in place with an artery forceps. The exit point of the guide pin should always be at the 3–4 portal. Beware not to entrap the extensor tendons.

We have employed the 2.7-mm BOLD cannulated screw for nonunion of the waist. As the bone graft is of cancellous nature, excessive compression should be avoided because this may cause collapse of the nonunion site and loss of the reduction (Fig. 35.25).

Percutaneous Multiple K-Wire Fixation

Multiple K-wires are used for scaphoid nonunion with relatively sizable bony defect and also particularly in proximal and distal one-third nonunion. The method is also indicated for persistent nonunion after previous screw fixation with screw loosening. The use of percutaneous screw under these situations can be too demanding technically to achieve the ideal position and with sufficient bone purchase. Surgical risk such as fragmentation of the nonunion parts or excessive compression force over the bone grafting site causing recurrence humpback deformity will be increased.

We routinely use three 1.1-mm K-wires. Position of the pins needs not be as exact as in guide pin insertion for compression screw. The first pin should aim at more a radial and proximal location across the nonunion site as described before. After bone graft impaction into the nonunion is completed, the remaining two wires can be inserted percutaneously from the same incision. A parallel or convergent placement of the three K-wires is more favorable than divergent placement. Transfixing the SL and scaphocapitate joints can also be considered for an unstable nonunion or in very proximal or distal nonunion (Fig. 35.26). The pins are cut short and buried underneath the skin and are kept in place up to 10–12 weeks. The wound is apposed with steristrips and no stitching is required (Fig. 35.27). The pin over the RL joint is left exposed outside the skin for early removal.

Early Scaphoid Nonunion Advanced Collapse Wrist

In cases with early SNAC changes, involving the radial styloid and distal scaphoid fragment, fixation of the nonunion is not contraindicated, provided that an adequate radial styloidectomy can be done at the same setting to reduce the subsequent impingement (Fig. 35.28–35.31). An advantage of arthroscopic

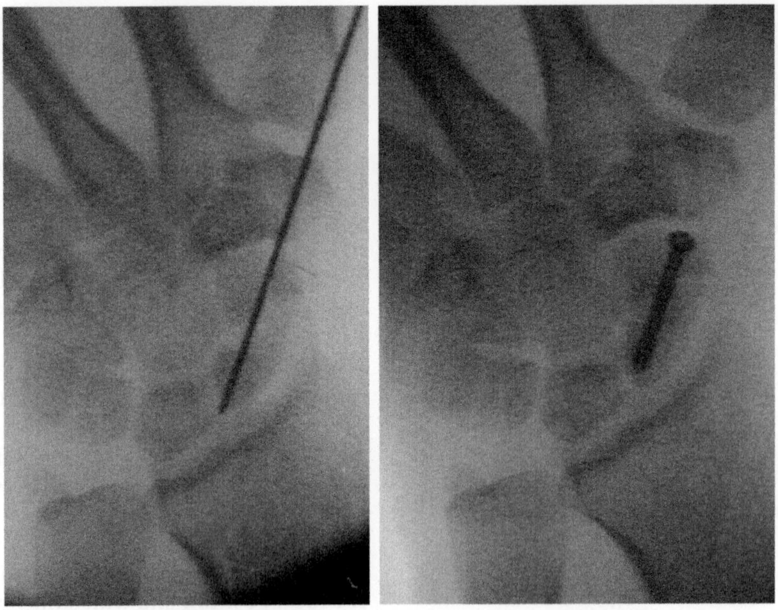

FIG. 35.25 Compression screw fixation of the nonunion.

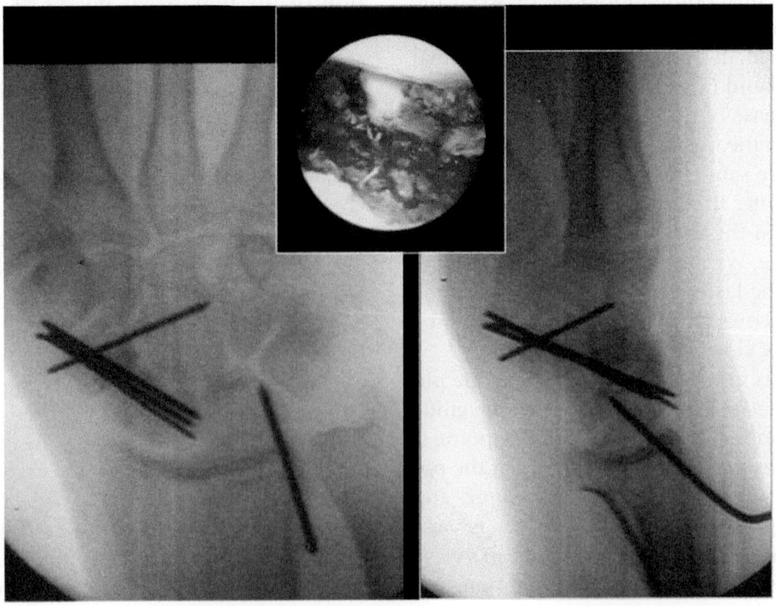

FIG. 35.26 Multiple K-wires fixation of the nonunion.

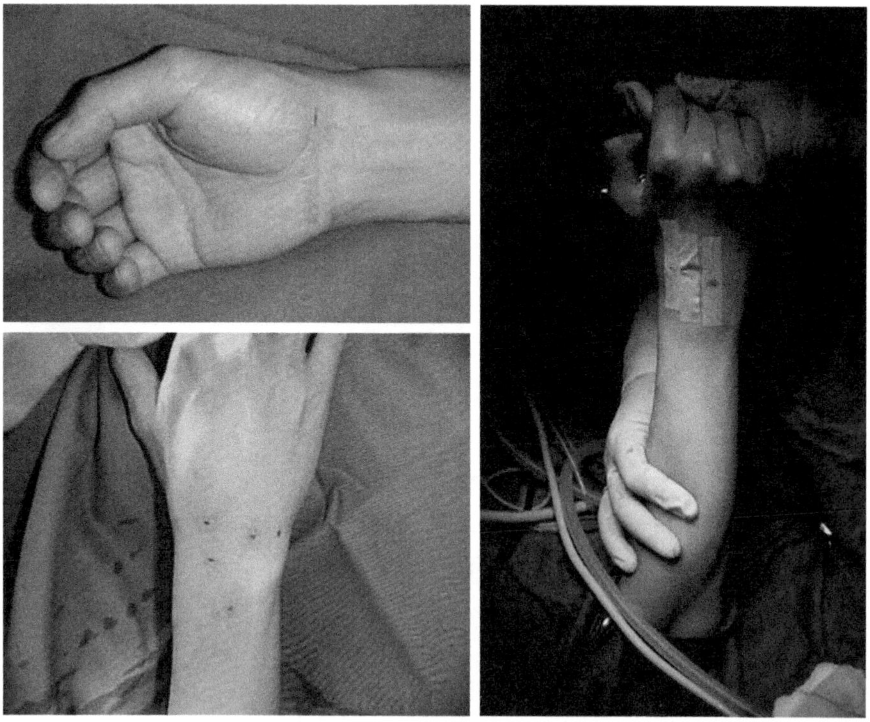

FIG. 35.27 The wounds were apposed with steristrips without stitch.

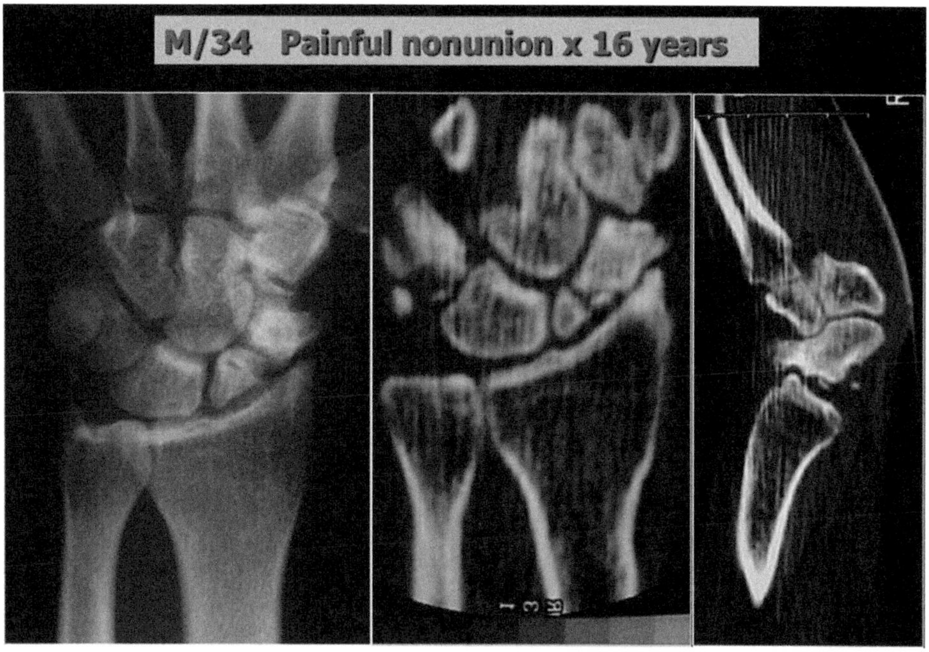

FIG. 35.28 A young male patient with scaphoid nonunion for 16 years developed radiologic signs of scaphoid nonunion advanced collapse wrist changes.

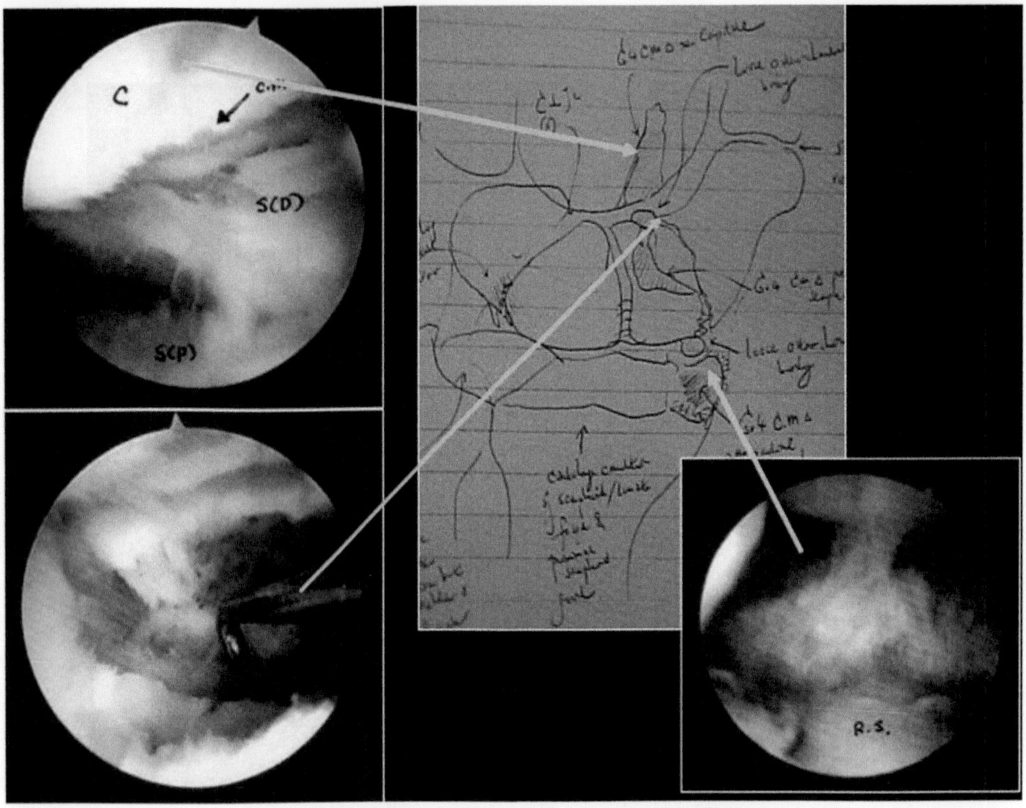

FIG. 35.29 Wrist arthroscopy showed the location of the cartilage damage and synovitis most severe at the radial styloid area. Cartilage damage at the midcarpal joint was relatively minor. The green arrows indicate the corresponding arthroscopic findings according to the schematic drawing.

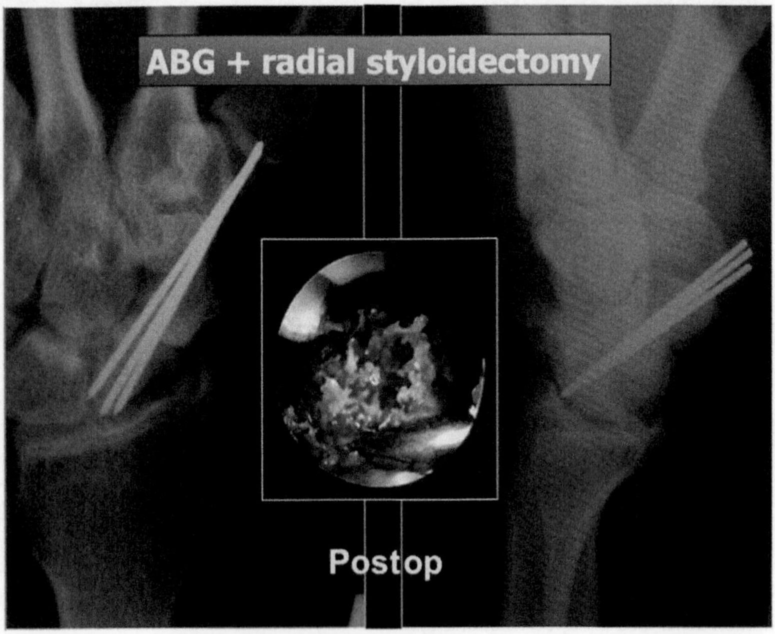

FIG. 35.30 Proceeded to nonunion fixation with percutaneous K-wires fixation, takedown of nonunion, arthroscopic bone grafting (ABG), and arthroscopic radial styloidectomy.

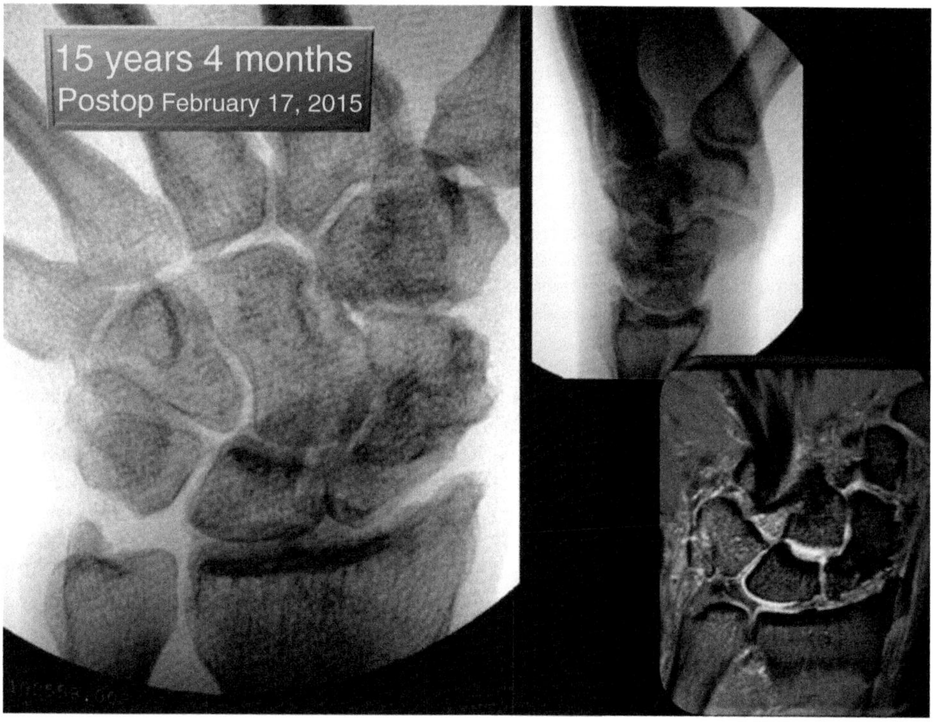

FIG. 35.31 Radiographs at 15 years 4 months postop showed solid union, sustained correction of scaphoid malalignment, and cessation of progression of scaphoid nonunion advanced collapse wrist changes.

radial styloidectomy lies on better visualization and therefore preservation of the important stabilizing structure of radioscaphocapitate ligament. With the arthroscope inserted from the 4–5 portal and directed toward the dorsal aspect of the radial styloid, a 2.9-mm burr can be introduced from the 3–4 portal and burr on the arthritic cartilage surface of the styloid region. The aim is to produce a defect of 5 mm depth. Caution should be exercised to prevent overburring of the rest of scaphoid fossa. Burring is continued at the radial border until a defect of even thickness is obtained. The volar aspect of the radial styloid can be spared because it is the important origin of the radio-scapho-capitate ligament and impingement symptom seldom arises from this area. Adequacy of radial styloidectomy can be confirmed by intraoperative fluoroscopy (Fig. 35.32).

Postoperative Care

A short-arm plaster slab is provided and maintained for 2 weeks. In cases with DISI deformity, the transfixing pin across the RL joint should be removed by 2 weeks. Delayed removal may result in iatrogenic breakage of the pin. A below elbow splint is then fabricated to provide protection to the nonunion site. Active mobilization of the wrist under supervision of hand therapist can be initiated as early as 2 weeks postoperation if the nonunion fixation is felt to be stable. This also applies to cases with K-wire fixation. X-ray is taken at regular intervals to monitor the progress of graft incorporation and healing of the nonunion. Once clinical and radiologic union is confirmed, the K-wires can be removed under local anesthesia, typically at 10–12 weeks postoperation. Any percutaneous screw flushed inside the bone needs not be removed. Passive mobilization of the wrist can be initiated once union is established, then strengthening of the hand and upper limb can follow, usually at 12–16 weeks postoperation.

PANEL 3
Case Scenario 2

A 23-year-old male medical student with right hand dominance presented with a 6-year history of left wrist scaphoid nonunion. He had history of multiple spraining episodes of his left wrist during football games. He had increasing pain on carrying heavy objects and doing strenuous exercise. Radiographs revealed a chronic left scaphoid nonunion with severe sclerosis at the fracture

Continued

PANEL 3
Case Scenario 2—cont'd

sites, marked humpback deformity with an SL angle nearly 90 degrees and CL angle larger than 30 degrees. (Fig. 35.15). He underwent arthroscopic takedown of the nonunion, reduction of the dorsal intercalated segment instability deformity and transfixing the radiolunate joint with a K-wire, arthroscopic bone graft using iliac crest autologous bone graft, and percutaneous fixation with multiple 1.1-m K-wires through the scaphoid nonunion and also at the scaphocapitate joint. The K-wires were removed at 12 weeks postoperation (Fig. 35.33).

At 13 years 9 months postoperation, he worked full-time as a radiologist. He maintained his regular football activities with no pain and disability. Clinical examination revealed no tender spot. Wrist grinding was smooth and painless. His scars were almost invisible. Comparing data preoperative and at latest follow-up, the wrist performance score increased from 36/40 to 40/40. Pain score reduced from 2/20 to 0/20. The DASH score was 0/100 and patient rated wrist evaluation was 0/100. Wrist flexion extension arc increased from 94.2% to 96.6% of the unaffected side. Radioulnar deviation range increased from 88.1% to 95.7% of the opposite side. Grip strength increased from 68.1% to 87.2%. Radiographs showed solid union of the fracture with normal SL and CL angles. There was some mild narrowing of the joint space between scaphoid and capitate (Fig. 35.34).

Results

In all cases, the procedure was accomplished arthroscopically without converting to open surgery. The mean operation time was 190 min (range 90–300 min). Ten patients had concomitant procedures, including distal radius fracture fixation (two), arthroscopic styloidectomy (two), Wafer procedure (one), scapholunate ligament (SL) thermal shrinkage (one), triangular fibrocartilage complex (TFCC) debridement (one), opponensplasty (one), thumb metacarpophalangeal joint (MCPJ) fusion (one), and arthroscopic curettage and bone grafting of lunate bone cyst (one). For osteosynthesis, we had employed cannulated screws in 26 cases and multiple K-wires for 43 cases. One patient lost follow-up 3 weeks after surgery. The average follow-up of the remaining 68 cases was 39.5 months (range 5–125 months). Overall union rate was 91.2% (62/68), including 7 cases of delayed union at 4–6 months. The average radiologic union time was 12 weeks (6–39 weeks). Poor intraoperative vascularity might predispose to persistent nonunion but did not preclude union entirely. Correlation of union status and vascularity of proximal scaphoid fragment was shown in Table 35.4. Poor intraoperative bleeding of proximal scaphoid still permitted union in 16 of 19 cases (84.2%), whereas good bleeding predicted union in 40 of 42 cases (95.2%).

At final clinical follow-up, there was no pain in 53 patients (78.2%) while the average pain score according to a 10-point Visual Analog Scale (VAS) in the remaining 15 patients was 1.8. There was significant improvement of ADL performance score increase from 33.4 to 39.0 on a 40-point scale, ADL pain score (decrease from 5.4 to 1.0 on a 20-point scale), exertion pain (decrease from 5.0 to 1.8 on a 10-point scale), and grip power (increase from 65.2% to 77.8% of the opposite hand) ($P < .05$). The average combined range of motion of the affected wrist adding extension, flexion, radial, and ulnar deviation range decreased from 82.2% to 74.4% of the opposite side ($P = .05$). All patients had inconspicuous scars left (Fig. 35.35). Carpal alignment was evaluated radiologically compared with nonaffected side. The average scapholunate angle was 62.3 degrees (range 49–76 degrees) and the average AP intrascaphoid angle was 34.5 degrees (range 27–50 degrees).

We had encountered one case of intraoperative complication where the tip of the screwdriver for inserting the mini-Acutrak cannulated screw was broken and being left attached to the end of the screw. The patients had no symptom of impingement or infection subsequently. Immediate postoperative complication included three cases of whole hand numbness, which resolved spontaneously after 2–5 days. They were presumably due to excessive and prolong traction of the fingers during the operation. Three patients had developed pin tract infection on follow-up. In all these cases, multiple K-wires fixation had been used and the K-wires were left protruded outside the skin. In one patient of distal scaphoid nonunion, where the infection was proven to be pseudomonas infection, the K wires had to be removed prematurely at 5 weeks. The wrist was then protected with cast and the nonunion subsequently healed at 6 months. For the other two patients, where the infection was caused by staphylococcus, the infection was successfully controlled through appropriate antibiotics and meticulous dressing of the pin tract. Bone union was not affected. Because of these complications in our early series, we have adopted the policy of burying the K-wire underneath the skin for later removal with small incision after fracture healing under local anesthesia. From then, there were no more infections. However, there were two cases with K-wire loosening and protrusion outside skin causing irritation. There was donor-site morbidity in three cases, including two cases of hematoma at the iliac crest and one case of lateral cutaneous nerve of thigh injury. All symptoms resolved spontaneously.

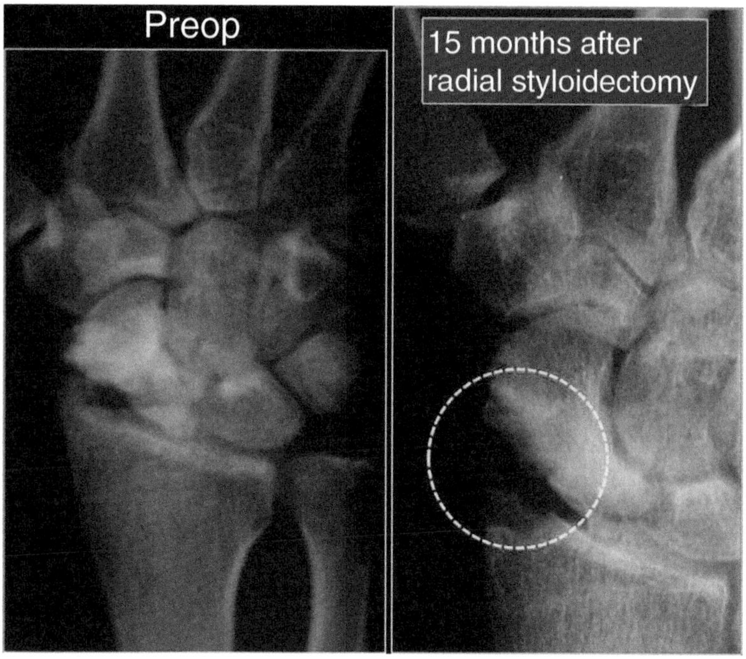

FIG. 35.32 Arthroscopic radial styloidectomy aimed to remove dorsal radial portion of the styloid while preserving the volar aspect to safeguard the important volar ligaments of the radiocarpal joint. The yellow dotted circle indicates the location of arthroscopic radial styloidectomy as depicted in radiological view.

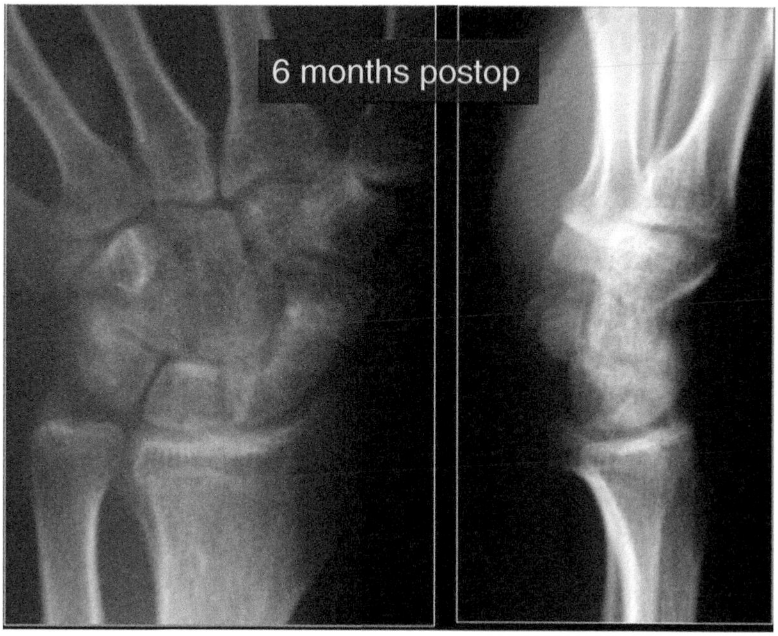

FIG. 35.33 Radiographs at 6 months postop.

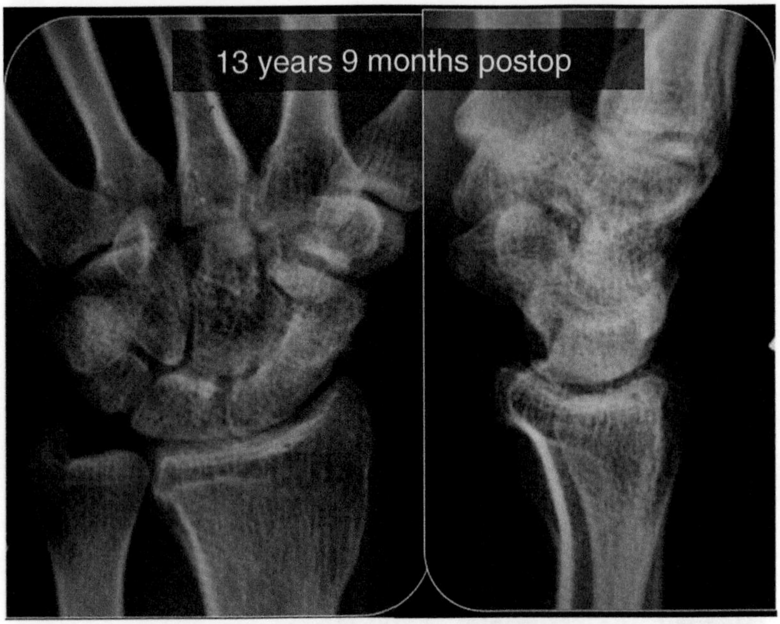

FIG. 35.34 Radiographs at 13 years 9 months postop.

TABLE 35.4
Correlation of Vascularity and Union

Vascularity of Proximal Scaphoid Fragment	Good	Fair	Poor
Union (55)	37	6	12
Delayed union >16 weeks (7)	3	0	4
Fibrous union (2)	1	1	0
Nonunion (4)	1	0	3
Overall union rate	95.2%	85.7%	84.2%

There were six failures in our series. Four patients received further surgery. One case required revision grafting with vascularized distal radius bone graft. Union was obtained at 13 weeks postop, and he was pain free and returned to full employment. In another case, because of the severe scaphoid collapse, scapholunate-capitate fusion was done and was augmented with vascularized distal radius bone graft. Fusion was obtained at 8 weeks postop and he had mild pain of 4 points in VAS scale at final follow-up. One patient was salvaged with radio-scapho-lunate fusion augment with vascularized bone graft. Fusion was achieved at 8 weeks. She remained painless with good hand function and later became a bronze medalist in track cycle racing at the 2012 London Olympics. Another patient received a revision arthroscopic bone grafting and finally got union after 12 months. He had no pain and could resume full employment. There was one case with proximal pole resorption but was clinically asymptomatic. The last case with progressive SNAC wrist changes refused further surgery all the time, although pain persisted at a level of 6 on a 10-point VAS scale.

Discussion

In 1998, we first reported on the technique of arthroscopic bone grafting in repairing osseous defects in 11 cases, including scaphoid nonunion, acute comminuted scaphoid fracture, bone cyst, and triscaphe fusion (Ho PC. Presented in 7th Congress of International Federation of Societies for Surgery of the Hand, Vancouver,

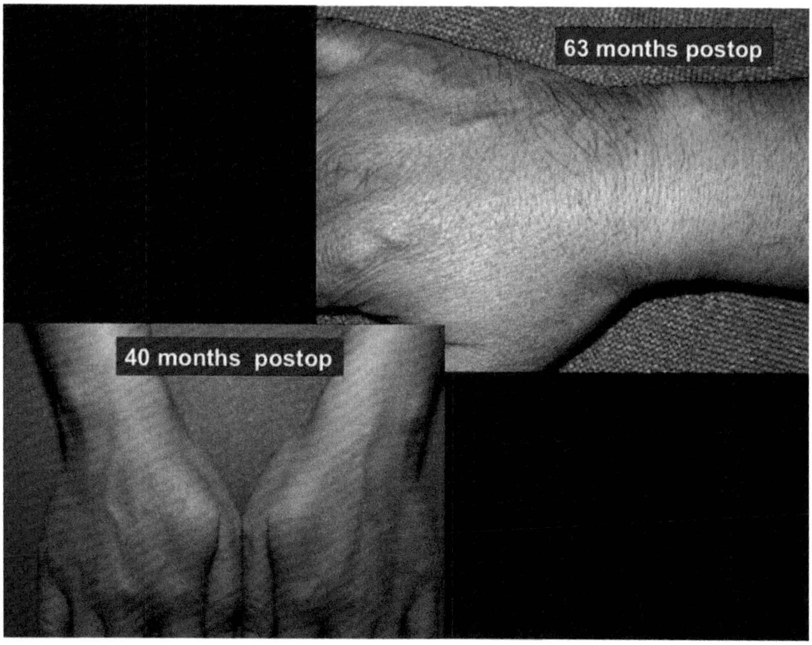

FIG. 35.35 Scars almost invisible at long-term follow-up.

Canada, 1998). We achieved union in all cases at an average of 3.4 months.

Since then it has become our primary treatment in all noncomplicated scaphoid delayed and nonunion cases. Our result of ABG over the past 20 years has been very encouraging. High union rate has been uniform at 91.2% and clinical outcome is highly satisfactory. Poor blood supply of scaphoid is not a contraindication to the technique as a union rate of 84.2% can still be expected. Literature on attempts to heal an avascular nonunion of proximal pole of scaphoid showed consistently poor outcomes. Vascularized bone graft used to be thought of as an ultimate solution for difficult scaphoid nonunion because of its sound principle of providing a living bone to the nonunion site. However, it was not without problems in actual clinical practice. Chang and Bishop evaluated the outcomes and complications of 1,2-intercompartmental supraretinacular artery (1,2-ICSRA) pedicled vascularized bone grafting of scaphoid nonunion in a large series of 50 scaphoid nonunions in 49 patients treated between 1994 and 2003 with 1,2-ICSRA-based vascularized bone grafts in a retrospective review of the clinical and radiographic information.[18] Two patients were lost to follow up in the study. 9 female and 38 male patients averaging 24 years of age were followed up for an average of 7.8 months. The result showed that 34 scaphoid nonunions (68%) went on to union at an average of 15.6 weeks after surgery. Complications occurred in eight patients and consisted of graft extrusion, superficial infection, deep infection, and failure of fixation. Univariate risk factors for failure included older age, proximal pole avascular necrosis, preoperative humpback deformity, nonscrew fixation, tobacco use, and female gender. They concluded that a successful outcome of vascularized bone grafts based on the 1,2-ICSRA was not universal, and it depended on careful patient and fracture selection and appropriate surgical techniques. Additional surgical trauma to the precarious vascularity with open arthrotomy is one of the contributing factors. The minimal disturbance of the carpal bone vascularity by this technique has probably contributed to the high union rate and the relative short duration of average 12 weeks for graft incorporation. Minimal disturbance of the ligamentous structures also allows earlier and more vigorous rehabilitation and therefore better clinical outcome. The results are particularly promising for those cases treated with implants previously and the fixation remains fairly stable. Under these circumstances, arthroscopic bone grafting would be a relatively simple and minimally invasive procedure. Another advantage of such technique is the provision of access to assess other intraarticular ligamentous or chondral lesions in addition to the scaphoid nonunion, which may potentially alter the course of healing and the choice of treatment. Associated SNAC wrist change can be addressed accurately by carefully inspecting both radiocarpal and midcarpal joint. Advanced degeneration may preclude the consideration for bone grafting and anatomic restoration. Concomitant treatment can be carried out in early stage of arthritis. In case of need for revision, other conventional treatment methods can still be applied. On the cost-benefit side, this operation requires no special instrument apart from the standard small joint arthroscopic instrument for the procedure.

Other authors described similar techniques with successful outcomes. In 2014, Teng et al. reported six patients with nonunion of the scaphoid waist treated with arthroscopic-assisted debridement of the sclerotic bone, percutaneous K-wire fixation, and arthroscopic autologous bone grafting between January 2011 and May 2012 in Ningbo, China.[19] According to the classification of Slade and Dodds,[20] there were one Grade 1, one Grade 2, two Grade 3, and two Grade 4 cases. All nonunions healed at an average of 13.7 weeks. The average follow-up was 7.5 months. Functional outcome was rated as excellent in 2, good in 3, and fair in 1 case according to the Modified Mayo Wrist Score.

Lee et al. in Korea also reported 20 patients with scaphoid nonunion treated with arthroscopically assisted bone grafting and percutaneous K-wires fixation from November 2008 to July 2012.[21] Time from injury to treatment was 74 months (range, 3–480 months) on average. There were one Grade 1, seven Grade 2, one Grade 3, seven Grade 4, and four Grade 6 cases. Autologous bone graft was harvested from the iliac crest. All nonunions healed successfully. The average radiologic union time was 9.7 weeks (range, 7–14 weeks). The average pain VAS score improved from 6.3 (range, 4–8) preoperatively to 1.6 (range, 0–3) at the last follow-up. The average Modified Mayo Wrist Score increased from 62.5 preoperatively to 85.7 at the last follow-up.

Kang and Choi et al. reported the result of 45 patients receiving arthroscopic bone grafting for symptomatic scaphoid nonunions without necrosis of the proximal fragment, severe deformities, or arthritis between 2008 and 2012.[22] They employed the iliac crest as the source of bone graft using a trephine technique for bone harvesting. The graft was introduced through the sheath of a 3.5-mm burr into the nonunion site at the midcarpal joint. The nonunion was fixed with either a headless screw or two terminally threaded pins. The wrists were immobilized for 8–10 weeks after the operations. CT scan was conducted at 8–10 weeks to evaluate for bone union. Thirty-three patients (73%) were followed up for at least 2 years. There were 5 distal third, 19 middle third, and 9 proximal third fractures. The mean follow-up was 33 months (range, 24–60 months). Thirty-two (97%) scaphoid nonunions healed successfully. The mean VAS pain score decreased from preoperative mean 4.5 (SD 1.8) to postoperative mean 0.6 (SD 0.8). The mean active flexion-extension angle increased from preoperative mean 100 degrees (SD 26) to postoperative mean 109 degrees (SD 16). The mean grip strength increased from preoperative mean 35 kg (SD 8) to postoperative mean 50 kg (SD 10). The mean Mayo Wrist Score increased from preoperative mean 56 (SD 23) to postoperative mean 89 (SD 8). The mean DASH score decreased from preoperative mean 25 (SD 18) to postoperative mean 4 (SD 3). There was no complication and no progression of arthritis at the last follow-up. Seventeen patients had coexisting intraarticular pathology, including 9 triangular fibrocartilage complex tears (7 traumatic and 2 degenerative), 17 intrinsic ligament tears, and 5 mild radioscaphoid degenerative changes. Concomitant arthroscopic treatments of these lesions were carried out. These patients generally achieved good results.

Other minimal invasive bone grafting technique has also been described. In 2006, Slade reported the technique of percutaneous bone graft in scaphoid nonunion with bone resorption at nonunion interface >1 mm with cyst formation and maintained scaphoid alignment. Core of cancellous bone graft was harvested from the distal radius using a 8G bone biopsy cannula.[20] The graft was delivered to the nonunion site through the reamer portal at the proximal scaphoid using the same cannula, before the nonunion was fixed with a screw. This technique was minimal invasive in nature, but comparing with the ABG technique, the amount of bone graft being inserted was limited.

In 2011, Chu and Shih in Taiwan reported the technique of arthroscopically assisted percutaneous internal fixation augmented by injection of a bone graft substitute performed between January 2006 and November 2007 in 15 consecutive patients of a mean age of 31 years (range, 20–45 years) with fibrous union or nonunions of the scaphoid with minimal sclerosis or resorption at the nonunion site.[23] There were three Schmitt stage I and 12 stage II cases. Nonunions with avascular necrosis, humpback deformity, severe carpal collapse, or arthrosis were excluded. The author utilized the approach similar to Slade but employed radiopaque bone graft substitute instead to be delivered into the nonunion site. The mean follow up was 33 months (range, 24–46 months). Union was obtained in 14 patients (93%) at a mean of 15.4 weeks according to clinical examinations and standard radiography.

According to the Mayo Modified Wrist Score, there were 10 excellent and 4 good results. Fourteen patients (93%) returned to work or sports activities at their preinjury level. Geissler et al. also achieved union in 14 of 15 cystic nonunion (Grade 4) using dorsal technique with arthroscopy combined with screw fixation and incorporating demineralized bone matrix.[24]

Limitations do exist for the ABG technique. Longstanding scaphoid nonunion with significant carpal collapse cannot be adequately corrected with closed percutaneous method, and ABG would become meaningless. Severe SNAC wrist changes will likely preclude good outcome from bone grafting. Avascular necrosis is not by itself a contraindication in our opinion, although the chance of persistent nonunion will be higher than those with good intraoperative bleeding. Significant arthrofibrosis that causes difficult access for the arthroscope also forms a relative contraindication. Nevertheless, with experience, patience and the use of smaller arthroscope such as 1.9 mm size, most fibrotic joint can be loosened up gradually by careful joint debridement and dilation to provide adequate working space for the bone work.

RECOMMENDATION

In patients with scaphoid nonunions, evidence suggests the following:

- Arthroscopic management of scaphoid nonunions without severe deformities or arthritis may lead to good results in terms of union and functional outcome (overall quality: low).
- The additional value is best considered by weighing advantages (minimal invasive character and quick rehabilitation) and disadvantages (complications/steep learning curve/technical challenges) (overall quality: very low).

CONCLUSION

Arthroscopic bone grafting has a definite role in managing difficult scaphoid delayed and nonunion. It represents a significant breakthrough in the history of arthroscopic surgery of the wrist. It allows thorough assessment and a comprehensive management approach for scaphoid fracture and its sequelae in a minimally invasive manner. With minimal surgical trauma to the vascularity of the carpal bone and its ligamentous connections, it provides a more favorable biologic environment for the nonunion to get repaired with quicker pacing of rehabilitation. With adequate training and experience, high union rates (over 90%) and highly satisfactory clinical outcome can be achieved. Poor blood supply of the scaphoid is not a contraindication to the bone grafting technique as a union rates over 80% have been reported, which is comparable with other existing surgical methods. In case of need for revision, other conventional treatment methods can still be applied. Although surgically demanding with a steep learning curve and extended initial operative times, no special instrument is required apart from standard arthroscopic instrument and therefore it can ultimately be considered cost-effective.

REFERENCES

1. Mack GR, Bosse MJ, Gerberman RH. The natural history of scaphoid nonunion. *J Bone Joint Surg Am*. 1984;66:504–509.
2. Ruby LK, Stinson J, Belsky MR. The natural history of scaphoid nonunion: a review of 55 cases. *J Bone Joint Surg Am*. 1985;67:428–432.
3. Lindstrom G, Nystrom A. Natural history of scaphoid nonunion, with special reference to "asymptomatic" cases. *J Hand Surg Am*. 1992;17:697–700.
4. Nagle DJ. Scaphoid nonunion. Treatment with cancellous bone graft and Kirscher-wire fixation. *Hand Clin*. 2001;17(4):625–629.
5. Fernandez DL. A technique for wedge shaped grafts for scaphoid nonunion with carpal instability. *J Hand Surg Am*. 1984;9:733–737.
6. Stark A, Brostom LA, Svartengren G. Scaphoid nonunion treated with the Matti-Russe technique; long term results. *Clin Orthop*. 1987;214:175–180.
7. Cooney III WP, Dobyns JH, Linscheid RL. Nonunion of the scaphoid; analysis of the results from bone grafting. *J Hand Surg Am*. 1980;5:343–354.
8. Christodoulou LS, Kitsis CK. Internal fixation of scaphoid nonunion: a comparative study of three methods. *Injury*. 2001;32(8):625–630.
9. Schuind F, Haentijens P. Prognostic factors in the treatment of carpal scaphoid nonunion. *J Hand Surg Am*. 1999;24(4):761–776.
10. Munk B, Larsen CF. Bone grafting the scaphoid nonunion: a systematic review of 147 publications including 5,246 cases of scaphoid nonunion. *Acta Orthop Scand*. 2004;75(5):618–629.
11. Nelson DL. Function wrist motion. *Hand Clin*. 1997;13(1):83–92.
12. Cheng HS, Hung LK, Ho PC, Wong J. An analysis of causes and treatment outcome of chronic wrist pain after distal radius fractures. *Hand Surg*. 2008;13(1):1–10.
13. Estrella EP, Hung LK, Ho PC, Tse WL. Arthroscopic repair of triangular fibrocartilage complex tear. *Arthroscopy*. 2007;23(7):729–737.
14. Clara W, Ho PC. Minimal invasive management of scaphoid fractures – from fresh to nonunion: acute scaphoid fracture, scaphoid delayed union and nonunion. *Hand Clin*. 2011;27:291–307.

15. Hung LK, Pang KW. Percutaneous screw fixation of acute scaphoid fractures. *J Hand Surg*. 1994;19(suppl 1):26.
16. Hung LK. Percutaneous screw fixation of acute scaphoid fractures. *HK J Ortho Surg*. 1998;2(1):54–57.
17. Hung LK, Pang KW, Ho PC. Anatomical guidelines for safe percutaneous screw fixation of scaphoid fractures. In: *International Proceedings, 6th Congress of IFSSH*; 1995: 797–800.
18. Chang MA, Bishop AT, Moran SL. The outcomes and complications of 1,2-intercompartmental supraretinacular artery pedicled vascularized bone grafting of scaphoid nonunions. *J Hand Surg Am*. 2006;31(3):387–396.
19. Xiaofeng T, Ruibin H, Hong C. Arthroscope assisted treatment of scaphoid nonunion: preliminary outcome analysis. *Chin J Hand Surg*. 2014;30(1):28–30.
20. Slade III JF, Dodds SD. Minimally invasive management of scaphoid nonunions. *Clin Orthop Relat Res*. 2006; 445:108–119.
21. Lee YK, Woo SH, Ho PC, Park JG, Kim JY. Arthroscopically assisted cancellous bone grafting and percutaneous K-wires fixation for the treatment of scaphoid nonunions. *J Korean Soc Surg Hand*. 2014;19(1):19–28.
22. Kang HJ, Chun YM, Koh IH, Park JH, Choi YR. Is arthroscopic bone graft and fixation for scaphoid nonunions effective? *Clin Orthop Relat Res*. 2016;474(1):204–212.
23. Chu PJ, Shih JT. Arthroscopically assisted use of injectable bone graft substitutes for management of scaphoid nonunions. *Arthroscopy*. 2011;27(1):31–37.
24. Geissler WB. Percutaneous and arthroscopic management of scaphoid nonunions. In: Capo JT, Tan V, eds. *Atlas of Minimally Invasive Hand and Wrist Surgery*. New York, NY: Informa Healthcare USA; 2008:105–115.

CHAPTER 36

Salvage Procedures for SNAC Wrist

MARC GARCIA-ELIAS, MD, PHD • DIANA M. ORTEGA HERNÁNDEZ, MD • RAÚL M. CASAS CONTRERAS, MD

KEY POINTS

- Scapholunate advanced collapse (SLAC) and scaphoid nonunion advanced collapse (SNAC) are not equivalent clinical conditions. The strategies that are reasonable for a symptomatic SLAC wrist may not be adequate to treat SNAC and vice versa.
- The ideal treatment for SNAC-I is to remove the impinging radial styloid and heal the nonunion. The goal is to normalize scaphoid kinematics. A salvage procedure should not be contemplated as an option unless the healing potential of the bone is unacceptably low.
- On theory, the best salvage option for a young individual with a SNAC wrist and a viable proximal scaphoid is to remove the distal portion of it and fuse the proximal scaphoid to the lunate and capitate. In practice, getting that fusion to heal is not easy.
- If the proximal scaphoid is not viable and the midcarpal joint is already osteoarthritic, complete scaphoidectomy plus lunocapitate fusion is the method of choice.
- No matter how tempting a proximal row carpectomy (PRC) may look, it should not be used in heavy manual workers under 35 years of age.

PANEL 1
Case Scenario

A 67-year-old male retired high school teacher with a sedentary lifestyle came to our office complaining of pain in his right wrist. Twenty-seven years before, he had a hyperextension injury to his wrist while rock climbing, but he didn't seek medical attention. At examination, we could see that the dorsolateral corner of the wrist was swollen and tender. Motion was slightly reduced and the anatomic snuffbox was particularly tender at palpation. Radiographs disclosed the presence of a chronic scaphoid nonunion (SNAC wrist stage I) (Fig. 36.1A). Informed about the different treatment options available, the patient requested to have the simplest and quickest solution to his pain. Grip strength was not a priority for him. What would be the preferred evidence-based management at this stage?

IMPORTANCE OF THE PROBLEM

The scaphoid plays a key role in carpal kinetics.[1] As a stabilizing bridge between the proximal and distal carpal rows, it ensures proper transmission of forces across the wrist. The presence of an unstable fracture of the scaphoid waist precludes that bridging effect and, therefore, the capacity of the joint to sustain physiologic loads. Once disconnected from its proximal counterpart, the unconstrained distal fragment moves as if it was a distal row bone; that is, it follows the capitate in all of its displacements, generating substantial shear forces at the fracture site and against the tip of the radial styloid.[2,3] The proximal fragment, by contrast, remains constrained by a relatively still lunate on a congruent cartilage-covered scaphoid fossa (Fig. 36.2). With time, the dysfunctional midcarpal joint evolves into a misaligned, osteoarthritic articulation, whereas the radiocarpal joint remains relatively intact.

In 1984, Mack et al.[4] analyzed the incidence and severity of the degenerative changes of 47 scaphoid nonunions in at least 5-year duration. Of those, 23 had sclerosis and/or bone resorption confined to the scaphoid fracture site, 14 had degenerative osteoarthritis (OA) between the distal scaphoid fragment and the radial styloid, and 10 generalized midcarpal OA. The average evolution time of the nonunion in the first group was 8 years, 17 years in the second group, and 32 years in the one with generalized OA.

Subsequent studies[4–8] further demonstrated that, in the presence of an unstable scaphoid fracture, the

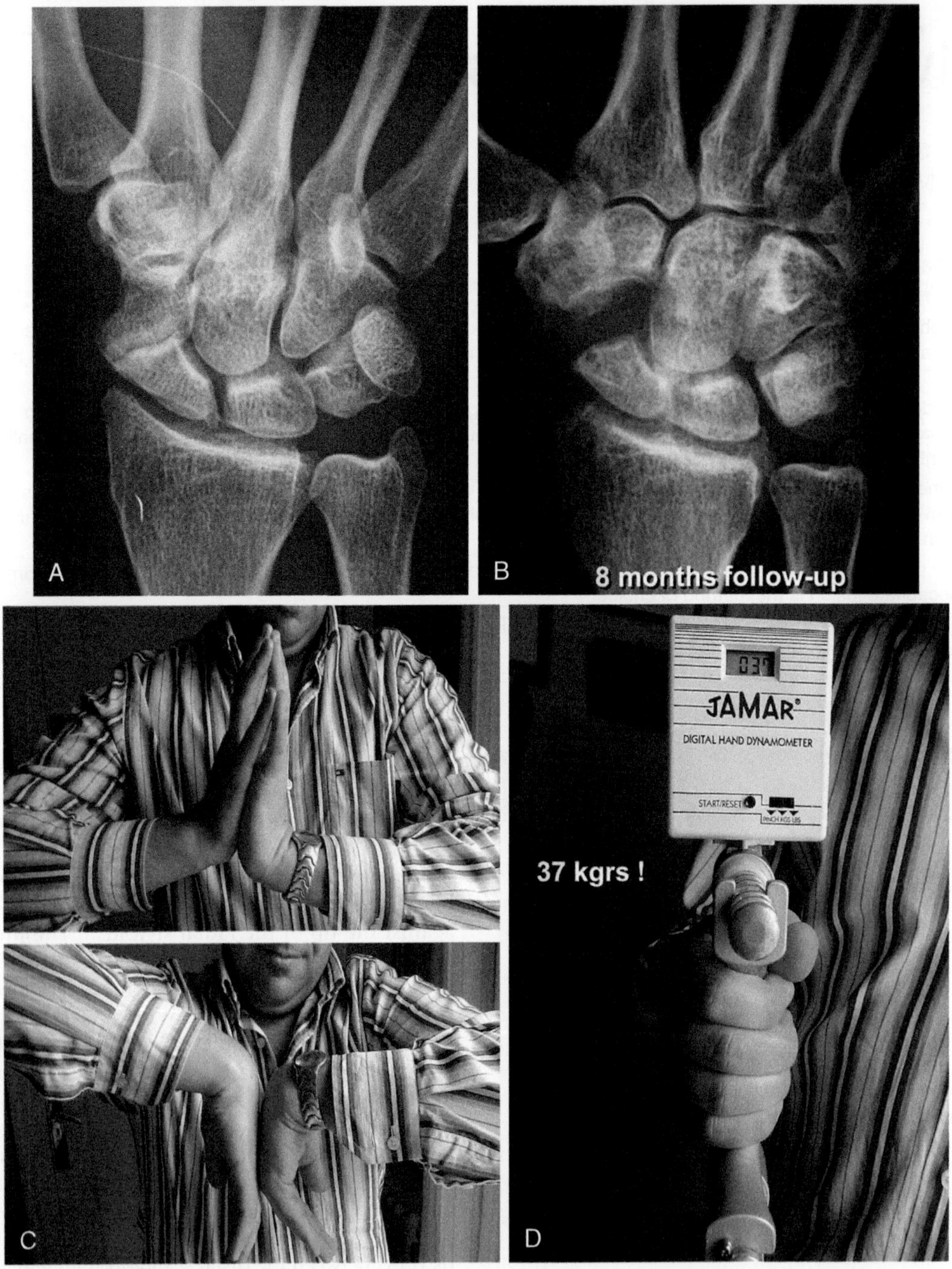

FIG. 36.1 **(A)** Posteroanterior (PA) view of a chronic scaphoid nonunion with degenerative changes at the tip of the radial styloid (scaphoid nonunion advanced collapse, stage I). **(B)** PA radiograph of the same wrist, 8 months after a distal scaphoid resection and radial styloidectomy. **(C)** The patient is satisfied with the procedure, for it allowed painless function, including total range of passive flexion-extension of 135 degrees (92%) and **(D)** 38 kg of grip strength (76% of the contralateral side).

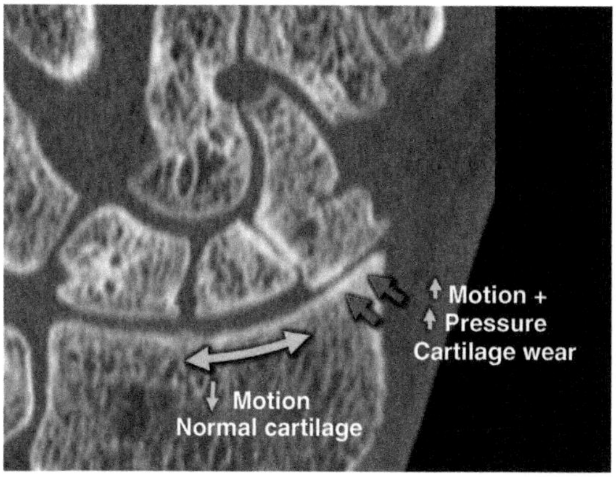

FIG. 36.2 Coronal view of a CT scan of a patient with chronic scaphoid nonunion with degenerative changes between the distal scaphoid and the radial styloid (scaphoid nonunion advanced collapse, stage I). Increased motion and high pressure explains the cartilage wear (*red arrows*) of both the tip of the radial styloid and the lateral aspect of the distal scaphoid, whereas decreased motion protects the cartilage of the proximal scaphoid (*yellow arrow*).

wrist undergoes a predictable pattern of joint degeneration. It always starts at the interval between the tip of the radial styloid and the distal scaphoid fragment (stage I), progresses toward the proximal scaphoid-capitate interval (stage II) and continues medially to affect the entire midcarpal joint (stage III) (Box 36.1) (Fig. 36.3). It is the so-called "scaphoid nonunion advanced collapse" (SNAC), an acronym proposed by Krakauer et al.[6] based on the similarities between this pattern and the one observed among patients with an untreated scapholunate dissociation (SLAC: "scapholunate advanced collapse").[7] According to Vender et al.,[8] it takes an average of 4.3 years for a waist scaphoid nonunion to evolve into SNAC stage I, 9 more years to reach stage II, and 15 years to exhibit complete midcarpal deterioration.

All the above only applies to scaphoid nonunions located in the waist of the bone, that is, distal to the insertion of the dorsal scapholunate ligament. As demonstrated by Moritomo et al.,[9] proximal pole nonunions evolve in a different manner and require specific treatment. Further discussion of the treatment of proximal scaphoid nonunions may be found in Chapter 14. This chapter will only discuss motion sparing procedures for the treatment of the symptomatic SNAC wrist. Wrist denervation, implant arthroplasties, and pancarpal fusions, although helpful in some cases of advanced wrist OA, will not be discussed.

BOX 36.1
Staging of "Scaphoid Nonunion Advanced Collapse (SNAC)"[6]

- **SNAC stage I** only affects the cartilage of the most distal end on the radial styloid and that of the dorsolateral corner of the distal portion of the scaphoid.
- **SNAC stage II** is the same as stage I with the addition of degeneration between the proximal portion of the scaphoid and the lateral corner of the capitate.
- **SNAC stage III** has degeneration of the radial styloid, scaphocapitate, and lunocapitate articular segments, plus substantial extension and ulnar translocation of the proximal row and dorsal subluxation of the capitate relative to the lunate.

THE QUESTION

What is the best treatment for the different stages of a symptomatic SNAC wrist?

Current Opinion

- The ideal treatment for scaphoid nonunion is the one that heals the bone and restores its normal kinematics. In the early stages of a SNAC wrist, this may be achieved through vascularized bone grafting, stable fixation, and radial styloidectomy.[10] If avoidable, rushing into salvage surgery is not recommended. Nothing compares the results of an anatomically reconstructed scaphoid.[10–12]
- If the scaphoid cannot heal, but the proximal portion of the nonunited scaphoid still is viable and large enough, a distal scaphoidectomy plus a "proximal scaphoid-lunate-capitate" (pSLC) arthrodesis as described by Viegas[14] is a reasonable alternative. The goal is to preserve as much radiocarpal articular contact as possible.[13–15]
- When the proximal portion of a nonunited scaphoid is not viable, the so-called "four-corner fusion" (4CF) is a reasonable option to alleviate pain and improve function of symptomatic SLAC and SNAC wrists (Fig. 36.4). Popularized by Watson and Ballet,[7] the technique consists on resecting completely the entire scaphoid and fusing the lunate, triquetrum, capitate and hamate bones to avoid midcarpal instability.[16–23]
- Some authors defend that fusing only the lunocapitate (LC) joint is enough to avoid the development of a "dorsal intercalated segment instability" (DISI). If properly executed, the stabilizing effect of that fusion is the same as with a 4CF, with similar nonunion rates.[24,25]

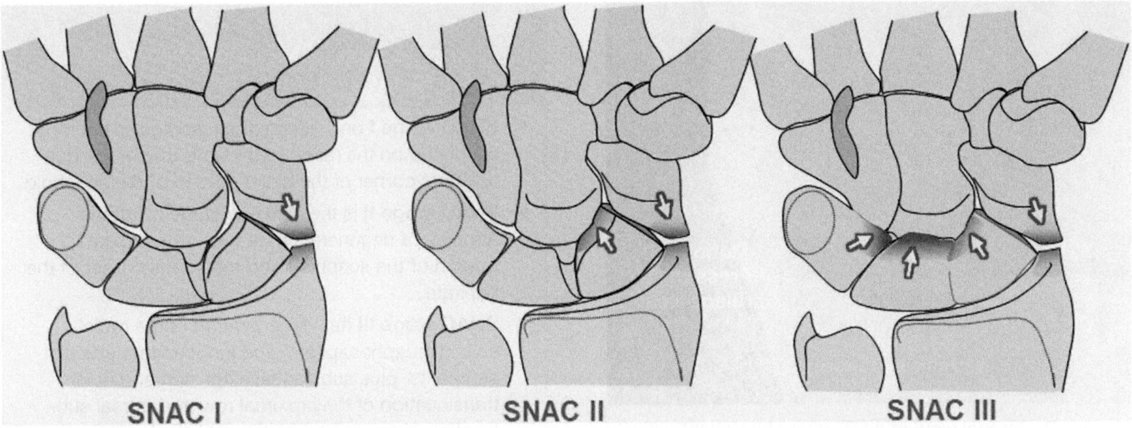

FIG. 36.3 The three stages of scaphoid nonunion advanced collapse (SNAC). Joint degeneration (*yellow arrows*), from localized radial styloid—distal scaphoid impingement (SNAC I), progresses toward the midcarpal joint, affecting first the proximal scaphoid-capitate joint (SNAC II) to affect all three joints facing the capitate (SNAC III).

- PRC is also frequently utilized in SNAC wrists stages I and II.[16–22,26] Reported to achieve similar results than a 4CF, PRC is a much less demanding procedure, requires little rehabilitation, and has lower complication rates than a 4CF.[16–22] PRC is only indicated when the cartilage of the lunate fossa and proximal capitate are in good condition.
- In low-demand patients with SNAC stage I, a distal scaphoid excision alone may obtain satisfactory results.[27,28] Implicit with the technique is the development of a DISI misalignment of the proximal row. Unlike complete scaphoidectomy, which always destabilizes the carpus, distal scaphoidectomy causes only mild DISI misalignment, usually well tolerated, particularly when associated with partial denervation of the posterior and anterior interosseous nerves.[28]

Finding the Evidence

Following PRISMA guidelines, both the "Cochrane Register of Controlled Trials" and Pubmed have been searched for all publications from January 1990 to December 2016 using all variations of the following key words: *"scaphoid nonunion advanced collapse"* OR"scaphoid nonunion" AND *"treatment."* To be eligible, a study had to report at least six patients being treated for a symptomatic SNAC wrist and followed for a minimum of 12 months.

The Cochrane registry only provided one systematic review of the outcomes of PRC and 4CF in SLAC and SNAC wrists.[17] Pubmed searching identified 244 SNAC-related publications. Of those, 35 dealt with the treatment of wrist OA.[10–19] Most papers did not differentiate SNAC from SLAC, so they were excluded. In total, we could evaluate 12 studies[14,29–39] (Levels II–IV: 174 wrists) discussing the results of six treatment alternatives for SNAC: (1) scaphoidectomy + 4CF (5 articles[29,33,34,36,38]: 87 patients), (2) scaphoidectomy + LC fusion (2 articles[30,35]: 20 patients), (3) distal scaphoidectomy + pSLC fusion (1 article[14]: 6 patients), (4) distal scaphoidectomy (3 articles[32,37,39]: 36 patients), (5) vascularized bone grafting + radial styloidectomy (1 article[31]: 12 patients), and (6) PRC (1 article[29]: 13 patients) (Table 36.1, Fig. 36.5).

Quality of the Evidence

As in most areas of wrist pathology, the existing levels of evidence concerning the treatment of the SNAC wrist are less than ideal. Of the 12 selected publications, only 1 was a prospective randomized study (evidence level II)[29] and 1 a Level III case-controlled study.[30] The rest were Level IV retrospective case series discussing a variety of treatments, each represented by a modest number of observations. The evidence being so weak, it is not possible to find a solid answer to the target question. What follows is an attempt to delineate what would be a reasonable answer to that question based on the available literature.

FINDINGS

- *The presence of minor degeneration at the radial styloid interval does not appear to be an obstacle to heal a nonunited scaphoid bone.*[10] The series by Malizos

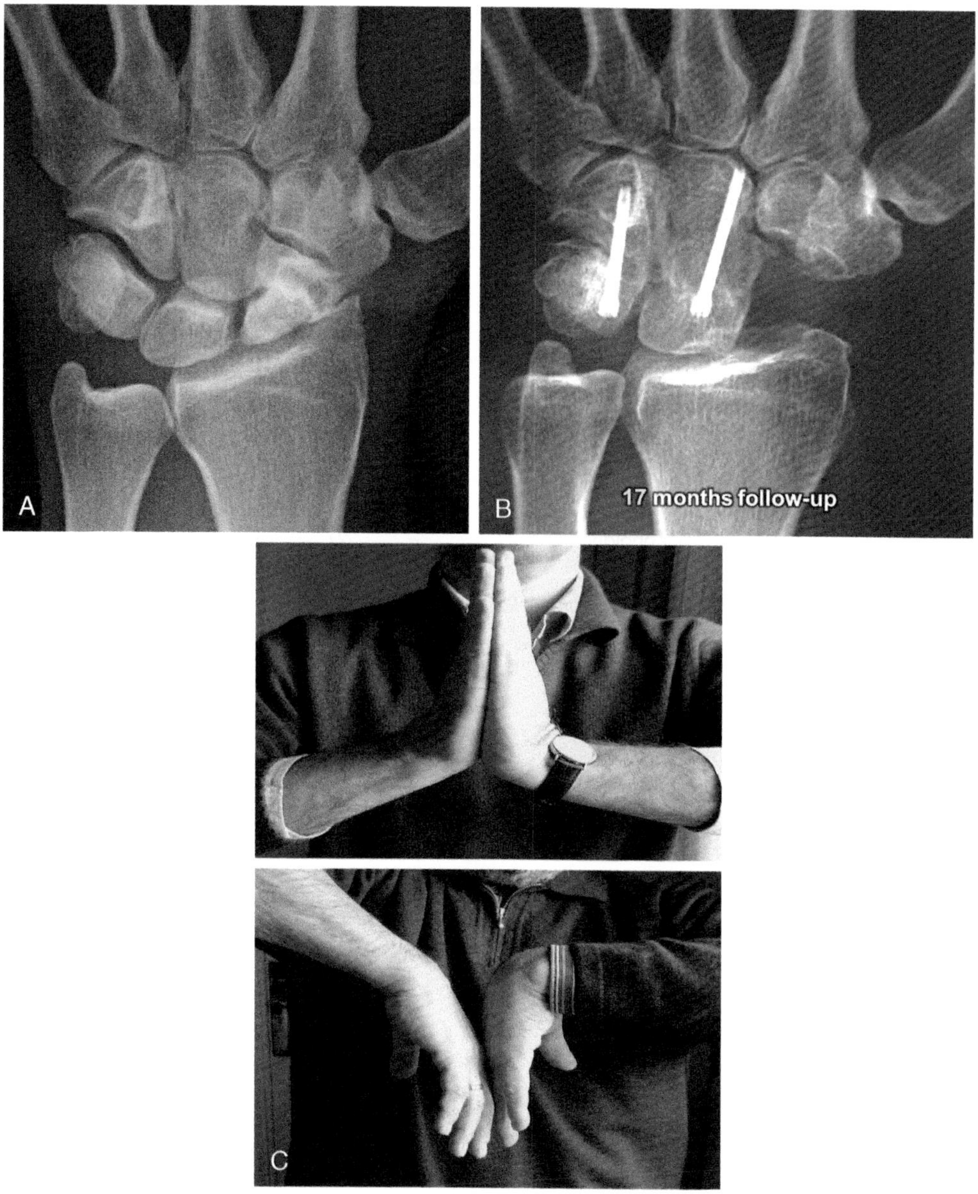

FIG. 36.4 Case example of a bicolumnar midcarpal arthrodesis, a variation of a four-corner fusion (4CF). **(A)** Posteroanterior view of a scaphoid nonunion advanced collapse II of a 44-year-old male stockbroker with a nonviable (necrotic) proximal pole of the scaphoid. **(B)** X-rays obtained 17 months after surgery. The two central and ulnar columns of the wrist have been fused. Because there is no motion between hamate and capitate, this bicolumnar fusion is to be regarded as a 4CF. **(C)** Despite a 45% reduction of his passive range of motion, the patient is satisfied.

TABLE 36.1
Results of Studies From the Cochrane Register of Controlled Trials and Pubmed

Authors		Evidence Level[a]	N	Technique	F-U (months)	Pain (VAS)[b]	ROM (%)[b]	Grip Strength (%)[b]	Return to Work (%)	DASH[b]	Mayo Score[b]
Aita et al.[29]	2016	II	14	Scaphoidectomy+4CF	73	2.9	58	65	84	13	–
			13	PRC	74	2.3	68	79	64	11	–
Hegazy[30]	2015	III	12	Scaphoidectomy+LC fusion	37	–	49	81	100	–	83
Malizos et al.[31]	2014	IV	12	Bone grafting+osteotomy	79	0.8	66	77	–	9	85
Malerich et al.[32]	2014	IV	19	Distal scaphoidectomy	180	0.9	79	83	–	–	–
Xu et al.[33]	2013	IV	11	Scaphoidectomy+4CF	21	–	27	44	–	–	–
Mahmoud et al.[34]	2012	IV	22	Scaphoidectomy+4CF	20	0.8	64	–	95	17	–
Giannikas et al.[35]	2010	IV	8	Scaphoidectomy+LC fusion	53	–	56	87	88	–	69
El-Mowafi et al.[36]	2007	IV	10	Scaphoidectomy+4CF	16	–	54	54	50	–	–
Drac et al.[37]	2006	IV	8	Distal scaphoidectomy	12	–	91	79	–	–	–
Dacho et al.[38]	2006	IV	30	Scaphoidectomy+4CF	47	–	56	87	–	–	–
Soejima et al.[39]	2003	IV	9	Distal scaphoidectomy	29	–	94	77	100	21	90
Viegas[14]	1994	IV	6	Distal scaphoidectomy+SLC fusion	18	–	50	51	–	–	–

[a]Levels of evidence from Sackett DL. Rules of evidence and clinical recommendations on the use antithrombotic agents. *Chest*. 1986;89 (2 suppl):2S–3S.
[b]Mean values at follow-up (F-U).
4CF, four-corner fusion; *DASH*, disability of the arm, shoulder and hand; *LC*, lunocapitate; *PRC*, proximal row carpectomy; *ROM*, range of motion; *SLC*, scaphoid-lunate-capitate; *VAS*, visual analog scale.

et al.[31] proves that healing a scaphoid nonunion in early stages of SNAC is feasible (12 cases; 100% union rate). It may require technically demanding techniques (lateral closing wedge osteotomy of the radius,[31] vascularized local bone grafting,[31] free medial femoral condyle vascularized bone grafting,[41] solid fixation with two 2.5-mm headless compression screws,[42] etc.) but the chances of union are as high as for nonarthritic scaphoid nonunions.

- *Healing the scaphoid of a SNAC wrist does not guarantee better long-term results than treating the case with a salvage procedure.* The series published by Malizos et al.[31] proves that healing the scaphoid is possible. Whether it is worth trying is debatable. Certainly, the long-term results obtained by those

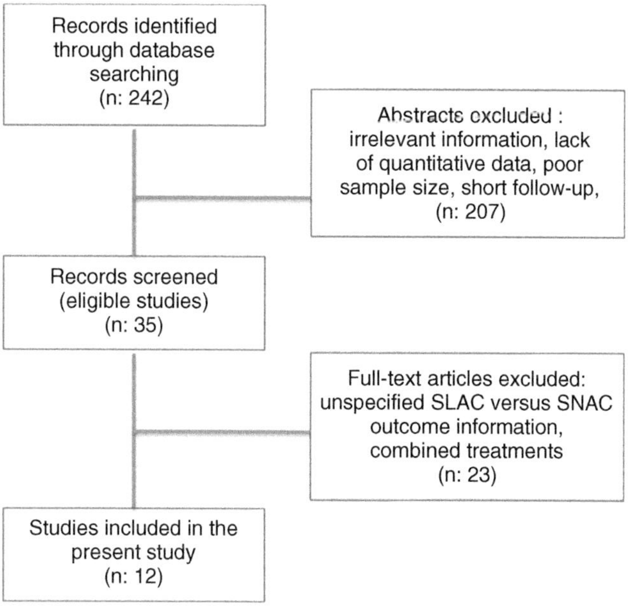

FIG. 36.5 Flowchart of the searches completed pertaining to the data in Table 36.1. *SLAC*, scapholunate advanced collapse; *SNAC*, scaphoid nonunion advanced collapse.

authors were outstanding, but not better than those attained by using a salvage procedure. With an average follow-up of 74 months, all 12 reconstructed wrists remained mostly asymptomatic, with a mean range of motion of 66%, an average grip strength of 77%, and an average DASH score of 9 points. The results published in the same period for the most commonly used salvage procedures for a SNAC wrist were essentially the same (Table 36.1).[29,32,38]

- *Complete scaphoidectomy + 4CF is a valid alternative for the treatment of SNAC wrists as it is for SLAC.* Since the early 1990s, five studies have analyzed the results obtained by completely excising the scaphoid and fusing the midcarpal joint in SNAC wrists (Table 36.1).[29,33,34,36,38] A total of 76 patients were followed for an average time of 49 months after surgery. There were 18 SNAC type II wrists and 58 SNAC stage III wrists. Except for the series by Xu et al.,[33] all other publications reported similar, acceptable results: in all the cases there was a substantial reduction in pain and excellent patient satisfaction; the average wrist motion and grip strength was 56% and 87% of the contralateral side, respectively; the union rate was 92%, and only 7 of 76 patients (9.2%) admitted failures requiring conversion to total arthrodesis. As stated above, the sample size is too small as to establish statistical comparisons, but the reported results do not seem different from those reported for other salvage options or when the same 4CF technique is used in SLAC wrists.[11,12]
- *The method used to stabilize the 4CF matters, but not as much as a careful decortication and the provision of good-quality cancellous bone graft to the fusion site.* To answer this question, we considered all papers, including those dealing with the treatment of SLAC wrists. The original technique involved stabilizing the 4CF with K-wires.[7,8] That implied prolonged immobilization periods and, in consequence, substantial joint stiffness. To improve stability at the fusion site and allow earlier postoperative mobilization, circular plates were introduced in the market, the first results being published in 2005.[43] Vance et al.[44] reported 58 patients who underwent 4CF either by plate fixation (n = 27) or by traditional fixation (n = 31). Failure to heal was seen in six wrists (26%) stabilized by a ring plate and only in one (3%) fixed with K-wires. In Kendall et al.[43] series, the nonunion rate was even worse: five of eight circular plates failed to heal the attempted midcarpal fusion. Similar failure rates were reported by Chung et al.[45] and De Smet et al.[18] Obviously, not only the plate design but also the surgical technique had to be revised to overcome that consolidation problem. Using better designed circular plates and making

emphasis on joint decortication and abundant provision of cancellous bone, Merrell et al.[46] reported a 100% fusion rate in a series of 28 wrists, followed for an average of 46 months with a grip strength of 82% and a range of motion of 45%. Similar acceptable union rates (24 of 27, 88%) were obtained by Iordache et al.[23] by crossing the fusing joint with two nonparallel headless compression screws. Indeed, when used properly, K-wires, circular plates, or compression headless screws are all useful fixation alternatives, provided that the key prerequisites for an uneventful bone fusion are met, namely: careful decortication of the bone surfaces to be fused, abundant provision of good-quality cancellous grafts, and solid stabilization of the fusing bones. Incidentally, it is important emphasizing that, although the number of observations does not allow proving it, correction of the DISI and not to overcorrect the frontal alignment of the central column of the wrist are also important issues to consider for a successful 4CF. If the DISI is not corrected, the neck of the capitate is likely to impact the dorsal rim of the radius, inducing pain and limited extension. If the lunate is excessively radialized relative to the capitate, the wrist will remain radial deviated forever.

In global terms, and taking all publications together (SLAC and SNAC wrists included), there is good evidence indicating that, when correctly indicated and executed, complete scaphoidectomy plus 4CF preserves 50%–60% of the total range of motion and allows 60%–80% of the normal grip strength. Moreover, 4CF reduces to a half the level of pain of those (about 50%) that cannot claim being painless at follow-up. Following well-known surgical guidelines the nonunion rate of 4CF is between 3% and 9%. Most fixation complications tend to occur in the first 2 years after surgery. Thereafter, little deterioration occurs except for radiolunate OA that is already present in about one-fourth of patients 10 years after surgery, most of these being asymptomatic.[11,12,16–23,29,30,34,36,38,44–47]

- *Once the scaphoid is completely resected, there is no need to fuse the four ulnar bones to stabilize the wrist; a LC fusion may be enough.* The notion that all four ulnar-side carpal bones needed to be included in the fusion to guarantee acceptable union rates was introduced in the early 1990s. The publication in 1993 by Kirschenbaum et al.[24] in which 6 of 18 (33%) capitolunate arthrodesis using K-wires went onto pseudoarthrosis was in part responsible for that recommendation. The introduction of more effective means of bone fixation (mostly compression headless screws) allowed revising that concept. Indeed, as demonstrated by Ferreres et al.[25] and Giannikas et al.,[35] LC fusion union rates (between 3% and 9%) do not differ from the rates reported for conventional 4CFs. A recent case-controlled study published by Hegazy[30] provides further evidence (Level III), supporting the concept of LC arthrodesis to consistently restore a stable functional wrist to patients with a SNAC wrist.
- *PRC, a widely utilized alternative for the treatment of SLAC wrists, may also be a valid solution for patients with a SNAC wrist, stages I or II.* Because of its simplicity, lack of complications, excellent functional outcome, and a 65% survival rate after more than 20 years, this apparently morbid procedure has become the treatment of choice of many hand surgeons Wall et al.[45] Of course, it cannot be used if the cartilages at both the lunate fossa and proximal aspect of the capitate are not intact. From a biomechanical perspective, PRC shortens the carpal height, slackens the tendons across the joint, removes most extrinsic ligaments, and accepts the incongruity of a convex capitate articulating with a shallow, almost flat, lunate fossa. Yet, PRC performs surprisingly well. Several long-term studies have demonstrated that this operation provides an average range of flexion-extension of 75 degrees (SD 10 degrees), a grip strength of 67% (SD 16%), a complication rate of 14%, and more than 80% patient satisfaction.[18,29]
- *Although apparently similar, there are differences between PRC and 4CF when it comes to treat patients with a SNAC wrist.* Several studies have looked at differences between PRC and 4CF.[16–22] There are no Level I prospective randomized and controlled studies to compare the two techniques in SNAC wrists. Aita et al.[29] published the only Level II study available based on SNAC wrists only. The authors randomly allocated 27 patients with a SNAC wrist into two treatments: (1) scaphoidectomy + 4CF (14 patients) and (2) PRC (13 patients). With a mean follow-up of 73 and 74 months, respectively, the differences between the two treatment modalities were not statistically significant. Yet, there was a clear tendency for PRC to produce better grip strength (79% vs. 65%), better range of motion (68% vs. 58%), and better chances to return to work (84% vs. 65%) than with a 4CF. The conclusions of two systematic reviews of studies comparing the results of PRC with those of 4CF in SLAC/SNAC wrists are similar but not exactly the same[14,18] In those studies, 4CF was found to provide better grip strength than PRC.
- *There are treatment options specific for SNAC wrists that cannot be used in SLAC wrists; vice versa, there are alternative treatments for a SLAC wrist that are too aggressive for a SNAC wrist.* Despite having similar patterns of joint degeneration, SLAC and SNAC are not identical entities. In SLAC wrists only the radiolunate

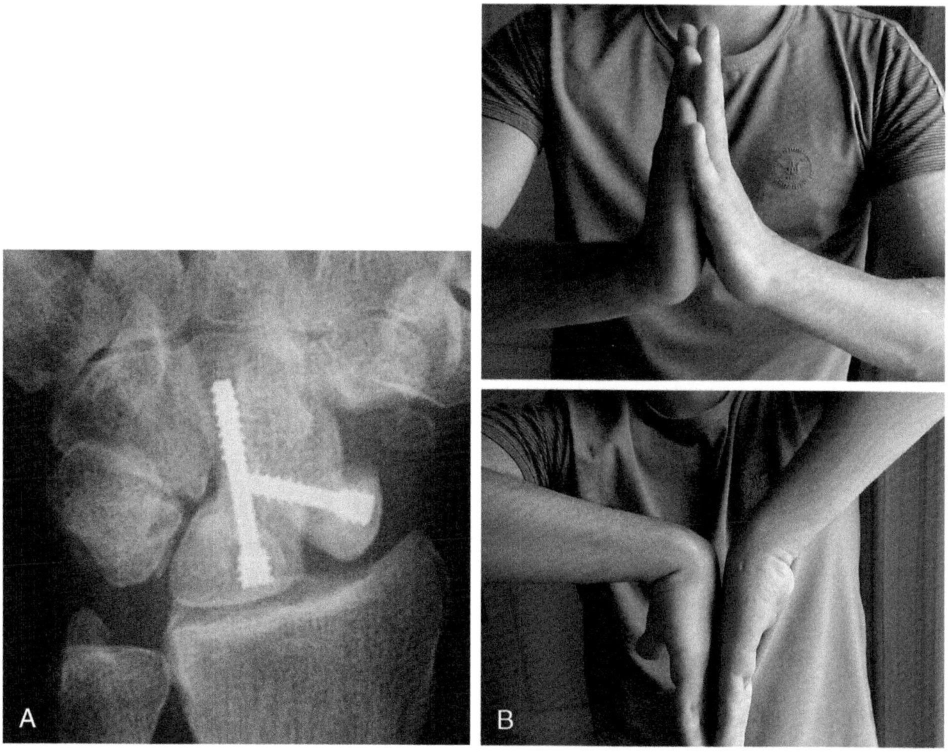

FIG. 36.6 **(A)** PA view of the wrist of a patient who underwent a proximal scaphoid-lunate-capitate fusion for the treatment of a scaphoid nonunion advanced collapse II. **(B)** As with other carpal fusion, the passive range of motion is substantially decreased when the midcarpal joint is fused.

articulation is spared from the joint deterioration process, whereas in SNAC both scaphoid and lunate have good proximal cartilages. To preserve as much radiocarpal joint as possible, some authors proposed excising the distal portion of the scaphoid and to fuse its proximal pole to the lunate and capitate (pSLC fusion). First described by Rotman et al. in 1993,[13] the idea of fusing both fragments of a nonunited scaphoid to the capitate and lunate never gained wide acceptance. Viegas[14] published a slightly different approach: distal scaphoid excision and fusion of the proximal pole of the scaphoid to the capitate and lunate (Fig. 36.6). Six patients with SNAC wrist underwent a pSLC fusion. The union rate was 100%, and good pain relief was obtained in all patients. At an average follow-up of 18 months, all patients were satisfied with their results, with a range of motion and grip strength of approximately half of the contralateral side. In 2012, Klausmeyer and Fernandez[15] reported on seven patients with a SNAC wrist treated by the pSCL technique. With a mean follow-up of 55 months, the range of flexion-extension was 70 degrees and the grip strength was 65%. Pain decreased in all patients, and the average DASH decreased from 44 preoperatively to 23 postoperatively.

- *Removal of the distal portion of a nonunited scaphoid results in a DISI pattern of malalignment, but this does not appear to be a problem: pain relief is optimal and the resultant dysfunction tends to be well tolerated.* It may not be a biomechanically sound operation, but it works. First described by Downing[48] in 1951, and revisited by Malerich et al.,[27,32] and again by Soeijima et al.[39] and Ruch et al.,[49] the distal scaphoid may be excised without paying substantial functional penalty. The prerequisites for this to happen are (1) the nonunion must be distal to radioscaphocapitate ligament, (2) the proximal fragment must not be vascularly compromised, (3) the proximal scapholunate attachments must be intact and functional, and (4) the lunate must not have a large distal facet for the hamate (lunate type II).[28,32,39,49] The best evidence supporting this conclusion is the series by Malerich et al.[32] 17 out of the 19 patients reported in 1999 were reviewed again in 2014, 10–25 years after surgery. Pain

(Visual Analog Scale score) at follow-up averaged 0.9 points; grip strength was 83%; and range of flexion-extension was 79% of the contralateral side. Based on that experience, the authors recommend that, in low-demand patients, distal pole excision is a valid alternative to partial wrist arthrodesis in recalcitrant scaphoid nonunions with mild OA.

RECOMMENDATION

Absence of evidence does not always mean evidence of absence. It would, if we had spent enough time and energy trying to find that evidence without success. But that is not the case here. We cannot provide a solid answer to the target question because the subject has not been searched well enough. Certainly, to know the most adequate treatment for the different forms of SNAC, we need large, prospective, carefully controlled, multicenter clinical trials specifically designed to address that question. Fortunately, we are not completely empty-pocketed in this. We have searched the subject long enough as to allow us some recommendations:

- SLAC and SNAC are not alike entities deserving the same treatment. The strategies that are reasonable for the treatment of SLAC may not be adequate to treat SNAC (overall quality: low).
- Excision of the distal fragment of the scaphoid (Downing's operation[48]) is indicated in low-demand patients with a SNAC wrist, stages I or II, provided that the proximal fragment is well vascularized and normally attached to the lunate and radius (overall quality: low).
- In young individuals with high functional demands, isolated distal scaphoidectomy is not recommended. In those cases, the distal scaphoidectomy is to be associated with a pSLC fusion (Viegas' operation[14]) (overall quality: low).
- Total scaphoidectomy + LC fusion is mostly recommended in SLAC III, when the proximal scaphoid is not viable from a vascular perspective, or when its proximal surface has poor proximal cartilage. Should the triquetral-hamate articular be also deteriorated, a total scaphoidectomy + 4CF would be indicated (overall quality: low).
- PRC has stood the test of time, it is simple, and involves little rehabilitation. Yet, owing to its tendency to deteriorate with time, PRC should not be used in patients younger than 40 years (overall quality: moderate).

CONCLUSION

The scaphoid is the bridge that interconnects the two carpal rows. When the two ends of the bridge are disconnected by a fracture, the dysfunctional midcarpal joint tends to become osteoarthritic. It's the so-called SNAC wrist. It is important emphasizing that SLAC and SNAC are not identical osteoarthritic conditions. The essential difference lies in the amount of normal radioscaphoid cartilage that is preserved. If the goal of treatment is to maintain as much radiocarpal articular contact as possible, most treatments suggested for a SLAC wrist would be too aggressive to be used in SNAC cases, and vice versa, SNAC wrists may benefit from strategies that are inappropriate in SLAC cases; yet, most articles discussing how to alleviate the symptoms of wrist OA include SNAC and SLAC into the same category. In other words, from an "Evidence-Based Medicine" viewpoint, there is no solid evidence behind any of the strategies suggested for the painful SNAC wrist.

PANEL 2
Case Scenario Continued

Because the gadolinium-enhanced MRI showed the proximal fragment to be viable from a vascular point of view, we decided a distal scaphoidectomy plus radial styloidectomy (Fig. 36.1B). The patient did very well: a quick recovery of an acceptable range of motion (Fig. 36.1C) and quite strong grip (Fig. 36.1D). If he had been a heavy manual worker, we would have added to the procedure a proximal scaphoid-lunate-capitate fusion.

PANEL 3
Authors' Preferred Techniques

- Scapholunate advanced collapse (**SLAC)-I**: Radial styloidectomy + standard scaphoid nonunion treatment strategy (volar/dorsal/arthroscopy approach + generous fibrous tissue excision + cancellous/vascularized bone grafting + solid fixation).
- **SLAC-II + viable proximal scaphoid** (*low-demand patients*). If the midcarpal dysfunction has persisted long enough, the damage to the scaphoid bridge may be unsolvable. In low-demand patients, removal of the distal end of the bridge usually suffices for the joint to be painless.
- **SLAC-II + viable proximal scaphoid** (*normal patients*): Distal scaphoid excision + proximal scaphoid-lunate-capitate fusion.
- **SLAC-II + necrotic and/or fragmented proximal scaphoid** (<45-year-old patients): Complete scaphoidectomy + LC arthrodesis
- **SLAC-II + necrotic and/or fragmented proximal scaphoid** (>45-year-old patients): Proximal row carpectomy.
- **SLAC-III**: Complete scaphoidectomy + LC arthrodesis

REFERENCES

1. Berdia S, Wolfe SW. Effects of scaphoid fractures on the biomechanics of the wrist. *Hand Clin*. 2001;17:533–540.
2. Smith DK, An KN, Cooney 3rd WP, et al. Effects of a scaphoid waist osteotomy on carpal kinematics. *J Orthop Res*. 1989;7:590–598.
3. Leventhal EL, Wolfe SW, Moore DC, et al. Interfragmentary motion in patients with scaphoid nonunion. *J Hand Surg Am*. 2008;33:1108–1115.
4. Mack GR, Bosse MJ, Gelberman RH, et al. The natural history of scaphoid non-union. *J Bone Joint Surg Am*. 1984;66:504–509.
5. Osterman AL, Mikulics M. Scaphoid nonunion. *Hand Clin*. 1988;4:437–455.
6. Krakauer JD, Bishop AT, Cooney WP. Surgical treatment of scapholunate advanced collapse. *J Hand Surg Am*. 1994;19:751–759.
7. Watson HK, Ballet FL. The SLAC wrist: scapholunate advanced collapse pattern of degenerative arthritis. *J Hand Surg Am*. 1984;9:358–365.
8. Vender MI, Watson HK, Wiener BD, et al. Degenerative change in symptomatic scaphoid nonunion. *J Hand Surg Am*. 1987;12:514–519.
9. Moritomo H, Tada K, Yoshida T, et al. The relationship between the site of nonunion of the scaphoid and scaphoid nonunion advanced collapse (SNAC). *J Bone Joint Surg Br*. 1999;81:871–876.
10. Kent ME, Rehmatullah NN, Young L, Chojnowski AJ. Scaphoid nonunion in the presence of a degenerate carpus: don't rush to salvage surgery. *J Hand Surg Eur Vol*. 2012;37:56–60.
11. Laulan J, Marteau E, Bacle G. Wrist osteoarthritis. *Orthop Traumatol Surg Res*. 2015;101(1 suppl):S1–S9.
12. Shah CM, Stern PJ. Scapholunate advanced collapse (SLAC) and scaphoid nonunion advanced collapse (SNAC) wrist arthritis. *Curr Rev Musculoskelet Med*. 2013;6:9–17.
13. Rotman MB, Manske PR, Pruitt DL, et al. Scaphocapitolunate arthrodesis. *J Hand Surg Am*. 1993;18:26–33.
14. Viegas SF. Limited arthrodesis for scaphoid nonunion. *J Hand Surg Am*. 1994;19:127–133.
15. Klausmeyer M, Fernandez D. Scaphocapitolunate arthrodesis and radial styloidectomy: a treatment option for posttraumatic degenerative wrist disease. *J Wrist Surg*. 2012;1:115–122.
16. Dacho AK, Baumeister S, Germann G, Sauerbier M. Comparison of proximal row carpectomy and midcarpal arthrodesis for the treatment of scaphoid nonunion advanced collapse (SNAC-wrist) and scapholunate advanced collapse (SLAC-wrist) in stage II. *J Plast Reconstr Aesthet Surg*. 2008;61(10):1210–1218.
17. Mulford JS, Ceulemans LJ, Nam D, et al. Proximal row carpectomy vs four corner fusion for scapholunate (SLAC) or scaphoid nonunion advanced collapse (SNAC) wrists: a systematic review of outcomes. *J Hand Surg Eur Vol*. 2009;34:256–263.
18. De Smet L, Deprez P, Duerinckx J, Degreef I. Outcome of four-corner arthrodesis for advanced carpal collapse: circular plate versus traditional techniques. *Acta Orthop Belg*. 2009;75:323–327.
19. Bisneto EN, Freitas MC, Paula EJ, et al. Comparison between proximal row carpectomy and four-corner fusion for treating osteoarthrosis following carpal trauma: a prospective randomized study. *Clinics (Sao Paulo)*. 2011;66:51–55.
20. Singh HP, Brinkhorst ME, Dias JJ, et al. Dynamic assessment of wrist after proximal row carpectomy and 4-corner fusion. *J Hand Surg Am*. 2014;39:2424–2433.
21. Saltzman BM, Frank JM, Slikker W, et al. Clinical outcomes of proximal row carpectomy versus four-corner arthrodesis for post-traumatic wrist arthropathy: a systematic review. *J Hand Surg Eur Vol*. 2015;40:450–457.
22. Berkhout MJ, Bachour Y, Zheng KH, et al. Four-corner arthrodesis versus proximal row carpectomy: a retrospective study with a mean follow-up of 17 years. *J Hand Surg Am*. 2015;40:1349–1354.
23. Iordache SD, Nam D, Paylan J, et al. Four-corner arthrodesis using two headless compression screws. *Acta Orthop Belg*. 2016;82:332–338.
24. Kirschenbaum D, Schneider LH, Kirkpatrick WH, et al. Scaphoid excision and capitolunate arthrodesis for radioscaphoid arthritis. *J Hand Surg Am*. 1993;18:780–785.
25. Ferreres A, Garcia-Elias M, Plaza R. Long-term results of lunocapitate arthrodesis with scaphoid excision for SLAC and SNAC wrists. *J Hand Surg Eur Vol*. 2009;34:603–608.
26. Chim H, Moran SL. Long-term outcomes of proximal row carpectomy: a systematic review of the literature. *J Wrist Surg*. 2012;1(2):141–148.
27. Malerich MM, Clifford J, Eaton B, et al. Distal scaphoid resection arthroplasty for the treatment of degenerative arthritis secondary to scaphoid nonunion. *J Hand Surg Am*. 1999;24:1196–1205.
28. Garcia-Elias M, Lluch A. Partial excision of scaphoid: is it ever indicated? *Hand Clin*. 2001;17:687–695.
29. Aita MA, Nakano EK, Schaffhausser HL, et al. Randomized clinical trial between proximal row carpectomy and the four-corner fusion for patients with stage II SNAC. *Rev Bras Ortop*. 2016;20(51):574–582.
30. Hegazy G. Capitolunate arthrodesis for treatment of scaphoid nonunion advanced collapse (SNAC) wrist arthritis. *J Hand Microsurg*. 2015;7:79–86.
31. Malizos KN, Koutalos A, Papatheodorou L, et al. Vascularized bone grafting and distal radius osteotomy for scaphoid nonunion advanced collapse. *J Hand Surg Am*. 2014;39:872–879.
32. Malerich MM, Catalano 3rd LW, Weidner ZD, et al. Distal scaphoid resection for degenerative arthritis secondary to scaphoid nonunion: a 20-year experience. *J Hand Surg Am*. 2014;39:1669–1676.
33. Xu YQ, Zhu YL, Wang Y. The memory plate for four-corner fusion of scaphoid non-union advanced collapse. *J Plast Surg Hand Surg*. 2013;47:442–445.

34. Mahmoud M, El Shafie S. Bicolumnar fusion for scaphoid nonunion advanced collapse without bone grafting. *Tech Hand Up Extrem Surg*. 2012;16:80–85.
35. Giannikas D, Karageorgos A, Karabasi A, et al. Capitolunate arthrodesis maintaining carpal height for the treatment of SNAC wrist. *J Hand Surg Eur Vol*. 2010;35:198–201.
36. El-Mowafi H, El-Hadidi M, Boghdady GW, et al. Functional outcome of four-corner arthrodesis for treatment of grade IV scaphoid non-union. *Acta Orthop Belg*. 2007;73:604–611.
37. Drac P, Manak P, Pieranova L. Distal scaphoid resection arthroplasty for scaphoid nonunion with radioscaphoid arthritis. *Biomed Pap Med Fac Univ Palacky Olomouc Czech Repub*. 2006;150:143–145.
38. Dacho A, Grundel J, Holle G, et al. Long-term results of midcarpal arthrodesis in the treatment of scaphoid nonunion advanced collapse (SNAC-wrist) and scapholunate advanced collapse (SLAC-wrist). *Ann Plast Surg*. 2006;56:139–144.
39. Soejima O, Iida H, Hanamura T, et al. Resection of the distal pole of the scaphoid for scaphoid nonunion with radioscaphoid and intercarpal arthritis. *J Hand Surg Am*. 2003;28:591–596.
40. Sackett DL. Rules of evidence and clinical recommendations on the use antithrombotic agents. *Chest*. 1986;89(2 suppl):2S–3S.
41. Larson AN, Bishop AT, Shin AY. Free medial femoral condyle bone grafting for scaphoid nonunions with humpback deformity and proximal pole avascular necrosis. *Tech Hand Up Extrem Surg*. 2007;11:246–258.
42. Garcia RM, Leversedge FJ, Aldridge JM, et al. Scaphoid nonunions treated with 2 headless compression screws and bone grafting. *J Hand Surg Am*. 2014;39:1301–1307.
43. Kendall CB, Brown TR, Millon SJ, et al. Results of four-corner arthrodesis using dorsal circular plate fixation. *J Hand Surg Am*. 2005;30:903–907.
44. Vance MC, Hernandez JD, Didonna ML, et al. Complications and outcome of four-corner arthrodesis: circular plate fixation versus traditional techniques. *J Hand Surg Am*. 2005;30:1122–1127.
45. Wall LB, Didonna ML, Kiefhaber TR, et al. Proximal row carpectomy: minimum 20-year follow-up. *J Hand Surg Am*. 2013;38:1498–1504.
46. Merrell GA, McDermott EM, Weiss AP. Four-corner arthrodesis using a circular plate and distal radius bone grafting: a consecutive case series. *J Hand Surg Am*. 2008;33:635–642.
47. Trail IA, Murali R, Stanley JK, et al. The long-term outcome of four-corner fusion. *J Wrist Surg*. 2015;4:128–133.
48. Downing FH. Excision of the distal fragment of the scaphoid and styloid process of the radius for nonunion of the carpal scaphoid. *West J Surg Obstet Gynecol*. 1951;59:217–218.
49. Ruch DS, Papadonikolakis A. Resection of the scaphoid distal pole for symptomatic scaphoid nonunion after failed previous surgical treatment. *J Hand Surg Am*. 2006;31:588–593.

Index

Note: Page numbers followed by "f" indicate figures, "t" indicate tables and "b" indicate boxes.

S

V

W

X

Printed and bound by CPI Group (UK) Ltd, Croydon, CR0 4YY
08/05/2025
01864759-0001